MW00674520

Second Edition

UROLOGIC COMPLICATIONS: MEDICAL AND SURGICAL, ADULT AND PEDIATRIC

SECOND EDITION

UROLOGIC COMPLICATIONS: MEDICAL AND SURGICAL, ADULT AND PEDIATRIC

Fray F. Marshall, M.D.
Professor of Urology
Director, Division of Adult Urology
The Johns Hopkins University School of Medicine
The Johns Hopkins Hospital
Baltimore, Maryland

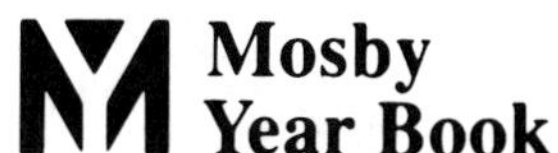

St. Louis Baltimore Boston Chicago London Philadelphia Sydney Toronto

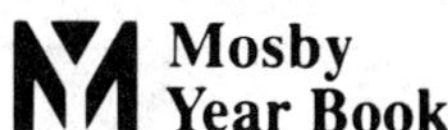

Dedicated to Publishing Excellence

Sponsoring Editor: David K. Marshall
Assistant Director, Manuscript Services: Fran Perveiler
Production Coordinator: Nancy C. Baker
Proofroom Supervisor: Barbara M. Kelly

Mosby-Year Book Inc.
11830 Westline Industrial Drive
St. Louis, MO 63146

1 2 3 4 5 6 7 8 9 0 Y R 94 93 92 91 90

Library of Congress Cataloging-in-Publication Data

Urologic complications/[edited by] Fray Marshall.—2nd ed.
p. cm.
Includes bibliographical references.
Includes index.
ISBN 0-8151-5761-4
1. Genitourinary organs—Surgery—Complications and sequelae.
2. Genitourinary organs—Diseases—Complications and sequelae.
I. Marshall, Fray F.
[DNLM: 1. Postoperative Complications. 2. Urogenital System—-surgery. 3. Urologic Diseases—complications. WJ 168 U749]
RD571.U695
617.4'601—dc20 90-12546
DLC CIP
for Library of Congress

To four men who have had a positive major influence in my urologic-training and personal development:
VICTOR FRAY MARSHALL—*my father, and a great urologist*
WYLAND F. LEADBETTER—*a charismatic teacher and surgeon*
W. HARDY HENDREN—*a phenomenal technical surgeon*
PATRICK C. WALSH—*a great intellect and urologic surgeon*

CONTRIBUTORS

Stephen C. Achuff, M.D.
Associate Professor of Medicine
Department of Medicine
The Johns Hopkins University School of Medicine
Director of Clinical Programs in Cardiology
The Johns Hopkins Hospital
Baltimore, Maryland

Alex F. Althausen, M.D.
Associate Clinical Professor
Department of Surgery
Harvard Medical School
Urologist, Massachusetts General Hospital
Boston, Massachusetts

John G. Bartlett, M.D.
Professor of Medicine
The Johns Hopkins University School of Medicine
Chief, Infectious Disease Division
The Johns Hopkins Hospital
Baltimore, Maryland

William R. Bell, Ph.D., M.D.
Professor of Medicine/Radiology
The Johns Hopkins University School of Medicine
The Johns Hopkins University Hospital
Baltimore, Maryland

Mark F. Bellinger, M.D.
Associate Professor
Department of Surgery
Division of Urology
The University of Pittsburgh
Chief, Pediatric Urology
The Children's Hospital of Pittsburgh
Pittsburgh, Pennsylvania

Donald R. Bodner, M.D.
Assistant Professor
Case Western Reserve University School of Medicine
University Hospital of Cleveland
Cleveland, Ohio

Charles B. Brendler, M.D.
Associate Professor of Urology
The Johns Hopkins University School of Medicine
The Johns Hopkins Hospital
Baltimore, Maryland

Kevin A. Burbige, M.D.
Assistant Professor of Urology
College of Physicians and Surgeons
Columbia University
Associate Director of Pediatric Urology
Babies Hospital
Columbia Presbyterian Medical Center
New York, New York

James F. Burdick, M.D.
Associate Professor
The Johns Hopkins University School of Medicine
The Johns Hopkins Hospital
Baltimore, Maryland

Chi Van Dang, Ph.D., M.D.
Assistant Professor of Medicine
The Johns Hopkins University School of Medicine
Attending Physician
The Johns Hopkins Hospital
Baltimore, Maryland

Charles J. Devine, Jr., M.D.
Professor of Urology
Eastern Virginia Medical School
Norfolk, Virginia

John P. Donohue, M.D.
Professor and Chairman of Urology
Indiana University
Indianapolis, Indiana

Michael J. Droller, M.D.
Professor and Chairman
Department of Urology
The Mount Sinai School of Medicine
Director of Urology
Attending Urologist
Mount Sinai Medical Center
New York, New York

Jack S. Elder, M.D.
Associate Professor of Surgery (Urology) and Pediatrics
Case Western Reserve University School
Director of Pediatric Urology
Rainbow Babies and Childrens Hospital
Cleveland, Ohio

William R. Fair, M.D.
Professor of Surgery/Urology
Cornell University Medical College
Chief, Urology Service
Memorial Sloan-Kettering Cancer Center
New York, New York

John P. Gearhart, M.D.
Assistant Professor of Pediatrics/Urology
The Johns Hopkins School of Medicine
The Johns Hopkins Hospital
Baltimore, Maryland

Terry W. Hensle, M.D.
Professor of Urology
Columbia University College of Pediatrics
Director of Pediatric Urology
Babies Hospital
New York, New York

C. Lee Jackson, M.D.
Associate Staff Urology
Cleveland Clinic Florida
Fort Lauderdale, Florida

Jonathan P. Jarow, M.D.
Assistant Professor of Surgery (Urology)
Bowman Gray School of Medicine
Winston-Salem, North Carolina

Robert D. Jeffs, M.D.
Professor of Pediatric Urology
The Johns Hopkins University School of Medicine
Director of Pediatric Urology
The Johns Hopkins Hospital
Baltimore, Maryland

Stephen A. Kramer, M.D.
Associate Professor of Urology
Mayo Clinic
St. Marys Hospital
Rochester, Minnesota

Arnon Krongrad, M.D.
Medical Lecturer
University of Texas Southwestern Medical School
Clinical Instructor
Division of Urology
University of Texas Southwestern Medical Center
Dallas, Texas

Herbert Lepor, M.D.
Associate Professor of Surgery and Pharmacology
Medical College of Wisconsin
Milwaukee, Wisconsin

Robin K. Levin, M.D.
Assistant Attending in Urology
Section of Pediatric Urology
Albert Einstein College of Medicine
Montefiore Medical Center
Bronx, New York

J. Keith Light, M.D.
Professor of Urology
Baylor College of Medicine
The Methodist Hospital
Houston, Texas

Thomas J. Maatman, D.O., F.A.C.S.
Assistant Clinical Professor of Urology
College of Osteopathic Medicine
Michigan State University
Chairman, Department of Surgery
Metropolitan Hospital
Lansing, Michigan

Terrence R. Malloy, M.D.
Professor of Urology
University of Pennsylvania
Chief, Section of Urology
Pennsylvania Hospital
Philadelphia, Pennsylvania

Fray F. Marshall, M.D.
Professor of Urology
Director, Division of Urology
The Johns Hopkins University School of Medicine
The Johns Hopkins Hospital
Baltimore, Maryland

Jack W. McAninch, M.D.
Professor of Urology
University of California at San Francisco
Chief of Urology
San Francisco General Hospital
San Francisco, California

David Mikkelsen, M.D.
Chief Resident
Washington University School of Medicine
Barnes Hospital
St. Louis, Missouri

Michael E. Mitchell, M.D.
Professor and Chief of Pediatric Urology
University of Washington School of Medicine
Children's Hospital and Medical Center
Seattle, Washington

Drogo K. Montague, M.D.
Head, Section of Urodynamics and Prosthetic Surgery
Department of Urology
Director, Center for Sexual Function
Cleveland Clinic Foundation
Cleveland, Ohio

James E. Montie, M.D.
Staff Urologist
Cleveland Clinic Florida
Fort Lauderdale, Florida

Jacek L. Mostwin, M.D., D.Phil.
Assistant Professor of Urology
The Johns Hopkins Medical Institutions
Baltimore, Maryland

H. Norman Noe, M.D.
Professor of Urology
University of Tennessee
Chief, Pediatric Urology
LeBonheur Children's Medical Center
Memphis, Tennessee

Andrew C. Novick, M.D.
Chairman, Department of Urology
Cleveland Clinic Foundation
Cleveland, Ohio

Martin I. Resnick, M.D.
Professor and Chairman
Division of Urology
Case Western Reserve University School of Medicine
Director, Division of Urology
University Hospitals of Cleveland
Cleveland, Ohio

Jerome P. Richie, M.D.
Elliott Carr Cutler Professor of Urological Surgery
Harvard Medical School
Chief of Urology
Brigham and Women's Hospital
Boston, Massachusetts

Richard C. Rink, M.D.
Assistant Professor
Chief, Pediatric Urology
Riley Hospital for Children
Indiana University Medical Center
Indianapolis, Indiana

Miriam P. Roger, R.N., M.N.
Oncology Clinical Nurse Specialist
Duke University Medical Center
Durham, North Carolina

Joseph W. Segura, M.D.
Carl Rosen Professor of Urology
Mayo Medical School
Mayo Clinic
Consultant in Urology
St. Marys Hospital
Rochester, Minnesota

Ellen Shapiro, M.D.
Associate Professor of Surgery (Urology)
The Medical College of Wisconsin
The Childrens Hospital of Wisconsin
Milwaukee, Wisconsin

Judith L. Stiff, M.D., M.P.H.
Associate Professor
Department of Anesthesiology and Critical Care Medicine
The Johns Hopkins University School of Medicine
Director, Department of Anesthesiology
Francis Scott Key Medical Center
Baltimore, Maryland

Donald L. Trump, M.D.
Professor of Medicine
Department of Medicine
Duke University School of Medicine
Durham, North Carolina

Bert Vorstman, M.D.
Attending Urologic Surgeon
Coral Springs Medical Center
Coral Springs, Florida

W. Gordon Walker, M.D.
Professor of Medicine
Division of Nephrology
The Johns Hopkins University School of Medicine
Baltimore, Maryland

Alan J. Wein, M.D.
Professor and Chairman
Division of Urology
University of Pennsylvania School of Medicine
Chief of Urology
Hospital of the University of Pennsylvania
Philadelphia, Pennsylvania

Boyd H. Winslow, M.D.
Associate Professor
Eastern Virginia Medical School
Chief, Department of Urology
Children's Hospital of the King's Daughters
Norfolk, Virginia

David P. Wood, Jr., M.D.
Fellow, Department of Urology
Memorial Sloan Kettering Cancer Center
Memorial Hospital
New York, New York

PREFACE

Anticipating urological complications is the best way to prevent them. It is hoped that this book will help urologists anticipate many of their clinical problems. Complications are not always addressed in detail in many publications but they remain as important as ever. I have maintained a broad interest in many areas of urology and it is for this reason that I initiated this book on urological complications. I hope it will be informative and helpful.

For the second edition all authors were asked to review their chapters and make any significant changes. Many of the chapters have been rewritten extensively. There are also entirely new chapters on the complications of cystectomy, shock wave lithotripsy, continence surgery in women, the management of erectile dysfunction, and complications of lasers. I would like to thank all of the authors who have contributed to this book. I also want to extend special thanks to my wife, Lindsay, and my children, Wheatley and Brooks, for being so patient. Mr. David Marshall and the entire staff at Mosby-Year Book have been excellent and helpful. Lastly, I am fortunate to have an excellent secretary in Mrs. Rosemary Rogers who has helped correct and organize this book.

FRAY F. MARSHALL, M.D.

CONTENTS

SECTION I

Medical Complications

CHAPTER 1

Cardiovascular Complications

Stephen C. Achuff, M.D.

This chapter addresses some of the clinical problems commonly seen jointly by urologists and internists/cardiologists. That these problems are of considerable frequency and magnitude is not surprising since a large proportion of patients undergoing urologic procedures are middle-aged or elderly and therefore likely candidates for cardiac complications. Optimal management of these potentially high-risk patients requires that the combined expertise of urologists, cardiologists, and anesthesiologists as well be brought to bear in as collaborative and collegial a manner as possible. While it would be inappropriate for the cardiologist to suggest which procedure the urologist should perform or which anesthetic agents the anesthesiologist should use, it *is* the cardiologist's prerogative and responsibility to provide clear and concise information in three areas: (1) expected surgical risk, (2) means of minimizing this risk preoperatively, and (3) specific problems to anticipate in the postoperative period and how to deal with them.[1, 2] More than anything else, he should perform and document a careful evaluation of the patient's preoperative cardiovascular status. This includes a complete history and physical examination, collation of pertinent past medical information and medication history, and ordering and interpreting of appropriate laboratory studies. Meticulous attention to these details will prove very rewarding to patients and physicians alike. It is not uncommon for a supposed cardiac patient to be found after careful evaluation to be remarkably healthy and free of important heart disease (e.g., a patient who has had previous overinterpretation of a heart murmur or an abnormal electrocardiogram [ECG]). By the same token, a seemingly fit and low-risk patient might have some signs of serious underlying cardiac disease detected by the astute internist and thereby receive the benefit of intensive hemodynamic monitoring that might not otherwise have been employed.

ESTIMATION OF SURGICAL RISK

Surgical risk is increased in several obvious patient groups: the elderly, the generally debilitated and medically unstable, those requiring emergency surgery, and those undergoing extensive intraabdominal procedures. Beyond these categories most perioperative morbidity and mortality relate to underlying cardiovascular disease. It has been known for many years, for example, that a recent myocardial infarction (MI) carries extraordinary risk for perioperative reinfarction and death. Two studies from the Mayo Clinic in the 1960s and 1970s showed a roughly 30% risk of reinfarction if the previous infarction occurred within 3 months, 15% if the previous infarction was 3 to 6 months prior to surgery, and 4% to 5% if more than 6 months had elapsed.[3, 4] Mortality for these recurrent infarctions was well above 50% in both studies. In addition—and this is important to bear in mind when deciding how long to monitor high-risk patients—only about 20% of perioperative MIs occurred within 24 hours of surgery, while 30% to 40% occurred between the fourth and sixth postoperative days.

Two recent studies suggest a much more favorable outcome can now be obtained in patients with a history of recent MI. Wells and Kaplan had no reinfarctions in a series of 48 patients at Emory University Hospital who had sustained prior MI within 3 months of surgery, although there was a 15% incidence of "significant" arrhythmias.[5] In the second study, Rao et al. reported perioperative infarction rates in patients with prior infarctions up to 3 months and 4 to 6 months preoperatively of 5.7% and 2.3%, respectively.[6] Presumably it is the current availability and frequent use of hemodynamic monitoring and vasoactive drugs that has improved the outlook for these patients.[7]

Apart from a history of recent MI, other cardiac abnormalities have been shown to identify patients at increased surgical risk. These findings have been documented extensively in the studies of Goldman and his colleagues in several recent publications.[2, 8, 9] Multivariate analysis of numerous potential risk factors was employed to develop what they termed a multifactorial index score for estimating cardiac risk in noncardiac surgery. Subsequent prospective studies in other institutions have confirmed the validity of these findings. In addition to a MI within the previous 6 months, signs of left ventricular decompensation (an S_3 gallop or jugular venous distention), ventricular ectopy (more than five premature ventricular beats per minute), and cardiac rhythms other than sinus were potent predictors of cardiac morbidity and mortality. Interestingly, other important aspects of patients' cardiac status were not independent predictors of complications. These included hypertension, stable angina, and history of cigarette smoking. It should be noted also that Goldman's study of over 1,000 operations which led to the development of the multifactorial risk index did not include minor operations under local anesthesia, endoscopies, or transurethral resections of the prostate. The last-named procedure has been well documented to be safe even in elderly patients with known coronary heart disease.[10, 11]

Table 1–1 presents the portion of Goldman's cardiac risk index scoring system dealing with specifically cardiac abnormalities. Additional points were assigned to problems of a more general medical nature (such as hypoxemia, hypercarbia, hypokalemia, and azotemia) and to type of surgery performed (e.g., intrathoracic, intraabdominal, and emergency or elective). Total point scores placed patients into one of four classes of risk, with those in class I having less than 1% incidence of cardiac death or life-threatening but nonfatal complications, those in class II, 7%; class III, 13%; and class IV patients, a staggering 22% incidence of serious complications and 56% incidence of death from cardiac causes.

TABLE 1–1.

Multifactorial Index Score to Estimate Cardiac Risk in Noncardiac Surgery*

Factors	Points
S_3 gallop or jugular venous distention on preoperative physical examination	11
Transmural or subendocardial MI in previous 6 mo	10
Premature ventricular beats, >5/min	7
Rhythm other than sinus or presence of PABs on last preoperative ECG	7
Age >70 yr	5
Aortic stenosis	3

*From Goldman L, et al: *N Engl J Med* 1977; 297:845. Used by permission.

MI = myocardial infarction; PABs = premature atrial beats.

This scoring system provides a very useful framework within which the surgeon, cardiologist, and anesthesiologist can estimate surgical risk in an individual patient, especially with regard to timing of surgery if an emergency procedure is not contemplated. It is clear that the most powerful predictors of cardiac risk (congestive heart failure and recent MI) are at least potentially modifiable. The remainder of this chapter will address some of the issues arising from this risk estimation approach, with particular attention to methods of minimizing risk and principles of management in specific cardiac conditions.

ISCHEMIC HEART DISEASE

Coronary atherosclerosis is extremely common in older patients undergoing urologic surgery and procedures, and its manifestations are complex, varied, and potentially treacherous. Any sign or symptom of ischemic heart disease must be heeded with great respect. It is not enough just to ask whether or not there has been a MI within the previous 6 months. One must ascertain the tempo of the disease, the complications it has already wrought, the level of compensation achieved by the individual patient, and the drugs necessary to establish or maintain that compensation. In addition to his own personal assessment, the cardiologist should seek out and review past records and evaluations. Old ECGs, stress tests, chest x-rays, and echocardiograms can be invaluable in answering some of these critical questions.

Assuming there has been no recent MI, careful questioning to determine the patient's New York Heart Association functional class should suffice to ascertain the stability of the ischemic heart disease. Where there remains a question as to the patient's ability to tolerate stress, I have no reservations about recommending a formal graded exercise test. Duration of exercise on the treadmill is a good measure of left ventricular function as well as the potential for myocardial ischemia. Exercise that is limited early by dyspnea should be further investigated by echocardiography or radionuclide ventriculography to document the presence and severity of left ventricular dysfunction (assuming the dyspnea is not explicable by noncardiac disease). An exercise test that is positive for ischemic ECG changes at a low workload should also lead to further investigation. If patients are already on a seemingly good regimen of β-blockers, long-acting nitrates, and/or calcium channel antagonists, consideration might be given to performing coronary angiography. If they are not on such a regimen, it should be instituted promptly and elective surgery should be deferred. If surgery cannot be postponed in this higher-risk patient, or if there was already a history of severe angina so that stress testing would be superfluous, the anesthesiologist should be consulted about using modern methods of hemodynamic monitoring (radial artery and pulmonary capillary wedge pressure measurements intraoperatively and postoperatively) and having available appropriate vasodilator drugs.

Patients who have undergone successful coronary artery bypass grafting appear to have considerably lower surgical risk for noncardiac operations than their extensive ischemic heart disease might predict.[12, 13] Actually this finding should not be surprising, since the revascularization places them in an entirely different category from patients with recent MI or even stable angina, for which surgery has not been performed. The same reasoning is applicable to patients who have undergone coronary balloon angioplasty procedures. What is required of the cardiologist, however, is that he document the extent of the prerevascularization coronary disease and the success of the procedure, both in terms of symptomatic improvement and, where possible, by objective parameters.

The proper handling of chronic preoperative medications in patients with angina or other forms of ischemic heart disease has been a source of confusion and contention, particularly between cardiologists and anesthesiologists. The most rational approach would seem to be the continuance of any and all medications that were required to keep the patient stable prior to surgery. It has been shown unequivocally that withdrawal of β-blockers can lead to acute ischemic events and probably the same is true for calcium antagonists.[14, 15] In the case of β-blockers the problem is one of rebound tachycardia and increased blood pressure, which lead to greater myocardial oxygen demands. With the calcium antagonists, abrupt withdrawal could lead to coronary spasm. Both drugs are not restricted to oral use alone. Intravenous propranolol and metoprolol are both available in the United States, and nifedipine can be administered sublingually. Alternatively, intravenously administered nitroglycerin can replace the calcium antagonist until the patient can take medications by mouth. Also cutaneous nitrates can be used—preferably the ointment form that is applied every 4 hours, rather than the questionably effective, once-daily patches.

CONGESTIVE HEART FAILURE

As was demonstrated by the data of Goldman and colleagues, signs of congestive heart failure are a very powerful predictor of increased surgical risk. The borderline or decompensated left ventricle can ill tolerate the hemodynamic stresses of even minor surgery, and where general anesthesia is required, a certain amount of myocardial depression from the anesthetic agents is inevitable. It is crucial, therefore, that the patient with congestive heart failure be treated vigorously preoperatively with diuretics, digitalis, and, where necessary, vasodilators. Ideally this therapy should begin days or more before surgery so that the patient's hemodynamic, fluid, and electrolyte status is stable. Recent aggressive diuresis can create its own serious problems, such as hypovolemia, hypokalemia, and contraction alkalosis. Likewise, it is prudent to ensure that blood levels of digoxin are well within the therapeutic range to avoid the risk of digitalis toxicity. Patients with a clear-cut history of congestive heart failure, especially recent, will benefit from the same type of hemodynamic monitoring used in patients with unstable or severe ischemic heart disease syndromes. For the former, intravenous nitroprusside or nitroglycerin may take the place of preoperative oral vasodilators such as captopril, prazosin, and long-acting nitrates.

Patients whose history suggests congestive heart failure, or whose initial evaluation reveals signs of left ventricular dysfunction, should undergo echocardiography or radionuclide ventriculography at some point, simply as a matter of good medical practice. Not only will this give quantitative information about the patient with a compromised left ventricle, but it will also reveal a remarkable number of patients who have been *labeled* as having congestive heart failure but do not have it at all. Too often patients are given a diagnosis of congestive heart failure because of dyspnea, or peripheral edema, or a slightly enlarged cardiac silhouette on chest x-ray film. What is especially harmful is that such patients are chronically treated with potent and entirely inappropriate medications. A typical scenario is the obese hypertensive patient with apparent cardiomegaly on his x-ray film who is given digitalis and diuretics for presumed poor left ventricular function but whose echocardiogram shows a thick and hypertrophied left ventricle with excellent function. A β-blocker would be the appropriate therapy, and digitalis and diuretics are relatively contraindicated. The knowledge of *not* having to deal with a compromised left ventricle and its attendant potential for complications should be very reassuring to the surgeon and anesthesiologist.

CARDIAC ARRHYTHMIAS

One of the most frequent reasons for preoperative cardiology consultation is the discovery of an arrhythmia on routine ECG or the detection of some pulse irregularity on examination. In the majority of patients these abnormalities are either intrinsically benign or are markers of some other problem—a correctible one, it is hoped. In the latter category are included ventricular ectopic beats (PVCs) due to diuretic-induced hypokalemia, or to relative excess of digitalis or some other arrhythmogenic drug, such as aminophylline. More worrisome are PVCs that are associated with left ventricular decompensation, severe angina, or a recent myocardial ischemic event, since the underlying cardiac problem may not be reversible or even readily controllable. In these situations it is always best to postpone surgery if at all feasible until the patient can be brought to as stable a condition as possible from every standpoint (hemodynamic, metabolic). The anesthesiologist should then be advised to have a "low threshold" for using intravenous antiarrhythmics such as lidocaine or procainamide perioperatively if frequent or complex ventricular ectopy is noted. Patients already on chronic oral antiarrhythmics, such as quinidine, procainamide, disopyramide, or β-blockers, should be maintained on their usual dosages that give standardized therapeutic blood levels up to the time of surgery and then have them reinstituted as promptly as possible postoperatively. It is the cardiologist's responsibility to try and document how compelling is the need for such intensive antiarrhythmic therapy since, as with virtually any drug, patients may have been placed on chronic therapy by previous physicians for trivial or long-since-irrelevant reasons. In fact, sometimes the preoperative cardiologic consultation provides an excellent opportunity for dispensing with unnecessary, bothersome, and potentially hazardous cardioactive drugs. Many patients are quite grateful for having previously complicated and troublesome medical regimens "tightened up." Furthermore, urologists need not be reminded about some of the side effects they see from cardiac drugs, such as impotence with β-blockers or bladder-emptying problems with disopyramide.

Supraventricular arrhythmias are also common but usually less problematic. Chronic atrial fibrillation is generally easily controlled with digoxin and the ventricular response is a reliable guide to the potential need for supplemental dosing perioperatively. Care must be taken, however, not to keep "pushing the dig." when a patient is appropriately tachycardic due to hypovolemia, fever, pain, or anxiety, lest a dangerous situation of digitalis toxic response develop. Sinus bradycardia and other variations of the sick sinus syndrome are frequently seen in the elderly, but these should not present significant problems for the patient undergoing operation unless they produce hypotensive symptoms beforehand. The same can be said about most asymptomatic conduction disturbances noted on a routine ECG. It has been adequately demonstrated that right or left bundle-branch block and bifascicular block (right bundle with left anterior or left posterior hemiblock) rarely progress to complete heart block intraoperatively, and these patients do not require prophylactic insertion of pacemakers.[16, 17] Obviously a history of syncope, near-syncope, or unexplained episodes of dizziness would warrant serious consideration of a pacemaker even when random ECGs do not document a high degree of conduction abnormality.

HYPERTENSION

This is another extremely common problem seen in the urologist's practice with middle-aged and elderly patients. Despite earlier concerns, it is now abundantly clear that stable and reasonably well-controlled hypertension and the drugs used to maintain this control should not present an important risk for patients undergoing surgery.[18, 19] Antihypertensive medication should *not* be discontinued, tapered, or omitted prior to surgery because of concern over interactions with anesthetic agents. As long as the anesthesiologist is aware of the medications the patient is taking chronically he should be able to deal effectively with intraoperative and postoperative swings in blood pressure with the judicious use of adrenergic agents, fluid challenges, intravenous vasodilators, and the like. Since the risks are analogous to the risks of withdrawing β-blockers in patients with ischemic heart disease, antihypertensive medications should not be stopped preoperatively, lest a hypertensive crisis occur intraoperatively or postoperatively. This situation may be disastrous in patients with borderline left ventricular function or extensive underlying coronary artery disease.

VALVULAR HEART DISEASE

The major complication one faces in dealing with patients having valvular heart disease is the potential for congestive heart failure. The same principles of preoperative evaluation and perioperative management apply as have been discussed earlier. The cardiologist needs to assess the functional level of compensation the patient has achieved, and this is most readily done by detailed history and examination, sometimes aided by simple tests, such as echocardiography. The patient with marginal compensation should be flagged as high-risk for perioperative complications, and the anesthesia team should be asked to provide invasive hemodynamic monitoring.

Two other problems should be mentioned that are nearly unique to the patient with valvular heart disease. First is the potential risk of endocarditis, particularly important in patients with prosthetic heart valves. Antibiotic prophylaxis should be given where there is even the slightest risk of bacteremia, as with a surgical procedure, or even diagnostic studies on the genitourinary tract when bacteriuria is present. The American Heart Association guidelines on antibiotic therapy are periodically reexamined and updated by a panel of infectious disease experts and represent the best currently available recommendations.[20]

The second area of specific concern in patients with valvular heart disease is the management of anticoagulation therapy. This applies primarily to patients with prosthetic heart valves, and mainly to those with mechanical valves rather than bioprosthetic or tissue valves. Thromboembolic complications are an inescapable hazard of artificial heart valves, even when anticoagulation is rigorously monitored and controlled. The potential is substantially greater when normal clotting status is maintained for more than 5 to 7 days, whatever the reason. Fortunately, the risk is relatively low if this time range is rigidly respected. The simplest strategy for managing warfarin in the face of upcoming surgery is to discontinue the drug 2 or 3 days preoperatively, then reinstitute administration on the second or third postoperative day, assuming the risk of surgical bleeding has subsided. With this scheme the patient is actually unanticoagulated for only 3 or 4 days beginning with the operation.[21] A more conservative approach, from the standpoint of preventing prosthetic valve thromboembolic complications, is to give heparin in full anticoagulating doses up to 6 hours preoperatively, and then again beginning 18 to 24 hours postoperatively, until warfarin can be given to achieve a therapeutic prothrombin time.[22]

SUMMARY

Patients with cardiac disease present the urologist with special problems and risks that often require the knowledge and expertise of an experienced cardiologist. Most of these findings are well appreciated, and effective methods of identifying and characterizing them fully are available. This management has occurred as a result of, and in conjunction with, the growth of cardiac noninvasive laboratories, catheterization laboratories, open heart surgery facilities, and intensive care units. We now have a much more complete understanding of cardiac pathophysiology and the tools with which to alter the balance in favor of maintaining life and health despite the stresses of anesthesia and surgery. There is still an important need, however, despite all the modern technology, for the consultant clinician to perform a detailed history and examination, synthesize the data, formulate specific recommendations, and follow the patient through the entire perioperative period.

EDITORIAL COMMENT

This lucid chapter covers cardiovascular complications of ischemic heart disease, congestive heart failure, cardiac arrhythmias, hypertension, and valvular heart disease. Dr. Achuff outlines in simple, concise terms the management of these cardiovascular problems. He has noted that careful management will result in markedly reduced morbidity and mortality of surgical patients with a history of recent myocardial infarction. Many higher-risk surgical patients can now be managed effectively with the aid of both the cardiologist and anesthesiologist (see Chap. 8 on respiratory complications).

REFERENCES

1. Wolf MA, Braunwald E: General anesthesia and noncardiac surgery in patients with heart disease, in Braunwald E (ed): *Heart Disease. A Textbook of Cardiovascular Medicine.* Philadelphia, WB Saunders, 1984, pp 1815–1825.
2. Goldman L: Cardiac risks and complications of noncardiac surgery. *Ann Intern Med* 1983; 98:504.
3. Tarhan S, Moffitt EA, Taylor WF, et al: Myocardial infarction after general anesthesia. *JAMA* 1972; 220:1451.
4. Steen PA, Tinker JH, Tarhan S: Myocardial reinfarction after anesthesia and surgery. *JAMA* 1978; 239:2566.
5. Wells PH, Kaplan JA: Optimal management of patients with ischemic heart disease for noncardiac surgery by complementary anesthesiologist and cardiologist interaction. *Am Heart J* 1981; 102:1029.
6. Rao TLK, Jacobs KH, El-Etr AA: Reinfarction following anesthesia in patients with myocardial infarction. *Anesthesiology* 1983; 59:499.
7. Rogers MC: Anesthetic management of patients with heart disease. *Mod Concepts Cardiovasc Dis* 1983; 52:29.
8. Goldman L, Caldera DL, Nussbaum SR, et al: Multifactorial index of cardiac risk in noncardiac surgical procedures. *N Engl J Med* 1977; 297:845.
9. Goldman L, Caldera DL, Southwick FS, et al: Cardiac risk factors and complications in noncardiac surgery. *Medicine* 1978; 57:357.
10. Thompson GJ, Kelalis PP, Connolly DC: Transurethral prostatic resection after myocardial infarction. *JAMA* 1962; 182:110.
11. Erlik D, Valero A, Birkhan J, et al: Pros-

tatic surgery and the cardiovascular patient. *Br J Urol* 1968; 40:53.
12. Mahar LJ, Steen PA, Tinker JH, et al: Perioperative myocardial infarction in patients with coronary artery disease with and without aorta-coronary artery bypass grafts. *J Thorac Cardiovasc Surg* 1978; 76:533.
13. Fudge TL, McKienon WMP, Schoettle P, et al: Improved operative risk after myocardial revascularization. *South Med J* 1981; 74:799.
14. Harrison DC, Alderman EL: Discontinuation of propranolol therapy. Cause of rebound angina pectoris and acute coronary events. *Chest* 1976; 69:1.
15. Goldman L: Noncardiac surgery in patients receiving propranolol. *Arch Intern Med* 1981; 141:193.
16. Pastore JO, Yurchak PM, Janis KM, et al: The risk of advanced heart block in surgical patients with right bundle branch block and left axis deviation. *Circulation* 1978; 57:677.
17. Bellocci F, Santorelli P, DiGennaro M, et al: The risk of cardiac complications in surgical patients with bifascicular block. *Chest* 1980; 77:343.
18. Goldman L, Caldera DL: Risk of general anesthesia and elective operation in the hypertensive patient. *Anesthesiology* 1979; 50:285.
19. Prys-Roberts C: Hypertension and anesthesiology—50 years on (editorial). *Anesthesiology* 1979; 50:281.
20. Shulman ST, Amren DP, Bisno AL, et al: Prevention of bacterial endocarditis. *Circulation* 1984; 70:1123A.
21. Tinker JH, Tarhan S: Discontinuing anticoagulant therapy in surgical patients with cardiac valve prostheses. *JAMA* 1978; 239:738.
22. Katholi RE, Nolan SP, McGuire LB: The management of anticoagulation during noncardiac operations in patients with prosthetic heart valves. *Am Heart J* 1978; 96:163.

CHAPTER 2

Acute Renal Failure in the Urologic Patient

W. Gordon Walker, M.D.

Acute renal failure complicating a preexisting urologic disorder is usually heralded by an acute reduction in urine output. The patient with normally functioning kidneys usually excretes at least 400 mL of urine a day even in the presence of severe hydropenia. For this reason oliguria is defined as a persistent urinary output of less than 15 mL/hr and represents abnormal suppression or reduction of urine output.[1-3] This minimum volume, in the hydropenic state with elevated circulating levels of antidiuretic hormone, is determined primarily by solute intake. The principal urinary solutes are sodium and potassium, their attendant anions, and the major metabolites associated with protein catabolism, i.e., urea, creatinine, and uric acid. The individual who is taking little or no food by mouth and is not receiving salt may thus have a urine output of less than 200 mL/day or less than 10 mL/hr and yet have perfectly normal renal function. This important fact must be kept in mind when evaluating hospitalized patients with presumed oliguria. Persistent reduction in urine output despite adequate hydration must be documented before a diagnosis of oliguria is made. Recognition of acute renal failure is made more difficult by the increasing frequency of nonoliguric acute renal failure that is associated with increasing clinical use of potentially nephrotoxic agents, particularly aminoglycosides.[4-8]

The causes of oliguria or anuria may be divided into three categories: (1) Oliguria due to *postrenal obstruction;* (2) oliguria due to *prerenal azotemia,* representing reduction in urine formation due to inadequate perfusion of kidneys with an anatomically and physiologically normal collecting system; and (3) oliguria due to *renal disturbances* associated with damage to the nephrons resulting in sharp reduction in urine formation, usually reversible.

Some of the more common disorders found in each of these three groups is listed in Table 2–1.

POSTRENAL OBSTRUCTION

Obstruction is a common feature of many urologic disorders as well as a potential complication of many of the usual urologic surgical procedures. It constitutes a particularly important problem in patients with only one functioning kidney. It is usually recognized promptly in urologic patients because of the generally high index of suspicion, but it nevertheless should be emphasized that complete anuria is much more likely to be associated with obstruction than with acute re-

TABLE 2–1.
Categories of Oliguria and Their Causes

Prerenal azotemia
Shock
Acute hypovolemia
Gastrointestinal fluid loss
Severe dehydration
Addisonian crisis
Postoperative antidiuresis
Segregated fluid accumulations ("third spaces")
Possibly reflex anuria
Acute renal failure
Nephrotoxic agents
Aminoglycosides
Radiographic contrast media
Heavy metals—Hg, As, Ur, Au, Pt
Ethylene glycol
CCl_4 and other organic solvents
Kanamycin, neomycin
Circulatory insufficiency
Blood loss and shock
Acute sodium depletion (sweating, diarrhea, etc.)
Trauma, crush injury, and shock
Transfusion reactions
Rhabdomyolysis
Burns
Glomerulonephritis
Bilateral renal cortical necrosis
Postrenal obstruction
Renal calculi
Acute pyelonephritis—rarely
Cancer of pelvic organs
Irradiation, edema, fibrosis
Surgical accidents
Prostate obstruction

nal failure. Even the patient who has had a manipulative procedure involving only one kidney should be considered as a most likely candidate for obstruction if he presents with *complete* anuria. Less than 1% of patients with oliguric acute renal failure present with total anuria, excluding patients who have had a surgical procedure in the aorta in the vicinity of the renal arteries or surgical procedures directly involving the renal arteries.

It is thus always imperative to establish that the collecting system leading to both kidneys is patent in the presence of anuria.

Relatively few conditions produce complete cessation of urine output resulting from urinary tract obstruction, so the list of differential diagnoses is not long. In practice it occurs most often in the individual who was not previously recognized as having only one functioning kidney, and the anuria is the result of complete obstruction of this remaining functional kidney. Simultaneous bilateral obstruction with anuria is rare; *prostatic obstruction* usually leads to overflow incontinence and inability to empty the bladder and often presents with very acute lower urinary tract discomfort, leading promptly to the correct diagnosis. *Bilateral ureteral obstruction* is rare but may be encountered with carcinoma of the bladder, prostate, colon, or cervix. Such obstruction may result directly from invasion by the tumor, from inflammation induced by focal irradiation, or from dense periureteric fibrosis most often seen with carcinoma of the prostate.[9, 10]

Obstruction as a cause of anuria must be excluded in all patients who exhibit complete anuria. Renal sonography is an invaluable aid in identifying collections of fluid within the calices resulting from obstruction. It is the most noninvasive procedure available for diagnosing or excluding obstruction. While diagnosis can only be established unequivocally by ureteral catheterization, it is doubtful that catheterization is ever indicated to exclude obstruction if sonography fails to identify any dilatation of the upper collecting system in either kidney. Sonography is also of great value in guiding percutaneous antegrade catheterization of the upper collecting system when retrograde catheterization of the ureter is unsuccessful.

Postobstructive diuresis may present a particularly acute and, at times, life-threatening problem in patients who have long-standing obstruction and who develop profuse diureses on correction of the obstruction.[9] Urine flow rates may approach 50% of the glomerular filtration rate under these conditions. This marked diuresis is frequently associated with profound natriuresis, rapidly developing sodium deficit, volume depletion, and resulting shock. Unless appropriately treated, this condition can lead to profound life-threatening vascular collapse. The histologic appearance of the kidneys of such patients suggests that this phenomenon is attributable to tubular atrophy resulting from the back-pressure associated with long-standing obstruction of the lower collecting system. The attendant solute load (mainly urea), which acts as an osmotic diuretic when flow is reestablished, cannot be modulated because of the tubular atrophy. This diuresis can produce such profound water and sodium losses that shock may supervene within minutes.

Appropriate fluid and sodium replacement at a rate that corrects for the excessive urinary losses alleviates the symptoms and signs of shock. The condition is usually reversible but weeks may be required before renal function is returned to normal. Appropriate management consists of hypotonic solutions such as 5% dextrose containing 75 mEq of sodium chloride or less. Rarely, it may be necessary to maintain this parenteral fluid therapy for several days to a week or more if the defect has reached a severity that requires a prolonged recovery period.[9] The general principles of management of this disturbance are listed in Table 2–2.

TABLE 2–2.
Management of Postobstructive Diuresis

1. Begin timed urine collection after hydronephrotic residual urine is removed
2. If urine flow <50 mL/30 min, patient may be managed with oral fluids and added salts po if there are no other contraindications to this approach; check blood pressure every 4 hr and 24-hr urine sodium output
3. If urine flow 50–100 mL/30 min, obtain sodium and potassium measurement in urine
   a. If rate of urine flow persists into second hour postobstruction, give solution of 0.075M NaCl in 5% dextrose at infusion rate equal to urine flow
   b. Continue infusion at this rate for first 24 hr postobstruction
   c. Monitor weight every 12 hr
   d. If weight stable and unchanging after 24 hr reduce infusion rate by 50%
   e. If weight decrease ≥1 kg, continue infusion for second 24 hr, then withdraw
4. If urine flow >100 mL/30 min, start infusion of 0.075M NaCl and 5% dextrose immediately at rate equal to rate of urine flow
   a. Measure sodium output in first urine collection before infusion; if [Na] >0.075M in urine, increase [Na] in infusate appropriately
   b. Continue infusion at this rate for first 48 hr
   c. After 48 hr, reduce infusion rate by 50% and observe urine flow and blood pressure carefully
   d. If urine flow decreased and blood pressure stable, continue regimen of progressive reduction
   e. If urine flow fails to decrease after 2 hr of infusate reduction, return to previous infusion rate and repeat
5. If initially measured urine flow rate >150 mL/30 min, proceed as outlined in 4 above but wait at least 96 hr before attempting reduction in infusion rate
   a. Monitor blood pressure and pulse at least every 30 min until stability is documented
   b. Monitor urinary potassium output and plasma electrolytes (particularly potassium and chloride) to ensure that replacement is adequate
   c. After 96 hr reduce infusion rate by no more than 25% and continue to follow patient very closely

OLIGURIA WITH PRERENAL AZOTEMIA

Oliguria with accompanying elevation of blood urea nitrogen (BUN) and creatinine may result from a variety of cardiovascular disturbances that lead to hypoperfusion of the kidneys. They may produce a temporary reduction in urine formation that persists sufficiently long to allow azotemia to develop. The most common causes for this disturbance are prolonged dehydration and sodium depletion. Such derangement in cardiovascular function may be produced from such diverse disturbances as congestive heart failure, heat exhaustion with severe sweat losses, severe diarrhea, diabetic acidosis, and excessive use of potent diuretic agents. Hemodynamically, the primary cause of the impaired renal function is volume depletion, which results from the dehydration and sodium loss. With adequate fluid and salt replacement, the azotemia usually disappears promptly, urine flow is readily reestablished, and no evidence of residual renal impairment can be detected. In individuals whose renal function was previously normal, the distinction between the prerenal oligurias and acute renal failure is readily made based on the rapidity with which the abnormalities are reversed with appropriate rehydration. When the disturbances producing the prerenal azotemia are correctly diagnosed and effectively treated, renal function is promptly restored to normal. Unless therapy is instituted promptly, however, persistence of this renal hypoperfusion may lead to damage of the nephron and the evolution of typical acute renal failure. For this reason prerenal causes should be sought in all cases of oliguria. *Urine sodium concentration* provides a useful diagnostic guide. A urine sodium concentration of less than 10 mEq/L or a urine osmolality greater than 500 mOsm/kg of water is much more likely to represent prerenal azotemia.[11] This approach to differentiation between prerenal azotemia and acute renal failure has been extended to the precise definition of a renal failure index: the ratio of urinary sodium to plasma sodium concentration divided by the corresponding urine-to-plasma ratio for creatinine (Cr), as illustrated by the following equation:

$$\frac{\text{Urine [Na]/plasma [Na]}}{\text{Urine [Cr]/plasma [Cr]}} \times 100$$

In the previously normal kidney, prerenal azotemia is usually associated with a value of less than 1 for this ratio and in acute renal failure the value exceeds 2. Although of great value in differentiating these two disturbances in the previously normal kidney, it is unreliable in patients who had substantial chronic impairment of renal function prior to the acute injury or insult. This most common circumstance in urologic patients renders the "renal failure index" nearly valueless in differentiating between prerenal azotemia and acute renal failure in the urologic patient with previously documented renal impairment. Similarly, examination of the urinary sediment is of limited value in these patients because of preexisting abnormalities of the urinary tract. In the absence of such local lesions that may be associated with an abnormal urinary sediment, the occurrence of renal tubular epithelial cells, tubular cellular casts, and granular casts is quite common in early acute renal failure but rarely seen in association with prerenal azotemia.

Practically, the differential diagnosis in patients with previously damaged kidneys must rest on clinical judgment and evaluation of the patient's response to corrective therapy directed toward hypovolemia and/or sodium depletion. The acute loss of more than 1.0 to 1.5 L of extracellular fluid is associated with profound hypotension, and hence in correcting presumed deficits one should use this as a guide for planning replacement. A treatment regimen designed to correct suspected hypovolemia as a cause of oliguria should consist of administration of no more than 1.5 L of saline (or Ringer's lactate) plus 500 mL of 5% dextrose solution over a span of 2 to 3 hours unless there is some readily identifiable source of continued fluid loss.

The use of agents to induce an osmotic diuresis is commonly recommended in this circumstance, and the two approaches that have been most extensively used are the administration of a strong loop diuretic such as furosemide or the administration of 40 to 50 g of mannitol whenever there is a suspicion of the impending development of acute renal failure. This approach is particularly useful in differentiating prerenal azotemia from acute renal failure, but its efficacy in preventing acute renal failure remains to be established.[12] *It must not be considered as a diagnostic or therapeutic intervention until the patient has received adequate fluids* (1 L of 0.155 M physiologic saline or Ringer's lactate solution plus an additional 500 mL of 5% dextrose or a volume of similar composition totaling about 30 mL/kg of body weight). If this hydration fails to overcome the oliguria, the use of furosemide is to be preferred, since administration of mannitol may be hazardous, particularly in elderly persons, because of its tendency to produce acute and relatively large increases in the vascular volume as a result of fluid shifts. If the patient does indeed have acute renal failure, mannitol presents an additional risk, namely, acute shifts of fluid from intracellular to extracellular space that may require removal of mannitol by dialysis for correction. Thus furosemide is the preferred agent for attempting to initiate an osmotic diuresis. If these therapeutic maneuvers fail to restore a normal urine flow rate, a presumptive diagnosis of acute renal failure should be made.

ACUTE RENAL FAILURE

Nephrotoxicity

In most general hospitals, nephrotoxic reactions attributable either to aminoglycoside damage or toxic effects of intravenous x-ray contrast media account for perhaps three fourths of the cases seen on the medical and surgical services.[6, 13–16] There are, however, numerous other causes of acute renal failure and these are listed in Table 2–1. The exact pathogenesis of acute renal failure remains an enigma, but there are clearly two categories of disturbance that lead to this clinical picture of profound oliguria and potentially reversible progressive renal failure. Virtually all of the categories of damage leading to acute renal failure listed in Table 2–1 may be classified either as nephrotoxic or as ischemic.

The histologic changes produced by specific toxic agents or chemicals are characterized primarily by necrosis of the epithelial lining of the renal tubules with relatively complete preservation of the tubular basement membrane.[17] The glomeruli usually appear quite normal. With appropriate treatment during this period of uremia, regeneration of the epithelial cells usually occurs within 2 to 3 weeks. When the tubular basement membrane is not damaged by the nephrotoxin, the epithelium grows to cover it completely, reestablishing continuity of the tubules and returning normal tubular function.[17] When the basement membrane is disrupted by the necrotic process, continuity is not reestablished during regeneration, and the tubule does not regain its function.

Ischemia

In the ischemic form of acute renal failure, the histologic findings are much less obvious than are those seen with nephrotoxins. The usual change in this category of disease is the conversion of the tubular epithelial cells to cells that are low-cuboid in appearance, with only minimal evidence of scattered foci of mild necrosis of tubular cells. In general, the intensity of the necrosis correlates quite well with the severity of the clinical manifestations of renal failure. Recent evidence suggests impairment may be more readily explained by obstruction of the tubules by casts than by this minimal evidence of focal necrosis.[18] The detailed pathogenesis of this disturbed state remains to be clearly defined.

Studies in humans with acute oliguric renal failure from various causes reveals total renal blood flow to be decreased and usually less than half of normal values.[19–21] Changes in intrarenal blood flow occur with marked reduction in cortical blood flow and increase in inner cortical or juxtamedullary flow. Afferent arteriolar vasoconstriction develops, and net filtration pressures fall to levels that are capable of producing only minimal amounts of glomerular filtrate. These early vascular changes have led to the designation of this disturbance as *vasomotor nephropathy*. It has been postulated that the reduced renal blood flow will not support the glomerular filtration but is in general adequate to prevent any extensive anoxic cellular necrosis of tubules. Though at times this disturbance is heralded by a well-documented bout of profound hypotension, it occasionally presents with minimal or no evidence of systemic shock. Humoral and local factors responsible for this persistent reduction in renal blood flow remain to be clearly identified. The renin-angiotensin system and catecholamines have been implicated, and some experimental evidence suggests that tubular obstruction could be the earliest identifiable event.

Clinical Course of Acute Renal Failure

The oliguria associated with this disturbance may be as short as 1 or 2 days or, rarely, may exceed 6 weeks. The severity of the oliguria provides a useful guide to the severity and duration that may be anticipated. In general, once blood pressure is stabilized and volume repletion is achieved, the persistence of oliguria with urine output less than 5 to 6 mL/hr usually means that the oliguric phase will be quite prolonged, and the patient will quite likely require support by some form of dialysis before recovery occurs.[1, 22] Typically, the vasomotor nephropathy is described as characterized by three phases: (1) the oligemic phase, (2) the oliguric phase, and (3) the diuretic phase.

As previously noted, the *oligemic* phase is associated with vascular instability. This early phase requires prompt stabilization of the blood pressure, and restoration of any volume deficits is mandatory if severe damage to the kidney is to be averted. Fluids used for volume replacement should reflect the pathogenesis of the disturbance. Optimal treatment of severe blood loss requires transfusions and plasma administration; fluid loss should be treated by appropriate isotonic fluid replacement that takes into account the nature and quantity of fluid lost. It is both unnecessary and unwise to give significant quantities of a dextrose-water solution that will ultimately represent excess solute-free water. Isotonic saline or isotonic Ringer's lactate should be administered with 1.0 to 1.5 L being given as replacement for presumed volume deficit unless losses of a greater magnitude have been documented. The addition of only a modest water load (500–1,000 mL of 5% dextrose) should be adequate to sustain a water diuresis if the volume expansion is successful in correcting renal hypoperfusion. If these maneuvers are unsuccessful in increasing urine flow, the presumptive diagnosis of acute renal failure should be made at this point, and management consistent with treatment requirements of the oliguric phase should be implemented.

The first and most important principal of management of the *oliguric-uremic* phase is prompt reduction in fluid intake. Fluid intake should be reduced to 400 mL daily plus *measured* losses. In the presence of profound oliguria, the "water of metabolism," or water resulting from the metabolism of carbohydrates and fats, is significant. Conversion of 100 g of carbohydrate to carbon dioxide and water generates 100 mL of water of metabolism. Similarly, combustion of fat yields approximately 1 mL of water per gram of fat oxidized. The body thus produces between 300 and 500 mL of water daily from metabolic activity. The persistence of tissue breakdown associated with the catabolic state further adds to water produced or "freed" by the patient, and thus there may be substantial sources of endogenous water production during the oliguric uremic phase. In addition, the preformed water of ingested food may contribute several hundred milliliters more. Limitation of fluid intake to 400 mL/day is in fact often associated with a total net fluid intake plus endogenous water release that exceeds 1,500 to 1,800 mL daily in these patients. Careful monitoring of fluid restriction is mandatory if the physician is to avoid fluid overload. *Accurate intake and output records and careful daily weights are the most essential data for adequate management of these patients.*

The patient should receive no sodium except that which is used to replace measured sodium losses. Similarly, potassium intake should be reduced to zero. In addition, in those individuals who have a urine output under 150 mL/day, Kayexalate (an ion exchange resin that will bind potassium in the gastrointestinal tract) should be given promptly and in doses of at least 25 to 30 g daily. One gram of Kayexalate (sodium polystyrene sulfonate) will bind 4 mEq of potassium, and hence a daily intake of 25 g of the resin is theoretically capable of binding 100 mEq of potassium. This insoluble potassium-resin complex is excreted via the gastrointestinal tract. In practice, exchange rarely exceeds 60% to 70%, so that 25 g of resin per day leads to excretion of 60 to 70 mEq of potassium via the gastrointestinal tract. Since this exchange, which leads to the conversion of the sodium polystyrene resin to the potassium polystyrene form, occurs mainly in the colon, there is about a 24-hour delay between oral administration of Kayexalate and its effect on an elevated extracellular fluid potassium pool. This nevertheless is adequate to prevent the development of hyperkalemia except in circumstances associated with marked catabolic activity or concealed hemorrhage. When hyperkalemia approaches 7 mEq/L, prompt dialysis is essential.

Attempts to minimize nitrogen catabolism should include the provision of at least 1,200 calories/day as carbohydrate and fat intake. In situations associated with severe systemic illness, extensive surgery, or other illnesses that are likely to be long-term, a sustained period of oliguria may require total parenteral nutrition. If this is undertaken in the uremic patient, *great care should be exercised in excluding calcium, phosphorous, and potassium from the administered solutions.* The most important elements of management of the oliguric uremic phase are summarized in Table 2–3.

The *diuretic phase* is variable in length and intensity and is most sharply defined in those individuals who have had a period of severe oliguria or anuria. When

TABLE 2–3.

Management of Oliguric Phase of Acute Renal Failure

Water

- Measure fluid intake and *total* fluid output
- Reduce fluid intake to 400 mL/day plus measured losses
- Weigh patient daily; if weight increases, reevaluate fluid intake
- Attempt to promote modest but continuing weight loss (¼–½ lb/day)

Sodium

- Place on sodium-free intake
- Sodium should be given only to replace measured sodium losses
- Measure sodium content of any urine excreted plus all other fluids

Potassium

- Place patient on potassium-free intake
- If plasma potassium exceeds 5 mEq/L, place on regimen of Kayexalate; if this cannot be taken orally, potassium of 5 mEq/L is indication for hemodialysis

Acidosis

- Acidosis should be prevented
- Reduce protein intake to minimal levels
- Replace sodium as Ringer's lactate or bicarbonate at earliest signs of acidosis
- Provide at least 1,200–1,500 calories/day

Dialysis

- Dialysis should be begun promptly for hyperkalemia, weight gain, acidosis, BUN >100 mg/dL (>50–60 mg/dL if patient is catabolic) urine output begins to increase, it usually does so over a period of 4 or 5 days during which the systemic manifestations of uremia and at times acidosis and other related pathophysiologic disturbances continue to worsen or fail to show improvement. In addition, urine that is formed as the kidney begins to recover from ischemic damage usually reflects marked limitation in tubular function. The most common abnormality that results from this tubular impairment is an obligatory natriuresis. The persistent tubular damage renders the tubule incapable of reabsorbing inadequate quantities of sodium so that sodium loss increases as urine volume increases. *For this reason it is important to monitor the daily sodium losses in the patient when the diuretic phase begins, and these losses should be replaced for at least the first 5 or 6 days of the recovery phase.* After the first week of recovery, this defect poses a less serious problem, and sodium administration should be gradually curtailed. Usually, if the patient is able to eat and take fluids orally the kidney is capable of maintaining homeostasis in reasonably adequate fashion after the diuretic phase has been present for 8 to 10 days.

INDICATIONS FOR HEMODIALYSIS IN ACUTE RENAL FAILURE

The principal objective of management during the oliguric stage should be the prevention of all clinical manifestations of uremia.[23–25] The measures recommended in the preceding section are designed to retard the development of uremic symptoms and to prevent fluid overload. These objectives should be vigorously pursued by including dialysis as standard medical therapy. *Early and frequent dialysis is the hallmark of a good therapeutic regimen for acute renal failure.* This is particularly true of patients in whom acute renal failure develops in the postoperative period or who have been subjected to extensive trauma of whatever type. In Table 2–4 are summarized data from relatively large series in the literature showing clearly that when acute renal failure complicates trauma, the prognosis is particularly poor. For that reason these patients with trauma-related acute renal failure should be subjected to dialysis very early in the course of their renal failure. Even the asymptomatic patient in this high-risk category should probably be dialyzed when the BUN reaches a level of about 75 mg/dL. Earlier dialysis should be instituted if there is any tendency for even modest elevation of the plasma potassium level. In trauma associated with extensive tissue injury and death, hyperkalemia is a particularly serious and frequently severe complication. Daily dialysis should be considered in such patients if there is a tendency for persistent hyperkalemia.

Patients requiring particular attention are those in whom acute renal failure complicates an illness that is already characterized by a sustained catabolic response and the patient is in need of total parenteral nutrition. Such patients should be dialyzed daily in order to allow adequate treatment without risking fluid overload or the production of acidosis or other manifestations of uremia.

The use of parenteral amino acid mixtures has been proposed as a means of minimizing catabolism and retarding the rate of development of uremia.[26] Hypertonic glucose plus essential amino acids has been reported to lessen the degree of renal failure; however, some experimental evidence suggests that this approach may have some adverse effects in animals. For that reason, such adjunctive therapy should only be undertaken when patients have been placed on a regular dialysis regimen.[27]

Hemorrhage, usually from the gastrointestinal tract, and infection are among the most common causes of death in patients with acute renal failure during

TABLE 2–4.
Prognosis in Acute Renal Failure

	Traumatic (Surgical)			Nephrotoxic (Medical)		
Source	No. of Cases	No. of Survivors	% Survival	No. of Cases	No. of Survivors	% Survival
Kleinkneckt et al.[22, 25]	296	142	50	229	146	64
Knepshield et al.[22]	62	19	30	95	67	71
University of Minnesota[22]	85	26	31	128	79	61
Cameron et al.[22]	73	28	38			
Composite reported experience, cited by Cameron[22]	1,994	836	42			

the oliguric phase. While prophylactic antibiotics are not warranted, very careful monitoring of the patient's condition is essential, with appropriate antibiotic therapy instituted at the first sign of significant infection. Because of the impaired excretory function of the kidney, careful attention to appropriate adjustment of antibiotic dosage schedules is mandatory. Early treatment of uremia with adequate dialysis reduces the likelihood of infection and of bleeding, and thus decreases morbidity and mortality. This approach yields extremely good results with the nephrotoxic cases of acute renal failure, which represent currently perhaps the leading cause of acute renal failure. When acute renal failure complicates traumatic injury, however, the mortality rate is substantial, despite even the optimal therapy illustrated in Table 2–3.

High-Risk Patients

Certain patients are at extremely high risk for the development of acute renal failure, and probably more of these patients reside on the urologic service than on other services in a general hospital. A large proportion of the urologic patients who are hospitalized have preexisting impaired renal function and thus exhibit increased susceptibility to nephrotoxic damage from both radiocontrast material and other nephrotoxic agents such as aminoglycosides, and that is why they are at such substantial risk. Many of the patients with nephrolithiasis and chronic pyelonephritis have organisms that are responsive to very few agents except the aminoglycosides, and for this reason these drugs must be used. When this becomes necessary, it is essential that adequate control be exercised by monitoring plasma levels of the drug. In individuals whose renal function has been reduced by 60% or more, daily measurements of these antibiotics is mandatory, with the dosage schedule being determined by these measurements. Should acute renal failure supervene and the gravity of the infection require that the treatment with aminoglycosides be continued, frequent and vigorous dialysis is mandatory during this period of sustained treatment. When this is done, prognosis in this group is usually favorable.

The individual who may be exposed to the greatest risk of aminoglycoside toxicity is the individual who received a course of aminoglycoside therapy and then has the drug restarted after an interval of 1 to 2 weeks. Experimental studies in animals have shown that the aminoglycoside is accumulated in the kidney and is only slowly excreted over a period of many weeks. Administration of a second loading dose to such an individual after only a short interval or drug-free period exposes that patient's kidneys to a very great risk of nephrotoxic damage. For this reason, the second loading dose under these circumstances should probably be no more than a third of the original loading dose.

Nonoliguric Acute Renal Failure

Some patients with acute renal failure never go through an oliguric phase yet manifest profound renal failure.[5, 7] When this clinical picture was first recognized, it was associated with severe trauma and a very rapidly rising uremia nitrogen level. For this reason it was considered that the condition was the result of a severe osmotic load being placed on the remaining functioning nephrons. More recently, this clinical picture has been associated with nephrotoxic damage to the kidney and is a particularly common feature of the acute renal failure produced by the aminoglycosides, most commonly gentamicin. Although no controlled trial has been reported, retrospective examination of these cases suggests that the prognosis may be somewhat better. For this reason, there has been great interest in trying to convert oliguric cases to nonoliguric cases by the use of diuretics, particularly furosemide.[12] If the individual with early oliguric renal failure exhibits a significant increase in urine output, there is a widely held view that such an individual should continue to receive doses of Lasix (furosemide) necessary to sustain this increased urine output. Whether this use results in an improved outcome remains to be determined. The prognosis in acute renal failure probably is more influenced by the underlying cause of the renal failure and associated illness. Those cases that are associated with trauma in general do quite poorly. The mortality rate in some series exceeds 60% (see Table 2–3). Nontraumatic cases usually exhibit a survival rate that exceeds 75%. It is difficult to separate causes of death directly attributable to acute renal failure from deaths related to the underlying or primary condition. Because of the efficacy of dialysis as a means of management of renal failure, it is likely that most deaths are attributable to the underlying or primary illness. Nevertheless, from the standpoint of management, it is essential that vigorous treatment of the renal failure with early dialysis is essential if deaths are to be kept to a minimum in patients with these complicated problems.

EDITORIAL COMMENT

Acute renal failure has confronted virtually all urologists at some time. Dr. Walker divides the discussion into the classic phases of postrenal, prerenal, and renal causes of acute renal failure. His tables provide excellent clinical guidelines for the management of the patient with acute renal failure. Postobstructive diuresis can be a difficult clinical problem and is secondary to the osmotic diuresis of the urea as well as the impairment of tubular function. Dr. Walker's suggestions need to be followed carefully, because overzealous intravenous fluid administration will often continue an iatrogenic phase of diuresis. If the patient is physically capable and alert and has a normal thirst mechanism, he will usually consume satisfactory quantities of fluid orally to maintain hydration. Another point worth stressing is the potential for aminoglycoside toxicity when the medication has been initiated again after a short interval following an earlier course. The loading dose should be approximately one third of the original loading dose.

REFERENCES

1. Swann RC, Merrill JP: The clinical course of acute renal failure. *Medicine* 1953; 32:215.
2. Whelton A, Donadio JV Jr: Post-traumatic

acute renal failure in Vietnam. *Johns Hopkins Med J* 1969; 124:95.

3. Bleumle LW, Webster GD Jr, Elkinton JR: Acute tubular necrosis: Analysis of 100 cases with respect to mortality, complications and treatment with and without dialysis. *Arch Intern Med* 1959; 194:180.
4. Vertel RM, Knochel JP: Non-oliguric acute renal failure. *JAMA* 1967; 200:598.
5. Anderson RJ, Linas SL, Berns AS, et al: Non-oliguric acute renal failure. *N Engl J Med* 1977; 296:1134.
6. Appel GB, Neu HC: Nephrotoxicity of antimicrobial agents. I, II, and III. *N Engl J Med* 1977; 296:663; 722; 783.
7. Meyers C, Roxe DM, Hano JE: The clinical course of nonoliguric acute renal failure. *Cardiovasc Med* 1977; 2:669.
8. Whelton A, Solez K: Aminoglycoside nephrotoxicity (editorial). *J Lab Clin Med* 1982; 99:148.
9. Bricker NS, Shwayri ER, Reardon JB, et al: Abnormality in renal function resulting from urinary tract obstruction. *Am J Med* 1957; 23:554.
10. Graham JR, Suby HI, LeCompte PR, et al: Fibrotic disorders associated with methysergide therapy for headache. *N Engl J Med* 1966; 274:359–368.
11. Miller TR, Anderson RJ, Linas SL, et al: Urinary diagnostic indices in acute renal failure: A prospective study. *Ann Intern Med* 1978; 89:47–50.
12. Levinsky NG, Bernard DB, Johnston PA: Enhancement of recovery of acute renal failure: Effects of mannitol and diuretics, in Brenner BM, Stein JH (eds): *Contemporary Issues in Nephrology: Acute Renal Failure.* New York, Churchill Livingstone, Inc, 1980, pp 163–179.
13. Swartz RD, Rubin JE, Leeming BW, et al: Renal failure following major angiography. *Am J Med* 1978; 65:31.
14. VanZee BE, Hoy WE, Talley TE, et al: Renal injury associated with intravenous pyelography in nondiabetic and diabetic patients. *Ann Intern Med* 1978; 89:51–54.
15. Ansari Z, Baldwin DS: Acute renal failure due to radiocontrast agents. *Nephron* 1976; 17:28.
16. Carvallo A, Rakowski TA, Argy WP, et al: Acute renal failure following drip infusion pyelography. *Am J Med* 1978; 65:38–45.
17. Oliver J, MacDowell M, Tracy A: The pathogenesis of acute renal failure associated with traumatic and toxic injury: Renal ischemia, nephrotoxic damage and the ischemic episode. *J Clin Invest* 1951; 30:1307.
18. Racusen LC, Finn WF, Whelton A, et al: Mechanisms of lysine-induced acute renal failure in rats. *Kidney Int* 1985; 27:517–522.
19. Lauson HD, Bradley SE, Cournand A: The renal circulation in shock. *J Clin Invest* 1944; 23:381–402.
20. Hollenberg NK, Adams DF, Oken DE, et al: Acute renal failure due to nephrotoxins: Renal hemodynamic and angiographic studies in man. *N Engl J Med* 1970; 282:1329.
21. Hollenberg NK, Epstein J, Rosen SM, et al: Acute oliguric renal failure in man: Evidence for preferential renal cortical ischemia. *Medicine* 1968; 47:455.
22. Friedman EA, Eliahou HE (eds): *Proceedings: Conference on Acute Renal Failure.* US Department of Health, Education, and Welfare publication (NIH) 74-608. Washington, DC, 1973.
23. Teschan PE, Baxter CR, O'Brien TF, et al: Prophylactic hemodialysis in the treatment of acute renal failure. *Ann Intern Med* 1960; 53:992.
24. Easterling RE, Forland M: A five-year experience with prophylactic dialysis for acute renal failure. *Trans Am Soc Artif Intern Organs* 1964; 10:200.
25. Kleinknecht D, Jungers P, Chanard J, et al: Uremic and non-uremic complications in acute renal failure: Evaluation of early and frequent dialysis on prognosis. *Kidney Int* 1972; 1:190.
26. Abel RM, Beck CH Jr, Abbott WM, et al: Improved survival from acute renal failure after treatment with intravenous essential 1-amino acids and glucose. *N Engl J Med* 1973; 288:695.
27. Schrier RW, Conger JD: Acute renal failure: Pathogenesis, diagnosis and management, in Schrier RW (ed): *Renal and Electrolyte Disorders,* ed 2. Boston, Little, Brown & Co, 1980, pp 376–407.

CHAPTER 3

Complications of Total Parenteral Nutrition

Terry W. Hensle, M.D.
Robin K. Levin, M.D.

Total parenteral nutrition, invaluable as it is in certain circumstances, has a number of clearly recognized complications. Some of these complications, especially the mechanical and infectious problems, are inherent in the placement and long-term maintenance of a central intravenous catheter. Other difficulties that are encountered, principally the metabolic ones, are almost unique to the administration of total parenteral nutrition.

TECHNICAL COMPLICATIONS OF CATHETER INSERTION

The technical complications of parenteral nutrition involve two potential dangers: first, the hazards of venipuncture and catheter placement in a central vein, and second, the harmful effects of long-term contact of a foreign body with the vessel wall. Technical complications have been reported to occur in 3% to 11% of patients receiving parenteral nutrition under the care of nutrition support teams.[1]

The hypertonicity of total parenteral nutrition (TPN) solutions requires the delivery of these substances through large veins. Most often the major central veins of the thorax or neck have been chosen for this purpose. (However, alternatives such as the saphenous system have been used successfully when the veins of the upper extremities are thrombosed).[1, 2] Several routes of access have been employed. The internal jugular insertion is technically fairly safe but is uncomfortable and is poorly tolerated by most patients, especially when long-term maintenance is required. As a result, the most common location for the insertion of a percutaneous central venous line has been the subclavian vein.

Introduced in 1951 in France and popularized in the United States in the early 1960s, the subclavian central venous catheter has been an extremely useful diagnostic and therapeutic tool. Among the most widely used indications have been rapid administration of fluid or blood, central venous pressure readings, and, relatively recently, nutritional therapy. Unfortunately, the anatomy of the subclavian area involves the complex intersection of major vessels, nerves, and organs. The potential for injury to neighboring structures during catheter insertion is great. The first rib forms the "floor" of the needle track as it advances cranially toward the subclavian vein. On an average of just 5 mm directly posterior is the pleura of the apex of the lung. For this reason, especially if the needle course is not kept parallel to the chest wall, pneumothorax is a common complication of subclavian vein puncture. Pneumothorax has been reported to occur in rates as high as 33% in patients not treated by a "nutrition support team."[2] There is an average overall incidence of 6%,[3] and pneumothorax is more common when tissue wasting is present. Thus, cachectic patients requiring parenteral nutrition are at a special risk. Fortunately, immediate pneumothorax can be easily diagnosed with a chest x-ray study and treated if necessary with a closed-tube thoracostomy.

Another pleural injury secondary to instrumentation that is becoming better recognized is delayed pneumothorax. In these cases, the postinsertion roentgenogram is normal. However, follow-up x-ray films taken several hours to days later, either because of the development of pleural symptoms or for unrelated reasons, show a pneumothorax on the side of the subclavian line. Multiple puncture attempts are a common predisposing feature. The pneumothorax is thought to be caused by a slow pleural air leak. Delayed chest x-ray studies as well as the immediate postinsertion roentgenogram are now recommended after a difficult subclavian insertion.

Hemothorax has been reported to occur in an incidence of 0.76% of all subclavian catheterizations.[3] It can occur after either a laceration of a major vessel at the time of venipuncture—usually the subclavian artery—or direct infusion of blood through a malpositioned catheter with its tip in the pleural cavity. Accidental puncture of the subclavian artery has been estimated to occur in 2% to 3% of subclavian venipuncture attempts. Because it is usually immediately recognized, local compression usually suffices to prevent further damage and formation of a hemothorax. However, if the patient is on anticoagulant therapy or the advancement of the catheter is difficult, a small, undetected arterial tear may occur, and close follow-up of the patient is warranted.

If the tear in the vessel wall is farther from the entrance site, for example in the superior vena cava, the subsequent collection of blood may cause hemomediastinum, which may be evident in a widened mediastinum on the postinsertion x-ray. This, however, depends on the size of the laceration and may not be evident clinically or radiographically for several hours.

Pericardial tamponade has been reported as a result of central venous catheterization, through cardiac perforation either at initial placement or with subsequent erosion of the catheter tip through the chamber wall. Of the 25 cases in the English-language literature, 75% have been fatal.

Air embolism is another potentially disastrous problem associated with central catheters. The consequences of the introduction of air into the circulatory system depends on the amount of air that enters and the rate of delivery. Death has been reported to occur after 100 mL of air entered an intravenous line suddenly.[4] Slower rates or smaller amounts result in hemodynamic compromise in the patient, usually manifested as dyspnea, hypotension, and a "null wheel" or machinery-like cardiac murmur. Neurologic symptoms are possible if a patent foramen ovale is present or cerebrovascular disease is preexisting.

TECHNICAL COMPLICATIONS OF CATHETER MAINTENANCE

Venous thrombosis is a serious, relatively common but largely preventable long-term complication of long-term TPN administration. "Virchow's triad" of risk for the thrombogenesis (venous stasis, hypercoagulable state, local trauma) is likely to be present in many TPN patients.

Ryan et al.[5] found that the superior vena cava and its main tributaries were thrombosed in eight out of 34 autopsied patients in their prospective study of 200 patients receiving TPN. Three of these had pulmonary emboli that appeared to have originated in the superior vena cava. The duration of parenteral nutrition therapy in the patients with thrombosis ranged from 3 to 95 days. All the catheters were made of polyethylene. Similarly, in a more recent study, subclavian vein thrombosis was estimated to be present in 71% of patients receiving TPN.[6]

A high incidence of thrombosis was documented by venography in up to 90% of the patients in whom a 16-gauge polyvinyl chloride (PVC) catheter was in place in a central vein from 1 to 35 days. Most often this finding consisted of thrombus adherent to the catheter ("sleeve thrombus"), but in 13% a mural thrombus was present, and in 7% complete occlusion of the vein was seen. Sleeve thrombi begin formation at the point of catheter entry into the vein and extend toward the tip. This process is thought to be complete within about 10 days of catheter placement. Although a sleeve thrombus may enter the circulation untethered after removal of the catheter, resulting in delayed thromboembolic consequences, most do not cause any serious sequelae.

The thrombogenicity of the catheter apparently depends on its composition. Silicone-based (SB or Silastic) catheters, such as those used in subcutaneous right atrial lines (Hickman/Brouviac) are reportedly less prone to causing thrombosis than PVC or polyethylene (PE) catheters. This is presumably due to the greater degree of endothelial damage caused by the stiffer PVC and PE lines. The silicone catheters, on the other hand, probably have less contact with the intima due to their greater propensity to float within the vessel. A significantly lower rate of thrombus formation has been documented by venography in SB catheters as compared to nonheparinized PE catheters.

Silicone catheters have two major drawbacks: their tendency to attract particulate matter and their fragility. Care must be taken to rinse gloves of talc and dust before handling the catheter. Such adherent particles are in part responsible for the phlebitis seen when catheters are in place in a vein. A somewhat greater incidence of catheter breakage has been reported in SB lines as opposed to lines composed of PVC or PE. Typically, rupture occurs with too vigorous flushing or with excessive traction on the line.

Once thrombosis has occurred, the extremity is elevated and a continuous heparin infusion is usually maintained for 7 to 10 days. However, there are indications that heparin may be less than effective in catheter-related thrombosis.[6] Fibrinolytic agents are being used in this situation with increasing frequency. With administration of dosages ranging from 25,000 units in 6 mL of saline over 20 minutes to 5,000 units/hr, streptokinase usually produces rapid clearance of the occlusion; however, hemorrhagic complications must be watched for closely.

METABOLIC COMPLICATIONS

Perhaps the most complex problems encountered during the administration of TPN are the metabolic complications that are directly related to the composition of the formula and the technique of delivery. The cause and effect of the metabolic derangement may not always be obvious; thus careful planning and vigilance is required of the clinician.

The most common metabolic abnormalities involve glucose and electrolytes. It seems logical that without close monitoring of blood glucose levels, administration of the high glucose loads of glucose-based TPN could result in hyperglycemia, especially in glucose-intolerant patients (e.g., those with diabetes mellitus, renal failure, or sepsis or those who are post trauma). Weinsier et al.,[7] in their prospective study of metabolic abnormalities in 100 patients on TPN, found that uncontrolled hyperglycemia (blood glucose level higher than 30 mg/dL after more than 48 hours on TPN) was present in 47 patients, making it the most common abnormality. Ryan et al.[5] noted glucose intolerance in 25% of the patients studied. Most often, this situation develops when the total calculated caloric requirement of the patient is delivered as soon as TPN is instituted. A lower starting concentration of glucose with a gradual increase, on the other hand, allows adaptation of endogenous insulin production. An alternative answer to the problem of hyperglycemia is to provide some of the caloric requirement as fat.

Total parenteral nutrition has the potential for causing a much less common but very serious abnormality of glucose metabolism: hyperosmolar nonketotic hyperglycemic coma. With a mortality rate reported as high as 40%, it may occur suddenly in patients receiving TPN.[8] The usual initial manifestations are neurologic: lethargy, confusion, focal neurologic signs, and focal or generalized seizures. Treatment consists of fluid replacement (hypotonic saline is usually recommended) and insulin in adequate amounts but at a gradual rate to prevent cerebral edema. Close monitoring of both serum and urine glucose levels as well as appropriate rates of delivery of TPN can help prevent this complication from occurring.

The osmotic load administered to the patient on TPN can be very high: from 2,930 to 5,000 mOsm in 1 day. The markedly expanded extracellular fluid volume may lead to changes in renal clearances with resulting electrolytic imbalances. An example is the hypouricemia seen in association with TPN administration.[8]

Another electrolyte abnormality seen relatively commonly in association with TPN is hypophosphatemia, and it may not be due to changes in renal clearance. It may be the most common electrolyte imbalance seen with TPN, occurring in up to 30% of patients. Hypophosphatemia can have profound effects on the metabolism of the red blood cell, causing a decrease in 2,3-diphosphoglycerate and resulting in impairment of tissue oxygenation. The clinical effects of hypophosphatemia are observed in many different organ systems including red blood cell, white blood cell, and platelet dysfunction, respiratory failure, muscle weakness, and seizures. Monitoring of serum phosphate levels with supplementation as necessary should be mandatory during TPN.

The elevation of alkaline phosphatase, serum glutamic oxaloacetic transaminase (SGOT), and serum bilirubin levels during the course of TPN is a well known and common phenomenon.[9] Weinsier et al.[7] found that 74% of patients studied had at least a 50% rise in one liver function test (LFT), while 35% had elevations in two or more tests, regardless of baseline liver function. Alkaline phosphatase was commonly affected: it rose in 63% of patients. Serum bilirubin and SGOT rose in 55% and 54% of patients, respectively. There was a return to normal LFT values during the course of TPN in about half of the patients.

Whether TPN can cause permanent hepatic damage in a subset of patients is unclear. To address this question, Bower et al.[10] followed the course of 60 adult patients with chronic gastrointestinal failure who were on home TPN. Fifty-one of the 60 had either no abnormality in liver enzymes or mild transient elevations. Nine out of 60 (15%) had LFT abnormalities that persisted for a median of 18 months. Three patients had prolonged jaundice, one died of hepatic encephalopathy, and one died after biliary tract exploration for protracted hepatic cholestasis.

Attempts at prevention of this problem have met with varying success. Liver function abnormalities may be lessened in patients receiving fat as one third of their caloric requirement as compared to patients receiving all glucose-based TPN. However, reversing the carbohydrate-fat ratio to 2:3 was shown to be associated with cholestasis. Timing of the infusion may also be important. There were fewer hepatic complications in patients when TPN was cycled during the day (in contrast to continuous TPN).

INFECTIOUS COMPLICATIONS

The use of TPN has been demonstrated to have a high incidence of catheter-associated sepsis ranging from 2% to 27%.[11] Catheter sepsis, when associated with a patient receiving TPN, has been defined as an episode of clinical sepsis for which no anatomical locus can be identified and which resolves on removal of the offending catheter.[12] Various routes for the initiation of infection have been postulated, including microbial colonization of the central venous catheter (CVC) from contaminated infusate, manipulation of the intravenous delivery system, hematogenous seeding of the intravascular segment of the CVC tip, and microbial contamination of the skin at the site of catheter insertion with subsequent colonization of the CVC. Confirmatory evidence of catheter sepsis is largely based on positive blood and/or catheter tip cultures, since other clinical and biochemical criteria frequently fail to identify CVC sepsis in the critically ill patients who remain at highest risk. The population of patients who are candidates for TPN are frequently debilitated and malnourished; they suffer from underlying diseases, including, inflammatory bowel disease, widespread burns, diabetes, renal or hepatic failure, and cancer, which predispose them to infection. In addition, a large number of these patients will be concurrently receiving broad-spectrum antibiotic therapy, chemotherapy, radiation therapy, or steroids, which further underscores the problem with immune compromise faced by these patients. In this setting, it comes as no surprise that sepsis is the most frequent and potentially the most serious complication that may be encountered in patients receiving TPN.

The main dilemma regarding CVC sepsis pertains to an ongoing controversy about the primary route of infection. Many studies have been carried out that support various alternatives. A review of the available literature supports the view that sepsis may be the end result of catheter seeding from several sites. Semiquantitative cultures of the catheter insertion site and catheter segments (i.e., subcutaneous and intravascular) have confirmed a significant correlation between the number of organisms recovered from the insertion site and colonization of the intravascular and/or subcutaneous catheter segments.[12] The organism most frequently isolated from the skin at the site of catheter insertion is *Staphylococcus epidermidis*, a component of indigenous skin flora. Previously considered a cutaneous nonpathogen, this organism has been identified as a potential pathogen regarding TPN, but it still remains the most common false-positive isolate.[13] Microbial skin growth appears to be related to several potential risk factors that have not been fully assessed. The duration of hospital stay prior to the institution of TPN, patient age, skin preparation technique, and insertion site maintenance, as well as violations of parenteral nutrition protocol, were all significantly associated with skin colonization.

Contaminated infusate is another potential source of CVC sepsis. Studies of solutions containing synthetic crystalline amino acids have noted that while yeast growth is possible, these solutions fail to support bacterial growth. In contrast, parenteral lipid emulsions, which became available in the United States in 1976, can support luxuriant growth of bacteria and yeast. Lipid emulsions gained rapid support because of their caloric density and isotonic nature. Various commercial products differ as to oil base and concentration, yet all provide equal support for bacterial and yeast growth. *Candida albicans* grows well regardless of the parenteral nutrition solution tested. Its growth in standard TPN has been attributed to the presence of glucose and nitrogen, two of its necessary growth factors. The growth of this particular yeast in lipid emulsion has been attributed to the organism's ability to substitute glycerol for glucose as a carbon source.[14] The clinical implications pertain to the establishment of strict guidelines for the utilization of lipid emulsions as part of a TPN regimen. A maximal 12-hour "hang time" is usually adequate for the standard 500-mL bottles. Smaller bottles are available but these are not usually cost-effective. Pediatrics is the one specific clinical area where small quantities of lipid emulsion are frequently used and where smaller bottles would be of benefit. Some hospitals repackage lipid emulsion but this practice could lead to augmented risks of emulsion contamination. In patients where CVC sepsis is of higher potential risk, thought should be given to TPN based solely on solutions of glucose and amino acids, which may afford the patient some protection against TPN-related infection. In young children, the inclusion of lipid emulsion may also predispose to infection by inducing reticuloendothelial system malfunction and derangement of immunologic defenses.[15]

Given that the diagnosis of CVC sepsis is difficult, it is important to mention that there appear to be a limited number of patients who demonstrate a noninfective, blood and catheter culture–negative, catheter-related fever, which normalizes within 24 hours of catheter removal and is probably secondary to a local reaction, thrombophlebitis, or hypersensitivity to the catheter material.[16] Available silicone rubber catheters are maximally inert[17] and may respond to antibiotic therapy without colonization in the face of presumptive sepsis, unlike the conventional PVC catheters.

The last major predisposing factor in the development of CVC sepsis is a break in technique. Such infractions include hub leakage, piggyback violation of the TPN lines, and inattentive line placement or local skin care. Newer techniques utilizing multiple-channel CVC systems and complete mixtures in larger plastic bags with laminar flow chambers are being explored in an attempt to decrease the risk of CVC sepsis.

In review, CVC sepsis is a potentially life-threatening complication in the administration of TPN to seriously ill and frequently immunocompromised patients. Sepsis is attended by a febrile episode, and CVC sepsis is a diagnosis of exclusion. The best predictors remain positive blood and/or catheter tip cultures, although semiquantitative skin cultures at the catheter insertion site have been helpful. The spectrum of organisms that have been recovered include *S. epidermidis* as the most common pathogen, with *C. albicans* as the most virulent. Other implicated organisms include: *Enterococcus, Staphylococcus aureus, Klebsiella pneumoniae, Acinetobacter anitratus,* diphtheroids, *Pseudomonas cepacia, Serratia marcescens, Escherichia coli,* and *Streptococcus* species. Recommendations designed to decrease CVC sepsis emphasize the value of rigid TPN maintenance protocols. Skin care at the insertion site should be given regularly by trained personnel. The use of antibacterial cleansing solutions and applications is unresolved; the use of sterile dressing changes with OpSite or Tegaderm is advised in order to permit visualization of the catheter and provide for the elimination of normal skin moisture via a semipermeable barrier. Suspicion or documentation of CVC sepsis when all other sources have been ruled out warrants removal of the catheter. Central venous catheter sepsis will usually clear spontaneously, but an established fungemia will require 6 weeks of systemic therapy. Reestablishment of TPN must await clearance of the fungemia and/or bacterial infection to prevent reseeding of the new CVC. Compromised patients of this class may harbor mycotic infection in aneurysmal vessels (i.e., retinal) or within septic thrombi, and these considerations must be reviewed in the face of recurrent sepsis. The duration of catheterization has been shown not to influence the risk of sepsis.[12] Given adherence to these general guidelines, TPN may be provided to high-risk patients with a low incidence of CVC sepsis.

EDITORIAL COMMENT

Nutrition is a frequently overlooked area in the management of surgical patients. Increasingly, urologic patients have become more demanding in preoperative and postoperative management. Surgery of great magnitude, older age, chemotherapy, or associated medical problems often mandate the use of total parenteral nutrition. Most of the severe complications are appropriately summarized in this chapter.

Pneumothorax is one of the most common complications and it may even be delayed. Although the diagnosis is usually made with a chest roentgenogram, auscultation of the chest immediately identifies the presence of pneumothorax.

REFERENCES

1. Daly JM, Long JM: Intravenous hyperalimentation: Techniques and potential complications. *Surg Clin North Am* 1981; 61:583–591.
2. Padberg FT, Ruggiero J, Blackburn GL, et al: Central venous catheterization for parenteral nutrition. *Ann Surg* 1981; 193:269–270.
3. Bernard RW, Stahl WM, Chase RM Jr: Subclavian vein catheterizations: A prospective study: I. Noninfectious complications. *Ann Surg* 1971; 173:184–190.
4. Coppa GF, Gouge TH, Hofstetter SR: Air embolism: A lethal but preventable complication of subclavian vein catheterization. *JPEN* 1981; 5:166–168.
5. Ryan JA, Abel RM, Abbot WM, et al: Catheter complications in total parenteral nutrition: A prospective study of 200 consecutive patients. *N Engl J Med* 1974; 290:757–761.
6. Bozzetti F, Scarpa D, Terno G, et al: Subclavian venous thrombosis due to indwelling catheters: A prospective study on 52 patients. *JPEN* 1983; 7:560–562.
7. Weinsier RL, Bacon J, Butterworth CE: Central venous alimentation: A prospective study of the frequency of metabolic abnormalities among medical and surgical patients. *JPEN* 1982; 6:421–425.
8. Greig PD, Baker JP, Jeejeebhoy KD: Metabolic effects of total parenteral nutrition. *Annu Rev Nutr* 1982; 2:179–199.
9. Krevitz B, Levine GM: Hepatic complications of TPN. *Nutr Support Serv* 1983; 3:11–14.
10. Bower RH: Hepatic complications of parenteral nutrition. *Semin Liver Dis* 1983; 3:216–224.
11. Bjornson HS, Colley R, Bower RH, et al: Association between microorganism growth at the catheter insertion site and colonization of the catheter in patients receiving total parenteral nutrition. *Surgery* 1982; 92:720–727.
12. Sitges-Serra A, Puig P, Jaurrieta E: Catheter-related sepsis during parenteral nutrition. *Surgery* 1983; 93:479.
13. Snydman DR, Pober BR, Murray SA, et al: Predictive value of surveillance skin cultures in total parenteral nutrition related infection. *Lancet* 1982; 2:1385–1388.
14. Melly MA, Meng HC, Schaffner W: Microbial growth of lipid emulsions used in parenteral nutrition. *Arch Surg* 1975; 110:1479–1481.

15. Berant A, Alon U: Pneumococcal meningitis following parenteral alimentation in infants. *J Pediatr Gastrointest Nutr* 1984; 3:312–314.
16. Colley R, Wilson J, Kapusta E, et al: Fever and catheter-related sepsis in total parenteral nutrition. *JPEN* 1979; 3:32.
17. Deitel M, Krajden S, Saldanha CF, et al: An outbreak of *Staphylococcus epidermidis* septicemia. *JPEN* 1983; 7:569–572.-

CHAPTER 4

Infectious Diseases

John G. Bartlett, M.D.

NOSOCOMIAL INFECTIONS

Definitions

Nosocomial infections refer to infections that develop within the hospital and are produced by microorganisms acquired during hospitalization. Epidemiologic patterns of a disease frequency may be expressed as sporadic, endemic, or epidemic. *Sporadic* indicates an irregular appearance of a microbe or disease with no specific pattern. *Endemic* indicates a level of frequency in a specific area, time, or population that exceeds the expected. *Hyperendemic* indicates an increase in the disease frequency beyond the expected number. *Epidemic* indicates a definite increase in the expected incidence. These terms refer to nosocomial infections in general and have proved valuable in epidemiologic investigations; they are especially important in urologic practice, since this has been a major source of nosocomial infections, often with multiply resistant gram-negative bacilli that may be endemic or epidemic on urologic services.

Mechanisms

There are three requirements for the spread of infection: a source of the infecting pathogen, a means of transmission, and a susceptible host. All microorganisms have a natural habitat or reservoir, which varies according to the growth requirements that are peculiar to a given species. The reservoir for most viruses and gram-positive bacteria are humans, including both hospital personnel and patients. For gram-negative bacilli, the reservoir may be either animate or inanimate. Some gram-negative bacilli are especially well adapted to survive in water such as *Pseudomonas aeruginosa,* other pseudomonads, *Serratia marcescens, Achromobacter, Flavobacterium, Acinetobacter,* and *Legionella* species. Three common methods of spread are by contact, through a common vehicle, or via the airborne route. The most important in urologic practice is contact spread, referring to person-to-person passage in which there is physical contact between the source of the microbe and the victim. The single most important factor in preventing this type of transmission is the physical separation of patients by barriers and rigid enforcement of handwashing procedures. The final component of the triad is the host. Hospitalized patients are often uniquely susceptible to infection as a result of associated disease states and a variety of diagnostic or therapeutic maneuvers. In urologic practice the most frequent predisposing factors are indwelling catheters and manipulations of the urinary tract. Current estimates are that at least half of nosocomial infections are preventable, so that methods to protect the host have become a major goal of hospital infection surveillance.

Types of Infection

Currently available data from acute care hospitals indicate that the incidence of hospital-acquired infections is approximately 3.3%.[1] The most frequent site is the urinary tract (1.3/100 patient discharges), surgical wound infections (0.7), lower respiratory tract infections (0.5), and primary bacteremia (0.2). The following is a brief review of general principles concerning infectious complications that commonly occur in patients in all hospital services as well as urology, including bacteremia, hospital-acquired pneumonia, wound infections, and infections related to intravenous lines; urinary tract infections will be discussed separately.

Bacteremia

Sepsis refers to a systemic disease caused by microorganisms or their products, and *septicemia* implies that these microorganisms are in the blood. *Bacteremia* indicates viable bacteria in the blood and requires positive blood cultures for documentation.

Classification.—Bacteremia may be classified as transient, intermittent, or sustained.

Transient bacteremia usually occurs with trauma to mucosal surfaces. The organisms recovered reflect the normal flora at the anatomical site that has been manipulated, and this is usually an occult episode with no demonstrable clinical evidence of sepsis. These episodes are rather frequent, they are self-limited, and they are of no concern except for the patient who is predisposed to endocarditis and possibly the patient with a prosthetic orthopedic device such as an artificial hip. With regard to urologic practice, previous studies indicate that the frequency of bacteremia is directly related to the extent of trauma. Thus, routine blood cultures have been positive in approximately 5% of patients who undergo catheterization, 25% of those who have cystoscopy, and 45% of patients undergoing a transurethral prostatectomy.[2] As mentioned, the great majority of these patients have a benign self-limited bout of bacteremia involving the organisms that colonize the urethra, primarily the same gram-negative bacilli and enterococci that are responsible for most urinary tract infections. Most patients have no overt symptoms, although occasional patients have a transient, self-limited bout of fever, sometimes associated with hypotension. These cases may be reminiscent of "catheter fever" as described 100 years ago by Sir Andrew Clark.[3] The American Heart Association[4] currently recommends prophylactic antibiotics directed against the enterococcus for patients undergoing genitourinary manipulation who are defined as being prone to endocarditis (Table 4–1). It should be noted that the prophylactic regimen is directed against the enterococcus, not because of its prevalence in transient bacteremia but because it is the only organism from this anatomical site that frequently causes endocarditis. Some authorities advocate a similar approach for patients with prosthetic orthopedic devices, although guidelines in this setting are not available from any authoritative source.

The most familiar form of bacteremia is *intermittent bacteremia* in which there is periodic hematogenous seeding. Blood cultures obtained in the appropriate temporal relationship to the fever curve is a critical factor for documenting the bacteremia episode. The preferred time is at the first indication of fever or on the ascending limb of the fever curve.

Sustained bacteremia is indicated by blood cultures that are repeatedly positive when obtained over extended periods regardless of associated clinical signs, and specifically suggests an endovascular infection, suppurative venous thrombophlebitis, or a mycotic aneurysm. In urologic practice, this bacteremia is most commonly seen as a complication of venous

TABLE 4–1.
Prophylactic Antibiotic Recommendations for Endocarditis-Prone Patients Undergoing Urologic Procedures*

Indications: cardiac conditions
- Prosthetic cardiac valves
- Most congenital cardiac malformations
- Surgically constructed systemic pulmonary shunts
- Rheumatic and other acquired valvular dysfunction
- Idiopathic hypertrophic subaortic stenosis
- Prior history of bacterial endocarditis
- Mitral valve prolapse with insufficiency

Indications: genitourinary procedures
- Cystoscopy
- Prostate surgery
- Urethral catheterization, especially in presence of infection ("in-and-out catheterization" with sterile urine is not an indication)
- Urinary tract surgery

Regimen
- Standard regimen: ampicillin, 2 g (50 mg/kg for children) IM or IV, plus gentamicin, 1.5 mg/kg IM or IV; the initial dose is given 30 min prior to the procedure and *may* be repeated at 8 hr
- Penicillin-allergic patients: vancomycin, 1 g for adults (20 mg/kg up to 1 g for children) given IV slowly over 1 hr, plus gentamicin given 1 hr prior to the procedure; this regimen *may* be repeated 8–12 hr later
- Oral regimen for minor or repetitive procedures in low-risk patients: amoxicillin, 3 g (50 mg/kg for children) orally 1 hr before the procedure, and 1.5 g (25 mg/kg for children) 6 hr later

*Adapted from Shulman ST, et al: *Circulation* 1984; 70:1123A–1127A.
IM = intramuscularly; IV = intravenously.

catheterization or as a result of a mycotic aneurysm at the site of vascular anastomoses in transplant recipients.

Breakthrough bacteremia is indicated by continued positive blood cultures despite appropriate antibiotic regimens according to sensitivity tests and, in urologic practice, is most frequent with closed-space infections of the genitourinary system.

Polymicrobial bacteremia indicates that two or more microbial species are recovered in blood cultures; in urology this is most frequently seen with an obstructed genitourinary tract.

Portals of Entry.—The most frequent portals of entry for bacteremia acquired in the hospital are the urinary tract, surgical wounds, lung, and soft tissue. The most prevalent bacteria are gram-negative bacilli, accounting for 70%, and the most frequent isolates in this category are *Escherichia coli, Pseudomonas aeruginosa, Klebsiella,* and *Enterobacter.*[5, 6] Forty percent of patients with gram-negative bacteremia develop septic shock as defined by a decrease in blood pressure to less than 90 mm Hg systolic, or a 70-mm Hg decrease in the systolic blood pressure of patients who were previously hypertensive. The classic presentation is chills, high fever, and prostration followed within 2 to 8 hours by hypotension. Other presentations of gram-negative bacteremia include fever alone, hypothermia, oliguria, hypotension, thrombocytopenia, tachypnea with a respiratory alkalosis, acidosis, or a change in mental status. One of the more deceptive findings noted is hypothermia or euthermia, which is found in approximately 15% of patients with documented gram-negative bacteremia and is especially common in those who are elderly, are receiving corticosteroids, or are uremic.[6]

Treatment.—Therapeutic recommendations that are almost universally endorsed include intravenous fluid support using colloid or crystalloid, aggressive antibiotic treatment, and careful monitoring of vital signs, renal function, serum electrolytes, and clotting parameters. Most authorities now regard dopamine as the preferred vasopressor if there is persistent hypotension despite an elevated central venous pressure or pulmonary wedge pressure. More controversial issues are the following:

Antibiotic Selection.—Repeated studies have shown that the prognosis is improved if the antibiotic initially selected shows in vitro activity against the isolated pathogen. The use of two drugs in the hopes of achieving synergy has been advocated by some but is not supported by the available evidence, with the possible exception of infections involving *P. aeruginosa* or infections in the immunocompromised host.[6] Another source of controversy concerns drugs that are bacteriostatic rather than bactericidal; despite theoretical differences, there is no clinical evidence that a bactericidal agent has any advantage in the usual patient with bacteremia. With regard to the initial selection, a recently isolated pathogen may be used as a guide to antibiotic selection. However, it is necessary to be cautious with respect to the urinary tract, since patients with recurrent urinary tract infections and those who have indwelling Foley catheters will often show rapid changes in the infecting flora even in the absence of antibiotic pressure.[7] Furthermore, it is often not possible to distinguish with confidence between bacteremia involving gram-negative and that involving gram-positive bacteria, according to the initial findings. Thus, drugs that are active against common gram-positive bacteria such as *Staphylococcus aureus* or the enterococcus may be important to include despite the clinical impression of gram-negative bacteremia.

Corticosteroids.—A controlled study of gram-negative bacteremia and septic shock in 172 patients by Schumer showed a mortality rate of only 12% in those treated with high doses of corticosteroids compared to 43% in control subjects.[8] Another well-controlled and highly publicized subsequent study failed to confirm these observations,[9] although a potential criticism is that the treatment was not initiated until an average of 17 hours after the onset of hypotension and a smaller sample size was examined. Thus, there is no definitive recommendation except that, if these agents are used at all, they should be given early in the course, pharmacologic doses should be employed (30 mg/kg of methylprednisolone or its equivalent), and only one or two doses should be given.

Nalaxone.—This is an opiate antagonist that may be used to reverse the activity of endorphins that are considered central in the pathophysiology of gram-negative shock. Efficacy of this agent has been shown with experimental animals, but the initial clinical trials have been disappointing.[10]

Antiserum Treatment.—Passive immunization with antisera to the core antigen of gram-negative bacteria is a promising new approach to therapy. The most extensively tested product is serum obtained from healthy donors following immunization with the J5 mutant of *Salmonella.*[11] An alternative and somewhat more readily available source of the hyperimmune globulin is sera obtained from blood donors that have been tested and found to have high titers of antibody to endotoxin, the common moiety of gram-negative organisms.[12]

Outcome.—It is easy to be skeptical about many of the current recommendations regarding the treatment of gram-negative bacteremia and septic shock, since the mortality rate tends to be persistently high. Nevertheless, there do appear to be major improvements during the past two decades. One of the most important factors in prognosis is the underlying or associated diseases classified as rapidly fatal (prognosis for survival of 1 year or less), ultimately fatal, or nonfatal. At the time that this classification was first described in 1962, the mortality rates were 91%, 66%, and 11%, respectively.[13] More recent analysis by the same investigators showed that the mortality rates for the respective groups are now 40%, 31%, and 15%.[6]

Pneumonia

The incidence of nosocomial pneumonia ranges from 5 to 50 cases per 1,000 admissions.[1] The major risk is for surgical patients, especially those who have undergone operations involving the chest or abdomen. Thus, the risk is magnified 14-fold for thoracic operations, 3-fold for abdominal incisions and 38-fold for a combined thoracoabdominal operation.

Bacteriology.—The bacteriology of nosocomial pneumonia is difficult to decipher due to the unreliability of the usual specimen source, expectorated sputum. Nevertheless, multiple studies, including the 82-hospital National Nosocomial Infection Study involving 1.6 million patients, indicate that the most frequent pathogens are gram-negative bacilli, the most frequent specific organisms being *Klebsiella* and *P. aeruginosa* followed by Enterobacteriaceae, *E. coli, S. marcescens,* and *Proteus.*[14] *Staphylococcus aureus* accounts for 10% to 30%. A Veterans Administration hospital study reviewed a smaller number of patients but was better in terms of the quality of microbiology, since nearly all study patients underwent a transtracheal aspiration. According to this report, gram-negative bacilli accounted for 47%, *Streptococcus pneumoniae* 31%, *S. aureus* 26%, and anaerobic bacteria 35%.[15] The total exceeds 100%, since about 60% of the patients had polymicrobial infections. More recent studies implicate *Legionella* species, especially *L. pneumophila* or *L. micdadei* in 4% of lethal cases of nosocomial pneumonia, and these organisms may be endemic or epidemic in some hospitals. The agents of legionnaires' disease have been a major problem for the compromised host, especially renal transplant recipients, other patients with compromised cell-mediated immunity, recipients of corticosteroids, or patients with acquired immunodeficiency syndrome (AIDS). An epidemic in one hospital was sufficiently severe to require that the renal transplant program be suspended.[16]

Pathophysiology.—The usual pathophysiologic mechanism for pneumonia is for entry into the lower airways by aspiration of bacteria that colonize the upper airways or by inhalation of aerosols containing viruses (especially influenza), mycobacteria, or *Legionella.* Most cases of hospital-acquired pneumonia appear to involve bacteria, and colonization of the upper airways by the implicated strain usually precedes pneumonia. Throat cultures of various patient populations indicate that the incidence of colonization of the upper airways by gram-negative bacilli, the major pathogens of nosocomial pneumonia, is directly correlated with the severity of associated medical conditions.[17] Thus, rates of abnormal colonization are low among housestaff, students, and psychiatric patients despite similar exposures in the hospital environment; colonization rates are substantially higher in patients who are judged to be moderately ill, and they are very high among patients hospitalized in the intensive care unit. The conclusion is that associated conditions are the most important variable for abnormal colonization, which represents a predisposing factor to gram-negative bacillary pneumonia acquired by microaspiration.

Diagnosis.—The diagnosis of pneumonia requires radiographic changes combined with clinical supporting observations such as fever, cough, and purulent sputum. The usual specimen source for most patients is the expectorated sputum sample, although there is considerable concern about the reliability of this specimen so that results must be interpreted with considerable caution. Two admonitions that are commonly advocated are that the Gram stain may be more reliable than culture and that cytologic screening to determine the cellular constituents of the specimen should be used as a method to screen specimens prior to culture.[18]

Treatment.—Assuming bacteriologic results are unknown, commonly recommended regimens for nosocomial pneumonia include administration of an aminoglycoside combined with a cephalosporin, an antipseudomonad penicillin, or sulfamethoxazole-trimethoprim. The initial regimen can be modified once cultures of expectorated sputum are available. Despite the comments noted earlier regarding the unreliability of this specimen, one redeeming value of the expectorated sample is that gram-negative bacilli, the organisms of paramount interest, are usually recovered and may be used to shape the antibiotic regimen; the major problems with sputum bacteriology are with false-positive cultures for gram-negative bacilli and failure to detect the pneumococcus or *Haemophilus influenzae* (common sources of false-negative cultures) and organisms that are not routinely sought, such as anaerobic bacteria, *Legionella*, viruses, and *Mycoplasma*.

Intravenous Therapy–Related Infections

Types of infections.—Infections related to intravenous cannulas usually result from microbial contamination at the insertion site. Four forms are recognized:

Purulent Thrombophlebitis.—This is severe but relatively infrequent. Patients with purulent thrombophlebitis usually have evidence of phlebitis with erythema, induration, swelling, and tenderness with or without a palpable cord at the intravenous (IV) line insertion site. The same findings may indicate mechanical or chemical irritation from the IV cannula or infusate, or they may represent simply cellulitis, which is a far more frequent form of infection. The difference is that purulent thrombophlebitis is associated with suppuration within the vessel lumen, many patients have persistently positive blood cultures despite appropriate antibiotic treatment, and surgical excision of the vein may be required.[19]

Cellulitis.—This is a relatively common complication and is characterized by similar findings, although pus is rarely detected at the site of infusion.

Occult IV Site Infection.—This refers to infections that do not produce local evidence of inflammation and appear to be the most frequent cause of IV-associated bacteremias. Evidence to support this portal of entry is the lack of another identifiable source coupled with the recovery of the blood culture isolate from cultures of the catheter.

Contamination of the IV Infusate.—This mechanism of infection is rare but important to recognize, since it may be responsible for epidemics of bacteremia. In most instances the level of contamination is not sufficient to detect by visual inspection of the bottles, many patients become hypotensive (endotoxic shock) during the infusion, and the diagnosis is established by discontinuing the infusion and culturing the bottle.

Bacteriology.—The usual organisms found in infections related to intravenous catheters are gram-negative bacilli, *Staphylococcus epidermidis, S. aureus,* and enterococci. Available evidence suggests that these organisms originate from the patient's skin. Frequent organisms involved with contaminated IV infusates are "waterborne bacteria" such as *Klebsiella, Serratia, Citrobacter freundii,* and *Pseudomonas cepacia* and other pseudomonads.

Prevention.—The recommended procedures for avoiding catheter-associated sepsis are the following: (1) use of stainless steel instead of plastic cannulas, (2) changing of peripheral cannulas every 48 to 72 hours, (3) insertion at one of the upper extremities (or jugular and subclavian site) instead of the lower extremities, (4) inspection and dressing of central cannulas every 48 to 72 hours, and (5) insertion of all lines using aseptic techniques, including washing hands with soap and water and applying tincture of iodine for the skin preparation.

Management.—If infection with phlebitis, cellulitis, or bacteremia is established or suspected, it is preferred to remove the entire IV system. The recommended procedure for culturing catheters is the semiquantitative method described by Maki et al.[19] to distinguish high-density colonization from contamination, which was a common problem using the previous method of culturing the catheter tip in broth media. With the semiquantitative method, a 5- to 7-cm segment of the catheter is rolled on the culture media, and the recovery of 15 colonies is considered "significant." Gram stains performed directly on the catheter that readily show microorganisms at ×1,000 magnification also indicate "line sepsis."[20]

INFECTION FOLLOWING RENAL TRANSPLANTATION

Historical Perspective

The first decade of renal transplantation from 1962 to 1972 was associated with frequent, severe, and often lethal infectious complications. At this time most reports indicate that 15% to 30% of all renal transplant recipients died due to infection, most deaths occurred within 3 months following the procedure, and opportunistic infections were a major problem.[21, 22] Common infectious agents encountered at that time reflected suppressed cell-mediated immunity such as *Nocardia, Pneumocystis carinii,* opportunistic fungi (*Candida* species, phycomycetes, *Aspergillus,* and *Cryptococcus*), *Listeria,* herpes simplex, herpes zoster, and cytomegalovirus (CMV). These infections presumably reflect the cumulative immunosuppressive effects of corticosteroid and azathioprine administration, thymectomy, splenectomy, antilymphocyte serum, and graft irradiation. These opportunistic pathogens continue to plague transplant recipients of other organs such as bone marrow, heart, lung, and liver. However, the situation has changed rather drastically for most renal transplant recipients since opportunistic infections other than CMV have become uncommon, and death due to infection now occurs in only 1% to 6% according to most reports.[23, 24] Several factors are credited with this improvement, perhaps the most important being better technical skill and improved methods of handling rejection, but also revised methods of immunosuppression and improved chemotherapeutic agents.

Infectious Complications

The data from the University of Minnesota are perhaps representative of the more recent experience.[23] Investigators from this center have tabulated their experience with 535 renal transplantations from 1977 to 1981 and found that 164 patients had infections sufficiently severe to prolong hospitalization or require rehospitalization (Table 4–2). The most frequently encountered infection was with CMV in 114 patients. The second largest category by type of microbe was bacterial infection involving the usual nosocomial pathogens such as enteric gram-negative bacilli, *P. aeruginosa,* and *S. aureus.* Systemic fungal infections were encountered in 28 patients, the most common pathogens being *Candida albicans* and *Aspergillus.* (It should be noted that the numbers do not equal 164 because polymicrobial infections were found in 33 patients.)

TABLE 4–2.
Infections in Renal Transplant Recipients*

Total transplant recipients	518
No. of patients with infection	164(32%)
Deaths due to infection	32(6%)
Infectious episode with established etiology	205
Viral infections	131(63%)
CMV	114
Varicella-zoster	11
Bacterial infection	82(40%)
Bacteremia	23
Urinary tract	22
Soft tissue/bone	17
Lung	15
Surgical wound	4
Fungal infections	28(14%)
Systemic candidiasis	12
Aspergillosis	14
Cryptococcosis	1
Rhinocerebral mucor	1
Parasitic infection	1(0.5%)
P. carinii	1

*Adapted from Peterson PK, et al: *Medicine* 1982; 61:360.

Analysis of the entire experience indicated that 32 patients (6%) died as a result of their infection. Analysis of data from the New York Hospital–Cornell Medical Service is similar except for an even lower mortality rate due to infection and a paucity of CMV infections.[24]

Fever

The Minnesota group has also analyzed their experience with 194 episodes of fever in 175 transplant recipients.[25] This showed that infections accounted for 74%, allograft rejection for 13%, malignancy (posttransplant lymphoma) for 4%, and drug fever for 2%, and there was no clearly established cause in 7%. Again, the most frequent cause was viral infection with CMV, which was identified as the exclusive cause in 53%, was associated with allograft rejection in 16%, and occurred in association with another systemic infection in 22%. The traditional definition of fever of unknown origin is a temperature of 38.8° C for 3 weeks. Restricting analysis to the 44 episodes that satisfied this definition, CMV was the single most common cause, accounting for 31 (70%).

Temporal Association of Infection and the Onset of Fever

The anticipated pathogens show considerable variation according to the time of clinical symptoms in relation to the time of renal transplantation. During the first postoperative month the most frequent pathogens are bacteria involved in the usual nosocomial infections. About two thirds of all febrile episodes occurring during the 2 weeks to 4 months following transplantation are caused by CMV infections, rejection, or reactions to antilymphocyte globulin. Febrile episodes occurring more than 1 year following transplantation are usually caused by bacterial infection, fungal infection, or malignancies.

Cytomegalovirus Infections

Cytomegalovirus is a member of the herpesvirus group that also includes herpes simplex virus, varicella-zoster virus, and Epstein-Barr virus. The characteristic properties of these viruses are that they cause an initial or primary infection that is usually asymptomatic followed by a prolonged period when the virus or viral genome resides in tissue cells. The latent viruses may become apparent after years of quiescence due to reactivation, particularly when cell-mediated immunity is compromised. Infection may also occur in patients who are previously seropositive (consequently considered immune) and in some persons who are reinfected from an exogenous source. Serologic studies in adults from high socioeconomic groups in industrialized countries show a seroprevalence rate of about 40%, although nearly 100% of persons in developing countries and lower socioeconomic groups in the United States have serologic evidence of previous infection.[26] The usual infection in otherwise well individuals is asymptomatic; occasional patients develop a nonspecific illness or, less frequently, there is a mononucleosis syndrome characterized by fever, lymphadenopathy, splenomegaly, hepatitis, and atypical leukocytosis.

Cytomegalovirus infections are a major cause of infectious diseases in immunocompromised patients, including organ transplant recipients, patients receiving hemodialysis, and patients receiving immunosuppressive drugs.[27] Studies of patients receiving renal transplants show that 40% to 96% have infections involving this virus, using the diagnostic criteria of a positive culture from any source or a fourfold rise in the complement fixation antibody within 7 months after renal transplantation.[28] The most frequent site of viral excretion is the urine; the buffy coat is another common source of the virus for cultivation in the laboratory, and many patients shed the virus from multiple sites. These infections are usually asymptomatic. However, one third to one half of the infections are associated with symptoms that depend to some extent on the severity of immunosuppression. The most frequent clinical expression is fever, often accompanied by a mononucleosis-like syndrome and pneumonia; other clinical syndromes include hepatitis, retinitis, encephalitis, and infections of the gastrointestinal tract.[26–29] The role of antibody to CMV in terms of severity of disease is controversial, but most reports indicate that patients with a primary infection following transplantation have a more severe disease.[29] Most studies have also shown that patients who are seropositive prior to transplantation have a higher incidence of CMV infection, and these infections are presumably due to reactivation of the latent virus during immunosuppression.[30] Patients who are seronegative prior to surgery have primary infections, and the transplanted kidney is now regarded as an important likely source of the virus.[31] Conceivably, this same mechanism could apply in seropositive patients if the transplanted organ contained a different strain of the virus.

Prognosis.—The consequences of CMV infection are considerable in renal transplant recipients. Serious illness or even death is reported in up to 30% of symptomatic patients.[29] Many investigators have also found that this infection has an adverse effect on renal allograft survival.[32] The latter observation has important clinical consequences, since treatment of the infection should be directed at a decrease rather than an increase in immunosuppressive drugs. Additionally, CMV infection has been implicated in causing suppression of cell-mediated immunity, presumably enhancing risk of other opportunistic infections as well.

Treatment and Prevention.—The most realistic preventive measure for potential renal transplant recipients who are seronegative is to use kidneys from seronegative donors. According to one study, CMV infections following transplantation occurred in 75% of seronegative recipients when the donor was seropositive compared to only 10% when the donor was seronegative. Patients who are seropositive are less likely to develop overt CMV infection. However, this protection is apparently ablated by the use of antithymocyte globulin for immunosuppression. Intensive research is now being conducted to develop vaccines for patients who are susceptible for primary infections[33] and for therapy using immunoglobulin (passive protection) or new antiviral agents such as 9(1,3-dihydroxy-2-propoxymethyl) guanine.[34]

URINARY TRACT INFECTIONS

Urinary tract infections are among the most frequent infections encountered in daily practice and are relatively easy to document with the routine urine culture, but there are few diseases in medicine so fraught with controversies regarding appropriate management strategies. No attempt will be made to review all facets of urinary tract infections, but efforts will be made to address the issues that are most controversial and important for urologic practice.

Terms

Significant bacteriuria indicates that the concentration of bacteria in voided urine exceeds the number that can be readily ascribed to contamination, e.g., 10^5 per milliliter. *Cystitis* has been used to describe the syndrome characterized by dysuria, frequency, urgency, and, sometimes, suprapubic tenderness. Similar symptoms may be caused by vaginitis, urethritis, or pelvic inflammatory disease so that some prefer to restrict the appellation to cases associated with significant bacteriuria. The *dysuria-frequency syndrome* is another term commonly applied to suspected cystitis, especially in young adult women. Approximately half of these patients have significant bacteriuria (cystitis), while the remainder have the *urethral syndrome,* presuming that vaginitis and sexually transmitted diseases have been excluded. *Chronic bacterial prostatitis* is a chronic infection of the prostate with focal nonacute inflammation that is frequently expressed clinically with perineal discomfort, low back pain, or dysuria, and periodic symptoms of urinary tract infections. The focus of bacterial infection can be demonstrated with the three-glass test using quantitative cultures as described by Meares and Stamey.[35] *Prostatosis* causes a similar syndrome without demonstrable bacteriuria or positive cultures in the three-glass test, and actually appears to be far more common than chronic prostatitis. *Acute pyelonephritis* is the clinical syndrome characterized by flank pain, flank tenderness, fever, lower urinary tract symptoms (dysuria, urgency, and frequency), and accompanied by significant bacteriuria. *Relapsing urinary tract infections* refer to the recurrence of bacteriuria with the same infecting microorganism that preceded therapy, as confirmed by speciation, serotyping, antibiotic sensitivity profile, plasmid profile, or combinations of these assays; the implication is that the nidus of infection has not been eliminated. Most of these patients have a residue of bacteria in the kidney (pyelonephritis), and a more sustained course of antibiotics is often required.[36, 37] *Reinfections* refer to recurrent urinary tract infections involving different microorganisms according to the previously defined criteria; this pattern is usually found in women with recurrent urinary tract infections and generally does not indicate that the course of treatment has been too short or that the upper tract is a source of persistent infection. *Chronic pyelonephritis* is a term commonly used by pathologists to describe asymmetric scarring with interstitial fibrosis and a chronic inflammatory response; however, multiple studies have shown little correlation between these histologic changes and documented urinary tract infections, so that many authorities now prefer the term *chronic interstitial nephritis* to account for the nonspecificity of the findings. *Papillary necrosis* indicates acute necrosis at the base of the corticomedullary junction that often progresses to sloughing of the necrotic papilla to produce a characteristic caliceal deformity that is demonstrable on x-ray film, and/or the finding of the sloughed portion in voided urine. This lesion is usually found in the presence of diabetes mellitus, obstruction of the urinary tract, sickle cell disease, or analgesic abuse.

Bacteria

Urine Culture Results.—Nearly all urinary tract infections are caused by bacteria, although occasional exceptions are cases involving viruses, especially adenovirus ("hemorrhagic cystitis") or fungi, especially *C. albicans. Escherichia coli* accounts for 75% to 95% of urinary tract infections in ambulatory patients. The majority of these patients are adult women, usually with the dysuria-frequency syndrome, and the strains tend to be pansensitive, indicating susceptibility to all antibiotics tested. The second most frequent gram-negative bacillus encountered in such patients is *Proteus mirabilis*. The gram-positive organisms most frequently encountered in this patient population are *Staphylococcus saprophyticus* (often misidentified as *S. epidermidis*) in 5% to 15% of cases, and *Streptococcus faecalis* (the enterococcus) in 5% to 10%.

The spectrum of bacteria in patients with complicated urinary tract infections and especially nosocomial acquired pathogens is far different. The National Nosocomial Infection Study involving 54 U.S. hospitals showed the following distribution of 13,165 pathogens recovered from the urinary tract in 1983: *E. coli*, 32%; the enterococcus, 15%; *P. aeruginosa*, 13%; *Klebsiella* sp., 8%; *Proteus*, 7%; and *Candida*, 5%.[1]

Associations.—Despite these overall observations, microbiologic patterns show considerable variation in selected settings, and they also cause different consequences. Urea-splitting organisms, especially *Proteus* species and *Klebsiella* species, are likely to produce calculi.[38] Calculi also enhance susceptibility to urinary tract infections, there is often polymicrobial bacteriuria, and the organisms presumably survive well within the depths of the calculi, making eradication especially difficult. *Staphylococcus aureus* is a relatively unusual cause of urinary tract infections and often indicates seeding of the kidney from a hematogenous source with an intrarenal or perinephric abscess. Miliary abscesses of the kidney are also common with disseminated candidiasis. *Candida albicans* and occasionally other *Candida* species may also cause colonization with or without bladder invasion in patients with indwelling catheters, especially those receiving antibiotics.[39] Anaerobic bacteria rarely cause cystitis or pyelonephritis, apparently due to the elevated oxidation-reduction potential of urine that is inhospitable to the replication of oxygen-sensitive forms. However, anaerobic bacteria have been frequently found in suppurative infections of the genitourinary system such as prostatic abscess, periurethral abscess, and perinephric abscesses.[40] Adenoviruses, especially type 11, appear to be responsible for most cases of hemorrhagic cystitis. Patients with chronic indwelling Foley catheters usually have bacteriuria and often have polymicrobial bacteriuria with frequent shifts in the infecting flora. One study of 619 weekly specimens obtained from 20 such patients showed that 98% had 10^5 bacteria per milliliter, the average specimen contained 2.6 different bacterial strains, and the average duration of persistence for a single strain was 1.8 weeks.[7]

Uropathogens.—Studies of bacterial-host interaction indicate somewhat intriguing variations in virulence factors for the organisms found in bacteriuria. One group of patients is young adult women who have anatomically normal genitourinary systems but are predisposed to urinary tract infections due to the short urethra in combination with the urinary stasis of pregnancy or the urethral massage associated with sexual intercourse.[41] The presumed mechanism of infection is retrograde transmission of bacteria through the urethra. The original source of the organism is the normal vaginal or fecal flora, the usual pathogens are gram-negative bacilli or *S. saprophyticus*, and the long-term prognosis in terms of renal function is excellent.[42, 43] The second group of patients who represent unique hosts may have similar bacteria that reach the genitourinary system by a similar mechanism, but they are distinguished by selective predisposing conditions such as catheterization, urinary stasis, or vesicoureteral reflux. A major difference in the second group is that the identified predisposing conditions play a decisive role in the pathogenesis of the infection, the bacteria anticipated are far more diverse, and the consequences in terms of upper tract involvement with eventual renal failure are substantially greater.[43] The organisms in the former group have attracted considerable attention since in these cases microbial virulence factors appear to supersede host factors in the pathogenesis of the disease.[44] Most infections in this group are caused by *E. coli* serotypes 01, 02, 04, 06, 07, and 075. These serogroups do not represent the dominant serogroups in the fecal flora that presumably are the original source, leading authorities to conclude that they are "uropathogenic *E. coli*," e.g., strains that possess specific virulence factors to promote colonization and invasion of the urinary tract. Recognized virulence factors include the restricted number of O and K antigen serogroups, resistance to the serum bactericidal action, production of hemolysin or colicin V, and the capacity to adhere to uroepithelial cells by proteins that bind receptors. Adhesions characteristic of uropathogenic *E. coli* are classified by receptor specificities as mannose-binding adhesions (type I pili that bind the Tamm-Horsfall glycoprotein in human urine), GAL-GAL binding adhesions (fimbriae that bind globoseries glycolipids on human uroepithelial cells), and X-binding adhesions that are heterogenous and agglutinate human red blood cells. Studies of uropathic strains from group 1 patients (asymptomatic bacteruria, cystitis, or pyelonephritis in women without anatomical abnormalities of the genitourinary system) show universal expression of the GAL-GAL binding adhesion and 75% were hemolytic. A gene probe for these properties hybridized with the DNA of the pyelonephritis strains. These properties were not found in most of the isolates from normal stool, supporting the concept that these organisms possess unique virulence properties that account for their prevalence in urinary tract infections among patients who do not have other predisposing conditions.

Laboratory Studies

Microbiology Studies.—The usual procedure is a quantitative culture, most frequently using a 0.001-mL loop that permits detection of 10^3 bacteria per milliliter or more. Interpretation is based on the observation that urinary tract infections generally show over 10^5 organisms per milliliter, while uninfected specimens contain less than 10^4/mL. The major problem with false-positive cultures is in women with asymptomatic bacteriuria who should have this test repeated for confirmation. Low colony counts or "false-negative cultures" may be found in patients who have specimens collected directly from the upper tract that are not subject to contamination (suprapubic bladder aspirates, catheterized specimens, or cystoscopy specimens), the urethral syndrome, the three-glass test for chronic bacterial prostatitis, fastidious organisms (anaerobic bacteria, *Candida*, mycobacteria, etc.), previous antibacterial treatment, complete obstruction, or inadvertent inclusion of antiseptic solutions in the specimen. A direct Gram stain of the uncentrifuged urine showing at least one bacterium per oil immersion field usually correlates with 10^5/mL by quantitative culture.[45] Numerous kit procedures are available that are simple, rapid, and relatively inexpensive. Reliability is 90% to 95% which is often adequate for screening purposes but does not match the reliability of the standard laboratory culture test.[45]

Localization Studies.—There is considerable interest in distinguishing upper from lower urinary tract infections, since this has potentially important implications in terms of prognosis and treatment. Nevertheless, there is no realistic method that can be recommended with enthusiasm for routine use.[46]

The most reliable method involves bilateral ureteral catheterization for quantitative culture.[47] Prior work using this technique indicates that approximately one half of patients with bacteriuria had infection restricted to the bladder and that the history and physical examination were of little predictive value in determining the site. Despite verified accuracy, this technique can obviously not be justified in most cases. The Fairley bladder washout procedure is also reasonably reliable, also involves catheterization, and results are not decisive in 10% to 20% of patients.[48] There has been periodic enthusiasm in detection of antibody coating of bacteria (ACB) in urine as a method to determine a renal source. Previous studies show a sensitivity of 72% to 100% and a specificity of 50% to 100%.[49] This test is not readily available to most physicians, the positive and negative predictive value is judged to be about 80%, and most authorities believe that the test does not play an important role in the routine management of urinary tract infections. Other tests that have received some attention include the measurement of elevated C-reactive protein, renal concentrating ability, urinary alkaline phosphatase isoenzymes, and renal excretion of β_2-microglobulin or gallium scans. However, none of these tests are considered sufficiently developed or specific for routine use.[46]

Another approach is the distinction between relapse and reinfection using speciation, serologic typing, biotyping, and the antibiotic sensitivity profile of organisms in the urine. Again, many regard this as too expensive for the average patient and advocate practical clinical observations as more realistic and equally useful. These include the reappearance of bacteriuria within a few days of abbreviated treatment courses, a delay in seeking medical consultation until 6 or more days after the inception of symptoms, or findings suggesting a complicated infection with fever, flank pain, or other clinical signs of upper tract infection.[46]

Urologic Studies.—Urologic studies, including intravenous pyelography, are not considered to be cost-effective for adult women with uncomplicated infections. These studies are advised for patients with complicated infections such as overt pyelonephritis, renal calculi, diabetes, or neurogenic bladder, and for patients who fail to respond to antibiotics.[50, 51]

SPECIAL CLINICAL SETTINGS

The Frequency-Dysuria Syndrome

A survey of women aged 20 to 64 years indicated that 22% experienced dysuria during the preceding year, 50% had dysuria at some point in their lifetime, and one half of the episodes led to a physician consultation.[52] There is no question that this is a health problem of major magnitude. A nominal number of these patients will have their symptoms explained by vaginitis or a sexually transmitted disease that is readily detected with the pelvic examination. The rest will have cystitis, as defined by significant bacteriuria, or the "acute urethral syndrome." Recent studies of patients with the acute urethral syndrome showed that about 70% had pyuria defined as 8 leukocytes per milliliter or more, and nearly 90% of these women had urinary tract infections with less than 10^5 coliforms or staphylococci per milliliter or with *Chlamydia trachomatis*.[53] The result of these observations is the recommended management strategy that includes a history and physical examination, a pelvic examination, examination of vaginal secretions for the agents of vaginitis, urinalysis, urine culture, treatment with antimicrobial agents, and follow-up assessment following completion of treatment.[54] Even streamlining the processing results in significant cost.[55] An alternative strategy is to simply recommend a 10-day course of trimethoprim-sulfamethoxazole without knowledge of the urinalysis, Gram stain, urine culture, or antimicrobial sensitivity tests.[56] It should be noted that this tactic is not advocated for patients who have anatomical disease of the genitourinary system, pregnancy, fever, flank pain, adverse reactions to sulfonamides, a urinary tract infection within the previous month, or evidence of vaginitis. The advantage of this approach compared to the single-dose treatment with a more elaborate diagnostic evaluation concerns the cost-benefit ratio and the reduced number of relapses. The disadvantage in this approach is the risk of diagnostic inaccuracies and the adverse reactions encountered with the usual 7- to 10-day course of treatment. Regarding adverse reactions, the most frequent are gastrointestinal intolerance, diarrhea, and vaginitis. These reactions are not usually severe, but their frequency with a single dose is only 5% to 10% compared to 30% to 40% with longer courses.[58]

Infection Stones

About 80% of renal calculi are composed of calcium oxalate that forms in sterile urine.[38] Most of the rest are composed of struvite and carbonate apatite that form in the presence of urea-splitting bacteria, primarily *Proteus* sp. The latter stones often herald a poor prognosis, since they are usually large staghorn calculi and cause renal insufficiency from infection and obstruction. A review of results of renal lithotomy for staghorn stones of various etiologies indicated recurrence rates of 20% to 50%. A more selective recent review of struvite stones by Silverman and Stamey showed that cultures of 46 struvite stones yielded bacteria in each of 46 cases and that *P. mirabilis* accounted for 40 of these.[38] More importantly, an aggressive and comprehensive therapeutic approach resulted in a recurrence rate of only 2.5% with a mean follow-up period of 7 years.

Urinary Tract Infections in Children

The prevalence of asymptomatic bacteriuria in girls is about 1.5% and in boys is about 0.03%. The incidence of infection during the newborn period is 0.1% to 1.4% and is actually higher among boys than girls. There are frequent problems with obtaining appropriate specimens in this patient population since bag cultures are of value only when they show sterile urine. Preferred methods include suprapubic aspiration or urethral catheterization. All children with documented urinary tract infections should be investigated, preferably at the time of initial presentation. For suspected obstruction, ultrasonography is suggested. Otherwise, an intravenous pyelogram and voiding cystourethrogram are advised. Many of these children have an anatomically abnormal genitourinary system. Many girls develop recurrent urinary tract infections, and, although the prognosis in this group is good, natural history studies indicate that they remain infection-prone.[58] About one third of children will have vesicoureteral reflux, but most (85%) will have low-grade reflux that usually resolves spontaneously.[59] Most authorities recommend prophylactic low-dose antimicrobial treatment for the lower grades of reflux to prevent recurrent infections.[60] The usual agents are nitrofurantoin, sulfonamides, and trimethoprim-sulfamethoxazole. The major indications for surgical intervention are grade 5 reflux, new renal scar formation during treatment, and breakthrough infections. Currently, grade 4 reflux may be managed by either medical or surgical means while awaiting more definitive recommendations from the International Reflux Study.[61] Renal scans are useful for following the course of children with reflux or for postsurgical correction since they minimize radiation exposure.[62]

Chronic Bacterial Prostatitis and Prostatosis

Chronic bacterial prostatitis is a chronic infection of the prostate, usually involving coliform organisms, that is often asymptomatic.[63] Symptoms, when present, include perineal discomfort, low back pain, and dysuria with periodic urinary tract infections. Needle biopsy of the prostate is unreliable, due to the focal nature of the disease, and the demonstration of leukocytes in prostatic fluid is nonspecific. The preferred method to establish the diagnosis is with the three-glass test of Stamey and Meares,[35] which includes a urethral urine (VB 1), a midstream urine (VB 2), prostatic secretions expressed by massage (EPS), and a voided urine immediately following massage (VB 3). These specimens must be cultured promptly, using a quantitative technique that will detect lower concentrations of bacteria than with routine urine cultures using a 0.001-mL loop. A Veterans Administration Cooperative Study of recurrent urinary tract infections in men showed that the antibody-coated bacterial test was positive in each of 46 cases and that 24 (52%) had evidence for prostate infection.[64] This group as well as others have found the infective nidus in the prostate to be extremely refractory to therapy, requiring long courses of antibiotics using drugs, such as trimethoprim, that penetrate the blood-prostate barrier well. Agents with established merit include trimethoprim-sulfamethoxazole (although only the trimethoprim component of the combination appears necessary), oral carbenicillin, and rifampin plus trimethoprim. Treatment is generally continued for 12 weeks. Prostatosis is a similar disease in terms of presenting complaints, although cultures of urine and the three-glass test are negative, so that no etiologic agent can be implicated. Postulated mechanisms include a fastidious organism or muscular spasm.[65-67]

Catheter-Associated Urinary Tract Infections

Mechanism.—Microorganisms gain access to the urinary bladder by three routes in catheterized patients: (1) meatal and urethral organisms may be pushed into the bladder at the time of catheter insertion, (2) bacteria contaminating the collecting system may reach the urine by retrograde migration through the catheter lumen, or (3) bacteria from the periurethral area may ascend through the periurethral mucosa external to the catheter.

Incidence and Consequences.—With a brief single catheterization the reported infection rate is 1% to 5%. The infection rate is 100% for patients with an indwelling urethral catheter using an open system for 4 days or longer. The closed urinary drainage method has markedly reduced this risk. Nevertheless, under the usual hospital circumstances, the risk of acquiring bacteriuria is 5% to 10% per day for each day of catheterization.[68] Host factors that magnify the risk are advanced age, debilitation, and the postpartum state. Most of the urinary catheter-associated infections are benign, asymptomatic, and detected only with routine urine cultures. However, these infections may also result in prostatitis, epididymitis, cystitis, pyelonephritis, and septicemia. The last-named is the most serious and, fortunately, occurs in less than 1% of catheterized patients.[6]

Prevention.—There are alternatives to the indwelling urethral catheter in some selected patient populations. The condom catheter may prove useful in incontinent male patients who have an intact voiding reflex without outlet obstruction. However, it should be emphasized that this technique requires meticulous nursing care to prevent local complications. Frequent manipulation of the catheter by agitated patients has been noted to actually increase the risk of urinary tract infections.[69] Suprapubic catheter drainage has been suggested to reduce infections, but clinical trials to verify efficacy have not been completed.[70] Intermittent catheterization is advocated for patients with bladder-emptying dysfunctions such as spinal cord injuries or for children with meningomyeloceles. Again, well-designed clinical trials to demonstrate efficacy are not available.[71]

Management.—Should the indwelling urethral catheter be necessary, it is important to use a sterile, continuously closed system for urinary drainage. Meatal care is theoretically attractive; however, controlled studies have not demonstrated that meatal care is an effective method to prevent urinary tract infections.[72] Systemic prophylactic antibiotics appear to delay the emergence of catheter-related infection, but this practice is not generally advocated, since the protection is transient and seems to select for antibiotic-resistant organisms. Continuous irrigation of the bladder with a nonabsorbable antibiotic has also been suggested. However, again, studies to date have not demonstrated this method to be effective. A concern is that the frequent interruption of the closed drainage system may actually prove detrimental.[73] Guidelines for the prevention of catheter-associated urinary tract infections as advocated by the Centers for Disease Control (CDC) are summarized in Table 4–3. Per tradition, these include the standard three categories: Category I indicates measures that are strongly recommended; category II, recommended with moderate enthusiasm; and category III, weakly recommended.

TABLE 4–3.
Guidelines for Prevention of Catheter-Associated Urinary Tract Infection*

Guidelines
Category I. Strongly recommended for adoption
Educate personnel in correct techniques of catheter insertion and care
Catheterize only when necessary and keep in place only as long as necessary
Emphasize hand washing.
Insert catheter using aseptic technique and sterile equipment
Secure catheter properly
Maintain closed sterile drainage; the catheter and drainage tube should be disconnected only for irrigation
Obtain urine samples aseptically, using the distal end of the catheter or the sampling port following cleansing with disinfectant
Maintain unobstructed urine flow; collecting bags should be below bladder level
Category II. Moderately recommended for adoption
Periodically reeducate personnel in catheter care
Use smallest-bore catheter suitable and minimize trauma
Avoid irrigation unless needed to prevent or relieve obstruction; the catheter tube should be disinfected before disconnecting; if the obstructed catheter requires frequent irrigations, it should be changed; continuous irrigation with antimicrobials should not be performed routinely
Daily meatal care is not recommended
Do not change catheters at arbitrary fixed intervals
Category III. Weakly recommended for adoption
Consider alternative techniques of urinary drainage before using an indwelling urethral catheter, e.g., condom catheter drainage, suprapubic catheterization, or intermittent urethral catheterization
Replace the collecting system when sterile closed drainage has been violated
Spatially separate infected and uninfected patients with indwelling catheters
Avoid routine bacteriologic monitoring

*Adapted from Clegg HW, et al.: *Guidelines for the Prevention and Control of Nosocomial Infections.* Atlanta, Centers for Disease Control, 1981, pp 1–5.

Urinary Tract Infections due to Candida albicans

Laboratory Observations.—The prevalence of *Candida* species in urine ranges from 0.2% to 4.8%.[39] In many instances, this range reflects improper collection of the urine sample. Alternative considerations are colonization of the genitourinary system, cystitis or pyelonephritis, or disseminated candidiasis. The number of organisms that signifies probable infection is disputed, since some authorities consider 10^3/mL significant whereas others require the traditional count utilized for bacteria, 10^5/mL. Perhaps most important is the consistency of recovery with repeated examinations or the recovery of *Candida* from alternative sources, such as a single catheterization or a suprapubic bladder aspiration, when there is confusion with urinary studies. The urine sediment in the presence of a *Candida* genitourinary infection of either the bladder or kidneys usually shows red and white blood cells mixed with yeast, pseudohyphae, and necrotic debris. The antibody-coated studies are of no value in localizing candidal urinary tract infections since these are often positive regardless of the site of invasion.

Predisposing Conditions.—These include diabetes mellitus, previous antibiotic treatment, corticosteroid therapy, and disturbance of urinary flow. Candidal cystitis is more frequent in women. Factors that specifically contribute to disseminated candidiasis include neutropenia and factors associated with disturbed cell-mediated immunity, such as corticosteroid treatment, lymphoma–Hodgkin's disease, cancer chemotherapy, or AIDS. Infections localized to the genitourinary system are more frequent with disturbance of urinary flow, as with congenital anomalies of the genitourinary tract, a neurogenic bladder, foreign bodies, indwelling catheters, renal calculi, or genitourinary surgery, particularly with reconstruction of ileal conduits. With candidal cystitis, the urethra is the usual portal of entry, and retrograde infection may result in infection of the renal pelvis and ureters, but the current consensus is that infection of the renal parenchyma in the absence of candidemia is unusual.[74] By contrast, renal parenchymal infection is a common sequela of candidemia, and the kidneys appear to be the most frequent site of infection in disseminated candidiasis.[75] Patients with abnormal systemic defense mechanisms as defined above with or without prolonged high-grade candidemia are prone to several forms of candidal urinary tract infections, including diffuse cortical abscesses, papillary necrosis, and/or fungus balls in the collecting system. The fungus ball represents a tangled mass of pseudohyphal forms of the organism that may cause obstruction.

Treatment.—*Candida* infections of the genitourinary system may be classified as asymptomatic infections in previously healthy individuals (group 1); patients with conditions predisposing to candiduria without evidence of disseminated disease (group 2), or candiduria with suspected disseminated candidiasis. The recommendation[39] for management of group 1 patients is an assessment using the same diagnostic guidelines advocated for patients with bacteriuria. For group 2 patients it is advised to observe the patient while predisposing factors are eliminated, if possible. This includes improvement of diabetes control, discontinuation of unnecessary antibiotics, discontinuation of immunosuppressive drugs, and elimination of foreign bodies such as indwelling catheters. If candiduria persists, there should be an attempt to detect associated anatomical lesions or a fungus ball with radiographic studies. The usual recommended treatment in the absence of evidence for systemic candidiasis, pyelonephritis, or ureteral obstruction is local application of amphotericin B in a concentration of 10 μg/mL with an infusate of 200 to 300 mL of sterile water, with the catheter cross-clamped for 60 to 90 minutes at regular intervals. This treatment should be continued for 5 to 7 days. For patients with suspected upper tract involvement or failure to respond to local irrigations or for whom the indwelling catheter for delivery seems ill-advised, an alternative is flucytosine given orally in a dosage of 150 mg/kg/day. This drug, unlike ketoconazole or amphotericin B, is selectively excreted in the urinary tract to provide high concentrations in bladder urine. It should be noted that the drug may accumulate to dangerous levels in patients with renal insufficiency and should probably be avoided for those patients. Approximately 25% of *C. albicans* strains are resistant to flucytosine, additional organisms that are susceptible at the initiation of treatment will develop resistance during the course of treatment, and serious side effects with this drug have been noted. Patients with disseminated candidiasis should be treated with amphotericin B given IV with or without the addition of flucytosine given orally.

Anaerobic Infections

The distal urethra and adjacent mucocutaneous surfaces are colonized by anaerobic as well as aerobic bacteria. These are the presumed sites of origin for most bacteria that are involved in the common forms of urinary tract infections, including both cystitis and pyelonephritis. Nevertheless, multiple attempts to recover anaerobic bacteria from voided urine have shown low yields, except for those cases in which low counts apparently reflect urethral contamination.[40] This observation has been so consistent that most laboratories will not perform anaerobic cultures on urine. The one possible exception is the case where organisms are seen on direct smear, but the routine cultures are negative, which suggests a fastidious organism. Even in this instance, the yield of anaerobes is extremely small.[76] The theoretical explanation is that the partial pressure of oxygen in the renal parenchyma and bladder urine is simply too high to support the growth of obligate anaerobes.

Despite sparse studies indicating a role of anaerobic bacteria in genitourinary infections of the usual type, these organisms appear to be highly prevalent in suppurative infections of the urinary tract. A review of 18 such infections by our group showed that anaerobic bacteria were recovered from 16, and the dominant isolate was *Bacteroides fragilis*, which was found in 11 patients.[40] The types of infections encountered were prostatic abscess, scrotal abscess, and perinephric abscess. Similar results have been noted by others. A comprehensive review of anaerobic infections reported between 1893 and 1975 showed 102 cases of urinary tract infections involving anaerobic bacteria; 78 (76%) of these infections were characterized by tissue necrosis or abscess formation.[77] The most frequent infections were periurethral gangrene, and periurethral, perinephric, or renal abscess. Drainage and debridement are the obvious mainstays for therapy. Antibiotic recommendations include the same regimens used for intraabdominal sepsis, such as an aminoglycoside combined with clindamycin, metronidazole, cefoxitin, carbenicillin (mezlocillin, ticarcillin, piperacillin), or chloramphenicol.

TREATMENT

Recommendations According to Patient Category

The antibiotic recommendations of Kunin are summarized in Table 4–4 for patients classified in six groups.[46] The groups show a progression in terms of simplicity of management, sensitivity of the anticipated pathogen, and long-range prognosis. Group 1 refers to female patients who have had a few previous episodes, are considered reliable for follow-up cultures, have a brief duration of symptoms prior to presentation, are likely to have a pansensitive *E. coli*, and in whom the risk of renal invasion is low, and the anticipated outcome with the most simplified form of treatment, a single dose, is likely to be successful. At the opposite extreme are group 6 patients, who have continuous catheter drainage, in whom management is difficult, the organisms are likely to be resistant, the probability of renal invasion is high, and antibiotics are recommended only during episodes of sepsis. Group 5 patients have an almost equally ominous prognosis for ease of management; these patients have a neurogenic bladder or a large residual volume, *E. coli* and other coliforms are the anticipated pathogens, the probability of renal invasion is high, and treatment is advocated only for symptomatic infections. Groups 3 and 4 are patients identified as having a fair prognosis based on previous episodes of urinary tract infections as well as associated conditions, and the recommended course of treatment for them is prolonged to 4 weeks or more. It should be noted that the considerations in the therapy column are restricted to the treatment of symptomatic urinary tract infections or the prophylactic use of antibiotics in patients who have multiple recurrences. With regard to asymptomatic bacteriuria, it should be noted that there is a consensus that only pregnant women and probably children should be treated.

Single-Dose Therapy

Single-dose regimens with established efficacy include amoxicillin, 3 g; sulfisoxazole, 2 g; and trimethoprim-sulfamethoxazole, 2 double-strength tablets.[57] This regimen is recommended for women with uncomplicated urinary tract infections characterized by dysuria and frequency; this is not recommended for patients who have symptoms of pyelonephritis, or for men, pregnant women, or patients who are not available for follow-up cultures.[46, 51, 57] The advantages of the abbreviated dose in-

TABLE 4–4.
Guidelines to Management of Urinary Tract Infections*

Group	Ease of Management	Patient	Findings	Anticipated Pathogen	Probability of Tissue Invasion	Treatment/ Prophylaxis
1	Excellent	Female	Few episodes, reliable 2 days since onset of symptoms	Sensitive *E. coli*	Low	Single dose
2	Good	Female	Few episodes, follow-up poor	Sensitive *E. coli*	Variable	3–10 days; prophylaxis for closely spaced episodes
3	Fair	Female or male	Multiple episodes, history of early recurrence, diabetes, or renal transplant	Variable; sensitivity tests necessary	High	4–6 wks; prophylaxis for closely spaced episodes
4	Fair	Male or female	Recurrent infections, underlying anatomical abnormality or chronic prostatitis	Variable; sensitivity tests necessary	High	4–6 wks, 12 wks for chronic prostatitis; prophylaxis for closely spaced episodes
5	Poor	Male or female	Neurogenic bladder, large residual urine	Variable; sensitivity tests necessary	High	Treat symptomatic episodes only; intermittent catheterization recommended
6	Very poor	Male or female	Continuous drainage required	Variable; sensitivity tests necessary	Very high	Treat for sepsis

*Adapted from Kunin CM: *Am J Med* 1981; 71:849.

clude convenience, high compliance, low cost, and reduced side effects. Efficacy using the regimens noted seems to be well verified by 12 properly controlled trials that show no significant difference between these drugs and the more conventional multidose therapy.[55, 77] However, it should be noted that some have quibbled with these results,[77] since the sample size in the studies was not sufficient to prevent type II error; moreover, by aggregating the data from all of the studies, there was a statistically significant difference favoring conventional multidose treatment (69% vs. 84% cure rates).

Prophylaxis

Prophylaxis is recommended by Kunin[46] for patients with recurrent infections at closely spaced intervals in groups 2, 3, and 4 (Table 4–4). Regimens recommended include trimethoprim-sulfamethoxazole, one-half tablet daily or three times weekly; nitrofurantoin, 50 mg daily; or trimethoprim, one half of a 100-mg tablet daily.[46, 51, 55] Prophylaxis is generally continued for 6 months. Patients who then resume the pattern of frequent reinfections may be given a prophylactic agent for 2 years. There is some concern with the long-term use of nitrofurantoin, due to the occasional serious side effect of pulmonary infiltrates. Alternative strategies for women with urinary tract infections associated with sexual intercourse is to reserve prophylaxis for a single dose at the time of susceptibility. Another approach is the self-administration of trimethoprim-sulfamethoxazole at the time of typical urinary symptoms, using four tablets in a single dose.[79]

Pyelonephritis

Patients with evidence of renal infection can often be treated with an oral agent, although parenteral treatment may be required for moderately ill patients, particularly before culture and sensitivity tests are available. Specific recommendations by *The Medical Letter* consultants for oral agents include ampicillin, amoxicillin, trimethorprim-sulfamethoxazole, or trimethoprim alone. When parenteral therapy is deemed necessary, it should consist of an aminoglycoside combined with either ampicillin or a cephalosporin; trimethoprim-sulfamethoxazole is another alternative. Treatment is generally continued for 10 to 14 days.[46, 52] Patients who suffer a relapse following treatment should receive a 4- to 6-week course of an effective antibiotic selected on the basis of in vitro sensitivity tests and given in full therapeutic dosage. By contrast, patients with recurrent urinary tract infections should be considered for chronic prophylaxis, using one of the previously noted regimens if the frequency of episodes is sufficient.

EDITORIAL COMMENT

Dr. Bartlett provides valuable, practical advice in the management of infections frequently found in patients with urologic disorders. As he indicates, many of the tests, such as antibiotic coating, are not always helpful. For the initial episode of cystitis in an otherwise healthy woman, a brief trial of antibiotics may be preferable to a more expensive evaluation with multiple urine cultures and radiographic studies. After evaluation, in the more complicated cases one antibiotic pill after intercourse has been very helpful in patients who can relate some of their urinary infections to sexual activity. It is also interesting to note that anaerobes are rarely found as urinary pathogens but can be found more commonly in prostatic, periurethral, scrotal, or perinephric abscesses. Although not strongly recommended in the chapter, intermittent catheterization has been a great boon to the urologist and patients with urologic disease. It has markedly reduced the incidence of urinary diversion. As long as the urinary tract is emptied on a regular basis, even in the presence of bacteria, sepsis is not common. Recently, eiprofloxacin has been a major addition in the oral treatment of resistant urinary tract infections.

REFERENCES

1. Jarvis WR, White JW, Munn VP, et al: Nosocomial infection surveillance, 1983. *MMWR* 1984; 33:95S–225S.
2. Sullivan NM, Sutter VL, Carter WT, et al: Bacteremia after genitourinary tract manipulation: Bacteriological aspects and evaluation of various blood culture systems. *Appl Microbiol* 1972; 23:1101–1106.
3. Clark A: Remarks on catheter fever. *Lancet* 1883; 2:1075–1077.
4. Shulman ST, Amren DP, Bisno AL, et al: Prevention of bacterial endocarditis. *Circulation* 1984; 70:1123A–1127A.
5. Weinstein MP, Murphy JR, Reller LB, et al: The clinical significance of positive blood cultures. *Rev Infect Dis* 1983; 5:35–53; 54–70.
6. Kreger BE, Craven DE, McCabe WR: Gram negative bacteremia. *Am J Med* 1980; 68:332–343; 344–355.
7. Warren JW, Tenney JH, Hoopes JM, et al.: A prospective microbiologic study of bacteriuria in patients with chronic indwelling urethral catheters. *J Infect Dis* 1982; 146:719–723.
8. Schumer W: Steroids in the treatment of septic shock. *Ann Surg* 1976; 184:333–341.
9. Sprung CL, Panagiota V, Caralis MD, et al: The effects of high-dose corticosteroids in patients with septic shock. *N Engl J Med* 1984; 311:1137–1143.
10. DeMaria A, Heffernan JJ, Grindlinger GA, et al: Naloxone versus placebo in treatment of septic shock. *Lancet* 1985; 1:1363–1365.
11. Ziegler EJ, McCutchan JA, Fierer J, et al: Treatment of gram-negative bacteremia and shock with human antiserum to a mutant *Escherichia coli*. *N Engl J Med* 1982; 307:1225–1230.
12. Baumgartner J-D, McCutchan JA, van Melle J, et al: Prevention of gram-negative shock and death in surgical patients by antibody to endotoxin core glycolipid. *Lancet* 1985; 2:59–63.
13. McCabe WR, Jackson GG: Gram-negative bacteremia. *Arch Intern Med* 1962; 110:847–855.
14. *National Nosocomial Infections Study Report. Annual Summary, 1979.* Atlanta, Centers for Disease Control, March 1982.
15. Bartlett JG, O'Keefe P, Talley FP, et al: The bacteriology of hospital-acquired pneumonia. *Arch Intern Med* (in press).
16. Meyer RD: *Legionella* infections: A review of five years of research. *Rev Infect Dis* 1983; 5:258–278.
17. Johanson WG Jr, Pierce AK, Sanford JP: Changing pharyngeal bacterial flora of hospitalized patients. *N Engl J Med* 1969; 281:1137–1140.
18. Bartlett JG, Brewer NS, Ryan KJ: Laboratory diagnosis of lower respiratory tract infections. *Cumitech* 1978; 7:1–15.
19. Maki DG, Weise CE, Harold WS: A semiquantitative culture method for identifying intravenous-catheter-related infection. *N Engl J Med* 1977; 23:1305–1309.
20. Cooper GL, Hopkins CC: Rapid diagnosis of intravasacular catheter-associated infection by direct gram staining of catheter segments. *N Engl J Med* 1985; 312:1142–1147.
21. Eikhoff TC: Infectious complications of renal transplant recipients. *Transplant Proc* 1973; 3:1233–1238.
22. Rifkind D, Marchioro TL, Waddell TR, et al: Infectious diseases associated with renal homotransplantation: I. Incidence, types and predisposing factors, *JAMA* 1964; 189:397–401.
23. Peterson PK, Ferguson R, Fryd DS, et al: Infectious diseases in hospitalized renal transplant recipients: A prospective study of a complex and evolving problem. *Medicine* 1982; 61:360–372.
24. Masur H, Cheigh JS, Stubenbord WT: Infection following renal transplantation: A changing pattern, *Rev Infect Dis* 1982; 4:1208–1219.
25. Peterson PK, Balfour HH, Fryd DSD, et al: Fever in renal transplant recipients: Causes, prognostic significance and changing patterns at the University of Minnesota Hospital. *Am J Med* 1981; 71:345–351.

26. Pass RE: Epidemiology and transmission of cytomegalovirus. *J Infect Dis* 1985; 152:243–248.
27. Jordan MC: Latent infection and the elusive cytomegalovirus. *Rev Infect Dis* 1983; 5:205–215.
28. Glen J: Cytomegalovirus infection following renal transplantation. *Rev Infect Dis* 1981; 3:1151–1178
29. Peterson PK, Balfour HH Jr, Marker SC, et al: Cytomegalovirus disease in renal allograft patients. *Medicine* 1980; 59:283–300.
30. Onorato IM, Morens DM, Martone WJ, et al: Epidemiology of cytomegaloviral infections: Recommendations for prevention and control. *Rev Infect Dis* 1985; 7:479–496.
31. Ho M, Suwansitikul S, Dowling JN, et al: The transplanted kidney as a source of cytomegalovirus infection. *N Engl J Med* 1975; 293:1109–1112.
32. Richardson WP, Colvin RB, Cheeseman SH, et al: Glomerulopathy associated with cytomegalovirus viremia in renal allografts. *N Engl J Med* 1981; 305:57–63.
33. Osborn JE: Cytomegalovirus: Pathogenicity, immunology and vaccine initiatives. *J Infect Dis* 1981; 143:618–630.
34. Shepp DH, Dandliker PS, de Miranda P, et al: Activity of 9-(2-hydroxy-1-[hydroxymethyl] ethoxymethyl) guanine in the treatment of cytomegalovirus pneumonia. *Ann Intern Med* 1985; 103:368–373.
35. Meares EM, Stamey TA: Bacteriologic localization patterns in bacterial prostatitis and urethritis. *Invest Urol* 1968; 5:402–412.
36. Turck M, Anderson KN, Petersdorf RG: Relapse and reinfection in chronic bacteriuria. I. *N Engl J Med* 1966; 275:70–73.
37. Turck M, Ronald AR, Petersdorf RG: Relapse and reinfection in chronic bacteriuria. II. *N Engl J Med* 1968; 278:422–433.
38. Silverman DE, Stamey TA: Management of infection stones: The Stanford experience. *Medicine* 1983; 62:44–51.
39. Fisher JF, Chew WH, Shadomy S, et al: Urinary tract infections due to *Candida albicans*. *Rev Infect Dis* 1982; 4:1107–1118.
40. Bartlett JG, Gorbach SL: Anaerobic bacteria in suppurative infections of the male genitourinary system. *J Urol* 1981; 125:376–378.
41. Nicolle LE, Harding GKM, Preiksaitis J, et al: The association of urinary tract infection with sexual intercourse. *J Infect Dis* 1982; 146:579–583.
42. Freedman L: Chronic pyelonephritis at autopsy. *Ann Intern Med* 1967, 66:697–701.
43. Freedman LR: Natural history of urinary tract infections in adults. *Kidney Int* 1975; 8:S96–S104.
44. O'Hanley P, Low D, Romero I, et al: GAL-GAL binding and hemolysin phenotypes and genotypes associated with uropathogenic *Escherichia coli*. *N Engl J Med* 1985; 313:414–420.
45. Barry AL, Smith PB, Turck M: Laboratory diagnosis of urinary tract infections. *Cumitech* 1975; 2:1–8.
46. Kunin CM: Duration of treatment of urinary tract infections. *Am J Med* 1981; 71:849–854.
47. Stamey TA, Govan DE, Palmer JM: The localization and treatment of urinary tract infections: The role of bactericidal urine levels as opposed to serum levels. *Medicine* 1965; 44:1.
48. Fairley KG, Carson NE, Gutch RC, et al: Site of infection in acute urinary tract infection in general practice. *Lancet* 1971; 2:615.
49. Thomas VL, Forland M. Antibody coated bacteria in urinary tract infections. *Kidney Int* 1982; 21:1.
50. Fowler JE, Pulaski ET: Excretory urography, cystography and cystoscopy in the evaluation of women with urinary tract infections. *N Engl J Med* 1981, 304:462–465.
51. Treatment of urinary tract infections. *The Medical Letter* 1981; 23:69–72.
52. Walters WE: Clinical significance of dysuria in women. *Br Med J* 1970; 2:754.
53. Stamm WE, Wagner KF, Amsel R, et al: Causes of the acute urethral syndrome in women. *N Engl J Med* 1980; 303:409–415.
54. Stamm WE, Running K, McKevitt M, et al: Treatment of the acute urethral syndrome. *N Engl J Med* 1981; 304:956–958.
55. Stamm WE: Is antimicrobial prophylaxis of urinary tract infections cost effective? *Ann Intern Med* 1981; 94:251.
56. Schultz HJ, McCaffrey LE, Keys TF, et al: Acute cystitis: A prospective study of lab-

oratory tests and duration of therapy. *Mayo Clin Proc* 1984; 59:391–397.
57. Souney P, Polk BF: Single-dose antimicrobial therapy for urinary tract infections in women. *Rev Infect Dis* 1982; 4:29–34.
58. Neu H: Urinary tract infections in the 1980's. *Semin Urol* 1983; 1:130–134.
59. Edwards D, Normand I, Prescod N, et al: Disappearance of vesicoureteral reflux during long-term prophylaxis of urinary tract infection in children. *Br Med J* 1977; 2:285–288.
60. Bickerton MW, Ducket JW: Diagnosis and treatment of pediatric UTIs. *Infections in Medicine*, May/June 1985, pp 150–161.
61. International Reflux Study Committee: Medical versus surgical treatment of primary vesicoureteral reflux. *J Urol* 1981; 125:277–283.
62. Gordon I: Renal diagnostic imaging, in Williams D, Johnston J (eds): *Paediatric Urology*. London, Butterworth Scientific, 1982, pp 11–26.
63. Meares EM: Prostatitis: A review. *Urol Clin North Am* 1975; 2:3.
64. Smith JW, Jones SR, Reed WP, et al: Recurrent urinary tract infections in men. *Ann Intern Med* 1979; 91:544–548.
65. Meares EM: Bacterial prostatitis vs. 'prostatosis.' A clinical and bacteriological study. *JAMA* 1973; 224:1372.
66. Mobley DF: Bacterial prostatosis. *Invest Urol* 1981; 19:31.
67. Segura JW, Opitz J, Green LF: Prostatosis, prostatitis or pelvic floor tension myalgia. *J Urol* 1979; 122:168.
68. Garibaldi RA, Burke JP, Dickman ML, et al: Factors predisposing to bacteriuria during indwelling urethral catheterization. *N Engl J Med* 1974; 291:215–218.
69. Hirsh DD, Fainstein V, Musher DM: Do condom catheter collecting systems cause urinary tract infection? *JAMA* 1979; 242:340–341.
70. Hodgkinson CP, Hodari AA: Trocar suprapubic cystostomy for postoperative bladder drainage in the female. *J Obstet Gynecol* 1966; 96:773–783.
71. Lapides J, Diokino AC, Gould FR, et al: Further observations on self-catheterization. *J Urol* 1976; 116:169–171.
72. Clegg HW, Cram S, DeGrout-Kosoleharoen J, et al: Guideline for prevention of catheter associated urinary tract infections, in *Guidelines for the Prevention and Control of Nosocomial Infections*, Atlanta, Centers for Disease Control, 1981, pp 1–5.
73. Warren JW, Platt R, Thomas KJ, et al: Antibiotic irrigation and catheter-associated bacteriuria. *N Engl J Med* 1978; 299:570–573.
74. Louria DB, Finkel G: Candida pyelonephritis, in Kass EH (ed): *Progress in Pyelonephritis*. Philadelphia, FA Davis Co, 1965, pp 179–184.
75. Lehner T: Systemic candidiasis and renal involvement. *Lancet* 1964; 1:1414–1416.
76. Segura JW, Kelalis PP, Martin WJ, et al: Anaerobic bacteria in the urinary tract. *Mayo Clin Proc* 1972; 47:30.
77. Finegold SM: *Anaerobic Bacteria in Human Disease*. New York, Academic Press, 1977, pp 314–349.
78. Philbrick JT, Bracikowski JP: Single-dose antibiotic treatment for uncomplicated urinary tract infections. *Arch Intern Med* 1985; 145:1672–1678.
79. Wong ES, McKevitt M, Running K, et al: Management of recurrent urinary tract infections with patient-administered single-dose therapy. *Ann Intern Med* 1985; 102:302–307.

CHAPTER 5

Hematologic Complications

Chi V. Dang, M.D., Ph.D.
William R. Bell, M.D.

PATHOHEMATOLOGIC CONDITIONS

The kidney, which is a major source of erythropoietin, and blood, which contains the carrier of oxygen and elements for effective hemostasis, are wedded in physiologic and pathophysiologic states. In this chapter we survey the pathohematologic conditions and their relationship with urologic complications.

Red Blood Cells

Normal erythropoiesis involves the orderly sequential maturation of erythrocyte precursors from the stem cell to pronormoblast, basophilic normoblast, polychromatophilic normoblast, orthochromatic normoblast, to the reticulocyte. The reticulocytes are released into circulating blood and constitute about 1% of peripheral red blood cells. The mature erythrocyte has a 120-day life span. The packed cell volume (PCV), designated hematocrit value, occupied by erythrocytes in whole blood is 48% ±6% for adult men and 42% ±4% for adult women. Erythropoietin, which is primarily made in the kidneys, stimulates the early commited cell to differentiate into the pronormoblast.

Ineffective erythropoiesis may result from various causes, including nutritional deficits. Deficiencies of iron, folate, vitamin B_{12}, or pyridoxine (vitamin B_6) result in a decreased red blood cell production, manifesting as anemia with a low reticulocyte count. Increased destruction or loss of red blood cells, as with bleeding or hemolysis, results in an increased reticulocyte count if bone marrow function is normal.

A sustained increase in red blood cell count (more than $6 \times 10^6/mm^3$) or hematocrit value (more than 55%) is called erythrocytosis. Polycythemia is the absolute increase in red blood cell mass, whereas erythrocytosis is an elevation of the red blood cell count or hematocrit value with a normal red blood cell mass. Polycythemia may result from myeloproliferative disorders or from ectopic production of erythropoietin by tumors, as in hypernephroma, Wilms' tumor, renal adenoma, or undifferentiated renal carcinoma.

The production of an effective erythrocyte may be hindered by the synthesis of abnormal hemoglobin due to mutations that result in amino acid substitutions or abnormal RNA splicing. One of the most common hemoglobinopathies in the United States is sickle cell anemia, which may present with various urologic manifestations.

White Blood Cells

The mature circulating neutrophil results from the sequential maturation of the myeloblast, promyelocyte, myelocyte, metamyelocyte, and the juvenile or band cell occurring over 7 days. The life span of the neutrophil is about 14 hours. About half of the neutrophils are marginated along venules and may demarginate in response to stress, corticosteroids, or epinephrine. An increase in the production of neutrophils, as reflected by an increase in the band cell count, usually occurs with infections. Neoplastic proliferation of the myeloid precursors may result in acute (AML) or chronic (CML) myelogenous leukemia. On the other hand, neutropenia can result from the depression of marrow function by toxins, drugs, radiation, infection, or nutritional deficits, or from sequestration at infection sites or increased immune-mediated destruction.

The lymphocyte originates from marrow-derived cells that migrate into the thymus and other lymphoid tissues. The thymus-derived cells enter the circulation as T lymphocytes, whereas germinal centers of lymphoid organs release B lymphocytes in response to antigenic stimulation. The plasma cells, which produce antibodies, are derived from B lymphocytes. Neoplastic proliferation of these lymphocytes may result in acute (ALL) or chronic (CLL) lymphocytic leukemia or the lymphomas. Neoplastic increase in plasma cells may result in multiple myeloma. Lymphocytosis is seen with acute or chronic infections. Severe lymphopenia may be encountered in patients with hypogammaglobulinemia, thymoma, chronic renal failure, or the acquired immunodeficiency syndrome (AIDS).

The monocytes and macrophages are phagocytic cells derived from marrow precursor cells, which also give rise to granulocytes. Monocytosis is associated with infections, neoplasms, connective tissue diseases, ulcerative colitis, or Crohn's disease.

Platelets

The platelet, a small cytoplasmic fragment of the megakaryocyte, is released from the bone marrow into circulation to number 150,000 to 400,000/mm^3 and has a life span of 10 days. Thrombocytosis is associated with infection, neoplasia, iron deficiency, and myeloproliferative syndromes. Thrombocythemia (more than 2×10^6/mm^3) is an idiopathic condition, probably due to abnormalities of the precursor stem cells. A decrease in platelet count or thrombocytopenia (to less than 100,000/mm^3) may be due to (1) decreased production secondary to radiation exposure, toxic injury, infiltrative diseases of bone marrow, ineffective hematopoiesis, or vitamin B_{12} or folate deficiency; or (2) removal of the platelets from the peripheral blood secondary to immune- or nonimmune-mediated destruction or to sequestration in hypersplenism. A large number of commonly used drugs may cause thrombocytopenia by either immune or nonimmune mechanisms.

Blood Clotting

The blood contains a number of glycoproteins that function as clotting factors (Table 5–1) whose intricate interactions (Fig 5–1) ultimately result in the conversion of soluble fibrinogen to insoluble fi-

TABLE 5–1.

Blood Coagulation Factors

Factor	Synonym	In Vivo Half-Life
I	Fibrinogen	3.0–4.5 days
II	Prothrombin	2–5 days
III	Thromboplastin	—
IV	Calcium	—
V	Proaccelerin	15–36 hr
VII	Proconvertin	2–6 hr
VIII	Antihemophilic globulin (AHG)	6–10 hr
IX	Christmas factor	8–12 hr
X	Stuart-Prower factor	32–48 hr
XI	Plasma thromboplastin antecedent	40–48 hr
XII	Hageman factor	48–52 hr
XIII	Fibrin stabilizing factor	5–12 days

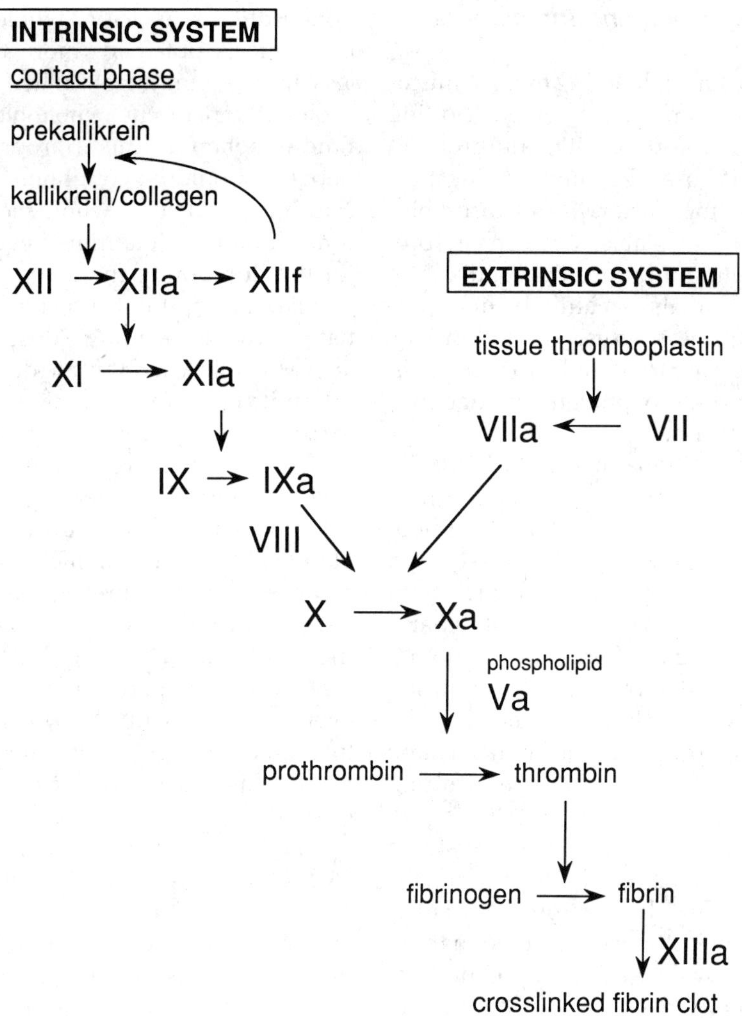

FIG 5–1.
Schematic representation of the coagulation system.

brin. Deficiencies of all known coagulation factors except Factors III (thromboplastin) and IV (calcium) have been described. The initial screening of patients with bleeding tendencies includes evaluation of platelet number and function and factor deficiency. The bleeding time is prolonged by a decrease in platelet number or because of platelet dysfunction. Prolongation of the prothrombin time (PT) reflects deficits in the extrinsic coagulation system (Factors II, V, VII, and X) (see Fig 5–1), and the partial thromboplastin time (PTT) reflects the intrinsic system (mainly Factors VIII, IX, XI, and XII). This technique is sensitive to the interaction of all the coagulation factors except VII. Bleeding abnormalities may result from circulating anticoagulants that are immunoglobulins directed against one or more components (factors) of the coagulation system. These circulating anticoagulants may occur in congenital (factor-deficient) patients undergoing replacement therapy or in patients with paraproteinemias, connective tissue diseases, in those exposed to drugs such as phenytoin, or in otherwise normal people.

Anticoagulation and Thrombolytic Therapy

Heparin, a sulfated anionic mucopolysaccharide, prolongs blood clotting by forming a complex with antithrombin III that binds to and inhibits serine proteases, including Factor X and thrombin. Commercially available heparin is prepared from lung and intestinal mucosa of a variety of animals—mainly bovine, porcine, and caprine species. The indications for the use of heparin result from the ability of this agent to prevent endogenous blood coagulation.

The dose of heparin should be designated in units, since 1 mg of heparin may contain between 100 and 170 units of heparin activity, depending on the tissue and animal source, preparation, formulation, and manufacturer. The amount of heparin needed for adequate therapeutic anticoagulation can be determined by measuring the whole-blood clotting time by the three-tube method or the nonactivated (PTT) or activated (APTT) partial thromboplestin time.

Aqueous heparin is best administered via the intravenous (IV) route and may be given continuously or intermittently. When possible, the continuous manner with a constant infusion pump is preferable. The subcutaneous route, because of erratic absorption, possible vessel puncture with bleeding, and discomfort, is not recommended. It should not be given intramuscularly.

The IV, continuous, constant infusion route is initiated by a loading dose (10,000 units IV) followed immediately by the constant infusion of heparin (300–375 units/kg in 250–500 mL of 5% dextrose to run 12 hours, or 600–750 units/kg in 1,000 mL of 5% dextrose to run 24 hours). A whole-blood clotting time should be checked 6 hours later. Depending on the whole-blood clotting time at 6 hours, the dose, concentration of heparin, and rate of infusion should be adjusted accordingly, and the whole-blood clotting time rechecked 6 hours later. This should be done until a satisfactory whole-blood clotting time is obtained (more than 20 and less than 35 minutes). When therapeutic prolongation of the whole-blood clotting time is obtained, the appropriate dose of heparin should be continued via constant infusion, and the whole-blood clotting time should be determined every 12 hours for the duration of therapy.

The intermittent infusion route is initiated by a loading dose (described above). Following this, a dose of 150 to 180 units/kg heparin should be given in 10 to 20 mL of 5% dextrose IV during a 10-minute period every 6 hours. During the first 24 hours of therapy, immediately prior to each 6-hour dose, the whole-blood clotting time should be determined, recorded, and the dose adjusted appropriately. Once the correct prolongation of the whole-blood clotting time is obtained, that dose of heparin should be given IV every 6 hours, with the whole-blood clotting time checked before the second and fourth dose each day for the duration of therapy.

The nonactivated (PTT) or activated (APTT) partial thromboplastin time also has been used to monitor heparin therapy. Neither of these tests has been demonstrated to be more helpful than the whole-blood clotting time in the management of patients on heparin therapy but these automated tests are inconvenient. If the APTT is employed for monitoring heparin, it should be maintained at 2.0 to 2.5 times the baseline normal APTT.

Administration of heparin impairs hemostasis and predisposes to hemorrhage that may be life-threatening. Patients receiving heparin should have daily examinations for abnormal bleeding, including tests of urine and stool for occult blood. Unusual care is required in performance of venipunctures, and prolonged (5 minutes) pressure should be applied to venipuncture sites. Invasive procedures in areas in which bleeding may be especially dangerous are contradindicated; for example, introduction of needles or catheters into neck veins should be avoided. In general, arterial punctures, lumbar punctures, and subcutaneous and intramuscular injections should not be performed on patients during heparin therapy because of the hazard of local hemorrhage.

If abnormal bleeding occurs at any time during heparin therapy, the heparin should be immediately discontinued. Should rapid reversal of heparin anticoagulation be necessary, 1 mg of protamine sulfate for every 100 units (USP) of heparin should be administered IV at a rate of 5 mg/min and to a maximum total dose of 50 mg. Clotting time should be checked 15 minutes after administration. The effect lasts 2 hours.

The warfarin (Coumadin) anticoagulants retard blood clotting by inhibiting glutamyl γ-carboxylation, which results in defective Factors II, VII, IX, and X. These factors require the second γ-carboxyl group for effective membrane binding through a calcium bridge. Initiation of oral anticoagulation may be achieved by giving 10 to 15 mg warfarin daily for 3 days, and subsequent doses are determined by the PT. Therapeutic anticoagulation is achieved at a prothrombin time of about 1.5 to 2.0 times baseline PT occurring at about 5 to 7 days after initiation of therapy. The PT should be checked chronically at intervals no longer than 4 weeks. Reversal of warfarin anticoagulation may be achieved with vitamin K_1 (AquaMEPHYTON) at small doses of 10 mg by IV infusion at a rate of 5 mg/min or less. Fresh frozen plasma or plasma factor concentrate may be used for immediate correction.

The two clinically available thrombolytic agents are streptokinase and urokinase. Streptokinase binds to plasminogen to form a complex that can promote the conversion of plasminogen to plasmin. Plasmin in turn digests fibrin and fibrinogen. Urokinase proteolytically cleaves plasminogen directly to plasmin. Systemic treatment with streptokinase is initiated by loading IV a dose of 250,000 units/20 min, followed by 100,000 units/hr for 24 to 72 hours. Urokinase is given as a loading dose of 4,000 IU/kg/20 min followed by 4,000 IU kg/hr for 12 to 24 hours. Systemic thrombolysis is achieved at a thrombin time (TT) of 1.5 to 5.0 times baseline. Tissue plasminogen activator, which has higher affinity for fibrin than fibrinogen in vitro, has been prepared by recombinant DNA technology and may be a promising new thrombolytic agent.

UROLOGIC COMPLICATIONS OF HEMATOLOGIC DISORDERS

A number of hematologic disorders may either complicate urologic therapy or may present primarily with urologic symptoms. In this section the management of patients with bleeding disorders and urologic manifestations of hematologic disorders are discussed.

Coagulation disorders.—Surgical candidates with bleeding disorders should be immediately recognized and thoroughly evaluated and supported to prevent catastrophic operative hemorrhage.

Preoperative screening includes a complete blood cell count (red blood cells, white blood cells, and platelets). Prolongation of PT suggests possible deficiencies of Factors II, V, VII, X, and fibrinogen. Prolongation of the activated partial thromboplastin time (APTT) suggests deficiency of Factors VIII, IX, X, or XII. The thrombin time (TT) may be prolonged with abnormalities in fibrinogen or in the presence of circulating anticoagulants or heparin. A bleeding time is performed when platelet dysfunction is suspected. Table 5–2 shows the laboratory findings expected for factor deficiencies.

Factor VIII.—Among the inherited factor deficiencies, hemophilia A or Factor VIII:C deficiency occurs in 1 in 10,000 persons. Most cases are inherited as a sex-linked recessive trait, and 20% of cases

TABLE 5–2.
Laboratory Findings in Factor Deficiencies*

Deficient Factor	PT	APTT	TT	Bleeding Time
I	↑	↑	↑	↑N
II	↑	↑	N	N
III*	—	—	—	—
IV*	—	—	—	—
V	↑	↑	N	N
VII	↑	N	N	N
VIII	N	↑	N	N
VIII:vWF†	N	↑	N	↑
IX	N	↑	N	N
X	↑	↑	N	N
XI	N	↑	N	N
XII	N	↑	N	N
XIII	N	N	N	N

*Deficiency affecting coagulation is unknown.
†von Willebrand's disease.
PT = prothrombin time; APTT = partial thromboplastin time; TT = thrombin time; ↑ = prolongation; N = normal time.

may be spontaneous mutations. In this disease the APTT is prolonged, while PT, fibrinogen level, TT, and platelet count are normal. In severe deficiency, there may be spontaneous bleeding, or in moderate deficiency there may be traumatic bleeding such as hemarthroses, hematomas, ecchymoses, or, rarely, gastrointestinal or genitourinary bleeding. The diagnosis is established by a reduction of factor VIII:C activity: mild is 5% to 20% normal; moderate is 1% to 5% normal; and severe is less than 1% normal. Factor VIII–related antigen (von Willebrand Factor) is more than 100% normal.

Patients with Factor VIII deficiency are treated with Factor VIII concentrate or fresh frozen plasma to achieve a level greater than 20% normal. Levels of 10% to 20% normal are usually adequate for hemostasis after minor trauma of the oral or genitourinary tracts. A level of more than 80% normal and the concomitant treatment with ϵ-aminocaproic acid (EACA) (0.1-g/kg IV bolus followed by 0.1 g/kg orally every 6 hours) is recommended for major surgery. Hemophiliac patients have undergone major urologic surgery without life-threatening hemorrhage.[1–3] Most patients require 2 to 3 weeks of postoperative support.[1–3] Factor IX deficiency, or Christmas disease, requires similar replacement therapy with Factor IX during and after urologic surgery.[3]

One unit of Factor VIII is defined as that amount present in 1 mL of normal plasma. Fresh frozen plasma (FFP) contains about 0.8 unit/mL, cryoprecipitate about 8 units/mL, and Factor VIII concentrate about 10 to 40 units/mL. Replacement therapy is calculated as follows: In order to achieve 50% normal activity in a patient with 0% activity, 50% of the patient's plasma volume must be replaced by fresh plasma. Plasma volume is estimated to be 40 mL/kg body weight. For a 60-kg patient the plasma volume is about 2,400 mL. To achieve 50% activity, 1,200 units of factor must be administered. Half of the initial dose should be administered every 8 hours to maintain the desired level.

von Willebrand's Disease.—This disease is seen as frequently as hemophilia A and is transmitted as an autosomal dominant or recessive trait. Characteristically, Factor VIII:C level is reduced, and Factor VIII–related antigen (VIII:vWF) is also low and reduced to the same degree as Factor VIII:C. The bleeding time may be prolonged, and ristocetin-dependent platelet aggregation is absent in 70% of patients with von Willebrand's disease. Bleeding may be mild and overlooked; however, serious gastrointestinal bleeding is common. Patients are treated preferably with cryoprecipitate but not with Factor VIII concentrates, since the latter contains only minimal amounts of Factor VIII:vWF.

Factor IX.—Clinically, Factor IX deficiency (Christmas disease) resembles hemophilia A with its recessive X-linked mode of inheritance, but it occurs in 1 in 100,000 persons. Replacement and duration of therapy is similar to Factor VIII deficiency.[3]

Factor X.—Inherited Factor X deficiency is autosomal recessive and rare. Acquired deficiency is associated with amyloidosis, presumably due to adsorption of Factor X by the β-pleated amyloid fibrils. Maintenance of plasma levels more than 40% normal may be achieved with plasma transfusion in preparation for surgery. Half of the initial dose is given every 24 hours to maintain the desired level.

Factor V.—Factor V deficiency is a very rare disorder in which the PT and APTT are prolonged. A Factor V–specific assay is available. One third of patients may have prolonged bleeding time. About 25% normal activity is maintained for surgery by giving 15 mL FFP per kilogram of body weight 12 hours before surgery, and therapy is maintained by a 10 mL/kg dose every 24 hours.

Factor VII.—Factor VII deficiency is uncommon and is inherited as an autosomal gene with intermediate penetrance. The PT is prolonged, while the APTT and TT are normal. Replacement is achieved by transfusing plasma (10 mL/kg of body weight) on the day of surgery, and half of the initial dose is given daily.

Factor II.—Hypoprothrombinemia is a very rare autosomal recessive disorder with prolonged PT and variably prolonged APTT. A specific assay is available.

Maintenance of more than 15% normal level should be adequate for surgery. Plasma transfusion (15 mL/kg of body weight) is performed 12 hours before surgery, followed by a dose that is half of the initial dose once every 24 hours.

Factor XI.—Factor XI deficiency is uncommon and is inherited in an autosomally dominant mode. A higher frequency of this deficiency has been noted in the Ashkenazic Jews. Patients with Factor XI deficiency may not have bleeding histories but commonly present with epistaxis. Severe bleeding may occur with trauma or major surgery. Patients can successfully undergo major urologic surgery with adequate FFP therapy.[4–6] A dose of 20 mL of plasma per kilogram of body weight is given 8 hours before surgery and then is maintained with a 10-mL/kg dose every 24 hours.

Factor XII and XIII.—Factor XII deficiency is not usually associated with bleeding manifestations. The APTT is prolonged. Orientals have significantly lower Factor XII levels than whites, among whom 10% have mild deficiencies. Therapy is not needed. A deficiency of the auxiliary contact factors Fletcher, Fitzgerald, Fleujac, Williams, Warren are also not predisposed to hemorrhagic complications. However, the Passovoy defect is associated with a bleeding disorder. Patients with the Passovoy defect may bleed excessively intraoperatively and require plasma transfusion.

Factor XIII stabilizes fibrin by cross-linking the noncovalently polymerized molecules into a covalent network. Coagulation studies in Factor XIII deficiency are normal except for fibrin stability. Patients with this disorder may present with ecchymosis, hematoma, or delayed traumatic bleeding. In some patients, bleeding may be delayed by 24 hours following trauma. Abnormal clot solubility and specific Factor XIII assay establish the diagnosis. Transfusion of plasma (3 mL/kg of body weight) is sufficient for hemostasis, which may last up to 1 month.

Fibrinogen.—Patients with congenitally deficient fibrinogen and/or abnormal fibrinogen (dysfibrinogenemia) are uncommon.[6a] The TT is prolonged. Abnormal fibrinogens polymerize slowly. Fresh frozen plasma or cryoprecipitate may be given to maintain a fibrinogen level of more than 100 mg/100 mL for normal hemostasis. A patient with dysfibrinogenemia underwent transurethral prostatectomy successfully with only the administration of EACA to prevent fibrinolysis.[7]

Circulating anticoagulants.—Circulating anticoagulants are usually gamma globulins directed against phospholipids or clotting factors. An equal mixture of normal plasma and plasma containing the circulating anticoagulant will result in a prolongation of the normal APTT or PT. Acquired anti-Factor VIII:C antibodies are probably most common and can result in devasting hemorrhage. These patients may have significant operative bleeding and in fact may present with internal or renal pelvic clots resembling an attack of nephrolithiasis.[8] Antiphospholipid antibodies are associated with a number of diseases, including systemic lupus erythematosus, and are elicited by certain drugs such as phenytoin. The antiphospholipid antibodies are usually not associated with pathologic bleeding.

Thrombocytopenia.—Thrombocytopenia is the decrease in platelet count below 100,000/mm^3 (normal range, 150,000–400,000/mm^3). In general, a platelet count of more than 50,000/mm^3 is adequate for hemostasis. Qualitative platelet disorders may be congenital or acquired and will not be discussed further.

Thrombocytopenia may result from diminished production,[9] enhanced destruction, or sequestration as seen in hypersplenism or splenomegaly. Defective or diminished platelet production may be congenital or acquired. Among the acquired causes, tumor infiltration of bone marrow, ionizing radiation, myelosuppressive drugs, and renal failure are relevant to the patient with urologic disease. Thiazides and estrogen may directly inhibit platelet production.

Nonimmune or immune-mediated drug-induced thrombocytopenia may be the most common cause of thrombocytopenia in the hospitalized patient.[6] Among the common offenders are sulfonamides, quinidine, quinine, heparin, and gold salts. Temporal relationships between initiation of drug therapy and the onset of thrombocytopenia may provide important clues to identify the offender(s). In general, the onset of drug-induced thrombocytopenia occurs within 1 to 7 days after exposure, and recovery of platelet count occurs about 10 to 14 days following removal of the drug.

Other causes of increased platelet destruction include disseminated intravascular coagulation, thrombotic thrombocytopenic purpura, immune thrombocytopenia, posttransfusion purpura, and sepsis. Each of these syndromes may be recognized with the appropriate laboratory studies.

The history provides clues for identification of possible offenders such as viral syndromes or recent drug ingestion as causes for thrombocytopenia.[10] The physical examination may reveal petechiae, ecchymoses, purpura, or splenomegaly. Examination of the peripheral blood smear confirms the automated platelet count and rules out pseudothrombocytopenia due to platelet aggregation in vitro. The blood smear may show microangiopathic hemolytic changes that are seen in disseminated intravascular coagulation or thrombotic thrombocytopenic purpura. Examination of the bone marrow shows decreased megakaryocyte numbers in the situation of marrow suppression or increased megakaryocytes associated with increased peripheral destruction. Megaloblastic changes indicate a nutritional deficiency of folate or vitamin B_{12} as a cause of thrombocytopenia. Detection of antiplatelet antibodies indicates immune thrombocytopenia either idiopathic or due to drugs, neoplasms, or infectious agents.

In chronic immune thrombocytopenia,[11] the thrombocytopenia may be treated with corticosteroids (1 mg/kg of body weight per day). The response may be seen as an increase in platelet count occurring over 1 to 2 weeks in 60% to 75% of patients. More recently, immunoglobulin infusion has been suggested to be efficacious for preoperative treatment of immune thrombocytopenia.[12] Should steroids and/or immunoglobulin therapy fail the patient, splenectomy may result in prolonged increase in platelet count (in 50% to 60% of patients).

When heparin-induced thrombocytopenia is recognized, either heparin therapy should be stopped or the type of heparin should be switched. A higher frequency of thrombocytopenia is seen with the bovine lung preparations (26%) as compared to porcine intestinal preparations (9%).[13] If another drug is suspected of causing thrombocytopenia, discontinuation or appropriate substitution should be promptly carried out.

In patients with marrow suppression and severe thrombocytopenia, as seen in cancer patients given chemotherapy or radiotherapy, platelet infusion is mandatory before surgery. This complication may be seen in patients with hemorrhagic cystitis secondary to cyclophosphamide therapy, which requires urologic intervention.

Aspirin Ingestion.—Qualitative platelet dysfunction resulting from acetylsalicylic acid (ASA) or aspirin ingestion may complicate surgery.[14–17] This may result in prolonged bleeding time and platelet dysfunction up to 2 weeks after the last dose. Several studies, however, suggest that post-ASA prolongation of bleeding times may not be predictive of surgical bleeding.[18–21] It is our opinion that post-ASA prolongation of the bleeding time is an indication of risk for bleeding during surgery. In fact, an apparent ASA-related surgical bleeding has been reported in a patient whose bleeding time shortened into the normal range after discontinuation of ASA.[22] Therefore, patients undergoing surgery should be specifically instructed to discontinue ASA and related medications (eg., dipyridamole and other nonsteroidal anti-inflammatory agents) at least 10 to 14 days prior to surgery. This is especially important in patients who are azotemic or uremic. In these patients, the effect of ASA greatly enhances the platelet dysfunction already present with azotemia and uremia.[23] A bleeding time should be obtained for patients with recent ingestion of ASA or related agents before surgery.[24,25] If the bleeding time is prolonged, surgery should be postponed. In the emergent setting, platelet transfusion in a nonuremic patient may be helpful. In the azotemic-uremic patient platelet transfusion plus cryoprecipitate or 1-deamino-8-D-arginine vasopressin (DDAVP) may be needed before surgery is performed. In both of these situations the amount of platelets to be transfused should provide the recipient with a circulating platelet mass 25% of which are transfused fresh nonacetylated platelets.

Uremic Bleeding.—The chronically uremic patient has a host of coagulation abnormalities. Impaired platelet function may result from urea, a protein catabolic product, guanidosuccinic acid, or intact parathyroid hormone. Platelet dysfunction does not appear to correlate with levels of serum calcium, phosphorus, or creatinine. Prolongation of the bleeding time, abnormal platelet aggregation, abnormal platelet release reactions, and abnormal platelet aggregation may be observed in uremic patients. Platelet dysfunction appears to abate immediately following dialysis.

The von Willebrand factor (Factor VIII:vWF) appears to be abnormally decreased in concentration and in molecular weight in severe uremia, probably as a result of proteolysis.[26] Treatment of uremic bleeding with cryoprecipitate can temporarily correct the bleeding tendency.[27] Infusion DDAVP causes a release of Factor VIII:vWF from storage sites and appears to shorten the bleeding time in uremic patients.[28] Patients with complicated uremia undergoing urologic surgery may require support by either of these modalities to achieve better hemostasis.

Management of Patients on Anticoagulation Therapy.—In the urologic patient, chronic anticoagulation therapy for pulmonary embolism, deep vein thrombosis, arterial thrombosis, artificial heart valves, atrial fibrillation, or cerebral thromboembolism presents an obstacle to effective hemostasis if preoperative preparation is not carefully undertaken. In fact, these patients may present with an iliacus hematoma with urologic manifestations of groin, flank, and thigh pain, groin tenderness, or hematuria.[29] Patients undergoing acute anticoagulation therapy for the above-mentioned and related thrombotic problems are likely to be poor surgical candidates. If surgical intervention is unavoidable, risks and benefits must be judged for the individual case.

Patients undergoing chronic warfarin therapy with an uncomplicated course should be instructed to stop warfarin therapy 3 to 5 days before admission. The prothrombin time and other tests of coagulation should be assessed before surgery. Patients with recurrent thromboembolic symptoms should stop warfarin therapy on admission and have heparin therapy started and continued until 6 hours before surgery. The PT and the APTT must be close to normal immediately before surgery. If emergency surgery is indicated, patients receiving warfarin therapy may require FFP immediately before, during, and after surgery. Use of excess vitamin K may complicate reinstitution of warfarin therapy and may not be recommended in this situation unless symptomatic fluid overload appears to be a salient feature of the patient.

Evaluation and Management of the Anemic Patient.—Anemias may be categorized into two very general classes of increased red blood cell loss and decreased red blood cell production. In general, the reticulocyte count is decreased when red blood cell production is impaired, while with increased red blood cell destruction the marrow compensates by increasing red blood cell production, and therefore results in an increased reticulocyte count.

Common causes of decreased red blood cell production are deficiency in iron, folate, and, rarely, vitamin B_{12}. Chronic diseases of all types (such as neoplasia, connective tissue disorders, and chronic infections, for example), including uremia, also suppress red blood cell production. The blood smear will usually show hypochromic microcytic red blood cells and the serum iron and ferritin are low while the total iron-binding capacity is high in iron deficiency. Absent bone marrow iron stores unequivocally establish iron deficiency. A workup to identify the site of bleeding is warranted if iron deficiency is established. In folate or vitamin B_{12} deficiency, there is characteristically hypersegmented polymorphonuclear white blood cells and macro-ovalocytes. Red blood cell folate and serum vitamin B_{12} studies may be helpful in the diagnosis. A Schilling test should be performed in suspected vitamin B_{12} deficiency.

Increased loss of red blood cells may occur with bleeding or hemolysis. Acute bleeding or hemolysis may result in an increased reticulocyte count, while depletion of iron stores due to chronic blood loss will result in a low reticulocyte count. Acute bleeding is usually readily detectable, except for cases of retroperitoneal bleeding or bleeding into the upper leg compartments. Chronic blood loss commonly occurs through the gastrointestinal tract but may also occur through the genitourinary system. Red blood cell hemolysis may result in decreased haptoglobin and hemopexin levels. Microangiopathic hemolysis characteristically shows fragmented and sheared cells on the blood smear. For the severely anemic patient in whom emergency surgery is necessary, transfusion to maintain a hematocrit value of 30% to 35% should be adequate for acceptable oxygen-carrying capacity. Anemic patients who are symptomatic with congestive heart failure, dyspnea, or angina should be transfused.

Hemoglobinopathies.—More than 200 structural variants of human hemoglobin have been reported. Some of these may present clinically with abnormal polymerization of hemoglobin (sickle cell anemia, sickle thalassemia, sickle-cell trait disease), unstable hemoglobin, hemoglobin with abnormal oxygen affinity, or hemoglobin M. We will only discuss sickle cell anemia with regard to the urologic patient. This problem may present to the urologist with hematuria or priapism.

The sickle hemoglobin (Hb S) is the result of a substitution of Val for Glu at the 6th residue of the hemoglobin β-chain. About 8% of black Americans are heterozygous for Hb S and 0.2% are homozygous. Hb S has the propensity to polymerize in the deoxygenated state. This results in tactoids of polymerized hemoglobin that distort the red blood cell. Occlusion of small vessels by these distorted or sickled red blood cells manifests clinically as painful crisis, hematoma, priapism, or neurologic compromises.

Patients with sickle cell trait may present with hematuria more commonly than the patient with homozygous disease. It is noteworthy that hematuria due to sickling is not restricted to the black patient.[30] Sickle cell thalassemia may occur commonly in Greek- or Italian-Americans. An abnormal hemoglobin electrophoresis is diagnostic of sickle hemoglobinopathy. Evaluation of hematuria includes the exclusion of infectious etiologies such as tuberculosis and tumors. An excretory urogram, urinary cytologies, cystoscopy, and urine acid-fast bacillus studies are performed. Other bleeding disorders should be kept in mind, since von Willebrand's disease in a sickle cell trait patient may present with gross hematuria.[31]

Histopathologically, sickling results in sludging and extravasation of blood into tubules and peritubular areas, including focal lesions and papillary necrosis. The left kidney, from which hematuria is more common, appears to be prone to venous stasis due to a longer left renal vein.[32] Hematuria due to hemoglobinopathies usually resolves spontaneously. However, intervention is necessary with marked persistent hematuria. Based on the pathophysiology of the sickling disorder, the following treatment modalities are suggested.[32, 33] Reducing the tonicity and acidity of the renal medulla and increasing its oxygen tension may avert sickling in the kidney. Oral fluid intake and furosemide (40 mg orally, twice daily) may effectively reduce renal medullary tonicity. Urinary alkalinization with sodium bicarbonate and/or acetazolamide is recommended. Inhalation of oxygen probably does not increase renal medullary oxygen tension and may adversely affect erythropoiesis, causing painful rebound episodes on discontinuation of oxygen therapy.[23]

The antifibrinolytic agent EACA (Amicar) has been advocated as a modality in controlling hematuria in sickle cell trait patients.[32] An oral loading dose of 5 g followed by 2 to 4 g four times a day until urine clears is recommended.

Priapism is persistent painful penile erection in the absence of sexual desire, which may be the presenting symptom of up to 40% of male sickle cell patients. Other common causes of priapism are trauma, local tumor infiltration, and leukemia. Priapism in most sickle cell patients resolves without aspiration, irrigation, or cavernosum-spongiosum shunting.[35, 36] Marked penile hypertrophy may result from multiple episodes of priapism.[37]

Management of priapism in the sickle cell patient includes nonsurgical modalities as outlined above for hematuria. In addition, analgesics and packed red blood cell transfusions to reduce the concentration of Hb S below 40% is recommended.

Persistent painful priapism may require a late shunting procedure, which has been claimed to be successful.[36] Thrombolytic therapy may be considered as an alternative modality of treatment.[38]

Leukemia, Lymphomas, and Myeloproliferative Disorders.—The acute leukemias may have urologic symptoms such as priapism, urate nephropathy, or bilateral ureteral uric acid stones.[39] Leukemic cell infiltration of the prostate[40, 41] is a potentially reversible cause of urinary obstruction; however, direct infiltration of the renal parenchyma is rarely a cause of renal failure.[42] The lymphomas may present as dysuria, gross hematuria, or decreased urinary stream as the result of local infiltration.[43] Metastasis to the ureter is reported with the common primary sites of breast, colon, lymphoma, and lung, in decreasing frequency of occurrence.[44]

The myeloproliferative diseases rarely present with urologic difficulties. Testicular infarction secondary to polycythemia has been reported in the neonate.[45] Some myeloproliferative disorders manifest with metastatic extramedullary hematopoietic deposits in the kidney.

Rare hematologic entities such as histiocytosis X may present as a primary penile lesion.[46] Eosinophilic cystitis with peripheral eosinophilia and eosinophilic infiltration of the bladder may present with weak stream, frequency, and dysuria.[47]

Primary or secondary amyloidosis may involve the bladder or ureter and present as gross hematuria, hydronephrosis, or, rarely, as priapism.[48–51]

HEMATOLOGIC COMPLICATIONS OF UROLOGIC DISORDERS

Surgical Bleeding

Prostatectomy usually results in significant hemorrhage with an estimated blood loss of about 0.5 to 1.0 L. Tranexamic acid (AMCA) and EACA are potent inhibitors of plasminogen activators and thereby decrease circulating plasmin activity. Using their antifibrinolytic activities, EACA and AMCA have been shown to be effective in reducing hemorrhage secondary to prostatectomy.[52, 53] Insoluble intravesical blood clots requiring surgical intervention have complicated the use of AMCA and EACA.[54] However, patients treated with antifibrinolytics are not at an increased risk for thromboembolism.[55] The use of furosemide in conjunction with EACA has been proposed to maintain diuresis effectively in order to prevent clot retention postoperatively.[52] The routine use of antifibrinolytic therapy in the urologic patient remains controversial. Our approach is to use this treatment modality only in patients with bleeding tendencies.

Another source of potential bleeding complication is perioperative prophylactic anticoagulation with low-dose heparin therapy. Several studies suggest that low-dose heparin does[56]and does not[57, 58] significantly increase bleeding complications in patients undergoing transurethral prostatectomy. In open prostatectomy low-dose heparin appears to result in more bleeding[59, 60] but it is also claimed to be relatively safe.[61] Thus, low-dose heparin therapy appears to be effective but may not be safe for patients undergoing prostatectomy.

Pulmonary Embolism

Pulmonary embolism is one of the most common causes of postoperative mortality and may account for 10% of all postoperative deaths.[62] Clinical signs of pulmonary embolism include tachypnea, chest pain, rales, increased P_2, tachycardia, low-grade fever, and, less frequently, S_3, S_4 gallop, diaphoresis, and cyanosis.[63] Patients may complain of dyspnea, coughing, pleuritic pain, hemoptysis, or syncope. Probably as much as 90% of pulmonary embolism originates from deep vein thrombosis, which is found in approximately 50% of postoperative patients by radioactive fibrinogen deposition studies.[64] However, in patients with pulmonary embolism, clinical evidence of deep-vein thrombosis is only found in about one third of patients. Preoperative and postoperative lung scanning revealed that 4 (8%) of 51 patients undergoing open prostatectomy had pulmonary embolism.[65] This is in contrast to a study showing 2.5% mortality among 2,015 patients undergoing transurethral prostate resection with 0.5% mortality due to pulmonary embolism.[66] According to some authors, pulmonary embolism is the most common cause of postprostatectomy mortality.[67] In a large prospective study including more than 4,000 patients undergoing all types of surgical procedures, 72 control patients and 52 low-dose heparin-treated patients were examined at necropsy. Acute massive pulmonary emboli were found in 16 (22%) of the control group and 2 (4%) of the heparin-treated group.[64] In a series of 300 patients undergoing open prostatectomies by a single surgeon, among the 150 receiving low-dose heparin (5,000 units, twice daily) 0% had postoperative pulmonary emboli, while 2.5% of the 160 control patients had clinical pulmonary embolism.[61] The criteria for the diagnosis of pulmonary embolism, however, were not indicated. Because of insignificant increase in bleeding complications with low-dose heparin therapy, it is recommended that patients undergoing prostatectomy who are at high risk for thromboembolism be prophylactically anticoagulated. Heparin may be administered at 5,000 units subcutaneously every 8 or 12 hours.[68]

Patients with documented pulmonary embolism should be treated with IV heparin (25,000–30,000 units/day) for 10 days and switch to oral anticoagulation for 6 months. In general, thrombolytic therapy should be reserved for patients without recent prior surgery and with cardiopulmonary compromise due to pulmonary embolism. If absolutely unavoidable, thrombolytic therapy may be initiated in postoperative patients as early as 3 days postoperatively, provided that all signs of bleeding are totally absent.

Other conditions predisposing to pulmonary embolism are underlying tumors,[69, 70] cryoprecipitate coagulum pyelolithotomy using thrombin,[71, 72] and antithrombin III deficiency.[73] Antithrombin III deficiency may be hereditary or acquired, as in prostate cancer estrogen therapy, which predisposes patients to thromboembolic events.[74]

Postoperative Thromboembolism

The frequency of postoperative deep vein thrombosis may be as high as 25% in a variety of different surgical procedures.[64] The most common site of thrombosis is in the midgastrocnemius area of the leg. The average frequency of thrombosis following prostate surgery, as determined by uptake of fibrinogen tagged with iodine 125, by phlebography, or by phleborheography in 15 different studies, is 38% for open prostatectomy and 11% for transurethral surgery.[75] The use of EACA or AMCA to control postoperative bleeding has been reported to result in thrombotic complications; however, in three prospective studies[55, 76, 77] and one double blind study of 515 prostatectomies, there was not an increased frequency of thrombosis in the group receiving EACA.[78]

A number of risk factors associated with an increased frequency of postoperative thrombotic events are identified: older age, prolonged surgery, immobilization, trauma, history of thromboembolic disease, varicose veins, malignancy (especially prostate cancer), obesity, cardiac insufficiency, infection, estrogens, oral contraceptives, pregnancy, and large amounts of crystalloid infusion during surgery.[75] A comparison between general and spinal anesthesia for prostatectomy showed no remarkable differences in frequency of thrombus formation by the uptake of ^{125}I-labeled fibrinogen.[79] Patients with high risk for thrombosis should be considered for thromboprophylaxis by a number of methods.

Thromboprophylaxis during the preoperative period has been comprehensively reviewed.[75] A mechanical modality, such as early mobilization and intermittent calf muscle compression, may be efficacious in reducing thrombosis; however, it is cumbersome and not readily available. Oral anticoagulation appears efficacious but is fraught with severe bleeding complications. Antiplatelet agents have not been demonstrated to be unequivocally effective as prophylactic agents. The role of low-dose ASA remains to be established.

Low-dose heparin therapy appears to be efficacious, especially in combination with dihydroergotamine (DHE).[80, 81] In combination with DHE, a lower dose of heparin may suffice and consequently decrease the risk of bleeding. Due to untoward vasospastic effects of DHE, this combination of DHE and heparin is not recommended.

It appears that in the urologic patient early ambulation and mobilization should be undertaken. In patients at high risk for thromboembolism, prophylaxis with low-dose heparin should be considered. With heparin therapy, intraoperative and postoperative bleeding may be significant but certainly supportable via blood transfusions, albeit with an increased risk for hepatitis.

Patients developing deep vein thrombosis may complain of calf pain or swelling. In decreasing frequency of occurrence, induration of calf muscles, unilateral edema, increased skin temperature, calf tenderness, and increased ankle circumference may be observed. Documentation by phlebography is the most sensitive and accurate technique for making the diagnosis when indicated. Patients with documented deep vein thrombosis necessitate treatment with heparin IV at 25,000 to 30,000 units/24 hr for 7 days, followed by oral anticoagulation for 3 months. Patients with proximal deep vein thrombosis above the popliteal area should be considered for thrombolytic therapy. This mode of therapy in the postoperative period may be complicated by bleeding, and one must carefully and thoughtfully weigh the risks against the benefits before instituting thrombolytic therapy.

Disseminated Intravascular Coagulation

Disseminated intravascular coagulation is an acquired coagulopathy secondary to an underlying systemic and usually severe disease process.[82, 83] It is not a primary disease entity. The mechanism of its pathogenesis remains unknown; however, the release of thromboplastic material into the circulation, the disruption of endothelial cells by endotoxin or fibrin (or fibrinogen) degradation products, and the inhibition of fibrin polymerization by fibrin (or fibrinogen) degradation products may play a role. The most probable etiologic factor is the release of a thromboplastic substance into circulation as a result of sepsis, neoplasms, trauma, hepatic disease, or a number of other conditions.[82]

In the urologic patient, bacterial sepsis and prostatic cancer are frequent causes of disseminated intravascular coagulation.[84] Aggressive treatment of metastatic prostate cancer with high-dose diethylstilbestrol has been reported to reverse it.[85] Bacterial sepsis may be the primary presentation or a result of urologic instrumentation. The manipulation of prostatic tumor or a prostatectomy may release thromboplastic material into the circulation, resulting in disseminated intravascular coagulation. In some patients with malignant tumor, a chronic form of this coagulopathy is evident with manifestations of thromboembolic events.[86] Patients with prostatic carcinoma may have a chronic form of disseminated intravascular coagulation with an overwhelming tendency to bleed.[86] Fibrinogen-fibrin degradation products are significantly elevated in patients with a number of urologic malignancies[87] and may serve as tumor markers.

In acute disseminated intravascular coagulation, spontaneous bleeding may present with petechiae or ecchymoses, acral cyanosis, hypoxemia, hypotension, or oliguria. The laboratory findings include thrombocytopenia, hypofibrinogenemia, elevated PT, APTT, and fibrinogen-fibrin degradation products, and a microangiopathic blood smear which are diagnostic of this disorder in the appropriate clinical setting. Thrombotic thrombocytopenic purpura may also present with similar laboratory findings, with the clinical constellation of fever, renal and/or neurologic impairment, thrombocytopenia, and a microangiopathic hemolytic anemia. Success in treatment of disseminated intravascular coagulation is dependent on the identification and control of the underlying disease process. If hemorrhage is excessive, replacement with packed red blood cells is advised. Platelet transfusion may be appropriate if the bone marrow is not producing platelets; however, transfused platelets are generally immediately consumed. In cases in which the underlying process is not immediately controllable, temporary control may be achieved with heparin infusion.[88] The use of heparin in disseminated intravascular coagulation is controversial[82, 88] and in fact may worsen bleeding.

Drug Interactions During Oral Anticoagulation

In patients requiring chronic warfarin therapy, especially those with artificial heart valves, the introduction of a new drug may result in undercoagulation or overanticoagulation. Reported interactions between warfarin and drugs that may be used in the urologic patient are shown in Table 5–3.

Anemia and Polycythemia in the Urologic Patient

Anemia may present as the manifestation of an underlying urologic problem. As with various other causes, reflux nephropathy may terminate with end-stage renal failure and anemia. Infiltration of the bone marrow with tumor, such as prostatic cancer, will result in anemia and ultimately pancytopenia. It is noteworthy that in patients who underwent radiotherapy for bladder carcinoma, vitamin B_{12} deficiency was observed in 10 of 41 patients.[89] Folate levels were normal, indicating that radiation-induced ileal damage may cause malabsorption of vitamin B_{12}. In the immediate postoperative period, massive hemolysis and possible renal

TABLE 5–3.
Drug–Oral Anticoagulants Interactions*

Drugs that increase the effect of oral anticoagulants:
Allopurinol
Antibiotics (cefamandole, moxalactam, cefoperazone)
Cimetidine
Quinine
Quinidine
Nalidixic acid
Salicylates (>1 g/day)
Sulfonamides
Drugs that decrease the effect of oral anticoagulants:
Antihistamines
Barbiturates
Cholestyramine
Diphenylhydantoin
Haloperidol
Oral contraceptives
Rifampin
Xanthines

*Selected common drugs and drugs used in the urologic patient.

failure may result from excessive intravascular uptake of the irrigating fluid that is used during transurethral surgery.[90] Drug therapy in the urologic patient may be complicated by drug-induced hemolytic anemia. Common drugs, such as nalidixic acid, nitrofurantoin, sulfamethoxazole, sulfanilamide, and phenazopyridine, are known to induce hemolysis in glucose-6-phosphate dehydrogenase (G6PD)–deficient patients.[91] Immunologic destruction of erythrocytes may occur with penicillins, cephalosporins, tetracycline, thiazides, and triamterene.[92] Autoimmune hemolytic anemias have been associated with neoplasia, commonly with lymphoid neoplasia, but also may be seen with renal tumors and seminoma.[93] A urologic source of bleeding rarely presents with anemia unless the bleeding is severe. Thus, an anemic urologic patient must be evaluated not only to identify the primary hematologic disorder but also to establish a possible connection to the underlying urologic disease or the treatment thereof.

The elevation of red blood cell mass or polycythemia usually presents with a higher-than-normal hematocrit value and may be associated with neoplasia.[94] Most of the neoplasias associated with polycythemia have been renal cell carcinoma or Wilms' tumor, the removal of which reverses polycythemia.[94, 95] Although polycythemia is associated with renal cell carcinoma, anemia is far more common in these patients.[95] The mechanism of erythrocytosis appears to be the inappropriate elaboration of erythropoietin by the tumor.[96] Polycythemia vera is an idiopathic myeloproliferative disorder that is probably due to an abnormality in the stem cell.[94] Unlike polycythemia vera, neoplasia-related polycythemia is usually not associated with thrombocytopenia, eosinophilia, basophilia, or leukocytosis. Patients with unexplained polycythemia should undergo radiographic evaluation for possible renal tumor.

EDITORIAL COMMENT

This well-referenced chapter provides basic information for any surgeon confronted by hematologic complications. The tables summarize blood coagulation factors, laboratory findings in factor deficiencies, and drugs that may affect oral anticoagulants. The chapter also provides basic information on coagulopathies and thrombocytopenia.

EDITORIAL COMMENT II

The authors address the problem of aspirin consumption in the surgical patient in a new section in this chapter. We now routinely tell patients not to take any aspirin for a least 2 weeks before considering any surgery and this caveat is included in our handout to patients undergoing outpatient surgical procedures.

REFERENCES

1. Kernoff PBA: Prostatectomy in haemophilia and Christmas disease. *Br J Urol* 1972; 44:51.
2. Miner GW, Wise HA, Bouroncle BA: Prostatectomy in hemophilia. *J Urol* 1976; 116:533.
3. Goldsmith JC, Unger HA, Fried FA: Successful prostatectomy in patients with inherited abnormalities of the factor VIII molecule. *J Urol* 1980; 124:570.
4. Kaufman JM: Prostatectomy in factor XI deficiency. *J Urol* 1977; 117:75.
5. Sidi A, Seligsohn U, Jonas P, et al: Factor XI deficiency: Detection and management during urological surgery. *J Urol* 1978; 119:528.
6. Jonas P, Sidi AA, Goldwasser B, et al: Prostatectomy in factor XI (plasma thromboplastin antecedent) deficiency. *J Urol* 1982; 128:1209.

6a. Dang CV, Bell WR, Shuman M: The normal and morbid biology of fibrinogen. *Am J Med* 1989; 87:567.

7. Forman WB, Kraus J: Transurethral resection in a patient with dysfibrinogen: Fibrinogen Cleveland I. *J Urol* 1977; 118:885.
8. Eisenberg RL, Clark RE: Filling defects in the renal pelvis and ureter owing to bleeding secondary to acquired circulating anticoagulants. *J Urol* 1976; 116:662.
9. Stoll DB, Blum S, Pasquale D, et al: Thrombocytopenia with decreased megakaryocytes. *Ann Intern Med* 1981; 94:170.
10. Hackett T, Kelton JG, Powers P: Drug-induced platelet dysfunction. *Semin Thromb Hemost* 1982; 8:116.
11. Burns TR, Saleem A: Idiopathic thrombocytopenia purpura. *Am J Med* 1983; 75:1001.
12. Bussel JB, Kimberly RP, Inman RD, et al: Intravenous gamma globulin treatment of chronic idiopathic thrombocytopenia purpura. *Blood* 1983; 62:480.
13. Bell WR, Royall RM: Heparin-associated thrombocytopenia: A comparison of three heparin preparation. *N Engl J Med* 1980; 303:902.
14. Merriman E, Bell WR, Long DM: Surgical postoperative bleeding associated with aspirin ingestion. *J Neurosurg* 1979; 50:682.
15. Torosian M, Michelson EL, Morganroth J, et al: Aspirin and Coumadin related bleeding after coronary-artery bypass surgery. *Ann Intern Med* 1978; 89:325.
16. Michelson EL, Morganroth J, Torosian M, et al: Relation of preoperative use of aspirin to increased mediastinal blood loss after coronary artery bypass graft surgery. *J Thorac Cardiovasc Surg* 1978;76:694.
17. Rubin RN: Aspirin and postsurgery bleeding. *Ann Intern Med* 1978;89:1006.
18. Amrein PC, Ellman L, Harris WH: Aspirin-induced prolongation of bleeding time and perioperative blood loss. *JAMA* 1981;245:1825.
19. Ferraris VA, Swanson E: Aspirin usage and perioperative blood loss in patients undergoing unexpected operations. *Surg Gynecol Obstet* 1983:156:439.
20. Ramsey G, Arvan DA, Stewart S, et al: Do preoperative laboratory tests predict blood transfusion needs in cardiac operations? *J Thorac Cardiovasc Surg* 1983;85:564.
21. Harris Wh, Salzman EW, Athansoulis CA, et al: Aspirin prophylaxis of venous thromboembolism after total hip replacement. *N Engl J Med* 1977;297:1247.
22. Hindman BJ, Koka BV: Usefulness of the post-aspirin bleeding time. *Anesthesiology* 1986;64:368.
23. Livio M, Benigni A, Vigano G, et al: Moderate doses of aspirin and risk of bleeding in renal failure. *Lancet* 1986;1:412.
24. Prager D: Aspirin and postoperative bleeding. *Ann Intern Med* 1979;90:123.
25. Harker LA, Slichter SF: The bleeding time as a screening test for evaluation of platelet function. *N Engl J Med* 1972;287:155.
26. Deykin K: Uremic bleeding. *Kidney Int* 1983; 24:698.
27. Janson PA, Jubelirer SJ, Weinstein MJ, et al: Treatment of the bleeding tendency in uremia with cryoprecipitate. *N Engl J Med* 1980; 303:1318.
28. Mannucci PM, Remuzzi G, Pusineri F, et al: Deamino-8-*d*-arginine vasopressin shortens the bleeding time in uremia. *N Engl J Med* 1983; 308:8.
29. Colapinto V, Comisarow RH: Urologic manifestations of the iliacus hematoma syndrome. *J Urol* 1979; 122:272.
30. Richie JP, Kerr WS: Sickle cell trait: Forgotten cause of hematuria in white patients. *J Urol* 1979; 122:134.
31. Weinger RS, Benson GS, Villarreal S: Gross hematuria associated with sickle cell trait and von Willebrand's disease. *J Urol* 1979; 122:136.
32. McInnes BK III: The management of hematuria associated with sickle hemoglobinopathies. *J Urol* 1980; 124:171.
33. Meyersfield SA, Morganstern SL, Seery W, et al: Medical management of refractory hematuria in sickle-cell trait. *Urology* 1976; 8:112.
34. Embury SH, Garcia JF, Mohandas N, et al: Effects of oxygen inhalation on endogenous erythropoietin kinetics, erythropoiesis, and properties of blood cells in sickle-cell anemia. *N Engl J Med* 1984; 311:291.
35. Nelson JH III, Winter CC: Priapism: Evolution of management in 48 patients in a 22-year series. *J Urol* 1977; 117:455.
36. Baron M, Leiter E: The management of priapism in sickle cell anemia. *J Urol* 1978; 119: 610.

37. Datta NS: Megalophallus in sickle cell disease. *J Urol* 1977; 117:672.
38. King LM, McCune DP, Harris JJ, et al: Fibrinolysin therapy for thrombosis of priapism. *J Urol* 1964; 92:693.
39. Rieselbach RE, Bentzel CJ, Cotlove E, et al: Uric acid excretion and renal function in the acute hyperuricemia of leukemia. Pathogenesis and therapy of uric acid nephropathy. *Am J Med* 1964; 37:872.
40. Mith WE Jr, Serpick AA: Leukemic infiltration of the prostate. A reversible form of urinary obstruction. *Cancer* 1970; 26:1361.
41. Garcia-Gonzales R, Bellas-Menendez C, Llorente-Abarca C, et al: Leukemic infiltration of the prostate causing acute urinary obstruction. *Eur Urol* 1984; 10:356.
42. Barakat AY, Mnaymneh LG: Acute lymphoblastic leukemia diagnosed by renal biopsy. *J Urol* 1977; 118:103.
43. Chaitin BA, Manning JT, Ordonez NG: Hematologic neoplasms with initial manifestations in lower urinary tract. *Urology* 1984; 23:35.
44. Cohen WM, Freed SZ, Hasson J: Metastatic cancer to the ureter: A review of the literature and case presentations. *J Urol* 1974; 112:188.
45. Jung AL, McGaughey HR, Mattak ME: Neonatal testicular infarction and polycythemia. *J Urol* 1980; 123:781.
46. Myers DA, Strandjord SE, Marcus RB, et al: Histiocytosis X presenting as a primary penile lesion. *J Urol* 1981; 126:268.
47. Rubin L, Pincus MB: Eosinophilic cystitis: The relationship of allergy in the urinary tract to eosinophilic cystitis and the pathophysiology of eosinophilia. *J Urol* 1974; 112:457.
48. Missen GAK, Tribe CR: Catastrophic haemorrhage from the bladder due to unrecognized secondary amyloidosis. *Br J Urol* 1970; 42:43.
49. Abramovici I, Chivatt S, Nussenson M: Massive hematuria and perforation in a case of amyloidosis of the bladder: Case report and review of the literature. *J Urol* 1977; 118:964.
50. Yazaki T, Iizumi I, Ogawa Y, et al: Renal autotransplantation for localized amyloidosis of the ureter. *J Urol* 1982; 128:119.
51. Lapan DI, Graham AR, Bangert JL, et al: Amyloidosis presenting as priapism. *Urology* 1980; 15:167.
52. Smart CJ, Turnbull AR, Jenkins JD: The use of furosemide and epsilon-aminocaproic acid in transurethral prostatectomy. *Br J Urol* 1974; 46:521.
53. Miller RA, May MW, Hendry WF, et al: The prevention of secondary hemorrhage after prostatectomy: The value of antifibrinolytic therapy. *Br J Urol* 1980; 52:26.
54. Ward MG, Richards B: Complications of antifibrinolysis therapy after prostatectomy. *Br J Urol* 1979; 51:211.
55. Hedlund PO: Postoperative venous thrombosis in benign prostatic disease. A study of 316 patients with ^{125}I-fibrinogen uptake test. *Scand J Urol Nephrol* 1975; 27(suppl):1.
56. Sleight MW: The effect of prophylactic subcutaneous heparin on blood loss during and after transurethral prostatectomy. *Br J Urol* 1982; 54:164.
57. Kass EJ, Sonda P, Gershon C: The use of prophylactic low dose heparin in transurethral prostatectomy. *J Urol* 1978; 120:186.
58. Tscholl R, Straub W, Zingg E: Electroresection of the prostate in patients treated with heparin. *J Urol* 1980; 124:221.
59. Allen NH, Jenkins JD, Smart CJ: Surgical hemorrhage in patients given subcutaneous heparin as prophylaxis against thromboembolism. *Br Med J* 1978; 1:1326.
60. Halverstadt DB, Albers DD, Kroovand RL, et al: Anticoagulation in urologic surgery. *Urology* 1977; 9:617.
61. Jasper WS Sr: Anticoagulants in open prostatectomies. *J Urol* 1977; 117:72.
62. Wessler S, Yin ET: Theory and practice of minidose heparin in surgical patients: A status report. *Circulation* 1973; 47:671.
63. Bell WR, Simon TL, De Mets DL: The clinical features of submassive and massive pulmonary emboli. *Am J Med* 1977; 62:355.
64. Kakkar VV, Corrigan TP, Fossard DP, et al: Prevention of fatal post-operative pulmonary embolism by low doses of heparin. An international multicentre trial. *Lancet* 1975; 2:45.
65. Salzman AJ, Axilrod HD: The value of preoperative lung scanning in the assessment of postoperative perfusion abnormalities. *J Urol* 1971; 106:581.

66. Holtgrewe HL, Valk WL: Factor influencing the mortality and morbidity of transurethral prostatectomy: A study of 2,015 cases. *J Urol* 1962; 87:450.
67. Antila LE, Markkula J, Iisalo E: Ten years experience of geriatric aspects in surgery of patients with benign prostatic hyperplasia. *Acta Chir Scand* 1966; 357:95.
68. Bell WR, Zuidema GD: Low-dose heparin—concern and perspectives. *Surgery* 1979; 85:469.
69. Seifter EJ, Bell WR: *Coagulation Disorders in the Cancer Patients.* Mt Kisco, NY, Futura Publishing Co, 1984.
70. Gore JM, Appelbaum JS, Greene HL, et al: Occult cancer in patients with acute pulmonary embolism. *Ann Intern Med* 1982; 96:556.
71. Pence JR II, Airhart RA, Novicki DE, et al: Pulmonary emboli associated with coagulum pyelolithotomy. *J Urol* 1982; 127:572.
72. Kalash SS, Campbell EW, Young JD: Further simplification of cryoprecipitate coagulum pyelolithotomy without thrombin. *Urology* 1983; 22:483.
73. Cosgriff TM, Bishop DT, Herhgold EJ, et al: Familial antithrombin III deficiency: Its natural history, genetics, diagnosis, and treatment. *Medicine* 1983; 62:209.
74. Eisen M, Napp HE, Vock R: Inhibition of platelet aggregation caused by estrogen treatment in patients with carcinoma of the prostate. *J. Urol* 1975; 114:93.
75. Bergqvist D: *Post-operative Thromboembolism.* New York, Springer-Verlag, 1983, pp 14–15.
76. Gordon-Smith IC, Hickman JA, El Masri SH: The effect of the fibrinolytic inhibitor epsilon-aminocaproic acid on the incidence of deep-vein thrombosis after prostatectomy. *Br J Surg* 1972; 59:522.
77. Becker J, Borgstrom S: Incidence of thrombosis associated with epsilon-aminocaproic acid administration and with combined epsilon-aminocaproic acid and subcutaneous heparin therapy. *Acta Chir Scand* 1968; 134:343.
78. Vinnecombe J, Shuttleworth KED: Aminocaproic acid in the control of haemorrhage after prostatectomy. Safety of aminocaproic acid—a controlled trial. *Lancet* 1966; 1:232.
79. Hassan MA, Rahman EA, Rahman IA: Prostatectomy and deep vein thrombosis in Sudanese patients. *Br J Surg* 1974; 61:650.
80. The Multicenter Trial Committee: Dihydroergotamine-heparin prophylaxis of post-operative deep vein thrombosis. *JAMA* 1984; 251:2960.
81. Multicenter Trial Committee: Prophylactic efficacy of low-dose dihydroergotamine and heparin in postoperative deep venous thrombosis following intra-abdominal operations. *J Vasc Surg* 1984; 1:608.
82. Bell WR: Disseminated intravascular coagulation. *Johns Hopkins Med J* 1980; 146:289.
83. Kursh ED, Ratnoff OD, Persky L: Current clotting concepts in urology. *J Urol* 1976; 116:214.
84. Pergament ML, Swaim WR, Blackard CE: Disseminated intravascular coagulation in the urologic patient. *J Urol* 1976; 116:1.
85. Goldenberg SL, Fenster HN, Perler Z, et al: Disseminated intravascular coagulation in carcinoma of prostate: Role of estrogen therapy. *Urology* 1983; 22:130.
86. Sack GH, Levin J, Bell WR: Trousseau's syndrome and other manifestations of chronic disseminated coagulopathy in patients with neoplasms: Clinical, pathophysiologic, and therapeutic features. *Medicine* 1977; 56:1.
87. Riedmiller H, Thuroff JW, Jacobi GH: Fibrinogen degradation products in urological malignant tumors. *Urol Int* 1984; 39:13.
88. Feinstein DI: Diagnosis and management of disseminated intravascular coagulation: The role of heparin therapy. *Blood* 1982; 60:284.
89. Kinn A-C, Lantz B: Vitamin B_{12} deficiency after irradiation for bladder carcinoma. *J Urol* 1984; 131:888.
90. Bird D, Slade N, Feneley RCL: Intravascular complications of transurethral resection of the prostate. *Br J Urol* 1982; 54:564.
91. Beutler E: Glucose-6-phosphate dehydrogenase deficiency and non-spherocytic congenital hemolytic anemia. *Semin Hematol* 1965; 2:91.
92. Garratty G, Petz LD: Drug-induced immune hemolytic anemia. *Am J Med* 1975; 58:398.
93. Canale D, Feldman R, Rosen M, et al: Autoimmune hemolytic anemia associated with seminoma. *Urology* 1975; 5:411.

94. Hocking WG: Pathophysiology, in Golde DW (moderator): Polycythemia: Mechanisms and management. *Ann Intern Med* 1981; 95:71.
95. Marshall FF, Walsh PC: Extrarenal manifestations of renal cell carcinoma. *J Urol* 1977; 117:439.
96. Sufrin G, Mirand EA, Moore RH, et al: Hormones in renal cancer. *J Urol* 1977; 117:433.

CHAPTER 6

Complications of Pharmacologic Agents in the Urologic Patient

Herbert Lepor, M.D.
David Mikkelsen, M.D.
Ellen Shapiro, M.D.

We are a pill-taking society. The average physician prescribes some pharmacologic agent for approximately 75% of his patients.[1] A recent study has shown that when objective tests examining the hazards of medications were administered to physicians, some scores were as low as 60%.[2] The consequences of this liberal use of drugs, and the lack of familiarity with the adverse effects of drugs, are staggering. One seventh of all hospital stays are devoted to the care of drug toxic effects at an estimated yearly cost of $3 billion.[3] Approximately 29,000 deaths annually are drug-related.[4] Severe adverse drug reactions are rarely caused by drugs prescribed by urologists. Digitalis, aspirin-containing compounds, steroids, antidiabetics, antihypertensives, antitumor agents, oral anticoagulants, and oral contraceptives accounted for 56% of the 260 drug reactions that required hospital admissions in 7,017 monitored patients.[5]

Adverse drug reactions can be categorized as reactions due to the action of drugs and reactions due to the interaction of drugs with other predisposing factors. Adverse reactions due to the action of drugs are usually predictable and dose-related and include overdosages, side effects, and cytotoxic effects. Predisposing factors that influence drug actions are constitutionally induced, disease-induced, drug-induced, and environmentally induced. Since approximately 80% of adverse drug reactions are secondary to the direct action of drugs, the vast majority of adverse drug reactions are predictable.[6]

The objective of this chapter is to review drug reactions that are specifically relevant to clinical urology. Urinary retention, impotence, infertility, hematuria, and priapism are adverse effects of drugs that are prescribed by our medical colleagues. Drugs that cause these specific genitourinary disorders will be presented. This chapter will also highlight the adverse drug reactions of pharmacologic agents commonly prescribed by the urologist. It is impractical to index all the adverse reactions of every drug with urologic indications. We have limited our review to drugs used to treat renal lithiasis (allopurinol, penicillamine, hydrochlorothiazide, orthophosphates, sodium cellulose phosphate, citrates, and hemiacidrin [Renacidin]), bacterial infections (sulfonamides, nitrofurantoin, ampicillin, carbenicillin, cephalosporins, tetracyclines, aminoglycosides, and quinolones), neurogenic bladder (propantheline bromide, phenoxybenzamine, imipramine, and bethanechol chloride), impotence (papavarine, phenoxybenzamine, and prostaglandin E_1), and benign prostatic hyperplasia (phenoxybenzamine, prazosin, and terazosin). Opioid analgesics (morphine), local anesthetics (lidocaine), and benzodiazepines (diazepam) will also be discussed. As the physiology and neuropharmacology of genitourinary function become more precisely elucidated, drugs will assume a more prominent role in the management of urologic disorders.

UROLOGIC COMPLICATIONS OF PHARMACOLOGIC AGENTS

Urinary Retention

The activity of the genitourinary tract is intimately controlled by the autonomic sympathetic (thoracolumbar) and parasympathetic (sacral) nervous systems. Norepinephrine and acetylcholine are released at postganglionic nerve terminals, and these neurotransmitters bind to specific adrenergic and muscarinic cholinergic receptors located on smooth muscle cellular membranes. In general, norepinephrine binds to α- and β-adrenoceptors, resulting in smooth muscle contraction and relaxation, respectively.[7]

Histochemical staining, in vitro isometric contraction, and radioligand receptor-binding experiments have demonstrated that neurotransmitter receptors are not homogeneously distributed between the bladder body and bladder neck.[8–12] The density of muscarinic cholinergic receptors is greater in the bladder body than in the bladder neck. Tissue strips obtained from the canine bladder body contract in the presence of muscarinic cholinergic agonists. Tissue strips obtained from the anterior canine bladder neck contract in the presence of muscarinic cholinergic agonists, whereas tissue strips from the remainder of the bladder neck and trigone are unresponsive to muscarinic cholinergic stimulation. α-Adrenoceptors are richly distributed in the bladder neck and are deficient in the bladder body. β-Adrenoceptors are richly distributed in the bladder body and are deficient in the bladder neck.

Micturition involves the simultaneous coordinated contraction of the bladder body under cholinergic (parasympathetic) control and the relaxation of the bladder neck under α-adrenergic (sympathetic) control. Theoretically, urinary retention should be precipitated by inhibiting muscarinic cholinergic and stimulating β-adrenoceptors in the bladder body (inhibition of detrusor contraction) and by stimulating muscarinic cholinergic and α-adrenoceptors in the bladder base (increased bladder outlet resistance). Clinically, urinary retention occurs following the administration of muscarinic cholinergic antagonists such as propantheline bromide and α-adrenergic agonists such as phenylephrine. Drugs that have relatively potent anticholinergic properties, such as the phenothiazines (chlorpromazine), tricyclic antidepressants (nortriptyline), and antispasmodics (oxybutynin chloride), may also promote urinary retention. Although the bladder body contains a rich β-adrenoceptor content, isoproterenol and other β-adrenergic analogues do not appear to cause urinary retention in man. The insensitivity of intravesical pressure to β-adrenergic analogues has been documented in the dog.[13] The apparent lack of correlation between physiologic and in vitro responsiveness of the bladder to β-adrenergic drugs may be explained by the physiologic and pharmacologic doses utilized in the respective studies.

Men with benign prostatic hyperplasia are susceptible to developing urinary retention following the administration of anticholinergic and α-adrenergic drugs. Tissue strips obtained from human prostatic adenoma and capsule contract in the presence of α-adrenergic agonists.[14] A moderate density of α-adrenergic receptors have been characterized in human prostate adenomas using radioligand receptor-binding methods.[15] α-Adrenergic drugs may promote urinary retention in men with benign prostatic hyperplasia (BPH) by increasing the tension of the smooth muscle in both the bladder neck and prostate adenoma.

Impotence

The ability to achieve an erection involves the coordinated interaction of endocrine, vascular, neurologic, and psychologic factors. The primary mechanical event that promotes an erection appears to be preferential redirection of increased arterial inflow into the corporal spaces. Maintenance of erection may involve active venous constriction.[16] The redistribution of blood flow is intimately regulated by the autonomic nervous system.

The neuropharmacologic regulation of erectile function is incompletely understood. Electrical stimulation of the parasympathetic nerves produces erections in the dog, cat, and monkey.[17–19] These electrically induced erections are inhibited by hexamethonium, a preganglionic blocking agent.[17] Muscarinic cholinergic receptors have been characterized in the penis using radioligand receptor-binding methods.[20] A direct role of muscarinic cholinergic receptors in mediating erection is unlikely since atropine, a muscarinic cholinergic antagonist, does not inhibit electrically induced erections,[17] and the intraaortic and intracorporal injection of acetylcholine does not produce erections.[17, 21, 22] In addition, histochemical studies demonstrate sparse cholinergic innervation of the corpora cavernosa, and human corporal tissue does not contract in the presence of cholinergic agonists.[23]

A rich distribution of adrenoceptors has been identified in the corpora cavernosa of various species, including man, using fluorescent microscopy and in vitro muscle contraction techniques.[23–25] The contractile properties of the corpora cavernosa to the α-adrenergic agonists norepinephrine and phenylephrine are dose-related. The phenylephrine-induced contractions of the corpora cavernosa are inhibited by pretreatment with phentolamine, an α-adrenergic antagonist. Despite the in vitro responsiveness of corporal tissue to α-adrenergic agonists, intraaortic infusion of norepinephrine does not produce erections or increase venous outflow.[17] The neurotransmitter receptors mediating erection are likely to be associated with vascular smooth muscle, and therefore in vitro isometric experiments using corpora cavernosa may be of limited value in defining the neurotransmitters mediating erection.

There is physiologic evidence supporting a primary role of β-adrenoceptors in the erectile mechanism. The response of strips of tissue obtained from the corpora cavernosa of various species to β-adrenergic agonists is relaxation.[25] Erections are produced following the intraaortic injection of salbutamol and terbutaline (β_2-adrenergic agonists) in the dog and cat.[21–26] These experimentally induced erections are abolished by propranolol, a β-adrenergic antagonist. Intraaortic and intracorporal injection of phenoxybenzamine, a nonselective α-adrenergic, produces erections in the cat,[21] and man,[27] respectively. Norepinephrine represents the in vivo neurotransmitter for both α- and β-adrenoceptors. Selective inhibition of α-adrenoceptors indirectly potentiates β-adrenoceptor-mediated responses. Phenoxybenzamine may induce erections by potentiating β-adrenoceptor activity.

Erections are also mediated by neuroreflexes controlled by the autonomic nervous system. Current experimental data and clinical observations suggest that norepinephrine is the neurotransmitter released at the effector sites. The peripheral pathways mediating erectile function are modulated by the central nervous system. Pharmacologic agents may interfere with erectile function by interfering with these central and peripheral neural pathways; blocking the release and/or binding of neurotransmitters at the tissue effector sites; and by directly altering vasomotor tone and penile blood flow. Drugs may also interfere with erections by altering libido.

Anticholinergic, antidepressant, antihypertensive, antipsychotic, antiandrogen, and narcotic classes of drugs have all been associated with impotence.

Anticholinergics.—Atropine sulfate, benztropine (Cogentin), diphenhydramine (Benadryl), and propantheline bromide (Pro-Banthine) are commonly prescribed drugs with anticholinergic properties. Anticholinergic drugs presumably cause erectile dysfunction by inhibiting preganglionic cholinergic receptors.[28] The effect of pharmacologic postganglionic muscarinic cholinergic receptor blockade on erectile function is equivocal.

Antidepressants.—Tricyclic antidepressant drugs such as amitriptyline, doxepin, nortriptyline, and imipramine interfere with the reuptake of norepinephrine at nerve terminals and antagonize acetylcholine receptors with variable affinities.[29] Penile blood flow may be diminished secondary to preganglionic cholinergic blockade and/or potentiation of adrenergic-mediated responses resulting from the inhibition of norepinephrine reuptake.

Antihypertensives.—Antihypertensive agents may interfere with erectile function by altering blood flow to the corpora cavernosa; interfering with androgen metabolism; and interfering with central and peripheral neural pathways that mediate erection.[30]

Spironolactone is a steroid analogue that competitively inhibits the binding of aldosterone to its receptor.[31] Spironolactone produces low serum testosterone levels, increases testosterone clearance, and elevates levels of estradiol and luteinizing hormone.[32] Spironolactone-induced endocrine dysfunction and competitive antagonization of testosterone binding to the androgen receptor may result in impotence.

The mechanism of thiazide-induced impotence is poorly understood. Thiazides may alter erectile function by interfering with vascular smooth muscle activity.[28] Thiazides are frequently prescribed together with other antihypertensive drugs. Impotence is usually attributed to the other coadministered drugs. Yendt and co-workers reported loss of libido in three of 67 patients treated with thiazides for prevention of renal calculi.[33]

Methyldopa reduces hypertension by antagonizing adrenergic receptors on vascular smooth muscle and by stimulating α-adrenoceptors in the brain. There is great variation in the reported incidence of erectile dysfunction in men treated with methyldopa. The incidence of impotence reported in the literature ranges between 1.3% and 50%.[34, 35] Clonidine, a selective α_2-adrenergic partial agonist, presumably reduces blood pressure through a centrally mediated mechanism. Clonidine has been associated with impotence in 10% to 20% of male patients.[36] α-Adrenoceptors have not been characterized in the penis. The intravenous administration of clonidine alters canine intraprostatic urethral resistance,[37] presumably by binding to α_2-adrenoceptors associated with prostatic smooth muscle. The human prostate contains a moderate density of α_2-adrenoceptors.[38] Clonidine may interfere with erections by directly altering the tone of penile smooth muscle or via a centrally mediated mechanism.

Propranolol is a commonly prescribed β-adrenergic antagonist and presumably causes erectile dysfunction by decreasing blood flow to the corpora. The Veterans Administration Cooperative Study on Antihypertensive Agents reported the development of impotence in six of 81 patients (7.4%) treated with propranolol alone.[39]

Hydralazine causes a direct relaxation of vascular smooth muscle. It is surprising that sexual dysfunction is rarely associated with this drug.[40] Hydralazine in doses greater than 200 mg/day has been associated with decreased libido.[28]

Prazosin is a selective α_1-adrenergic antagonist. One of its major advantages is its freedom from effects on sexual dysfunction.[40]

Cardioselective β-blockers, calcium antagonists, and angiotensin converting enzyme (ACE) inhibitors are several new classes of antihypertensive agents that have recently come into use. The new β-adrenergic cardioselective blocking agents include atenolol (Tenormin), labetalol (Normodyne), and metoprolol (Lopressor). Although erectile dysfunction appears less commonly with these newer agents compared to propranolol (Inderal), several reports of impotence secondary to these agents have been documented.[41–43] Peyronie's disease has been associated with the use of metoprolol in approximately 1 in 10,000 cases.[44] Priapism has been associated with the use of labetalol.[45]

The calcium antagonists interfere with calcium transport in the heart muscle and in the vascular smooth muscle cells.[46, 47] This class of antihypertensive agents includes verapamil (CALAN), nifedipine (Procardia), and diltiazem (Cardizem). Although impotence is rarely associated with these agents, several case reports have documented the association of impotence following administration of verapamil.[48, 49] The incidence of verapamil-induced impotence has been estimated to be 1 in 10,000 cases.[44]

The ACE inhibitors enalapril (Vasotec) and captopril (Capoten) decrease blood pressure by lowering peripheral resistance, decreasing aldosterone-mediated extracellular fluid volume expansion, and by limiting angiotensin II–stimulated activation of sympathetic nervous system activity. Impotence has not been associated with these agents.[45] ACE inhibitors are becoming first-line therapy for essential hypertension and may represent a suitable substitute when confronted with a presumed case of drug-related impotence. ACE inhibitors may actually exacerbate chronic renal insufficiency.[50] This may be pertinent in the impotent patient who is both hypertensive and diabetic.

Antipsychotics.—Phenothiazines such as chlorpromazine and thorazine cause erectile and ejaculatory dysfunction secondary to peripheral anticholinergic and antiadrenergic effects. Sexual function has been shown to be affected by the central monoamine neurotransmitters serotonin and dopamine.[30] The dopaminergic blocking properties of the phenothiazines and butyrophenones may alter sexual behavior, presumably by depleting central monoamine neurotransmitters.[51]

Narcotics.—Morphine, meperidine (Demerol), and codeine result in impotence, presumably by depressing central nervous system activity.[28]

Antiandrogens.—Drugs with antiandrogenic properties may impair erectile function, libido, and fertility. The antiandrogens will be discussed later in the chapter as a potential cause of infertility.

Hematuria

Drugs that interfere with the function of the coagulation factors and platelets may cause hematuria. A complete prescription and nonprescription drug history is therefore an essential component of preoperative screening interviews and the evaluation of hematuria.

Platelets, and the conversion of coagulation factors to thrombin and fibrin, are primarily responsible for hemostasis. The unique feature of platelets is their ability to adhere to foreign surfaces, forming aggregates. Hemostasis begins with the adherence of platelets to the exposed connective tissue of injured blood vessels. The adherence of platelets promotes the release of adenosine diphosphate (ADP) from storage organelles of the adherent platelets. The released ADP causes other platelets to aggregate to the already adherent platelets.[52]

Aspirin and the nonsteroidal anti-inflammatory drugs interfere with platelet function through several mechanisms. Phenylbutazone[53] and aspirin[54] interfere with the aggregation of platelets promoted by collagen. Aspirin[55] and nonsteroidal anti-inflammatory drugs[56] inhibit ADP-mediated platelet aggregation. The endogenous release of ADP by platelets promotes secondary platelet aggregation.

Aspirin and nonsteroidal anti-inflammatory drugs inhibit the biosynthesis of cycloendoperoxides from arachidonic acid by competitively blocking the enzyme prostaglandin synthetase (cyclooxygenase).[57] Thromboxanes are biologically active products of the arachidonic cascade that promote platelet aggregation.[58] Aspirin and the nonsteroidal anti-inflammatory agents block thromboxane synthesis. The unique feature of aspirin is its ability to acetylate the enzyme cyclooxygenase.[59]

A single dose of 300 mg of aspirin doubles the mean bleeding time of a normal person between 4 and 7 days.[56] Although indomethacin is more potent than aspirin, the effects of a single dose of indomethacin last approximately 6 hours.[60] The life span of a platelet is between 4 and 7 days. Aspirin appears to irreversibly impair platelet function, presumably through acetylation of prostaglandin synthetase (cyclooxygenase).[61]

Nonsteroidal anti-inflammatory agents have been associated with "idiopathic" hematuria. An etiology for microscopic and gross hematuria was not identified in 21% of 116 consecutive patients undergoing complete urologic evaluation. Fifty-four percent of these patients with idiopathic hematuria were receiving nonsteroidal anti-inflammatory drugs on a routine basis. One third of these patients received ibuprofen, one third received aspirin, and the remainder received naprosin and indomethacin.[61]

Microscopic and gross hematuria are commonly associated with anticoagulation therapy. The coagulation parameters are frequently within accepted therapeutic range in those anticoagulated patients presenting with hematuria. Eighty-two percent of anticoagulated patients evaluated urologically for hematuria were found to have vesicoureteral reflux, urethral strictures, ureteritis cystica, calculus disease, or carcinoma of the bladder and prostate.[62] Although identification of a specific urologic etiology for hematuria in patients on anticoagulation regimens in this series exceeds our personal experience, a thorough urologic evaluation is justified in these patients.

Infertility

The identification of pharmacologic agents interfering with male fertility is complicated by the lack of a definitive quantitative indicator of fertility. The paucity of observations on the effects of drugs on human fertility is not a result of negative study but, rather, reflects the absence of studies. Drugs can alter male fertility by inhibiting spermatogenesis, altering sperm motility, and impairing the function of the reproductive tract. The precise effect of a drug on male fertility can be ascertained only in a group of men actively trying to initiate a pregnancy. Although a semen analysis provides an indication of fertility potential,[63] men are unlikely to volunteer for drug protocols requiring repeated semen analysis. An alternative to clinical trials is to examine the effects of drugs on fertility in experimental animals. Unfortunately, owing to appreciable species variability, the toxic effects of drugs on fertility in laboratory animals cannot consistently be extrapolated to man.[64]

The effects of single-agent chemotherapeutic drug regimens on male fertility has been investigated in men with lymphoma and testicular carcinoma. It is difficult to ascertain in these men the role of malignant disease and chemotherapeutic agents as the cause of infertility since only 23% of men with lymphoma and testicular carcinoma were judged to have pretreatment semen quality adequate for initiating a pregnancy.[65]

Richter et al.[66] demonstrated that the degree of testicular damage in men with lymphoma was related to the dose of chlorambucil administered. As the dose of chlorambucil approached 400 mg, severe oligospermia occurred. Testicular biopsies in these men showed only Sertoli cells and peritibular fibrosis. Recovery of testicular function was also dose-dependent.

The cumulatative effect of 11 g of cyclophosphamide in adult men with nephritis resulted in azoospermia.[67] Some degree of testicular recovery eventually occurred in men receiving as much as 17 g of cyclophosphamide. Buchanan et al.[68] demonstrated that the recovery of testicular function was not significantly dependent on the interval of treatment and total drug dose received. Prolonged intervals were required for the return of testicular function in many circumstances. Three azoospermic men fathered children when the cyclophosphamide was withdrawn. Other antineoplastic drugs, such as busulfan (Myleran)[69] and triethylenemelamine (TEM),[70] have been shown to alter spermatogenesis in laboratory animals.

Timmermans[71] investigated the effects of 10 antibiotics on spermatogenesis in the rat at doses adjusted for human physiology. Gentamicin sulfate, *N*-5-nitrofurylidene)-1-aminohydantoin, oxytetracycline, spiramycin, sodium-7-(thiophene-2-adetamido) cepholosporanate, colistimethate (Coly-Mycin), penicillin G potassium, chloromycetin succinate, and trimethoprim all altered germ cell mitotic and meiotic division so that metaphase was never achieved.[71] Biopsies of human testis from men receiving preoperative gentamicin prior to prostatic surgery showed arrest of spermatogenesis with increased numbers of primary spermatocytes.[71] The current widespread use of antibiotics and the concentration of some antibiotics in the seminal fluid justifies further investigation of the clinical significance of Timmermans' observations.

Nitrofurantoin is a urinary-specific antibiotic that is frequently used for long-term bacterial suppression. Nitrofurantoin reversibly inhibits spermatogenesis in animals[72] and man,[73] presumably by inhibiting protein synthesis of the spermatogonia and primary spermatocyte.[74] Nitrofurantoin administered at a dose of 10 mg/kg/day for 14 days temporarily suppressed the sperm count in 13 of 34 men.[73] Prophylactic levels of nitrofurantoin most likely do not contribute to male infertility.

A case report described a man who became azoospermic while receiving colchicine; recovery of testicular function was demonstrated when colchicine was withdrawn, and azoospermia recurred when the colchicine was reinstituted.[75] Bremner and Paulsen did not demonstrate changes in testicular function in seven men between the ages of 20 and 25 years receiving therapeutic doses of colchicine.[76] Colchicine is used in chromosomal studies to arrest meiosis at the spindle stage. Inhibition of cellular division by colchicine may contribute to impaired maturation of spermatocytes. Hamsters and mice receiving colchicine developed azoospermia. However, the dose when adjusted for body weight was 40 times clinically administered doses.[77]

Diphenylhydantoin (Dilantin) is excreted into the seminal plasma.[78] Semen analysis obtained from three men receiving phenytoin identified one specimen with abnormal morphology and motility.[78] Phenytoin may have a direct toxic effect on spermatogenesis. Dilantin was noted to depress follicle-stimulating hormone (FSH) levels in eight of 24 patients receiving chronic treatment.[79] The depressed levels of FSH suggests that phenytoin may affect gonadotropin releasing hormone rather than directly interfering with spermatogenesis.

Sulfasalazine, a drug indicated for the management of ulcerative colitis, has been associated with infertility. Six of 10 men with presumed infertility secondary to sulfasalazine, who tolerated discontinuing the drug, initiated pregnancy within 3 months.[80] Oligospermia dramatically improved in four of four infertile men with ulcerative colitis when sulfasalazine was withdrawn.[81] Several other investigators have confirmed the reversibility of altered sperm motility and morphology in men taking sulfasalazine.[82, 83]

Aspirin in large quantities is associated with decreased levels of prostaglandins E and F in seminal fluid.[84] Aspirin is a potent inhibitor of the enzyme prostaglandin synthetase. The clinical significance of the altered seminal prostaglandins is unknown.

All aspects of male reproduction are keenly dependent on androgens. Steroidal and nonsteroidal compounds that inhibit androgen synthesis and antagonize the effects of androgens on target tissues may alter fertility. Circulating androgens may be decreased secondary to disturbances of the hypothalamic-pituitary-gonadal axis.

Estrogens inhibit gonadotropin activity.[85] Cyproterone acetate depresses the uptake of androgens, lowers plasma testosterone levels, decreases nuclear retention of dihydrotestosterone, and decreases the binding of dihydrotestosterone to cytosol receptors.[85, 86] Flutamide, a nonsteroidal antiandrogen, lacks hormonal activity.[85, 87] Flutamide inhibits the retention of dihydrotestosterone receptor complex by target cell nuclei, thereby interfering with the events mediated by the androgen receptor complex.

Cimetidine, a histamine (H_2) receptor antagonist, interferes with endocrine function and the binding of androgens to the androgen receptor. Cimetidine inhibits the response of luteinizing hormone to clomiphene and luteinizing hormone–releasing factor.[88] Despite the inhibitory effect on the hypothalamic-pituitary axis, basal testosterone levels are elevated in men following treatment with cimetidine.[88] Cimetidine also binds to cytoplasmic androgen receptors and blocks nuclear uptake of dihydrotestosterone.[89] The clinical significance of cimetidine as a cause of infertility remains unclear. The administration of cimetidine to a group of men was associated with a significant reduction in sperm concentration.[88]

Male reproductive function requires antegrade transport of semen through the urethra. The release of seminal fluid into the prostatic urethra (seminal emission) represents active discharge from the vas deferens, seminal vesicles, and prostatic ducts. Langley and Anderson demonstrated that electrical stimulation of the sympathetic lumbar outflow, contained within the hypogastric nerve, resulted in contraction of the vas deferens and the seminal vesicles.[90] The unidirectional transport of semen through the urethra (ejaculation) requires contraction of the periurethral striated muscles and closure of the bladder neck or proximal prostatic urethra. Cinefluoroscopic studies in the ram have shown that retrograde ejaculation does not occur following the separation of the bladder neck from the proximal prostatic urethra.[91] The preprostatic sphincter, under control of the autonomic nervous system, presumably prevents retrograde ejaculation. The seminal content is propelled antegrade by contraction of the striated periurethral musculature, which is under somatic control derived from the pudendal nerve.[92] Emission appears to be under sympathetic control and ejaculation under sympathetic and somatic control.

Neurohistochemical studies have identified a prominent adrenergic innervation of the vas deferens, seminal vesicle, and bladder neck.[93] Pharmacologic and biochemical studies have demonstrated that these structures are under α-adrenergic control.[14, 94] α-Adrenergic antagonists such as phenoxybenzamine would be expected to result in retrograde ejaculation and altered emission. Retrograde ejaculation and altered emission are not consistently associated with α-adrenergic blocking drugs. Guanethidine blocks the reuptake of norepinephrine at sympathetic postganglionic nerve endings, thereby depleting intraneuronal norepinephrine. Guanethidine is associated with retrograde ejaculation.

A comparative study of muscarinic cholinergic receptors in the rabbit's genitourinary tract by Lepor and Kuhar demonstrated that the density of muscarinic cholinergic receptor was twofold greater in the vas deferens compared to the bladder.[20] The functional role of muscarinic cholinergic receptors in the vas deferens is unknown.

Priapism

Priapism is a painful, persistent erection, unaccompanied by sexual pleasure. The corpora cavernosa are engorged and the corpus spongiosum is not turgid. The corpora cavernosa are drained by the deep dorsal vein and Santorini's plexus, whereas the venous outflow of the corpus spongiosum is provided by the superficial dorsal vein[95] The etiology of priapism appears to be the selective obstruction of the venous outflow of the corpora cavernosa.

The etiology of priapism is categorized according to primary (idiopathic) and secondary causes. Nelson and Winter[96] observed that sickle cell disease, leukemia, trauma, and solid tumors accounted for 28 of 48 patients treated for priapism. In the remaining 20 patients with presumed idiopathic priapism, three were therapeutically heparinized and four were on chronic phenothiazines.[96] In another recent review, four of 29 patients with priapism were on phenothiazines, whereas no patients were anticoagulated.[97]

Phenothiazines affect the autonomic nervous system by directly antagonizing cholinergic and adrenoceptor binding.[29] α-Adrenergic antagonists such as phenoxybenzamine produce erections when administered intraarterially to laboratory animals[26] and intracorporally to man.[27] An overdose of prazosin, a selective α-adrenergic antagonist, has been reported to cause priapism.[98] The α-adrenergic antagonist properties of phenothiazines most likely produce priapism. The selective effect of phenothiazines on the corpora cavernosa is perplexing.

ADVERSE REACTIONS OF DRUGS WITH UROLOGIC INDICATIONS

Nephrolithiasis

Thiazides.—Hypercalciuria may be resorptive, absorptive, or renal, depending on whether the principal derangement of calcium metabolism is excessive bone resorption, enhanced intestinal absorption, or impaired renal tubular reabsorption (renal leak) of calcium, respectively. Thiazides are indicated for the treatment of renal leak hypercalciuria, since the renal loss of calcium is diminished and normal parathyroid function is restored. Although thiazides do not alter intestinal absorption of calcium in individuals with primary absorptive hypercalciuria, thiazides may reduce stone formation in these patients.[99]

Rare cases of hypersensitivity reaction

secondary to thiazides have been described. Serum potassium should be carefully monitored since potassium loss may become clinically significant. Potassium is replaced with preparations of potassium chloride or potassium citrate. The toxicity of digoxin is dramatically enhanced in the presence of hypokalemia. Thiazides may produce hyperglycemia and may aggravate preexisting diabetes mellitus. Thiazide-induced hyperuricocemia is not associated with hyperuricosuria, and therefore individuals are not at greater risk for developing uric acid lithiasis. Thiazides may cause impotence by affecting vasomotor smooth muscle.[28] The side effects of thiazides when administered for prevention of renal calculi are, in order of frequency, weakness, increased thirst, lightheadedness, constipation, loss of libido, increased urination, arthralgia, and rash.[33]

Calcium Binders.—There is no available treatment regimen that corrects the basic abnormality leading to absorptive hypercalciuria. Nevertheless, several drugs may act to restore normal calcium excretion. Sodium cellulose phosphate (Calcibind), when given orally, acts as a nonabsorbable ion exchange resin which binds calcium and inhibits calcium absorption.[100] The mechanism of action accounting for the therapeutic action of sodium cellulose phosphate also accounts for the adverse reactions associated with its therapy. Sodium cellulose phosphate may cause a negative calcium balance and parathyroid stimulation when used in patients with normal intestinal calcium absorption. Sodium cellulose phosphate may also cause magnesium depletion by binding magnesium. Finally, sodium cellulose phosphate may produce secondary hyperoxaluria by binding divalent cations in the intestinal tract, reducing divalent cation-oxalate complexing, and making more oxalate available for absorption.[101] These drug actions may be overcome by using the drug sodium cellulose phosphate only in documented cases of absorptive hypercalciuria, administering oral magnesium supplementation, and imposing dietary restriction of oxalate.

Orthophosphates.—Orthophosphates (neutral or alkaline salts of sodium and/or potassium, 0.5 g phosphorus) have been shown to inhibit 1,25-(OH)2D synthesis.[101] There is convincing evidence that orthophosphates restore normal intestinal absorption of calcium. Orthophosphates presumably reduce urinary sodium by directly impairing the renal tubular reabsorption of calcium.[101] Since the administration of orthophosphates is associated with markedly elevated urinary phosphorus levels, the urinary saturation of calcium oxalate is decreased, whereas the urinary saturation of calcium phosphate (brushite) is increased.[102] The urinary inhibitor activity of orthophosphates is reduced owing to increased excretion of citrate with pyrophosphate. Finally, soft tissue calcification and parathyroid stimulation have recently been reported following orthophosphate administration.[103]

Citrate.—Citrate lowers the urinary saturation of calcium salts by forming soluble complexes with calcium, thereby inhibiting the crystallization of calcium salts.[101] A low urinary concentration of citrate prevents the nucleation and growth of calcium salts. Historically, alkali therapy has been the treatment of choice for patients with distal renal tubular acidosis. Alkali therapy may be administered either in the form of sodium bicarbonate or Shohl's solution (a combination of sodium citrate and citric acid).

Citrate is available as sodium citrate (Bicitra) or potassium citrate (Polycitra). Potassium citrate may be preferable in certain clinical situations when sodium restriction is important. In addition, a recent report suggests that sodium alkali may increase the risk of calcium stone formation.[104] Theoretically, urinary calcium excretion remains unchanged owing to the excess sodium load created by the use of sodium alkali. The use of potassium citrate is contraindicated in patients with renal impairment or severe myocardial damage.

Allopurinol.—Allopurinol is indicated for the management of hyperuricosuria associated with uric acid and calcium nephrolithiasis. Allopurinol is an inhibitor of xanthine oxidase, an enzyme required for the biosynthesis of uric acid from hypoxanthine. Alloxanthine, the metabolite of allopurinol, is also an inhibitor of xanthine oxidase.

Allopurinol may interfere with hepatic inactivation of phenylbutazone and oral anticoagulation agents by inhibiting microsomal cytochrome P-450.[105] Although limited clinical trials have not demonstrated changes in phenylbutazone levels or prothrombin times following warfarinization, coagulation parameters should be carefully monitored in patients when allopurinol is initiated.

The most common adverse effect of allopurinol is hypersensitivity reaction. The reaction may occur several months or years after initiating therapy. The cutaneous reaction is predominantly a pruritic, erythematous, or maculopapular eruption. Allopurinol may cause transient leukopenia, leukocytosis, and eosinophilia. Sporadic cases of hepatomegaly, peripheral neuritis, bone marrow depression, and cataracts have been reported. Undesirable side effects include headache, drowsiness, nausea, vomiting, vertigo, diarrhea, and gastric irritation.[52]

Penicillamine.—Penicillamine is a chelator of copper, mecury, lead, and zinc. Penicillamine in a dose of 30 mg/kg/day lowers urinary cystine and prevents further stone development in patients with cystinuria.[106] Penicillamine binds to cystine via a disulfide bond, the resulting complex being 50 times more soluble in urine than cystine.

The major toxicity of penicillamine is limited to the *l* and *dl* isomers. The toxic effects resemble pyridoxine deficiency and are managed by administration of pyridoxine.[107] Acute hypersensitivity reactions are manifested by fever, rashes, leukopenia, eosinophilia, and thrombocytopenia. Anorexia, vomiting, and the loss of taste for salt and sweet rarely occur. Nephrotoxicity from the *d* isomer of penicillamine results presumably from a hypersensitivity reaction. Penicillamine-linked nephrotic syndrome regressed following cessation of the drug. Individuals who are allergic to penicillin may have a similar reaction to penicillamine.[107]

Hemiacidrin.—Hemiacidrin (10%) contains several multivalent organic acids buffered to a pH of 4.7 and magnesium ions at a concentration of approximately 0.6M. Hemiacidrin irrigation may dissolve struvite and apatite calculi.[108] The drug was withdrawn by the Food and Drug Administration (FDA) for the dissolution of calculi in the renal pelvis following four reported deaths.[109–111] In retrospect, all four patients showed evidence of sepsis prior to death, and cessation of treatment and appropriate antibiotic management likely would have prevented these deaths.

Sterilization of the urine, a maximum irrigation rate of 120 mL/hr, and cessation of irrigation in the presence of flank pain and fever resulted in no major complications in 35 consecutive patients undergoing hemiacidrin irrigation.[108] Magnesium levels should be monitored owing to the potential toxic effects of systemic absorption.

Antibiotics

Sulfonamides.—The sulfonamides were the first agents employed systematically for the prevention and cure of bacterial infections. The overall incidence of adverse reactions to sulfonamides is about 5%. The etiology of acute hemolytic anemia is either a hypersensitivity reaction or a manifestation of glucose-6-phosphate dehydrogenase (G6PD) deficiency. Hemolysis may be associated with nausea, fever, vertigo, jaundice, pallor, hepatosplenomegaly, and shock. There is a marked decrease in erythrocyte levels, and leukocytosis, reticulocytosis, bilirubinemia, and hemoglobin casts commonly occur.[112]

Agranulocytosis, aplastic anemia, and thrombocytopenia have been related to sulfonamides. Nephrotoxicity rarely occurs and may be secondary to hypersensitivity reactions or the formation and deposition of crystalline aggregates. Hypersensitivity reactions frequently present with skin or mucous membrane manifestations. Morbilliform, scarlatiniform, urticarial, erysipeloid, pemphigoid, purpuric, and petechial rashes represent sensitization reactions. Erythema nodosum, erythema multiforme, Behçet's syndrome, exfoliative dermatitis, and photosensitivity may also occur. A serum sickness syndrome may appear several days after sulfonamide exposure. Hepatitis occurs in less than 0.1% of patients. Anorexia, nausea, and vomiting occurs in 1% to 2% of persons receiving sulfonamides. Goiter, hypothyroidism, peripheral neuritis, arthritis, and neuropsychiatric disturbances are other rare untoward side effects.[112]

Trimethoprim-Sulfamethoxazole.—Trimethoprim and sulfamethoxazole act on sequential steps in an obligate enzymatic bacterial reaction. The complications of this drug combination are primarily secondary to the complications associated with sulfamethoxazole.

Ampicillin.—Ampicillin is a semisynthetic compound derived from 6-amino penicillanic acid. The incidence of hypersensitivity reactions to the penicillins ranges between 0.7% and 10%.[113] Hypersensitivity reactions manifest as skin rashes of all degrees of severity, oral lesions, fever, and interstitial nephritis. Skin rashes occur in approximately 9% of patients receiving ampicillin. The most serious hypersensitivity reactions produced by the penicillins are angioedema, serum sickness, anaphylaxis, and the Arthus phenomenon. The incidence of anaphylactic reaction is between 0.015% and 0.04%, and 0.002% of patients receiving penicillins die from anaphylactic reactions.[113] Agranulocytosis with peripheral monocytosis and bone marrow histiocytosis has been observed.

Cephalosporins.—The most common adverse reactions to the cephalosporins are rash, drug fever, and the development of a positive Coombs' test. Approximately 5% of patients with known penicillin hypersensitivity develop clinically evident allergic reactions to cephalosporins. A history of an allergic reaction to penicillin is not a contraindication for the use of cephalosporins.[114] The rare case of renal toxicity from cephalothin (Keflin) represents an allergic reaction that pathologically resembles interstitial nephritis. Cephaloridine in high doses may cause acute tubular necrosis. Intravenous injections of cephalosporins are frequently associated with phlebitis owing to local irritation.

Carbenicillin.—Carbenicillin is a penicillinase-susceptible derivative of 6-amino penicillanic acid that is effective against pseudomonads and other gram-negative organisms that are characteristically resistant to penicillin. Hypersensitivity reactions such as anaphylaxis are exceedingly rare.[115] The parenteral form of carbenicillin is administered as a disodium salt and contains 4.7 mg of sodium per gram of drug. The recommended daily dose of carbenicillin for serious infections may exceed 30 g. This substantial sodium load (120 mEq/day) may exacerbate symptoms of congestive heart failure. The large amount of nonreabsorbable anion delivered to the distal tubule may cause hypokalemia.[115]

Carbenicillin alters platelet aggregation in a dose-related phenomenon by binding to ADP.[116] Neutropenia has been reported in patients receiving carbenicillin. Pseudomembranous colitis due to *Clostridia difficile* has been described. Hepatic toxicity manifested by the elevation of liver function enzymes has been reported. Carbenicillin may inactivate aminoglycoside activity at high doses.[117]

Aminoglycosides.—Untoward effects of aminoglycosides include nausea, vomiting, headache, transient proteinuria, and elevation of liver function enzymes. Allergic reactions such as eosinophilia, rash, and fever have been reported in 1% to 3% of patients.

Ototoxicity is a serious side effect and occurs in 2% of patients. Ototoxicity is potentiated by ethacrynic acid, furosemide, mannitol, and other diuretics. Vestibular function is more susceptible to toxicity than auditory function. Vestibular and ocular function testing should be performed at frequent intervals.

The frequency of aminoglycoside nephrotoxicity varies from 2% to 10%.[118] Elderly, debilitated individuals and patients with preexisting renal disease and depleted intravascular volumes are at greater risk for nephrotoxicity. There is reasonable evidence that long duration of therapy and high doses are risk factors for nephrotoxicity.[119] The nephrotoxicity usually becomes clinically evident within 5 to 7 days and manifests as mild proteinuria, granular cylindruria, and declining renal function. Aminoglycosides cause proximal tubular dysfunction. The presence and resolution of urinary cast excretion is the best method for detecting and following the progression and resolution of proximal tubular injury.

Nitrofurantoin.—Nitrofurantoin is urinary tract–specific since the drug is rapidly cleared by the kidneys and effective plasma levels are not achieved. Nausea, vomiting, and diarrhea are the more common untoward effects, and these effects are diminished by dose reduction and administration of the drug with milk or food. These gastrointestinal side effects are less common with macrocrystalline preparations. Hypersensitivity reactions occasionally occur and are manifested by rash, urticaria, angioneurotic edema, fever, pneumonitis, cholestatic jaundice, and arthralgia. Hemolytic anemia occurs in association with G6PD deficiency.

Allergic pneumonitis has been observed and usually resolves within hours of discontinuing the drug. Interstitial pulmonary fibrosis can occur in patients on chronic suppression. Vertigo, drowsiness, and nystagmus may occur, and these symptoms are readily reversible when the drug is discontinued. Severe polyneuropathies presenting with ascending sensorimotor defects, such as paresthesias, may be progressive. The polyneuropathy is more common in patients with renal failure, the elderly, and patients receiving prolonged drug courses. Nitrofurantoin has been associated with decreased sperm counts in men receiving doses of 10 mg/kg/day.[73]

Tetracyclines.—Nausea, vomiting, and abdominal pain are commonly associated with oral tetracyclines. Irritative diarrhea and candidal overgrowth occur more commonly with conventional tetracyclines than with minocycline and doxycycline, since tetracycline is poorly absorbed.

Fatty infiltration of the liver is associated with parenteral tetracycline administered in doses exceeding 2 mg/day.

All of the tetracycline preparations, with the exception of doxycycline, are contraindicated in patients with renal failure. Doxycycline is inactivated by a complex process of backdiffusion in the large intestine and therefore its dose is not adjusted for renal failure.

Tetracyclines may induce nephrogenic diabetes insipidus in a dose-dependent reversible fashion.[120] Phototoxicity may occur with tetracycline and minocycline. Tetracyclines should be avoided in pregnancy and in children younger than age 8 years, since they discolor deciduous teeth. Tetracyclines may also temporarily inhibit bone growth.

Vestibular toxic reaction is unique to minocycline. The lipid-laden cells of the vestibular apparatus concentrate the drug, producing vertigo. Reversible nausea and vertigo may occur in up to 90% of patients receiving minocycline.[121]

Quinolones.—Norfloxacin and ciprofloxacin are members of the quinolone carboxylic acid group of compounds which have become widely used oral antibiotic agents. The concentration of these agents in the urine exceeds the minimal inhibitory concentrations of all common urinary pathogens several times.[122] The low protein binding, high lipid solubility, and zwitterion nature favor entrapment of these antibiotics in the human prostatic tissue.[123] Norfloxacin and ciprofloxacin are active agents against *Pseudomonas aeruginosa* and many other gram-negative rods including *Escherichia coli, Klebsiella* species, *Enterobacter* species, and *Proteus*. These agents have poor activity against anaerobic strains and somewhat lowered activity against gram-positive organisms, though enterococcus and some staphlococcal strains are highly sensitive.

The most common adverse effects of these drugs are related to the gastrointestinal and central nervous (CNS) systems.[124] The gastrointestinal toxicity is manifestated primarily by nausea, vomiting, and diarrhea. The CNS toxicity is manifested primarily by dizziness, headache, tremors, and restlessness.

The quinolones alter theophylline metabolism thereby prolonging and raising plasma theophylline concentrations.[125] The early signs of theophylline overdose such as nausea and vomiting may easily be overlooked or attributed to the side effects of the antibiotic. The plasma theophylline concentrations should be monitored when these antibiotics are coadministered with theophylline.

Crystalluria has also been associated with the administration of these agents.[126, 127] Crystalluria appears to be related to dose (>1000 mg ciprofloxacin and >1200 mg norfloxacin), pH (>7.3), and the time of urinary collection (shortly after administration). Increasing fluid intake has a negligible impact on this phenomenon.[128] Avoidance of foods and other conditions that produce an alkaline urine has been suggested.

Finally, the inhibition of growth in the limb buds of experimental animals represents the basis for the warning against use of these agents in children whose skeletal growth is incomplete.[129, 130]

Neurogenic Bladder

Propantheline Bromide.—The muscarinic cholinergic receptors are ubiquitous. The side effects of muscarinic cholinergic agonists and antagonists reflect the lack of tissue selectivity of these agents. Therapeutic doses of muscarinic cholinergic antagonists are associated with accelerated heart rates, mydriasis, impaired visual accomodation, decreased salivary and gastric secretion, inhibition of gastric and bladder contractions, and impaired sweating.[131]

Synthetic muscarinic cholinergic antagonists with appreciable tissue selectivity have not been developed. Propantheline bromide, a commonly used anticholinergic agent for the treatment of detrusor instability, is a quaternary ammonium substitute for atropine. Central side effects of propantheline bromide are less common than those of atropine, owing to the inability of propantheline bromide to cross the blood-brain barrier. The side effects of the various synthetic anticholinergic drugs reflect relative antimuscarinic and ganglionic blocking properties. Propantheline bromide has substantially less ganglionic blocking properties compared to other quaternary ammonium analogues. Impotence is therefore rarely associated with propantheline bromide.

Bethanechol Bromide.—Bethanechol bromide is a very selective muscarinic cholinergic agonist that virtually lacks ganglionic and nicotinic properties. The usual cholinergic effects of vasodilation, decreased heart rate, and decreased contractility of the heart are not observed with bethanechol bromide at the usual clinical doses. Bethanechol bromide is relatively selective for increasing contractions of the smooth muscle of the urinary bladder and gastrointestinal tract.[132] The gastrointestinal toxicity of bethanechol bromide includes nausea, belching, and vomiting. Impaired visual accomodation, headache, and salivation may accompany bethanechol bromide administration.[132]

The major contraindications to the use of cholinergic agonists are asthma, hyperthyroidism, coronary insufficiency, and peptic ulcer disease.

Imipramine.—The common side effects of imipramine reflect the prominent anticholinergic properties, which include dry mouth, constipation, dizziness, tachycardia, palpitations, blurred vision, and urinary retention. Weakness and fatigue are attributed to central effects. Headaches, muscle tremors, and epigastric distress are not uncommon side effects.

The tricyclic antidepressants compete with norepinephrine reuptake at postganglionic nerve terminals. Cardiac abnormalities, including arrhythmias and electrocardiographic changes, occur most commonly in older patients with underlying cardiac disease. The overall effect of antidepressants on adrenergic activity is not clear, since interference with the reuptake mechanism may result in depletion of norepinephrine in the storage granules while increasing levels of circulating norepinephrine.[133]

Hallucinations and delusions may occur. A persistent fine tremor occurs in 10% of patients. High doses of imipramine may produce grand mal seizures and a mild parkinsonian syndrome.

Imipramine has been associated with an allergic type of obstructive jaundice. Skin rashes, photosensitivity, eosinophilia, and agranulocytosis are hypersensitivity reactions reported with imipramine.[29]

Phenoxybenzamine.—Phenoxybenzamine antagonizes the responses mediated by α-adrenoceptors. Postural hypotension and reflex tachycardia occur because of loss of vasomotor control. These vasomotor effects are more profound in association with hypovolemia. Miosis and impaired ejaculation have been associated with phenoxybenzamine.

Impotence

Major advances in the understanding of the physiology of penile erection and the pathophysiology of impotence have led to innovative approaches for the treatment of impotence. The injection of vasoactive drugs into the corpus cavernosum of experimental animals mimics the action of endogenous neurotransmitters and induces erections. This observation has led to the use of vasoactive intracavernous pharmacotherapy for the treatment of impotence.

There are several drugs which, when administered directly into the corpus cavernosum, induce hemodynamic changes in man similar to those occurring during normal erection. Currently, papavarine hydrochloride alone or in combination with phentolamine mesylate is the most commonly used agent for vasoactive intracavernous therapy.

Papavarine Hydrochloride.—Papavarine hydrochloride is the salt of a benzylisoquinoline alkaloid.[134] Papavarine hydrochloride is a potent, nonspecific smooth muscle relaxant that directly alters muscle tone regardless of its innervation. Mechanisms of action include an inhibition of oxidative phosphorylation with blocking of cyclic adenosine monophosphate phosphodiesterase and interference with calcium flow during muscle contraction.[135]

The primary complications secondary to intracavernous injection therapy include priapism, hematoma, cavernositis, inadvertent injection of the urethra, paresthesia, corporal fibrosis, swelling, and penile deviation.[134]

The most serious local complications of vasoactive intracavernous therapy are sustained erections and localized induration at the injection site. Sustained erections usually occur during the dose-determining period and are most common in those patients with neurogenic impotence. Early intervention is mandatory because tissue damage from ischemia may occur in as little as 4 hours.

Local nontender induration at the injection site occurs presumably secondary to the repeated trauma from needle insertion, faulty injection technique, reaction to the pharmacologic agent, organized hematoma, or ischemia. Extensive scarring may interfere with the quality of the erection and with subsequent attempts to implant a penile prosthesis.[136]

The most significant short-term complication following the use of papavarine is prolonged erection, which may develop into priapism.

Peyronie's disease secondary to cavernosal fibrosis may be the limiting factor of papavarine use since the acidic pH of this agent will cause tissue sclerosis.[137]

Systemic complications associated with the use of papavarine include vasovagal reactions manifested by bradycardia, hypotension, dizziness, and facial flushing.[138] These vasovagal reactions can be easily treated with atropine. Finally, several cases of reversible liver toxicity have been reported following papavarine use.[137, 139, 140]

Phentolamine Mesylate.—Phentolamine induces smooth muscle relaxation by blocking the α-adrenoceptors on cell membranes. Phentolamine mesylate has a minimal effect on the venous outflow from the corpora cavernosa; however, it potentiates the action of papavarine.[141] The coadministration of phentolamine and papavarine allows for a smaller dose of papavarine to be administered, thereby reducing the incidence of priapism and possibly the corporal fibrosis associated with papavarine. Although side effects secondary to phentolamine injection are rare, it is a potent α-blocking agent and systemic absorption may create a hypotensive episode.

Phenoxybenzamine.—Phenoxybenzamine, like phentolamine, is an α-adrenergic antagonist. Phenoxybenzamine was the initial agent used for intracavernosal injection.[142] The use of phenoxybenzamine was tempered somewhat by reports of mutagenic activity in mice.[143]

Prostaglandin E_1.—Prostaglandin E_1 is another agent that has recently been shown to be effective as an injectable vasoactive preparation.[144] Prostaglandin E_1 is a natural constituent of many mammalian tissues. Prostaglandin E_1 is found in high concentrations within human seminal vesicles and seminal plasma.[145] Intracavernous injection of prostaglandin E_1 appears to relax the cavernous and arteriolar smooth muscles.

Waldhauser and Schramek recently reported their experience with intracavernous injections of prostaglandin E_1.[146] Prostaglandin E_1 was associated with a much lower incidence of systemic reactions and priapism compared to papavarine, presumably owing to the rapid metabolism of prostaglandin E_1. Sustained erections of greater than 10 hours have been reported with the use of prostaglandin E_1.[146] Fibrosis of the cavernosa was reduced since the pH of the prostaglandin solution is more physiologic. However, it remains uncertain whether fibrosis and angulation are attributed to the properties of the drug or the repeated trauma of injection with organized hematoma formation. Approximately 75% of patients experience a burning pain with prostaglandin injection.

Benign Prostatic Hyperplasia (BPH)

Phenoxybenzamine.—Caine and associates observed in 1975 that the human prostate adenoma contracted in the presence of norepinephrine, an α-adrenergic agonist.[147] The contractile response to norepinephrine was abolished by pretreatment with phenoxybenzamine, a nonselective α-adrenergic antagonist. Several clinical trials subsequently demonstrated the efficacy of phenoxybenzamine for the treatment of symptomatic BPH.[148–151] The toxicity of phenoxybenzamine has limited its widespread use for the treatment of prostatism secondary to BPH. Caine et al. reported a double blind placebo-controlled study of phenoxybenzamine for the symptomatic treatment of benign prostatic obstruction.[149] Fifty patients suffering from BPH were randomized to receive either phenoxybenzamine 10 mg or an identical-looking placebo for 14 days. Statistically significant evidence of an improvement in both peak and mean flow rates was observed. Side effects were reported in 11 of the 25 patients receiving phenoxybenzamine. The side effects associated with phenoxybenzamine generally consisted of tiredness or slight dizziness. Two patients reported impaired ejaculation, two, nasal stuffiness or dryness; and one, difficulty with visual accomodation. The medication was not discontinued in any of these patients; however the clinical trial was only 2 weeks in duration. Boreham et al. reported their experience with phenoxybenzamine for the treatment of symptomatic BPH.[148] Side effects were observed in 19 of the 30 patients. Three patients withdrew from the study owing to the adverse reactions to the drug.

Prazosin.—The contractile properties of the human prostate adenoma are mediated primarily by the α_1-adrenoceptor.[152, 153] Prazosin (Minipress) is a selective α_1-adrenergic antagonist presently marketed for the treatment of hypertension. Several clinical trials have documented the efficacy of prazosin for the treatment of symptomatic BPH.[154–156] Prazosin is far better tolerated than phenoxybenzamine when used for the treatment of symptomatic BPH. Kirby et al. recently reported a double blind parallel study of prazosin versus placebo in 80 patients with BPH.[156] Mean maximum flow rates increased significantly more in patients treated with prazosin than in those treated with placebo. The incidence of side effects was low and differed little between prazosin and placebo. It was concluded that prazosin is a safe and effective drug in the treatment of prostatic outflow obstruction.

Terazosin.—Terazosin (Hytrin) is a long-acting selective α_1-adrenergic antagonist which recently was approved by the FDA for the treatment of hypertension.[157]

Dunzendorfer recently reported a preliminary clinical experience of terazosin for the treatment of symptomatic BPH.[158] The daily dose of terazosin was increased sequentially (2 mg, 5 mg, 10 mg) until there was evidence of a therapeutic response to treatment or until a maximum daily dosage of 10 mg terazosin was reached. A total of 15 men participated in this preliminary clinical trial. Terazosin was associated with a significant improvement in peak and mean urinary flow rates, and improvement in obstructive symptoms. A single episode of mild headache, dizziness, asthenia, and dysuria were reported.

We have administered terazosin to over 40 normotensive men with symptomatic BPH. Our preliminary experience with this pharmacologic approach for the treatment of BPH has been very satisfactory. Orthostatic hypotension was observed in only one patient. Mild tiredness has been observed sporadically. A single patient developed a macular rash and alopecia requiring discontinuing the medication. It is premature to make meaningful conclusions regarding the long-term efficacy of terazosin. The majority of men with symptomatic BPH in our experience have elected to continue on terazosin therapy since it was generally well tolerated and clinically effective.

Miscellaneous Drugs

Lidocaine.—Local anesthetics prevent the generation and conduction of nerve impulses. Lidocaine is one of the most widely used local anesthetics, since its effects are prompt, long-lasting, and intense. Hypersensitivity reactions are infrequently associated with locally administered lidocaine. Hypersensitivity reactions manifest as allergic dermatitis, asthmatic attacks, and fatal anaphylaxis.[159]

Systemic toxicity of locally administered anesthetics are determined by the absorption and degradation of these agents. Lidocaine is degraded by the liver, and therefore hepatic insufficiency may enhance its toxicity.[160] Absorption of lidocaine is reduced by coinjection of vasoconstricting agents such as epinephrine. The absorption of these vasoconstrictor agents may cause untoward reactions, such as restlessness, increased heart rate, palpatation, and chest pain. The coinjection of vasoconstrictor agents should be avoided in individuals with coronary artery disease.

Toxic levels of lidocaine may cause seizures, which are best managed by diazepam. Systemic absorption may decrease the electrical excitability of the myocardium, decrease the conduction rate, and decrease the force of contraction of the heart. The administration of small quantities of lidocaine has resulted in cardiovascular collapse. The mechanism for the sudden death is unknown and may simply reflect inadvertent injection of lidocaine parenterally.

The maximal safe topical use of lidocaine (5 to 7 mg/kg) in a healthy 70-kg adult is 500 mg (100 mL of a 0.5% solution).

Opioid Analgesics.—Morphine and related opioids produce their major effects on the CNS and the bowel. The primary effects of the opioids include analgesia, drowsiness, changes in mood, respiratory depression, decreased gastrointestinal motility, nausea, vomiting, and alterations of the endocrine and autonomic nervous systems.

Morphine directly depresses respiratory activity via its actions on the brainstem. Direct stimulation of the chemoreceptor trigger zone by morphine produces emesis. The emetic effect of morphine is countered by phenothiazines. Nausea and vomiting are relatively uncommon in recumbent patients, which suggests that the opioids produce increased vestibular sensitivity.

Morphine and related agonists dilate resistance and capacitance vessels, thereby decreasing the ability of the cardiovascular system to respond to gravitational fields, resulting in orthostatic hypotension.[161]

The opioids dramatically increase the tone of the antrum of the stomach, resulting in decreased motility. In the small and large intestine, propulsive contractions are markedly decreased. The tone of the bladder muscle is augmented by morphine, occasionally resulting in urinary urgency. The tone of the bladder neck is increased, promoting urinary retention.

The above-mentioned undesirable effects of the opioids occur with such frequency that they cannot be considered idiosyncratic. Allergic phenomena occur infrequently with opioids. Skin rashes and anyphylactoid reactions are rare.

The depressant effects of opioids may be exaggerated and prolonged by phenothiazines, monoamine oxidase inhibitors, and trycyclic antidepressants. These effects must be recognized especially in patients with decreased respiratory reserve.

Benzodiazepines.—The primary effects of benzodiazepines result from actions on the CNS. In man, the most prominent effects are sedation, hypnosis, decreased anxiety, muscle relaxation, and anticonvulsant activities.

Hypnotic doses of benzodiazepines cause varying degrees of lightheadedness, lassitude, increased reaction time, motor incoordination, ataxia, impairment of mental and psychomotor functions, disorganization of thought, confusion, dysarthria, retrograde amnesia, dry mouth, and a bitter taste. Interaction with ethanol may be especially serious.

Relatively uncommon side effects of benzodiazepines are weakness, headache, blurred vision, vertigo, nausea and vomiting, epigastric distress and diarrhea, joint pains, chest pains, and incontinence.

CONCLUSION

A complete drug history is a mandatory aspect of the urologic workup of urinary retention, impotence, infertility, hematuria, and priapism. This pertinent information may obviate the need for expensive and invasive diagnostic evaluations and unnecessary surgical intervention.

The maximum efficacy of drugs is achieved when the physician is aware of the precise indications and untoward side effects of the drugs prescribed. It is the responsibility of physicians to know both the common and subtle untoward reactions of the drugs they prescribe. This chapter serves a reference for the untoward reactions of drugs with urologic indications.

REFERENCES

1. Melman KL: Preventable drug reactions—causes and cures. *N Engl J Med* 1971;284:1361.
2. Markowitz JS, Pearson G., Kay BG, et al: Nurses, physicians and pharmacist: Their knowledge of hazards of medications. *Nurs Res* 1981;30:366.
3. United States Department of Health, Education and Welfare, Task Force on Prescription Drugs: *Final Report.* Washington, DC, Government Printing Office, 1969.
4. Jick H: Drugs—remarkably nontoxic. *N Engl J Med* 1974;291:824.
5. Boston Collaborative Drug Surveillance Program: Hospital admissions due to adverse drug reactions. *Arch Intern Med* 1974;134:219.
6. Ogilvie RI, Ruedy J: Adverse drug reac-

tions during hospitalization. *Can Med Assoc J* 1967;97:1450.

7. Ahlquist RP: A study of the adrenotropic receptor. *Am J Physiol* 1948:153:586.
8. El-Badawi P, Schwenk EA: A new theory of the innervation of bladder musculature. *J Urol* 1974;111:613.
9. Khanna OP, Barbieri EJ, McMichael RF: The effects of adrenergic agonists on vesicourethral smooth muscle of rabbits (abstract 275). Abstracts of the American Urological Association, 75th Annual Meeting, San Francisco, 1980, p 155.
10. Raezer DM, Wein, AJ, Jacobowitz D: Autonomic innervation of canine urinary bladder: Cholinergic and adrenergic interaction of sympathetic and parasympathetic nervous systems in bladder function. *Urology* 1983;2:211.
11. Awad S, Bruce AW, Carro-Ciampi G, et al: Distribution of alpha and beta adrenoreceptors in human urinary bladder. *Br J Pharmacol* 1974;50:525.
12. Levin RM, Shofer FS, Wein AJ: Cholinergic, adrenergic, and purinergic response of sequential strips of rabbit urinary bladder. *J Pharmacol Exp Ther* 1980;212:536.
13. Khanna OP, Heber D, Gonick P: Cholinergic and adrenergic neuroreceptors in urinary tract of female dogs. *Urology* 1975;5:616.
14. Caine M, Raz S, Zeigler M: Adrenergic and cholinergic receptors in the human prostate, prostatic capsule and bladder neck. *Br J Urol* 1975;47:193.
15. Lepor H, Shapiro E: Characterization of the $alpha_1$ adrenergic receptors in human benign prostatic hyperplasia. *J Urol* 1984;132:1226.
16. Lue TF, Zeineh SJ, Schmidt RA, et al: Physiology of penile erections. *World J Urol* 1983;1:194.
17. Dorr LD, Brady MJ: Hemodynamic mechanism of erection in the canine penis. *Am J Physiol* 1967;213:1526.
18. Semans JH, Langworthy OR: Observations on the neurophysiology of sexual function in the male cat. *J Urol* 1938;40:836.
19. Nikolsky W: Ein Beitrag zur Physiologie der Nervi erigentes. *Arch Anat Physiol (Leipzig)* 1879; 209.
20. Lepor H, Kuhar MJ: Characterization of muscarinic cholinergic receptor binding in the vas deferens, bladder, prostate, and penis of the rabbit. *J Urol* 1984;132:392.
21. Domer FR, Wessler G, Brown RL, et al: Involvement of the sympathetic nervous system in the urinary bladder internal sphincter and in penile erection in the anesthetized cat. *Invest Urol* 1978;15:404.
22. Penttila O: Acetylcholine, biogenic amines and enzymes involved in their metabolism in penile erectile tissue. *Ann Med Exp Biol Fenn* 1966;44:9.
23. Benson GS, McConnell J, Lipshutz LI: Neuromorphology and neuropharmacology of the human penis: An in vitro study. *J Clin Invest* 1980;65:506.
24. McConnell J., Benson GS, Wood J: Autonomic innervation of the mammalean penis: A histochemical and physiological study. *J Neurol Transm* 1979;45:227.
25. Klinge E, Sjostrand NO: Comparative study of some isolated mammalian smooth muscle effectors of penile erection. *Acta Physiol Scand* 1977;100:354.
26. Krane RJ, Siroky MB: Neurophysiology of erection. *Urol Clin North Am* 1981;8:91.
27. Brindley GS: Cavernosal alpha-blockade: A new technique for investigating and treating erectile impotence. *Br J Psychiatry* 1983;143:322.
28. Vliet LW, Meyer JK: Erectile dysfunction: Progress in evaluation and treatment *Johns Hopkins Med J* 1982;151:246.
29. Byck R: Drugs and the treatment of psychiatric disorders, in Goodman LS, Gilman A (eds): *The Pharmacological Basis of Therapeutics*. New York, Macmillan Publishing Co, 1975, pp 469–476.
30. Goldstein J, Krane RJ: Drug-induced sexual dysfunction. *World J Urol* 1983;1:239.
31. Soyka LF, Mattison DR: Prescription drugs that affect male sexual function. *Drug Ther* 1981;46–58.
32. Rose LI, Underwood RH, Newmark SR, et al: Pathophysiology of spironolactone-induced gynecomastia. *Ann Intern Med* 1977;87:398.
33. Yendt ER, Guay GF, Garcia DA: The use of thiazides in the prevention of renal calculi. *Can Med Assoc J* 1970;102:614.
34. Johnson P, Kitchin AH, Lowter CP, et al:

Treatment of hypertension with methyldopa. *Br Med J* 1966;1:133.
35. Mewman RJ, Salerno HR: Sexual dysfunction due to methyldopa. *Br Med J* 1974;4:106.
36. Onesti G, Martniez EW, Fernandes M: Alpha-methyldopa and clonidine: Antihypertensive agents with action on the central nervous system, in Onesti G, Lowenthal TD (eds): *The Spectrum of Antihypertensive Drug Therapy*. New York, Biomedical Information Corp, 1976, p 61.
37. Shapiro E, Tsitlick JE: $Alpha_2$ adrenergic receptors in canine prostate: Biochemical and functional correlations. *J Urol* (submitted for publication).
38. Shapiro E, Lepor H: $Alpha_2$ adrenergic receptors in hyperplastic human prostate: Identification and characterization using [^{3}H] Rauwoscine. J Urol (in press).
39. Veterans Administration Cooperative Study Group on Antihypertensive Agents: Propranolol in the treatment of essential hypertension. *JAMA* 1977;237:2302.
40. Papadopoulos C: Cardiovascular drugs and sexuality. *Arch Intern Med* 1980;140:1341.
41. Ambrosioni E, Costa FU, Montebugnoli L, et al: Comparison of antihypertensive efficay of atenolol, oxprenolol and pindolol at rest and during exercise. *Drugs* 1983;25 (suppl):30.
42. Greminger P, Vetter HH, Boerlin HJ, et al: A comparative study between 100 mg atenolol and 20 mg pindolol slow release in essential hypertension. *Drugs* 1983;25(suppl):36.
43. Heel RC, Brodgen RM, Speight TM, et al: Atenolol: a review of its pharmacological properties and therapeutic efficacy in angina pectoris and hypertension. *Drugs* 1979;17:425.
44. *Physicians Desk Reference*. 1988.
45. Abramowicz M (ed): Drugs that cause sexual dysfunction. *Med Lett Drugs Ther* 1987;29:65.
46. Aoki K, Sato K, Kawguchi Y: Increased vascular responses to norepinephrine and calcium antagonists in essential hypertension compared with normotension in humans. *J Cardiovasc Pharmacol* 1985;7(suppl):182.
47. Laragh JH: Calcium antagonists in hypertension—focus on verapamil. A symposium. *Am J Cardiol* 1986;57:1D.
48. Fogelman J: Verapamil caused depression, confusion and impotence (letter). Amer J Psychiatry 1988;145:P380.
49. Fogelman J: Verapamil may cause depression, confusion and impotence (letter). *Texas Med* 1987;83:8.
50. Weinberger MH: Angiotensin-converting enzyme inhibitors. *Med Clin North Am* 1987:71:983.
51. Shader RI, Elkin R: The effects of antianxiety and antipsychotic drugs on sexual behavior. *Med Probl Pharmacopsychiatry* 1980;15:19.
52. Woodbury DM, Fingl E: Analgesic-antipyretics, anti-inflammatory agents, and drugs employed in the treatment of gout, in Goodman LS, Gilman A (eds): *The Pharmacologic Basis of Therapeutics*. New York, Macmillan Publishing Co, 1975, pp 325–358.
53. Packham MA, Warrior ES, Glynn MF, et al: Alteration of the platelets to surface stimuli by pyrazole compounds. *J Exp Med* 1967;126:171.
54. Evans G, Packham MA, Nishizawa A, et al: The effect of acetylsalicylic acid on platelet function. *J Exp Med* 1968;128:877.
55. Zucker MB, Peterson J: Inhibition of adenosine diphosphate–induced secondary aggregation and other platelet function by acetylsalicylic acid. *Proc Soc Exp Biol Med* 1967;127:547.
56. O'Brien JR: Effect of anti-inflammatory agents on platelets. *Lancet* 1968;1:894.
57. Flower RJ: Drugs which inhibit prostaglandin biosynthesis. *Pharmacol Rev* 1974;26:33.
58. Hamberg M, Swensson J, Samuelsson B: Thromboxanes: A new group of biologically active compounds derived from prostaglandin endoperoxides. *Proc Natl Acad Sci USA* 1975;72:2994.
59. Roth GJ, Stanford N, Majerus PW: Acetylation of prostaglandin synthetase by aspirin. *Proc Natl Acad Sci USA* 1975;72:3073.
60. Vane JR: The mode of action of aspirin-like drugs. *Agents Actions* 1978;8:439.
61. Kraus SE, Siroky MB, Babayan RK, et al: Hematuria and the use of nonsteroidal

anti-inflammatory drugs. *J Urol* 1984;132:228.

62. Antolak SJ, Mellinger GT: Urologic evaluation of hematuria occurring during anticoagulation therapy. *J Urol* 1969;101:111.
63. Sherins RM, Brightwell D, Sternthal PM: Longitudinal analysis of semen of fertile and infertile men, in Troen P, Nankin H (eds): *New Concepts of the Testis in Normal and Infertile Men: Morphology, Physiology,* and *Pathology.* New York, Raven Press, 1977, pp 473–488.
64. daCunha MF, Mesitrich ML, Ried HL: Spermatogenesis following cancer chemotherapy with doxorubicin (Adriamycin). Presented at the Annual American Society of Andrology, New Orleans, March 14, 1981.
65. Sanger WG, Armitage JO, Schmidt MA: Feasibility of semen cryopreservation in patients with malignant disease. *JAMA* 1980;244:789.
66. Richter P, Calamera JC, Morgenfeld MC, et al: Effect of chlorambucil on spermatogenesis in the human with malignant lymphoma. *Cancer* 1970;25:1026.
67. Qureshi MSA, Goldsmith HJ, Pennington JH, et al: Cyclophosphamide therapy and sterility. *Lancet* 1972;2.
68. Buchanan JH, Fairley KF, Barrie JU: Return of spermatogenesis after stopping cyclophosphamide therapy. *Lancet* 1975;2:156.
69. Jackson H, Partlington M, Fox BW: Effect of busulfan (Myleran) on the spermatogenic population of the rat testis. *Nature* 1962;194:1184.
70. Bock M, Jackson H: The action of triethylinemelamine on the fertility of male rats. *Br J Pharmacol* 1957;12:1.
71. Timmermans L: Influence of antibiotics on spermatogenesis. *J Urol* 1974;112:348.
72. Nelson WO, Steinberger E: Effects of nitrofuran compounds on the testis of the rat. *Fed Proc* 1953;12:103.
73. Nelson WO, Bunge RG: The effect of therapeutic dosages of nitrofurantoin (Furadantin) upon spermatogenesis in man. *J Urol* 1957;77:275.
74. Prior J, Ferguson J: Cytotoxic effects of a nitrofuran on the rat testis. *Cancer* 1950;3:62.
75. Merlin HE: Azoospermia caused by colchicine: A case report. *Fertil Steril* 1972;23:180.
76. Bremner MJ, Paulsen CA: Colchicine and testicular function in man. *N Engl J Med* 1976;294:1384.
77. Poffenbarger PL, Brinkley BK, Goldfinger SE: Colchicine for familial Mediterranean fever: Possible adverse effects. *N Engl J Med* 1974;290:56.
78. Swanson BN, Leger RM, Gordon WP, et al: Excretion of phenytoin into semen of rabbits and man. *Drug Metab Dispos* 1978;6:70.
79. Stewart-Bentley M, Virgi A, Chang S, et al: Effects of Dilantin on FSH and spermatogenesis. *Clin Res* 1976;24:101.
80. Levi AJ, Fisher AM, Hughes L, et al: Male infertility due to sulfasalazine. *Lancet* 1979;2:276.
81. Toth A: Reversible toxic effect of salicylazosulfapyridine on semen quality. *Fertil Steril* 1979;31:538.
82. Toovey S, Hudson E, Hendry WF, et al: Sulfasalazine and male infertility: Reversibility and possible mechanism. *Gut* 1981;22:445.
83. Cosentino MJ, Chey WY, Takihard H, et al: The effects of sulfasalazine on human male fertility potential and seminal prostaglandins. *J Urol* 1984;132:682.
84. Collier JG, Flower RJ: Effect of aspirin on human seminal prostaglandins. *Lancet* 1971;2:852.
85. Liao S, Fang S, Tymoczko JL, et al: Androgen receptors, antiandrogens, and uptake and retention of androgens in male sex accessory organs, in Brandes D (ed): *Male Accessory Sex Organs: Structure and Function in Mammals.* New York, Academic Press, 1974, pp 238–265.
86. Walsh PC, Korenman SG: Mechanism of androgen action effect of specific intracellular inhibitors. *J Urol* 1971;105:850.
87. Sufrin G, Coffey DS: Mechanism of action of a new nonsteroidal antiandrogen. *Invest Urol* 1976;13:429.
88. Van Thiel DH, Gavaler JS, Smith WI Jr., et al: Hypothalamic-pituitary-gonadal dysfunction in men using cimetidine. *N Engl J Med* 1979;300:1012.
89. Winters SJ, Banks JL, Loriaux DL: The histamine H_2 antagonist cimetidine is an

antiandrogen. *Gastroenterology* 1979;76:504.
90. Langley JN, Anderson HK: The innervation of the pelvic viscera and adjoining viscera: IV. The internal generative organ. *J Physiol* 1895;19:122.
91. Essenhigh DN, Chir M, Ardran GM, et al: The vesical sphincters and ejaculation in the ram. *Br J Urol* 1969;41:190.
92. Siroky MB, Krane RJ: Physiology of sexual function, in Krane RJ, Siroky MB (ed): *Clinical Neurology-Urology.* Boston, Little, Brown & Co, 1979, pp 45–62.
93. Baumgarten HG, Holstein AF, Rosengren G: Arrangement, ultrastructure and adrenergic innervation and noradrenaline content of smooth muscle layers of the human epididymis and ductus deferenes. *J Anat* 1971;109:348.
94. Ventura WP, Freund M, Davis J, et al: Influence of norepinephrine on the motility of the human vas deferens: A new hypothesis of sperm transport by the vas deferens. *Fertil Steril* 1973;24:68.
95. Fitzpatrick TJ: Spongiosograms and cavernosograms: A study of their value in priapism. *J Urol* 1973;109:843.
96. Nelson JH, Winter CC: Priapism: Evolution of management in 48 patients in a 22-year series. *J Urol* 1977;117:455.
97. Wasmer JM, Carrion HM, Mekras G, et al: Evaluation and treatment of priapism. *J Urol* 1981;125:204.
98. Robbins DN, Crawford D, Lackner H: Priapism secondary to prazosin overdose. *J Urol* 1983;130:975.
99. Pak CYC: Medical management of nephrolithiasis. *J Urol* 1982;128:1157.
100. Pak CYC, Delea CS, Bartler FC: Successful treatment of recurrent nephrolithiasis (calcium stones) with cellulose phosphate. *N Engl J Med* 1974;290:175.
101. Preminger GM: Pharmacologic treatment of calcium calculi. *Urol Clin North Am* 1987;14:328.
102. Pak CYC, Galose RA: Propensity for spontaneous nucleation of calcium oxylate. Quantitative assessment of urinary FPR-APR discriminant score. *Am J Med* 1980;69:681.
103. Dudley FJ, Blackburn CRB: Extraskeletal calcification complicating oral neutral phosphate therapy. *Lancet* 1970;2:628.
104. Preminger GM, Khashagar S, Pak CYC: Alkali action on the urinary crystallization of calcium salts: Contrasting responses to sodium citrate and potassium citrate. *J Urol* 1988;139:240.
105. Rawlins MD, Smith SE: Influence of allopurinol on drug metabolism in man. *Br J Pharmacol* 1973;48:693.
106. MacDonald WB, Fellers FX: Penicillamine in the treatment of patients with cytinuria. *JAMA* 1966;107:396.
107. Levine WG: Heavy metal antagonists, in Goodman LS, Gilman A (eds): *The Pharmacologic Basis of Therapeutics.* New York, Macmillan Publishing Co, 1975, pp 912–923.
108. Nemoy NJ, Stamey TA: Use of hemiacidrin in management of infection stones. *J Urol* 1976;116:693.
109. Fostvedt GA, Barnes RW: Complications during lavage therapy for renal calculi. *J Urol* 1963;89:329.
110. Kohler FP: Renacidin and tissue reaction. *J Urol* 1963;87:102.
111. Auerbach S, Mainwaring R, Schwarz F: Renal and ureteral damage following clinical use of renacidin. *JAMA* 1963;183:61.
112. Weinstein L: Antimicrobial agents: Sulfonamides and trimethoprim-Sulfamethoxazole, in Goodman LS, Gilman A (eds): *The Pharmacologic Basis of Therapeutics.* New York, Macmillan Publishing Co, 1975, pp 1113–1129.
113. Idsoe O, Guthe T, Willcox RR, et al: Nature and extent of penicillin side reactions with particular references to fatalities from anaphylactic shock. *Bull WHO* 1968;38:159.
114. Quintiliani R, French M, Nightingale CH, et al: First and second generation cephalosporins. *Med Clin North Am* 1982;66:183.
115. Neu HC: Carbenicillin and ticarcillin. *Med Clin North Am* 1982;66:61.
116. Brown CH III, Natelson EA, Bradshaw MW, et al: The hemostatic defect produced by carbenicillin. *N Engl J Med* 1974;291:265.
117. Richardson AG, Spittle CR, James KW, et al: Experience with carbenicillin in the treatment of septicemia and miningitis. *Postgrad Med* 1968;44:844.

118. Ristuccia AM, Cunha BA: The aminoglycosides. *Med Clin North Am* 1982;66:303.
119. Smith TR, Smith CR: Risk factors for aminoglycoside nephrotoxicity, in Welton A (ed): *The Aminoglycosides.* New York, Marcel Dekker, Inc. 1981, pp 401–415.
120. Whelton A, et al: Pharmacokinetic characteristics of doxycycline accumulation in normal and severely diseased kidneys. *J Infect Dis* 1975;132:467.
121. Brogen RN, Speight TM, Avery GS: Minocycline: A review of its antibacterial and pharmacokinetic properties and therapeutic use. *Drugs* 1975;9:251.
122. Hanno P: Therapeutic principals of antimicrobial therapy and new antimicrobial agents. *Urol Clin North Am* 1986;577.
123. Bergeron MG, Thabet M, Roz R, et al: Norfloxacin penetration into human renal and prostatic tissues. *Antimicrob Agents Chemother* 1985;28:349.
124. Arcieri M, Griffeth E, Gruenwalt G, et al: Ciprofloxacin: an update on clinical experience. *Am J Med* 1987;82(suppl):381.
125. Ho G, Tiernez MG, Dales RE: Evaluation of the effect of norfloxacin on the pharmacokinetics of theophylline. *Clin Pharmacol Ther* 1988:44:35.
126. Preheim LC, Cuevas TA, Roccaforte JS, et al: Oral ciprofloxacin in the treatment of elderly patients with complicated urinary tract infections due to trimethoprim/sulfamethoxazole resistant bacteria. *Am J Med* 1987;82(suppl):285.
127. Raoof S, Wollschlager C, Khan F: Treatment of respiratory tract infections with ciprofloxacin. *J Antimicrob Chemother* 1986;18(suppl):139.
128. Thorsteinsson SB, Bergan T, Oddsclottir S, et al: Crystalluria and ciprofloxacin: Influence of urinary pH and hydration. *Chemotherapy* 1986;32:408.
129. Smith CR: The adverse effects of flouroquinolones. *J Antimicrob Chemother* 1987;19:709.
130. Barley RR, Natale R, Linton AL. Nalidic acid arthralgia. *Can Med Assoc J* 1972;107:604.
131. Innes IR, Nickerson M: Atropine, scopolamine and related antimuscarinic drugs, in Goodman LS, Gilman A (eds): *The Pharmacological Basis of Therapeutics.* New York, Macmillan Publishing Co, 1975, pp 514–532.
132. Koelle GB: Parasympathomimetic agents, in Goodman LS, Gilman A (eds): *The Pharmacological Basis of Therapeutics.* New York, Macmillan Publishing Co, 1975, pp 469–476.
133. Raisfield IH: Cardiovascular complications of anti-depressant therapy. *Am Heart J* 1972;83:129.
134. Sidi AA: Vasoactive intracavernous pharmacotherapy. *Urol Clin North Am* 1988;15:95.
135. Macht DI: A pharmacologic and clinical study of papavarine. *Arch Intern Med* 1916;17:786.
136. Sidi AA, Duffy LM, Wasserman W: Short and long term complications of vasoactive intracavernous pharmacotherapy (VIP) for impotency (abstract). *J Urol* 1987;137:203A.
137. Nelson RP: Pathophysiology, diagnosis and management of erectile dysfunction, in Rous S (ed): *Urology Annual.* Norwalk, Conn, Appleton & Lange Publishing, 1987, vol 1, pp 139–169.
138. Nelson RP: Nonoperative management of impotence. *J Urol* 1988;139:2.
139. Zorgniotti AW, Lefleur RS: Autoinjection of the corpus cavernosum with a vasoactive drug combination for vasculogenic impotence. *J Urol* 1985;133:39.
140. Abber JC, Lue TF, Orvis BR, et al: Diagnostic tests for impotence: A comparison of papavarine injection with the penile brachial index and nocturnal penile tumescence monitoring. *J Urol* 1986;135:923.
141. Juenemann K-P, Lue TF, Fournier GR Jr, et al: Hemodynamics of papavarine- and phentolamine-induced penile erections. *J Urol* 1986;136:158.
142. Brindley GS: Cavernosal alpha-blockade: a new technique for investigating and treating erectile impotence. *Br J Psychiatry* 1983;143:332.
143. Caine M: The present role of alpha-adrenergic blockers in the treatment of benign prostatic hypertrophy. *J Urol* 1986;136:1.
144. Stackle W, Hasun R, Marberger M: Intracavernous injection and prostaglandin E1 in impotent men. *J Urol* 1988;140:66.

145. Piper PJ: Distribution and metabolism, in Cutlbert MF (ed): *The Prostaglandins: Pharmacological and Therapeutic Advances.* Philadelphia, JB Lippincott Co, 1973, p 125.
146. Waldhauser M, Schramek P: Efficiency and side effects of prostaglandin E1 in the treatment of erectile dysfunction. *J Urol* 1988;140:525.
147. Caine M, Raz S, Ziegler M: Adrenergic and cholinergic receptors in the human prostate, prostatic capsule, and bladder neck. *Br J Urol* 1975;47:193.
148. Boreham PF, Braithwaite P, Milewoki P, et al: Alpha-adrenergic blockers in prostatism. *Br J Surg* 1977;64:756.
149. Caine M, Perlberg S, Meretyk S: A placebo-controlled double-blind study of the effect of phenoxybenzamine in benign prostatic obstruction. *Br J Urol* 1978;50:551.
150. Abrams PH, Shah PJR, Stone R: Bladder outflow obstruction treated with phenoxybenzamine. *Br J Urol* 1982;54:527.
151. Gerstenberg T, Blaabjerg J, Nielsen ML, et al: Phenoxybenzamine reduces bladder outlet obstruction in benign prostatic hyperplasia. *Invest Urol* 1980;18:29.
152. Hieble JP, Boyce AJ, Caine M: Comparison of the alpha-adrenoceptor characteristics in human and canine prostate. *Fed Proc* 1986;45:2613.
153. Lepor H, Gup DI, Baumann M, et al: Laboratory assessment of terazosin and $alpha_1$ blockade in prostatic hyperplasia. *Urology* 1988;32(suppl):21.
154. Hedlund H, Andersson K-E, and Ek A: Effects of prazosin in patients with benign prostatic obstruction. *J Urol* 1983;130:275.
155. Martorana G, Giberti C, Damonte P, et al: The effects of prazosin in benign prostatic hypertrophy, a placebo controlled double-blind study. *IRCS Med Sci* 1984;12:11.
156. Kirby RS, Coppinger SWC, Corcoran MV, et al: Prazosin in the treatment of prostatic obstruction. *Br J Urol* 1987;60:136.
157. Ruoff G: Comparative trials of terazosin with other antihypertensive agents. *Am J Med* 1986;80(suppl):42.
158. Dunzendorfer MV: Clinical experience with symptomatic management of BPH with terazosin. *Urology* 1988;32(suppl):21.
159. Ritchie JM, Cohen PJ: Cocaine, procaine, and other synthetic local anesthetics, in Goodman LS, Gilman A (eds): *The Pharmacological Basis of Therapeutics.* New York, Macmillan Publishing Co, 1975, pp 379–403.
160. Selden RO, Sasahara AA: Central nervous system toxicity induced by lidocaine: Report of a case in a patient with liver disease. *JAMA* 1967;202:908.
161. Jaffe JH, Martin WR: Narcotic analgesics and antagonists, in Goodman, LS, Gilman A (eds): *The Pharmacological Basis of Therapeutics.* New York, Macmillan Publishing Co, 1975, pp 245–283.

CHAPTER 7

Complications of Cytotoxic and Biologic Agents Used in the Treatment of Genitourinary Malignancies

Donald L. Trump, M.D.
Miriam P. Rogers, R.N., M.N.

The use of cancer chemotherapeutic agents in patients with testicular cancers yields results which may be classified as truly spectacular. Intravesical chemotherapy for superficial transitional cell carcinoma (TCC), systemic cytotoxic chemotherapy of advanced TCC, and several old and new hormonal therapies for advanced prostate cancer offer substantial potential for improvement of quality of life and enhanced survival. Progress in the therapy of advanced renal cell carcinoma (RCC) has been scanty. While much excitement surrounds the apparent activity of biologic agents such as interleukin-2 plus lymphokine-activated killer (LAK) cells and the interferons in advanced RCC, the precise impact of this class of agents on length and quality of survival remains to be elucidated. This chapter will review the major toxic effects of the drugs most often used in the treatment of genitourinary cancers and will briefly summarize the therapeutic expectations of these treatments.

TESTIS CANCER

Testis cancer is one of the few advanced epithelial neoplasms occurring in adults that the physician can approach with truly curative intent. Significant improvement in survival of patients with advanced testis cancer is evident not only from the reports of institutional and cooperative group trials in selected patients but also in the population-based data summaries enumerated by the National Cancer Institute.[1] Advanced testis cancer has been recognized to be responsive to chemotherapy since the mid-1950s.[2] However, it is the work of Golbey[3], Samuels et al.,[4] and Einhorn,[5] and their colleagues that has led to the development of curative combination chemotherapy programs for patients with testicular as well as extragonadal germ cell tumors.

PVB/VAB6 Regimens

Chemotherapy in germ cell tumors clearly requires the use of combinations of effective agents. There is *no* role for single-drug therapy in patients with germ cell cancers. The two combinations which have been most studied are the PVB regimen, studied carefully by Einhorn and colleagues, and the VAB6 regimen, developed by workers at Memorial Sloan-Kettering Institute[6, 7] (Table 7–1). The "backbone" of the VAB6 regimen is PVB—platinum (cisplatin), vinblastine, and bleomycin. While doses and schedules of drugs differ somewhat between these two regimens, there are no data indicating either the therapeutic superiority of PVB or VAB6 or important differences in side effects. Recent results of a randomized trial clearly indicate that the BEP regimen (bleomycin, etoposide, and cisplatin) causes less neuromuscular toxicity than PVB. BEP is now accepted as standard therapy, and preferable to PVB due to reduced toxity. The regimens are generally administered for only 3 to 6 months. If complete tumor regression is obtained or can be completed with surgical resection of residual disease, prolonged chemotherapy is not needed.[8]

TABLE 7–1.
The PVB, BEP, and VAB6 Regimens

PVB regimen	
Cisplatin	20 mg/m^2 IV days 1, 2, 3, 4, 5
Bleomycin	30 μm IV days 2, 9, 16
Vinblastine	0.15 mg/kg days 1 and 2
Cycles repeated every 21 days	
BEP regimen	
Bleomycin	30 units IV days 2, 9, 16
Etoposide (VP-16)	100 mg/m^2 IV days 1, 2, 3, 4, 5
Cisplatin	20 mg/m^2 IV days 1, 2, 3, 4, 5
VAB6 regimen	
Cisplatin*	120 mg/m^2 IV day 4
Bleomycin	20 μm/m^2 continuous infusion, IV days 1, 2, 3
Vinblastine	4 mg/m^2 IV day 1
Cyclophosphamide	600 mg/m^2 IV day 1
Actinomycin D	1 mg/m^2 IV day 1
Cycles repeated every 21–28 days	

*With mannitol, furosemide, and saline diuresis.
IV = intravenous.

Cisplatin is a planar coordination complex of the metal platinum that appears to exert its anticancer effect by reacting with DNA and forming intrastrand and interstrand DNA cross-links in a manner similar to that of the alkylating agents. Vinblastine is a plant alkaloid that interacts with microtubular structures in dividing cells and results in arrest of cells in metaphase. Bleomycin is a fermentation product and causes scission of single-stranded DNA, hence preventing cell replication. The two additional drugs in the VAB6 regimen are actinomycin D (AMD) and cyclophosphamide (CTX). Actinomycin D is an antibiotic that interacts with ribosomal proteins and inhibits protein synthesis. Cyclophosphamide is an alkylating agent which produces DNA inter- and intrastrand cross-links. Etoposide is a podophyllotoxin derivative which appears to exert its cytotoxic effects through inhibition of DNA synthesis by interacting with topoisomerase II. These regimens may have toxic effects upon the blood, kidneys, nervous system, gastrointestinal organs, lungs, skin, gonads, and circulation.

Hematologic Toxicity.—PVB, BEP, and VAB6 employ appreciable doses of myelosuppressive drugs. Leukopenia and thrombocytopenia invariably occur. Potentially life-threatening leukopenia (white blood cells less than 1,000/mm^3) or thrombocytopenia (platelets less than 20,000/mm^3) occurs in approximately 10% of patients receiving these regimens. Myelosuppression occurs 8 to 12 days following initiation of therapy and resolves by days 16 to 18 of treatment. Myelosuppression is often more prominent in patients who have suffered greater weight loss with their disease or have received radiation therapy to areas of active bone marrow production. Transient bone marrow suppression is a serious complication, and its management requires careful patient education and close observation. However, since marrow suppression is transient and techniques for controlling infection and/or bleeding are readily available, death from myelosuppression *should not occur* in carefully followed, appropriately managed, well-informed, and compliant patients.

Renal Toxicity.—A potentially life-threatening effect of cisplatin is renal toxicity. Prior to recognition of renal damage prevention, cisplatin was almost discarded as too toxic a drug. However, it is now clear that cisplatin nephrotoxicity can be largely averted by ensuring that patients are well hydrated prior to treatment and then by maintaining generous hydration during and following administration for several hours. Data suggest that the risk of nephrotoxicity is related to the dose of cisplatin and the peak blood level of cisplatin. Consequently, cisplatin administered in the PVB and BEP regimens requires only generous daily hydration (normal saline, 3 L/day, for 20 mg/m^2 cisplatin five times daily) whereas the VAB6 regimen, which administers cisplatin as a large single dose (120 mg/m^2), requires hydration plus mannitol and furosemide diuresis to prevent nephrotoxicity. Both techniques are successful, and clinically significant increases in serum creatinine or decrements in creatinine clearance are seen in fewer than 5% to 10% of patients carefully treated with these regimens.

The site of toxic effect of cisplatin in the kidney is the renal tubule. While significant alterations in serum creatinine are uncommon in patients treated with PVB, BEP, or VAB6, more subtle alterations in tubular function are very common. The most common manifestation of this effect is renal magnesium wasting.[9] Hypomagnesemia is seen in 30% to 50% of patients receiving these regimens. Clinical manifestations of hypomagnesemia are those of hypocalcemia, since the homeostatic mechanisms for these divalent cations are closely linked. Carpopedal spasm, acral and circumoral paresthesias, seizures, and cardiac arrhythmias (prolonged QT interval, ventricular irritability, ventricular fibrillation) may occur if the physician is unaware of the potential for the development of hypomagnesemia. Prevention of magnesium wasting is not possible. Chronic oral magnesium supplementation is also difficult. Assessment of serum magnesium two or three times per month during therapy and parenteral supplementation if serum levels fall below 1.5 to 1.8 mg/dL seem judicious. With this plan we rarely see clinically significant examples of hypomagnesemia.

Neurologic Toxicity.—Both vinblastine and cisplatin cause neurologic toxicity. The most troublesome neurotoxicity of vinblastine is an enteric visceral neuropathy which leads to abdominal bloating, pain, and constipation. This generally occurs 7 to 10 days after therapy and resolves in 5 to 7 days. This acute syndrome may also be associated with diffuse myalgias and on occasion severe, lancinating jaw or extremity pain. "Prophylactic" laxatives and stool softeners are indicated in patients receiving vinblastine. While seldom life-threatening, this toxicity can be quite uncomfortable and difficult to avert entirely. Vinblastine may also cause a mild to moderate peripheral neuropathy, manifested by diminished distal extremity fine touch, two-point discrimination, and paresthesias. This manifestation of vinblastine neuropathy develops after 2 to 3 months of therapy and may persist for 6 to 8 months following treatment.

Cisplatin neuropathy may also be a clinical problem. Peripheral neuropathy may be dose-limiting at high doses of cisplatin. While peripheral neuropathy that is specifically related to cisplatin is uncommon following 2 to 4 months of therapy with standard doses of cisplatin, prolonged cisplatin therapy or very high doses of cisplatin (150 mg/m^2 course or more) may be limited by the development of severe neuropathy (see below).

Auditory toxicity is also seen following cisplatin therapy. This is mediated through damage to the cochlear hair cells and is manifest first as tinnitus and high-frequency hearing loss. While audiographic studies will delineate high-frequency hearing loss in most patients treated with VAB6, BEP, or PVB, it is uncommon for hearing loss to be clinically manifest. However, following very large single doses or cumulative doses of cisplatin, clinically apparent hearing loss may be dose-limiting.

Gastrointestinal Toxicity.—Nausea and vomiting are prominent acute toxicities of cisplatin-based chemotherapy. The severity of nausea and vomiting that was seen following cisplatin slowed its wide acceptance in clinical practice. However, at this time, effective antiemetic regimens based on the use of high-dose metoclopramide (1–2 mg/kg) and dexamethasone, as well as the recognition that nausea and vomiting are reduced with prolongation of cisplatin infusion time (avoiding high peak blood levels), make nausea and vomiting a generally manageable toxicity of PVB and VAB6 regimens.[10] Sedation from these aggressive antiemetic regimens is appreciable and may require that the patient be hospitalized during therapy. Occasionally, patients receiving high doses of metroclopramide may experience extrapyramidal symptoms such as facial dystonia or restlessness of the arms and legs. These vary in severity and are immediately reversible with intravenous diphenhydramine.

Oral ulceration is a possible side effect of bleomycin and actinomycin D. Earlier regimens employed 5 to 7 days of continuous infusion schedules of bleomycin and were complicated by severe oral ulceration in 30% to 60% of patients.[11] Such ulcers involve the lateral borders of the tongue and buccal mucosa and begin 5 to 8 days after initiation of therapy. This complication can be debilitating and is potentially dangerous if it coincides with substantial leukopenia. However, the PVB and VAB6 regimens rarely are a cause of oral ulceration.

Pulmonary Toxicity.—Drug-induced pneumonitis is a complication of bleomycin therapy. While basilar pulmonary infiltrates, pleural-based plaques, and diminished diffusing capacity may be seen in patients treated with PVB, BEP, or VAB6 regimens, symptomatic pneumonitis is uncommon if cumulative bleomycin doses are kept to less than 200 $units/m^2$.[12] Two exceptions to this generalization require emphasis: (1) Patients who have received mediastinal radiation therapy are at a substantially higher risk of symptomatic and occasionally fatal pneumonitis after bleomycin therapy. Bleomycin and radiation exert synergistic effects experimentally even if the interval between administration of these treatments is a month or more. Great care should be taken if these two treatment modalities must be used in the same patient. (2) Oxygen appears to potentiate bleomycin pulmonary damage. Several examples of fatal pneumonitis have been reported in patients who have received standard doses of bleomycin (cumulative dose less than 200 $units/m^2$) and then have been exposed to high concentrations of inspired oxygen (FIO_2) during a surgical procedure. Pneumonitis is of particular concern, since 10% to 20% of patients treated for advanced testis cancer may require a major surgical procedure following chemotherapy to remove residual tumor masses. Caution should be exercised in such cases that the minimal FIO_2 necessary to maintain physiologic oxygenation is employed.[13]

Dermatologic Toxicity.—Patients receiving PVB, BEP, or VAB6 frequently note mild pruritus and xeroderma. Hyperpigmented streaks along lines of trauma or scratching, especially on the back and arms, are also common. These skin changes are related to bleomycin. Reversible alopecia of a moderate degree invariably accompanies these therapies.

Allergic Reactions.—In addition to the cutaneous reactions noted above, severe allergic reactions including anaphylaxis have been observed with the use of bleomycin, cisplatin, and etoposide. Such reactions are rare and should be managed with standard anaphylactic treatment.[14]

Gonadal Toxicity.—Damage to germinal epithelium as well as Leydig's cells may occur following PVB or VAB6 therapy. Such damage may result in temporary abnormalities of sex steroid secretion, which can cause gynecomastia or mastodynia.[15] Azoospermia and infertility may also occur. Theoretically, one might predict that the VAB6 regimen would be more likely to produce azoospermia, since alkylating agents such as cyclophosphamide are the cytotoxic drugs with greatest potential for gonadal damage. Dragsa and co-workers have shown that adequate sperm counts and evidence of compensated Leydig's cell damage are present in 50% of men treated with PVB.[16] Similar studies have not yet been reported for patients treated with VAB6. At the present time, the possibility that PVB is less damaging to gonadal function is only theoretical. Clear-cut abnormalities in gonadotropin and sex steroid secretion have been described following both regimens. There is no evidence that such combinations are teratogenic for the offspring of men who receive them.

Vascular Toxicity.—Raynaud's phenomenon has recently been reported to develop in as many as 40% of patients treated with PVB.[17] Interestingly, other findings which may be related to altered arterial reactivity such as hypertension and myocardial ischemia have also been described. It has been suggested that hypomagnesemia, which enhances smooth muscle contractility and is common in patients receiving PVB or VAB6, may contribute to these changes. No definitive data exist linking these chemotherapies with any abnormality of arterial function other than Raynaud's phenomenon.

Hypotension.—Etoposide may cause significant hypotension during infusion. These episodes may be prevented by keeping the patient recumbent during infusion and avoiding rapid infusion rates.[18]

Very High-Dose Cisplatin Regimens

In experimental and clinical models there is persuasive evidence for a steep dose-response curve for cisplatin. Ozols et al. showed that there is *no* renal toxicity following the administration of cisplatin 40 mg/m^2/day for 5 days if cisplatin is administered with vigorous (6 L/24 hr) saline diuresis with infusion of hypertonic (3%) sodium chloride solution.[19] The relative contribution of the 3% saline vehicle and the intense saline diuresis in averting renal damage following the administration of cisplatin 40 mg/m^2/day for 5 days is uncertain. Since the demonstration that very high-dose cisplatin is feasible, studies have been carried out exploring the use of this dose schedule of cisplatin together with vinblastine, bleomycin, and etoposide. Ozols et al. have described the use of the PVeBV (platinum, vinblastine, bleomycin, etoposide) regimen as initial therapy for poor-prognosis testis cancer,[20] and Trump and Hortvet have reported the use of etoposide combined with very high-dose cisplatin as a salvage regimen for patients failing PVB.[20, 21]

These regimens produce profound myelosuppression. White blood cell and platelet nadirs of 100 to 200/mm^3 and 5,000 to 15,000/mm^3, respectively, are to be expected. Fever with leukopenia is very common. Nephrotoxicity has not been seen in either experience with cisplatin 40 mg/m^2/day for 5 days. Neurotoxicity is the dose-limiting toxicity of these regimens. Disabling peripheral neuropathy and overt hearing loss are expected side effects of these regimens in patients who have previously received standard doses of cisplatin. The role of very high-dose cisplatin in the therapy of germ cell tumors is uncertain. While the ability to administer such treatments is demonstrated, they should be undertaken only with care and by physicians experienced in managing profound myelosuppression.

BLADDER CANCER

Intravesical Therapy of Superficial Disease

Intravesical chemotherapy for superficial transitional cell carcinoma (STCC) offers several potential chemotherapeutic advantages over therapies for most other human cancers: (1) STCC has a high propensity for multifocal recurrence, and data suggest that local control of superficial disease may delay or prevent the development of invasive, truly life-threatening disease. (2) The therapeutic ratio for intravesically administered drugs may be enormous. There is relatively little systemic absorption of drugs administered intravesically; hence, high intravesical doses may be administered with little danger of systemic toxicity. The extent to which drugs are absorbed from the bladder is related to molecular weight; little if any absorption occurs from an intact bladder if the molecular weight exceeds 200.[22] It is said that the extent of involvement of the bladder, recent transurethral resection, and the presence of ureteral reflux all enhance drug absorption from the bladder, but little data critically evaluating these issues are available. Similarly, the biochemical parameters of drug, vehicle, and urine (e.g., urine pH) which might influence systemic absorption are unclear.

Thiotepa.—Thiotepa is a polyfunctional alkylating agent that is active on reconstitution of the desiccated form of the drug with sterile water. Thiotepa exerts its antiproliferative effect through alkylation of biologically active molecules, primarily nucleic acids. Thiotepa has been used intravesically in the treatment of superficial transitional cell carcinomas since the late 1950s.[23] The molecular weight of thiotepa is 189, and hence some systemic absorption is to be expected. In fact, severe systemic toxicity of intravesically administered thiotepa is uncommon. The National Bladder Cancer Group (NBCG) studied thiotepa at both 30 mg and 60 mg/week over 8 weeks and found a 2% and 13% incidence of leukopenia (less than 3,000/mm^3) for 30-mg and 60-mg doses. Treatment cessation was required in four of 95 patients due to myelosuppression.[24] Life-threatening myelosuppression may occur following the intravesical administration of thiotepa, especially in poor-performance-status patients with compromised bone marrow reserves. Weekly monitoring of white blood cell and platelet counts is indicated, but dangerous toxicity is uncommon. No other systemic toxicity has been reported following intravesical administration of thiotepa. Local irritation of the bladder is the primary toxicity of intravesical thiotepa. Urgency, frequency, and dysuria occurred in 17% of patients in the NBCG study. No patients required interruption of therapy because of irritative symptoms. Thiotepa is a well-tolerated drug that causes little limiting toxicity and is effective in destroying multiple superficial TCC and delaying the recurrence of new tumors.

Mitomycin (Mutamycin) and Doxorubicin (Adriamycin).—Neither of these drugs is found in the plasma following intravesical administration.[25, 26] While mitomycin, an alkylating agent, and doxorubicin, an anthracycline that intercalates DNA, cause important myelosuppression, alopecia, and renal (mitomycin) or cardiac (doxorubicin) damage following intravenous administration, no systemic toxicity has been described following intravesical administration. Toxicity is confined to cystitis of mild to moderate degree in 10% to 15% of patients following the administration of 40 mg mitomycin weekly for 8 weeks and in 30% of patients who received 60 mg doxorubicin every 3 weeks. In 10% to 20% of patients receiving mitomycin, a scaling, erythematous, pruritic eruption develops on the hands, soles of the feet, penis, or perineum. This dermatitis appears likely to be related to the local irritative effects of mitomycin with which these parts of the body are soiled with urine following intravesical instillation.

Bacillus Calmette-Guérin.—Several reports note the substantial tumor-ablating effect seen following the intravesical application of bacillus Calmette-Guérin (BCG).[27, 28] This attenuated mycobacterial species has been used for many years as a vaccination against *Mycobacterium tuberculosis* as well as a nonspecific means of "augmenting" host immunity. It is unclear to what extent the tumor-ablating effect of BCG is related to nonspecific irritative changes of BCG or to augmentation of immune mechanisms.

Intravesical BCG (120 mg/wk for 6 weeks) results in transient hematuria, dysuria, and urinary frequency in almost all patients. When higher doses of drug are employed, systemic syndromes indicating systemic reaction may be seen—fever, arthralgias, nausea, vomiting, and pulmonary infiltrates. These findings are like those seen in 10% to 20% of patients following injection of BCG into cutaneous tumors. This constellation of findings suggests "systemic BCGosis," and, while uncommon, it is an indication for interruption of therapy. Such patients require careful observation and, at times, the administration of antimycobacterial antibiotics.

Systemic Therapy for Disseminated Disease

The agents most useful for the systemic therapy of metastatic transitional cell carcinoma are (1) cisplatin (response rate 30%–40%), (2) methotrexate (20%–30%), (3) doxorubicin (15%–20%), (4) vinblastine (20%–30%), and (5) cyclophosphamide (20%).[29] As a single agent, cisplatin is clearly the most useful drug; however, the modest response rate, the rarity of complete response (2%–5%), and the relatively short duration of response (4–6 months) indicate the small overall impact that cisplatin and other single agents have on patients with advanced transitional cell carcinoma.

Methotrexate.—A drug not previously discussed, methotrexate (MTX) is a folate antagonist whose primary mechanism of action is inhibition of the enzyme dihydrofolate reductase. This inhibition impairs the single-carbon transfer reactions necessary for the synthesis of the nucleic acid components thymidine and purines. The toxic effects of MTX are most pronounced in rapidly dividing cells and cell populations in which a large fraction of cells are in active cell cycle. The efficacy and toxicity of MTX are markedly enhanced if the drug is administered as a prolonged infusion (6–24 hours) or on a four-to-six-times-daily or weekly schedule. The simplest explanation for this observation is that this schedule provides a greater opportunity for the drug to reach different cells entering the cell cycle. Methotrexate is excreted almost entirely through renal mechanisms. Even apparently mild abnormalities in renal function may substantially increase the toxicity of MTX by delaying excretion and prolonging exposure of dividing cells to the drug. *Any* degree of renal compromise is a strong contraindication to the use of MTX in the palliative therapy of advanced cancer. Important drug interactions between MTX and commonly prescribed over-the-counter (OTC) medications have been noted which may result in significantly enhanced MTX toxicity. Trimethoprim-sulfamethoxazole and a variety of nonsteroidal anti-inflammatory agents may interfere with renal tubular excretion of MTX. Concomitant use of these drugs and MTX should be avoided.[30]

The toxicities of the standard doses of MTX (30–60 mg/m^2 every 1–2 weeks) are myelosuppression and oral ulceration. These toxicities appear 5 to 7 days following the administration of a toxic dose of MTX. Since MTX blocks the formation of reduced folates (tetrahydrofolate), it is possible to bypass the effects of MTX by directly supplying tetrahydrofolate (leucovorin factor). This maneuver allows an antidote to be given simultaneously with or immediately following MTX and averts or reduces toxicity (and perhaps therapeutic effect). This concept is employed in the use of high-dose MTX (200–1,500 mg/m^2) plus leucovorin rescue. This investigational technique is not routinely indicated in any genitourinary neoplasm.[31] Unfortunately, once toxicity is manifest, the administration of leucovorin does little to speed recovery, since the biochemical event has passed by the time toxicity is recognized.

The toxicities of the other single agents have been discussed previously.

Combination Chemotherapy of Advanced Bladder Cancer

It has been difficult to demonstrate a superiority of combination chemotherapy over single-agent treatment in metastatic bladder cancer. While there have been enthusiastic reports of response rates approaching 80% with the use of cisplatin, cyclophosphamide, doxorubicin combinations, randomized comparative trials have failed to demonstrate a survival advantage or a striking response rate advantage of combination chemotherapy compared to cisplatin alone.[32, 33] Two recent trials, carefully conducted and analyzed, do *suggest* a substantial advantage for combination chemotherapy. Workers at the Memorial Sloan-Kettering Institute and the Northern California Oncology Group have each reported studies in which the *complete* response rates were high and the 95% confidence limits of overall response rate were clearly outside those reported in prior single-agent trials (Table 7–2).[34, 35] Trials testing these treatments in direct comparison to cisplatin alone are beginning. It must be emphasized that while the response rates seen in these two trials were high, toxicity was also appreciable. Toxicities were those expected for these drugs, and no striking or unusual evidence of drug interaction or potentiation of toxicity was noted. The following side effects were noted in these trials and are to be anticipated with these treatment plans: (1) fever and granulocytopenia, 15% to 20%; (2) thrombocytopenia (less than 50,000/mm^3), 15% to 20%; (3) renal dysfunction (creatinine more than 2 mg/dL), 10% to 15%. Drug deaths have been reported in both series. Overall response rates (more than 50% reduction in measurable tumor masses) in both studies were 60% to 70%, and pathologically confirmed complete regression of tumor was seen in 15% to 20%.

One application of a chemotherapy

TABLE 7–2.

New, Potentially Superior Combination Chemotherapy Regimens for Bladder Cancer

Study	Cisplatin	Methotrexate	Vinblastine	Doxorubicin
Memorial Sloan-Kettering Institute	70 mg/m^2, day 2	30 mg/m^2, days 1, 15, 22	3 mg/m^2, days 2, 15, 22	30 mg/m^2, day 2
Northern California Oncology Group	100 mg/m^2, day 2	30 mg/m^2, days 1, 8	3 mg/m^2, days 1, 8	—

regimen with a high response rate in advanced disease would be to use such treatment as initial therapy immediately preceding definitive therapy for locally advanced bladder cancer ("neoadjuvant") or as postcystectomy surgical adjuvant therapy. While theoretically attractive, such approaches must be considered investigational and appropriate only in the context of a carefully controlled clinical trial. One must anticipate potentiation of the expected toxicities of the treatments by the concomitant therapy when closely integrating systemic and optimal local therapy. Many urologists employ radiation therapy before cystectomy; some patients have undergone definitive radiation therapy for localized bladder cancer prior to the need for "salvage cystectomy." Such radiation therapy may interact with cytotoxic therapy to cause enhanced bone marrow toxicity or radiation sensitization or "recall."

Enhanced Bone Marrow Toxicity.—Two thousand rad in five fractions or 4,000 rad in 4 weeks administered to the whole pelvis or a substantial portion of the pelvis will result in bone marrow suppression. The pelvis contains approximately 30% of active bone marrow in adults, and radiation to these areas may severely compromise marrow function. Previous radiation may lead to pronounced myelosuppression following cytotoxic chemotherapy. Either attenuation of *initial* doses of myelosuppressive drugs (by 20%–25%) or careful observation of patients after administration of full doses to manage dangerous myelosuppression should be carried out if adjunctive or "neoadjunctive" chemotherapy is contemplated.

Radiation Sensitization or Recall.—A number of cytotoxic drugs interact with irradiated cells to produce exaggerated or synergistic responses. Cisplatin is a potent radiosensitizer and is being investigated in combination with radiation therapy in head and neck, brain, bladder, and lung tumors.[36] Doxorubicin is even more potent in its ability to enhance damage in previously irradiated tissues. Doxorubicin not only enhances the toxic effects of radiation when administered with or immediately before radiation, but it can interact with irradiated tissue and "recall" an acute inflammatory response in fields irradiated weeks or months earlier. The additive effects of doxorubicin and ionizing radiation that may occur are dramatically illustrated by the lethal esophageal toxicity and dangerous cardiac effects noted after simultaneous doxorubicin and chest radiation for lung cancer.[37] The possibility of a radiation-doxorubicin interaction must be remembered if one contemplates the adjunctive or neoadjunctive use of combination chemotherapy, radiation, and surgical therapy for local or regionally advanced bladder cancer.

ADENOCARCINOMA OF THE KIDNEY

While the possible toxicities following cytotoxic therapy for advanced renal cell carcinoma are numerous, none merit discussion, since no standard cytotoxic drug has ever been shown to have substantial activity in renal cell carcinoma. A great deal of enthusiasm has arisen recently regarding the apparent antitumor activity of the interferons in advanced renal cell carcinoma.[38–40]

Interferons

Interferons are a class of polypeptides produced naturally by a wide variety of mammalian cells. These substances were discovered by virtue of their ability to be produced in mammalian cells and to interfere with and limit intracellular viral replication; hence the name interferon.[41] Three separate classes of interferon are known: (1) interferon-α (INF-α), derived from peripheral blood leukocytes; (2) interferon-β, produced by monocytes and fibroblasts; and (3) interferon-γ, or immune interferon, produced by activated thymus-dependent lymphocytes (T cells). Each of these classes is structurally, biochemically, and physiologically distinct. Thirteen separate subclasses of INF-α have been recognized in nature.

Recombinant DNA techniques now make possible the isolation of substantial quantities of pure interferons. The INF-α, both natural and recombinant, subclass types, have been the most widely tested in renal cancer at the time of this report. Response rates of 20% to 30% are reported, and well-documented complete regression of widespread metastases has been seen. The Eastern Cooperative Oncology Group (ECOG) has conducted chemotherapy trials in more than 450 patients with different agents and has not seen an agent with a response rate exceeding *10%*. The ECOG pilot study of lymphoblastoid interferon (Wellferon) was conducted in patients similar in all respects to those studied in prior ECOG trials and observed a 15% response rate.[39] While modest, these response rates *seem* to represent a clear improvement in the therapy of advanced renal cell cancer.

Interferons must be administered parenterally, and most schedules of administration utilize prolonged treatment—daily for 30 days or daily for 10 days, every 21 days. These schedules are chosen based on experimental data indicating that continuous exposure of cancer cells is more growth-inhibitory than intermittent treatment. Doses of interferons are measured in standardized antiviral units. The dose range of INF-α utilized has been 1 to 30 $\times$ 10^6 units/day.

Interferon Toxicities

While these substances are "natural products," they are not innocuous. The toxicities of INF-α are dose-dependent and vary somewhat with different products.

High Fever.—Temperature elevations to 104° to 105° F may occur, and in almost everyone some fever develops within 4 to 6 hours of the interferon injection. Antipyretics are routinely indicated to reduce the hyperpyrexia which follows interferon administration. In vitro data suggest that cyclooxygenase inhibitors (aspirin) and corticosteroids may antagonize the antiproliferative effects of interferons; hence acetaminophen is the indicated antipyretic. Despite continued interferon administration, fever and chills abate after 3 to 4 days of therapy. The explanation for this tachyphylaxis is unknown. Headache may accompany fever and chills but is generally mild.

Neurotoxicity.—A striking and occasionally dose-limiting effect of interferons is the development of fatigue. Generalized fatigue may rarely be of such proportions that patients become confined to bed. This symptom resolves in 3 to 7 days following cessation of interferon. Those patients most debilitated from their cancer are those most likely to be seriously impaired by fatigue. However, asymptomatic individuals may have their functional capacities limited by the development of fatigue.

Infrequently neurotoxicity may be dose-limiting, particulary with high-dose interferon therapy. The effects range from mood changes and somnolence to frank psychosis necessitating discontinuation of therapy. This toxicity is usually reversible, but may require a considerable recovery period.[42,43]

Increase in SGOT.—Mild to moderate increase in serum glutamic oxaloacetic transaminase (SGOT) is frequently seen with interferon therapy. This increase occurs within 3 to 6 days of initiation of interferon and resolves within 3 to 7 days of ceasing interferon administration. Only rarely has hyperbilirubinemia or clinically apparent hepatic dysfunction occurred.

Granulocyte and Platelet Decrease.— Diminution in circulating granulocyte and platelet count is seen in 30% to 40% of patients treated with interferon. Platelet counts less than 100,000/ mm^3 are uncommon, but granulocyte counts of less than 1,000/mm^3 have been reported in 15% to 20% of patients.[44] These depressions in blood counts are unlike those seen following the administration of cytotoxic drugs in that they occur within 3 to 5 days of beginning treatment. Granulocyte counts recover within 24 to 48 *hours* of cessation of interferon. This pattern suggests changes in the distribution of granulocytes between circulating and "marginated" pools rather than the destruction of granulocytes. Infections complicating interferon-associated granulocytopenia are very uncommon, despite occasionally substantial decreases in peripheral granulocyte counts (less than 250/mm^3). At the present time, myelosuppression, while meriting careful attention, has not been a serious clinical problem even with very high doses of interferons.

Other Cytokines

Much attention has been focused on a new approach to cancer therapy—the use of populations of immune effector cells which are capable of killing cancer cells. These cells have been used with the T cell growth factor, interleukin-2 (IL-2). The greatest experience in this area has been with isolation of lymphocytes from the peripheral blood of individuals with cancer, expansion of the number of cells by incubation with IL-2 and reinfusion with simultaneous intravenous IL-2 infusion to maintain these cells. This does result in tumor regression in animal models and humans. Cells so treated in vitro are called lymphokine-activated killer cells, or LAK cells. These cells are similar to naturally occurring killer (NK) lymphocytes.

In the initial studies of IL-2 plus LAK cells carried out by Rosenberg and colleagues, 44% of patients treated responded.[45] This study included three patients with advanced renal cell carcinomas, each of whom responded. All patients had failed conventional therapy or were patients for whom there was no conventional therapy available. In a recent update of this experience a complete/partial response rate of 30% was seen among 36 patients with advanced renal cell carcinoma.[46] Research in this area is developing rapidly. Among the variables being explored to optimize therapy are (1) the use of IL-2 alone, as LAK cells may not be a prerequisite for activity; (2) the use of effector cells isolated from the patient's tumor (tumor-infiltrating lymphocytes, TIL cells); (3) optimizing the dose of IL-2; (4) the use of IL-2 and other cytokines as well as cytotoxics. In this rapidly changing area, all treatment approaches are experimental.

Toxicities related to IL-2 and IL-2 plus LAK cells can be significant, dose-limiting, and on occasion have been fatal. Most of the toxicity of IL-2 plus LAK cells is related to the IL-2 rather than the LAK cells. IL-2 toxicity is dose-related with greatest toxicity seen following very high-dose IL-2 infusions. Malaise is common. Fever is an invariable occurrence during IL-2 infusion, but can often be prevented with prophylactic antipyretics, and cyclooxygenase inhibitors (e.g., indomethacin). Elevated hepatic enzymes and hyperbilirubinemia occur in 85%, but resolve when IL-2 is discontinued. Nausea and vomiting are present but manageable in most patients and resolve with discontinuation of therapy. Neurotoxicity, which may progress in rare instances to coma, has been seen. In the most recent update of IL-2 and IL-2–LAK therapy, 50% of courses were complicated by somnolence, disorientation, or coma. Overt or clinically occult hypothyroidism has been reported in 20% of patients treated in one series.[47] This maybe related to activation of auto immune mechanisms which are targeted against thyroid.

By far the most serious complication is the enhanced capillary permeability and decreased peripheral vascular resistance associated with IL-2 administration. These hemodynamic alterations are similar to those seen in early septic shock. Resultant fluid shifts into extravascular compartments may result in a number of clinical problems: hypotension may require both pressors and fluid replacement. Many patients have experienced significant renal dysfunction as a result of hypovolemia and hypotension. Interstitial pneumonitis with respiratory distress requiring intubation may occur. Weight gain associated with fluid accumulation (ascites, pleural effusion, peripheral edema) is common. After discontinuation of IL-2, resolution of all these manifestations of increased capillary permeability generally occur.[48]

The most common hematologic effect of IL-2 is anemia. The mechanism of anemia is not clearly defined. Neither thrombocytopenia nor neutropenia are serious problems following IL-2 administration. Lymphokines, including IL-2, interferon, and other agents, have been implicated in occasional instances of cardiac toxicity. Both atrial and ventricular arrthythmias have been reported as well as acute myocardial infarction. In a recent series, cardiac toxicity other than hypotension was noted in approximately 13% of 123 patient treatments. Cardiac toxicity responded to medical management. It has been suggested that the genesis of these cardiac effects is related to the hemodynamic effects on peripheral blood vessels. Careful screening for patients for significant pretreatment cardiac dysfunction or prior treatment with cardiotoxic chemotherapy has been suggested as a means of reducing the incidence of cardiotoxicity.

The role of therapy with IL-2 or IL-2 and LAK cells in advanced genitourinary malignancy, particularly renal cell cancer, remains to be defined. It is clear, however, that antitumor effect is seen with IL-2 or IL-2 plus LAK cells in renal carcinoma. Complete responses have been noted. Toxicity is substantial, but efforts to reduce toxicity and learn better use of these agents are underway. Better understanding of the genesis of toxicity and its management will allow for a thorough evaluation of these exciting new cancer chemotherapeutics.

PROSTATE CANCER

The standard systemic therapy for disseminated or regionally advanced prostate cancer is orchiectomy. For some patients orchiectomy is an unacceptable option. Several new approaches to ablation of testicular and/or adrenal androgen secretion also merit consideration.

Diethylstilbestrol (DES)

Diethylstilbestrol is the standard alternative to orchiectomy. Anorchic plasma concentrations of testosterone are achieved within 2 to 3 weeks of beginning DES therapy. Administration of pharmacologic doses of DES results in the suppression of release of luteinizing hormone (LH), which results in a decrease in testicular androgen secretion. Despite years of use, the dose of DES utilized for the treatment of prostate cancer still varies greatly. Five milligrams of DES administered daily results in dependable suppression of testosterone secretion but a high incidence of complications and inordinate mortality.[49] Three milligrams of DES per day is less often associated with complications and is a dependable dose with which to lower plasma testosterone.[50] One milligram of DES per day may be even less toxic but may result in less dependable suppression of plasma testosterone.[51]

The complications of DES are well known and include nausea and vomiting, salt and water retention, and thromboembolic disease. It is also widely acknowledged that the randomized Veterans Administration Cooperative Studies demonstrated no survival advantage for asymptomatic patients with stages C and D prostate cancer with the use of 5 mg DES daily. In part, failure of early hormone therapy was the result of increased cardiovascular mortality. Whether these studies still justify the delayed application of less toxic hormonal manipulations, in view of the demonstrated activity of lower doses of DES, improved techniques for recognizing and managing cardiovascular morbidity, and new hormonal therapies available (see below), is arguable.

Antiandrogens

In human breast cancer, relatively specific and clinically effective antiestrogens are available. The most widely used drug, tamoxifen, blocks the action of estrogens at peripheral target tissues. A drug with a similar ability to inhibit testosterone secretion and block testosterone activity would be very useful. An ideal antiandrogen has not yet been synthesized. Several drugs exist that disrupt androgen metabolism by inhibiting testicular and adrenal androgen synthesis, blocking gonadotropin secretion, or interfering with activation and binding of testosterone in target tissues. Flutamide is a nonsteroidal substance that antagonizes the effect of androgens on peripheral target tissues but does not inhibit gonadotropin secretion. Flutamide may cause less impotence, infertility, and thromboembolic disease than DES does. However, flutamide does induce gynecomastia in 30% to 40% of men. While flutamide is clearly active in untreated advanced prostate cancer and may cause fewer side effects than DES, the results of rigorous comparative trials are not yet available. It is suggested that flutamide may have activity in patients whose tumors have progressed despite DES or orchiectomy. This response rate may be 15% to 30%.[52, 53] The precise role of flutamide in the therapy of advanced prostate cancer is uncertain.

Cyproterone acetate and megestrol acetate are both potent progestational agents. They suppress plasma testosterone by reducing gonadotropin secretion and also may antagonize the activation of androgens in sensitive target tissues. Both drugs reduce libido and may cause gynecomastia and fluid retention. Thromboembolic complications and salt retention comparable to that seen with DES are not seen. Both drugs are active in untreated prostate cancer but are only occasionally beneficial in patients whose tumors have progressed despite DES or orchiectomy.[54, 55] None of the other agents with antiandrogenic activity or with the property of inhibiting adrenal androgen secretion (aminoglutethimide, spironolactone, ketaconazole) has been shown to have widespread clinical application at this time.[56–58]

Luteinizing Hormone–Releasing Hormone Analogues

Guillemin and Schally shared the Nobel prize for Medicine and Physiology in 1977, with Rosalyn Yalow, for their work in characterizing substances present in the hypothalamus that exert important influences on the pituitary secretion of thyroid-stimulating hormone, prolactin, growth hormone, luteinizing hormone (LH), and follicle-stimulating hormone (FSH). These hypothalamic substances generally, but not invariably, act to stimulate pituitary release of these hormones. While it was initially believed that FSH and LH were released by different substances, it subsequently has not been possible to distinguish two separate factors. The releasing factor that stimulates FSH and LH release is called gonadotropin-releasing hormone (GnRH) but is also often still referred to as LH-releasing hormone (LHRH). This decapeptide is released by hypothalamic cells directly into blood vessels, which then carry GnRH to the pituitary and stimulate gonadotropin release. Normal, pulsatile GnRH secretion is essential for gonadotropin secretion and normal testicular function. When adequate quantities of GnRH and related analogues became available for clinical trials, it was noted that frequent parenteral treatment with pharmacologic doses of GnRH analogues resulted in *suppression* of LH and FSH secretion and diminution of gonadal function.[59] Continuous exposure of the pituitary to pharmacologic concentrations of GnRH analogues results in the loss of GnRH receptors on pituitary cells and decrease in FSH and LH secretion.[60] This unexpected result suggested that these substances may be useful in suppressing gonadal function in hormone-sensitive malignancies such as prostate and breast cancer. Recent studies indicate that GnRH analogues are quite effective in reducing plasma testosterone concentrations and causing regressions of prostate cancer.[61–63] A randomized trial has recently been completed comparing DES, 3 mg/day, and leuprolide, a GnRH analogue produced by Abbott Laboratories. This trial indicates that these two treatments are therapeutically indistinguishable. The DES-treated patients more often had painful gynecomastia, nausea and vomiting, fluid retention, and thromboembolic disease. The side effects reported with leuprolide were hot flashes and diminished libido.[64] A disadvantage of these initially used GnRH analogues has been the necessity that they be administered daily subcutaneously or as a frequent daily nasal spray. Trials are now underway in Europe and the United States with a depot formulation of GnRH analogue. Preliminary data indicate that anorchic plasma levels of testosterone and clinical remission may be obtained with a single monthly subcutaneous injection.[65]

The initial experience with GnRH analogues suggests that a widely acceptable, safe, and virtually nontoxic mode of treatment for advanced prostate cancer is at hand. If these data withstand more extensive clinical trials, then several avenues of clinical research may be opened. For example, the question of early adjunctive hormonal therapy for B_2- and C-stage prostate cancer must be reconsidered. Labrie and co-workers have already reported success with the use of antiandrogens and GnRH analogues; the latter prevent "gonadotropin-override," which accompanies antiandrogen use.[66] This combined treatment offers the potential for complete androgen ablation in a safe and well-tolerated manner.

Recent reports of a randomized trial of LHRH analogues with or without flutamide indicate a small but significant survival advantage for the combined approach.[67]

Cytotoxic Drugs

Cytotoxic drugs have not been shown to be dependably effective in advanced prostate cancer refractory to hormonal therapy. While a priori one might expect adenocarcinoma of the prostate to be modestly responsive to cytotoxic drugs, the age of patients who develop prostate cancer and the difficulties in evaluating bone metastases have made the evaluation of cytotoxic therapy difficult.

Doxorubicin (Adriamycin), cyclophosphamide, and methotrexate have all been shown to have real though modest activity in advanced prostate cancer. None of these drugs causes objective antitumor responses in more than 25% to 30% of patients. The toxic effects of these agents have been discussed earlier.[68]

The drug estramustine phosphate (Emcyt) merits brief consideration. This "rationally synthesized" antineoplastic is composed of an estradiol steroid nucleus joined to an alkylating moiety, nonnitrogen mustard, by a carbamate linkage. This drug and others like it were synthesized with the hope that the steroid nucleus would bind to hormone-dependent cells and "deliver" an alkylating moiety. Much work has been done with such agents and some antineoplastic activity is evident. Estramustine phosphate does bind to rat and human prostate tissue; the binding protein involved has not been characterized. However, the cytotoxic effects of estramustine phosphate seem neither entirely related to its alkylating ability nor its estrogenic effects. The latter effects are quite evident, since estramustine phosphate is readily hydrolyzed to estrone and estradiol.[69]

Estramustine phosphate appears to have antineoplastic activity similar to that seen with DES in previously untreated patients with prostate cancer. While antitumor responses have been reported following estramustine phosphate administration to patients who have failed to respond to DES or orchiectomy, the duration and survival impact of such responses is unclear.

The adverse effects of estramustine phosphate are similar to those seen with DES. Cardiovascular and thromboembolic complications have been reported with similar frequency. Painful gynecomastia, abnormal liver function tests, and nausea and vomiting severe enough to limit drug acceptance are also reported. Estramustine phosphate is also many times more expensive than DES, a drug to which it does not appear to be superior.

EDITORIAL COMMENT

This chapter provides an excellent summary of the chemotherapeutic complications of genitourinary malignancies. The complications of chemotherapy in patients with testis tumor can be very high, but most patients are cured. Fortunately, in bladder cancer intravesical chemotherapy is very well tolerated. In patients who do manifest myelosuppression with thiotepa, we have used mitomycin, because it is a larger molecule with less systemic absorption. On the other hand, we are increasingly utilizing BCG, which appears to have improved response rates. In the future, use of the laser and chemotherapeutic photoactivation with such substances as hematoporphyrin appear to hold promise. Some of the new systemic regimens for metastatic transitional cell carcinoma also appear increasingly effective. Unfortunately, renal cell carcinoma has remained resistant to chemotherapeutic efforts. In prostatic carcinoma many agents have been utilized over the years, and newer agents are studied each year, but no new chemotherapeutic agent has any obvious therapeutic efficacy greater than diethylstilbestrol.

EDITORIAL COMMENT II

There has been increasing refinement of the protocols for testicular carcinoma with the use of bleomycin, etoposide, and cisplatin. There appears to be less toxicity with this regimen. Immunotherapy has been developed for carcinoma of the kidney, but the protocols employing interleukin-II (IL-2) and LAK cell therapy have had very significant toxicity. In the future, combinations of biologic response modifiers and chemotherapeutic agents may have more efficacy and less toxicity than some of the present regimens.

REFERENCES

1. Li FP, Connelly RR, Myers M: Improved survival rates among testis cancer patients in the United States. *JAMA* 1982; 247:825–826.
2. Li MC, Whitmore WF, Golbey RB, et al:

Effect of drug therapy on metastatic cancer of the testis. *JAMA* 1960; 174:1291.
3. Golbey RB: The place of chemotherapy in the treatment of testicular tumors. *JAMA* 1970; 213:101–103.
4. Samuels ML, Lanzotti VJ, Holoye PY, et al: Combination chemotherapy in germinal cell tumors. *Cancer Treat Rev* 1976; 3:135–204.
5. Einhorn LH: Testicular cancer as a model for a curable neoplasm: The Richard and Hinda Rosenthal Foundation Award Lecture. *Cancer Res* 1981; 41:3275–3280.
6. Einhorn LH, Donohue J: Cis-diamminedichloroplatinum, vinblastine, and bleomycin combination chemotherapy in disseminated testicular cancer. *Ann Intern Med* 1977; 87:293–298.
7. Vugrin D, Herr HW, Whitmore WF Jr, et al: VAB-6 combination chemotherapy in disseminated cancer of the testis. *Ann Intern Med* 1981; 95:59–61.
8. Einhorn LH, Williams SD, Troner M, et al: The role of maintenance therapy in disseminated testicular cancer. *N Engl J Med* 1981; 305:727–731.
9. Schilsky RL, Anderson T: Hypomagnesemia and renal magnesium wasting in patients receiving cisplatin. *Ann Intern Med* 1979; 90:929–931.
10. Seigel LJ, Longo DL: The control of chemotherapy-induced emesis. *Ann Intern Med* 1981; 95:352–359.
11. Reynolds TF, Vugrin D, Cvitkovic E, et al: VAB-3 combination chemotherapy of metastatic testicular cancer. *Cancer* 1981; 48:888–898.
12. Pascual RS, Mosher MB, Sikand RS, et al: Effects of bleomycin on pulmonary function in man. *Am Rev Respir Dis* 1973; 108:211–217.
13. Goldiner PL, Carlon GC, Cvitkovic E, et al: Factors influencing postoperative morbidity and mortality in patients treated with bleomycin. *Br Med J* 1978; 1:1664–1667.
14. Weiss RB, Brumo S: Hypersensitivity reactions to cancer chemotherpeutic agents. *Ann Intern Med* 1981; 94:66–72.
15. Trump DL, Anderson SA: Gynecomastia following cytotoxic therapy for testis cancer: A potentially favorable prognostic sign? *J Clin Oncol* 1983; 1:416–420.
16. Dragsa RE, Einhorn LE, Williams SD, et al: Fertility after chemotherapy for testicular cancer. *J Clin Oncol* 1983; 1:179–184.
17. Vogelzang NJ, Bosl GJ, Johnson K, et al: Raynaud's phenomenon: A common toxicity after combination chemotherapy for testicular cancer. *Ann Intern Med* 1981; 95:288–292.
18. Valdiviesco M, Pazdur R, Flaherty L, et al: Intensive chemotherapy (int-rx) of small cell lung cancer (sclc) with weekly etoposide (e), cyclophosphamide (c), hydroxyurea (h), and oncovin (O)—echo. *Proc Annu Meet Am Soc Clin Oncol* 1988; 7:A848.
19. Ozols RF, Corden BJ, Jacob J, et al: High-dose cisplatin in hypertonic saline. *Ann Intern Med* 1984; 100:19–24.
20. Ozols RF, Deisseroth AB, Javadpour N, et al: Treatment of poor prognosis nonseminomatous testicular cancer with a 'high dose' platinum combination chemotherapy regimen. *Cancer* 1983; 51:1803–1807.
21. Trump DL, Hortvet L: Etoposide (VP16) and very high dose cisplatinum in refractory testis cancer. *Cancer Treat Rep* 1985; 69:259–262.
22. Bessman JD, Johnson RK, Goldin A: Permeability of normal and cancerous rat bladder to antineoplastic agents. *Urology* 1975; 6:187–193.
23. Jones HC, Swinney J: Thiotepa in the treatment of tumours of the bladder. *Lancet* 1961; 2:7–11.
24. Koontz WW Jr, Prout GR Jr, Smith W, et al: The use of intravesical thio-tepa in the management of non-invasive carcinoma of the bladder. *J Urol* 1981; 125:307–312.
25. Mishina T, Watanabe H: Mitomycin-C bladder instillation therapy for bladder tumors, in Carter SK, Crooke ST (eds): *Mitomycin-C: Current Status and New Developments.* New York, Academic Press, 1979, pp 193–203.
26. Jacobi GH, Kurth K: Studies on the intravesical action of topically administered G ^{3}H-doxorubicin hydrochloride in men: Plasma uptake and tumor penetration. *J Urol* 1980; 124:34–37.
27. Brossman SA: Experience with bacillus Calmette-Guérin in patients with superficial bladder carcinoma. *J Urol* 1982; 128:27–29.

28. Morales A: Adjuvant immunotherapy in superficial bladder cancer. *Natl Cancer Inst Monogr* 1978; 49:315–319.
29. Harker WG, Torti FM: The chemotherapy of bladder carcinoma: Systemic therapy. *Recent Results Cancer Res* 1983; 85:37–49.
30. Balis FM: Pharmacokinetic drug interactions of commonly used anticancer drugs. *Clin Pharmacokinet* 1986; 11:223–235.
31. Frei III E, Blum RH, Pitman SW, et al: High dose methotrexate with leucovorin rescue. Rationale and spectrum of antitumor activity. *Am J Med* 1980; 68:370–376.
32. Khandekar JD, Elson PJ, DeWys WD, et al: Comparative activity and toxicity of cis-diamminedichloroplatinum (DDP) and a combination of doxorubicin, cyclophosphamide, and DDP in disseminated transitional cell carcinomas of the urinary tract. *J Clin Oncol* 1985; 3:539–545.
33. Soloway M, Einstein A, Corder M, et al: A comparison of cis-platinum and the combination of cis-platinum and cyclophosphamide in advanced urothelial cancer. A National Bladder Cancer Collaborative study. *Cancer* 1983; 52:767–772.
34. Sternberg CN, Yagoda A, Scher HI, et al: Preliminary results of M-VAC (methotrexate, vinblastine, doxorubicin and cisplatin) for transitional cell carcinoma of the urothelium. *J Urol* 1985; 133:403–407.
35. Harker WG, Freiha FS, Shortliffe LD, et al: Cisplatin, methotrexate, and vinblastine (CMV) chemotherapy (CT) for metastatic cancer of the uroepithelium. *Proc Am Soc Clin Oncol* 1983; 2:135.
36. Douple EB, Richmond RC: A review of interactions between platinum coordination complexes and ionizing radiation: Implications for cancer therapy, in Prestayko AW, Crooke ST, Carter SK (eds): *Cisplatin: Current Studies and New Development*. New York, Academic Press, 1980, pp 125–147.
37. Ruckdeschel JC, Baxer DH, McKneally MF, et al: Sequential radiotherapy and Adriamycin in the management of bronchogenic carcinoma. The question of additive toxicity. *Int J Radiat Oncol Biol Phys* 1979; 5:1323–1328.
38. Quesada JR, Swanson DA, Trindade A, et al: Renal carcinoma: Antitumor effects of leukocyte interferon. *Cancer Res* 1983; 43:940–943.
39. Trump DL, Harris J, Tuttle R, et al: Phase II trial of high dose human lymphoblastoid interferon (Wellferon) in advanced renal cell carcinoma. *Proc Am Soc Clin Oncol* 1984; 3:153.
40. Neidhart JA, Gagen MM, Young D, et al: Interferon therapy of renal cancer. *Cancer Res* 1984; 44:4140–4143.
41. Isaacs A, Lindemann J: Virus interference: I. The interferon. *Proc R Soc Lond (Biol)* 1957; 147:258–267.
42. Adams F, Quesada JR, Gutterman JU: Neuropsychiatric manifestations of human leukocyte interferon therapy in patients with cancer. *JAMA* 1984; 252:938–941.
43. Figlin RA, deKernion JB, Malduzys J, et al: Treatment of renal cell carcinoma with alpha (human leukocyte) interferon and vinblastine in combination: A phase I-II trial. *Cancer Treat Rep* 1985; 69:263–367.
44. Ernstoff MS, Kirkwood JM: Changes in the bone marrow of cancer patients treated with recombinant interferon alpha-2. *Am J Med* 1984; 76:593–596.
45. Rosenberg SA, Lotze MT, Muul LM, et al: Special report: Observation on the systemic administration of autologous lymphokine-activated killer cells and recombinant interleukin-2 to patients with metastatic cancer. *N Engl J Med* 1985; 313:1485–1492.
46. Rosenberg SA, Lotze MT, Muul LM, et al: A progress report on the treatment of 157 patients with advanced cancer using lymphokine-activated killer cells and interleukin-2 or high dose interleukin-2 alone. *N Engl J Med* 1987; 316:879–905.
47. Atkins MB, Mier JW, Parkinson DR, et al: Hypothyroidism after treatment with interleukin-2 and lymphokine-activated killer cells. *N Engl J Med* 1988; 318:1157–1563.
48. Gaynor ER, Vitek L, Stricklin L, et al: The hemodynamic effect of treatment with interleukin-2 and lymphokine-activated killer cells. *Ann Intern Med* 1988; 109:953–958.
49. Veterans Administration Co-operative Urological Research Group: Carcinoma of the prostate: Treatment comparisons. *J Urol* 1967; 98:516.
50. Bailar JC III, Byar DP, and Veterans Administration Co-Operative Urological Research Group: Estrogen treatment for can-

cer of the prostate: Early results with 3 doses of diethylstilbestrol and placebo. *Cancer* 1970; 26:257.

51. Kent JR, Bischoff AM, Arduino LJ, et al: Estrogen dosage and suppression of testosterone levels in patients with prostatic carcinoma. *J Urol* 1973; 109:858.
52. Stolear G, Albert DJ: SCH 13521 in the treatment of advanced carcinoma of the prostate. *J Urol* 1974; 111:803.
53. Narayana HS, Loening SH, Culp DH: Flutamide in the treatment of metastatic carcinoma of the prostate. *Br J Urol* 1981; 53:152.
54. Jacobi GH, Altwein JE, Kurth KH, et al: Treatment of advanced prostatic cancer with parenteral cyproterone acetate: A Phase III randomised trial. *Br J Urol* 1980; 52:208–215.
55. Geller J, Albert J, Yen SS: Treatment of advanced cancer of prostate with megestrol acetate. *Urology* 1978; 12:537–541.
56. Block M, Trump DL, Rose DP, et al: Aminoglutethimide treatment of stage D prostate cancer: Clinical and pharmacologic studies. *Cancer Treat Rep* 1984; 68:719–722.
57. Walsh PC, Siteri PK: Suppression of plasma androgens by spironolactone on castrated men with carcinoma of the prostate. *J Urol* 1975; 114:254.
58. Trachtenberg J, Halpern N, Pont A: Ketoconazole: A novel and rapid treatment for advanced prostatic cancer. *J Urol* 1983; 130:152.
59. Labrie F, Cusan L, Seguin C, et al: Antifertility effects of LHRH agonists in the male rat and inhibition of testicular steroidogenesis in man. *Int J Fertil* 1980; 25:157–170.
60. Labrie F, Auclair C, Cusan L, et al: Inhibitory effect of LHRH and its agonists on testicular gonadotropin receptors and spermatogenesis in the rat. *Int J Androl* 1978; 2:303–318.
61. Borgmann V, Nagel R, Al-Abadi H, et al: Treatment of prostatic cancer with LH-RH analogues. *Prostate* 1983; 4:553.
62. Koutsilieris M, Tolis G: Gonadotropin-releasing hormone agonistic analogues in the treatment of advanced prostatic carcinoma. *Prostate* 1985; 4:569.
63. Smith JA: Androgen suppression by a gonadotropin releasing hormone analogue in patients with metastatic carcinoma of the prostate. *J Urol* 1984; 131:1110.
64. The Leuprolide Study Group: Leuprolide versus diethylstilbestrol for metastatic prostate cancer. *N Engl J Med* 1984; 311:1281.
65. Ahmed SR, Grant J, Shalet SM, et al: Preliminary report on use of depot formulation of LHRH analogue ICI 118630 (Zoladex) in patients with prostatic cancer. *Br Med J* 1985; 290:185–187.
66. Labrie F, Dupont A, Belanger A, et al: New approach in the treatment of prostate cancer: Complete instead of partial withdrawal of androgens. *Prostate* 1983; 4:579.
67. Crawford ED, Mcleod D, Door A, et al: A comparison of leuprolide with flutamide and leuprolide in untreated stage d2 prostate cancer. Presented at International Symposium on Endocrine Therapy, Nov 19–21: Monaco, A35a, 48.
68. Torti FM, Carter SK: The chemotherapy of prostatic adenocarcinoma. *Ann Intern Med* 1980; 92:681–689.
69. Murphy GP, Slack NH, Mittelman A, et al: Experiences with estramustine phosphate (Estracyt, Emcyt) in prostate cancer. *Semin Oncol* 1983, 10:34–42.

CHAPTER 8

Respiratory Complications and Complications of Anesthesia

Judith L. Stiff, M.D.

INFORMED CONSENT

Anesthesia complications range from the minor, such as nausea and vomiting, to the full disaster of cardiac arrest and death. Surgeons need to be aware of potential anesthetic complications, especially complications related to their specific procedure, so that they can adequately answer patients' questions. Discussion of the risk of a procedure can be difficult, especially when the surgeon or anesthesiologist believes that such a discussion will be upsetting to a patient in the face of the need for an operation. However, because of the recognized necessity for a patient to participate in the decision to undergo a procedure or treatment, risks must be discussed. Much of the burden of answering a patient's questions about anesthesia rests upon the surgeon, since the patient's questions start as soon as the operation is proposed, and the anesthesiologist usually does not have the opportunity to meet the patient until the night before the operation. That time, so close to the operation itself, is a poor time to be presenting great quantities of sobering information about risks and complications. Sometimes the patient will not be really listening or understanding what is being said.

THE RISK OF ANESTHESIA AND OPERATION

The risk of anesthesia (actually, the risk of perioperative mortality) can be put into a realistic framework, with numbers and percentages, for patients who want to have it expressed in those terms. The overall risk of perioperative mortality is usually related to the physical status of the patient (Table 8–1).[1, 2] This assignment of physical status began in the 1950s, and the mortality associated with the various classifications has remained relatively unchanged since then.

Anesthesia or operative risk in the healthy patient ought to be exceedingly small and be that due to drug interaction or unrecognized concomitant disease. Elimination of the risk of error or equipment problems has always been the goal, and newer monitoring techniques are be-

TABLE 8–1.
Physical Status Classification and Associated Perioperative Mortality

Classification	Physical Status	Mortality Rate (%) Marx et al.[1]	Farrow et al.[2]	Warner et al.[3]
I	A normal, healthy patient	0.06	0.3	0.0
II	A patient with a mild to moderate systemic disease	0.47	0.9	0.03
III	A patient with a severe systemic disease that limits activity but is not incapacitating	4.4	5.3	
IV	A patient with an incapacitating systemic disease or a systemic disease that is very poorly controlled	23.5	25.9	
V	A moribund patient who is not expected to survive 24 hr with or without operation	50.8	57.8	

ing used to reach that goal. A recent study looked at the mortality for healthy patients undergoing operations since 1985, in whom pulse oximetry was used to monitor oxygen saturation. Perioperative mortality was found to be less than earlier studies (see Table 8–1).[3]

To relate this classification to numbers that nonmedical people might understand better, anesthesia mortality can be compared to motor vehicle accidental death: In 1985, the death rate for motor vehicle accidents for all ages was 0.0192% for all ages, but as high as 0.0531% for males 15 to 24 years old.[4] Thus, the risk of anesthesia and operative death for a healthy patient is in the same range as his risk of dying in an automobile accident during a single year.

However, for patients with significant preexisting conditions, the perioperative risk can be much higher. One area of preexisting disease for which some data are available is recent myocardial infarction (see Chap. 1, Cardiovascular Complications). Most anesthesiologists would prefer not to administer anesthesia within 6 months of a myocardial infarction. This is based upon studies such as those from the Mayo Clinic,[5, 6] which showed the same reinfarction rate in 1975 as in 1968, with a significant decrease in this rate if the myocardial infarction was more than 6 months old (Table 8–2). However, a more recent study has shown a dramatic decrease in those reinfarction rates.[7] These authors suggest this decrease may be due to more sophisticated anesthesia care, involving invasive hemodynamic monitoring. If these new numbers are reliable, then recent myocardial infarction becomes a less-feared entity. However, are all myocardial infarctions alike, or is a simple subendocardial infarction different from one that was accompanied by complex arrhythmias and/or congestive heart failure? Most would agree that the patient who had the myocardial infarction accompanied by complications or who now requires multiple medications for control of his cardiac conditions is at a much higher risk, and that the mere history of myocardial infarction is only part of the story.

TABLE 8–2.
Risk of Perioperative Reinfarction

Previous Myocardial Infarction (%) <3 mo	3–6 mo	>6 mo	Study
37.0	16.0	5.0	Tarhan et al. (1972)[5]
27.0	11.0	4.0–5.0	Steen et al. (1978)[6]
5.8	2.3	1.0	Rao et al. (1983)[7]

EVALUATION OF THE PULMONARY SYSTEM

Respiratory complications following anesthesia and operation are a major concern. Patients with preexisting pulmonary disease would be expected to have a higher risk of pulmonary complications. It has been shown that patients with chronic obstructive lung disease requiring regular treatment with bronchodilators who undergo operations have up to three times the rate of postoperative respiratory complications as those without pulmonary disease.[8] The actual rate of complications is influenced by age, type of operation, and type of anesthesia. The preoperative evaluation of patients should have two goals: (1) establishing a baseline of respiratory function so that patients at risk can be identified, and (2) optimizing the conditions of patients with treatable respiratory disease.

Tests to Determine Respiratory Function.—Routine preoperative chest x-ray studies are rapidly declining in use as a screening tool. The procedure has been shown to be of little benefit in routine admissions to the hospital,[9] and many anesthesiology departments are dropping the chest x-ray requirement, except in patients with pulmonary or cardiac history. In a group of 368 patients with no risk factors, only one chest x-ray film (0.3%) was abnormal and did not affect surgery. In 504 patients with risk factors, 114 (22%) had significant abnormalities.[10] An x-ray study also should be obtained in instances where it might be useful as a comparison with possible postoperative films. Arterial blood gases are not a useful screening or predictive tool, because they tend to remain in the normal range until pulmonary status is significantly compromised, and because they only reflect a momentary point of respiratory function. However, they are useful and should be obtained preoperatively to determine a baseline for postoperative management of any patient with respiratory problems who is to undergo a major operation with potential pulmonary complications.

Prediction of Respiratory Insufficiency.—The tests that are the best predictors of postoperative respiratory difficulties for patients who have signs and symptoms of pulmonary disease are simple pulmonary function tests. Although some difference of opinion exists as to what battery of tests should be done, a vital capacity measurement (VC) and the 1-second forced expiratory volume (FEV_1) is sufficient in most cases to define problems of restrictive and obstructive disease. Response to bronchodilators should be added in cases of bronchospastic diseases. It may be necessary to add tests of diffusion for those few patients with disease that impairs gas exchange.

The predictive value of pulmonary function tests relates to the degree of impairment and the site of operation. The effect of site of operation on postoperative respiratory function was first noted more than 50 years ago and more recently has been confirmed by other articles.[11, 12] Upper abdominal operations will cause a 60% to 75% reduction in vital capacity; lower abdominal operations, 40% to 50%; and flank, 30% to 40%. The maximum impairment is not immediate, but develops over the first 8 to 12 hours, and gradually resolves over the next several days. For patients with normal respiratory function, this reduction is not a problem. However, in order to cough, clear secretions, and avoid atelectasis, a patient needs an adequate vital capacity, in the range of 15 cc/kg or about 1,000 cc. If a patient starts preoperatively with a diminished vital capacity such that the reduction caused by the operation will bring his vital capacity below that necessary level, he runs a high risk of pneumonia, atelectasis, and respiratory failure. Similarly, an adequate expiratory flow is also necessary for clearing of secretions, which is usually thought to be an FEV_1 of 800 cc or more. Combining these guidelines with the site of operation, patients at risk can be identified: for example, with a patient who has only 30% of his predicted vital capacity, or one who has only 50% of his predicted vital capacity plus an FEV_1/VC of 50%, certainly there is a high risk for respiratory failure following a major abdominal operation. Patients who meet these criteria for possible respiratory failure, or come close to them, should be cared for postoperatively where they can be closely watched, especially since the time of maximum difficulty will be during the first postoperative night.

Optimizing Respiratory Condition.— It is also important to optimize the condition of patients whose respiratory status can be improved. Obviously, infection should be treated, and patients should be encouraged to stop smoking. Moderate to heavy smoking has been shown to double the incidence of postoperative respiratory complications.[13] Forty-eight hours of abstinence can be expected to return carboxyhemoglobin levels to the normal range. However, the effects of smoking on mucus clearance and small airway narrowing is not rapidly reversible. Patients can be taught the postoperative respiratory maneuvers they will be asked to perform, so that in the haze of postoperative pain and pain relievers, these maneuvers are understood. However, those patients who will benefit most by preoperative improvement of their respiratory conditions are those who have bronchospastic disease and are not optimally treated. If an asthmatic patient is actively wheezing, or if the pulmonary function tests of a patient with chronic obstructive pulmonary disease show a significant improvement when bronchodilators are administered, then it is wise to postpone the operation long enough to add to the patient's medical regimen and reassess his condition after institution of therapy.

The question of whether to cancel an operation when a patient has, or is recovering from, an upper respiratory infection (URI) is difficult to answer. There are problems in the actual definition of what signs and symptoms constitute a significant URI, as well as in determining the significance of some of the complications. For example, in 25 children with signs of URIs who underwent general anesthesia for otolaryngologic procedures, five had oxygen saturations below 95% in the recovery room while none of the 20 without URIs had low saturations.[14] However, neither group had any further increased or new respiratory symptoms. In patients up to 20 years of age undergoing general anesthesia for a variety of procedures, the group with URI symptoms had a similar intraoperative complication rate (laryngospasm, bronchospasm) as those with no symptoms.[15] However, there was an increased rate of these intraoperative events in patients who had recently recovered from a URI. It does seem prudent to postpone a purely elective general anesthetic in the face of a current or recent URI and to carefully assess patients with URIs who need urgent procedures to be sure that one is dealing with a mild viral disease only.

RENAL DISEASE AND ANESTHESIA

The patient with renal compromise presents a twofold problem to the anesthesiologist: avoiding further renal compromise in the patient who has some remaining function and limiting the potential for altered drug excretion. Renal damage can be caused by drugs; however, in present anesthesia practice this damage is rarely a problem. An inhalational agent, methoxyflurane (Penthrane), has been implicated in high-output renal failure caused by one of its metabolic products, free fluoride ion. However, this agent is rarely used. Knowledge of this complication has led to the very careful use of enflurane (Ethrane) in patients in whom renal disease is already present or may occur in the perioperative period. Enflurane does have free flouride ion as one of its metabolic products, but in quantities many times less than methoxyflurane. Since there are other inhalational agents and techniques available, enflurane can usually be avoided or used in very low doses in patients at risk.

A more threatening situation to poorly functioning kidneys is further damage due to poor renal perfusion. General anesthesia has some depressant effect on renal blood flow and glomerular filtration. However, of greater consequence would be any further reduction in perfusion caused by prolonged hypotension.

The only class of anesthetic drugs seriously affected by altered excretion are the nondepolarizing neuromuscular blocking agents. Two, gallamine and decamethonium, are totally excreted by the kidney and are not given to patients with renal dysfunction. Two older agents, pancuronium bromide (Pavulon) and curare and its derivatives, are excreted renally in normal patients but have an alternative pathway of hepatic metabolism and can be used on patients with little or no renal function, provided they are used with caution. The two newer agents, atracurium besylate (Tracrium) and vecuronium bromide (Norcuron), are less of a problem. The first does not depend upon the kidney or liver for its degradation, and the latter is 50% metabolized by the liver, making both drugs easy to use in the patient with little or no renal function.

Overall, it is important not to impose additional hazards upon poorly functioning kidneys at the time of operation. Therefore, doses of nephrotoxic drugs, such as gentamicin, should be carefully monitored, dehydration must be avoided, and patients having studies involving the administration of hypertonic contrast materials should have their renal function carefully monitored, so that multiple factors which might combine to produce postoperative renal failure are avoided.

PREEXISTING DRUG THERAPY

Preexisting drug therapy has consequences for anesthetic management. Monoamine oxidase (MAO) inhibitors are the one class of drugs that should be discontinued, if possible, prior to anesthesia. These drugs can cause very exaggerated swings in blood pressure. However, stopping them should only be done in consultation with the patient's psychiatrist. All other drugs can safely be continued.

The most frequent hazard of preexisting drug therapy is discontinuance. This loss of medication leads to the possibilities of exacerbation of medical conditions. In general, patients should continue with their drug regimens up to and including the morning of operation, especially when the medications are short-acting agents for control of such conditions as arrhythmias, angina, hypertension, bronchospasm, and seizures.

SPINAL VS. GENERAL ANESTHESIA

Urologic procedures can be done under either general or regional (spinal, epidural, or caudal) anesthesia. Frequently, the opinion of cardiologists and internists is that regional anesthesia is "safer." Overall, there is little difference in risk. A comparison of the overall perioperative mortality found regional to be 0.9% and general to be 1.8%, but the difference was due to very few regionals being done on the higher-risk class IV and V patients.[1] Risk for class II patients was 0.4% for regional and 0.5% for general.

Currently, many centers are looking

at the regional vs. general anesthesia debate. In a group of patients greater than 90 years of age undergoing hip replacement or transurethral prostatic resection (TURP), no difference between the two forms of anesthesia was found in either perioperative mortality or long-term outcome.[16] However, in a study of patients undergoing major intrathoracic, intraabdominal or major vascular operations, those having epidural plus light general anesthesia and receiving postoperative epidural narcotics had fewer cardiovascular complications and lower hospital costs than patients who underwent purely general anesthesia.[17] Yet, in another group of patients who underwent vascular operations, those having epidurals had more episodes of myocardial ischemia.[18] The fact that consistent conclusions cannot be drawn is due to the difficulties in performing such studies well and dealing with all the confounding factors. The decision for the type of anesthesia must be based upon surgical needs, specific risks to the individual patient, and the patient's opinion once the options and risks have been presented.

Complications of Regional Anesthesia

Neurologic Complications.—From a patient's viewpoint, the most feared complications are those of neurologic deficit, and many patients claim to know of a case where someone was paralyzed by spinal anesthesia. However, neurologic deficits attributable to regional anesthesia are rare, and complete paralysis of one or more extremities is exceedingly rare. In a comprehensive review of the literature encompassing several large series of patients, an incidence of deficits of 0.00% to 0.077% following spinal anesthesia, and 0.000% to 0.168% for epidural anesthesia, was found; however, among these were many minor deficits consisting of paresthesias only.[19] Some of these reports are older, and in years past some of the damage may have been due to factors that are no longer a threat, such as the preservatives in the drugs.

Hypotension.—Of greater threat is the hypotension that can be caused by spinal or epidural anesthesia due to the sympathetic blockade that is established along with the sensory and motor block. In dealing with a patient with significant cardiac or cerebral vascular disease, this complication can have serious consequences, because the sympathetic block can have a very rapid onset. If a patient has an adequate intravascular volume, hypotension is usually rapidly reversed by the administration of a vasopressor and additional intravenous fluids. As the block wears off some hours later, those additional fluids may be difficult to manage in the patient with diminished cardiac function.

Post–Lumbar Puncture Headache.—More worrisome rather than serious are the complications of nausea and vomiting during spinal or epidural anesthesia and post–lumbar puncture headache. Nausea and vomiting may be due to reflexes from the operative field or the use of some intravenous sedation agents. Post–lumbar puncture headache following spinal anesthesia or inadvertent dural puncture during epidural anesthesia has a reported incidence of 11%.[20] However, Vandam and Dripps showed that the incidence was lower in older patients and related to needle size.[20] The greatest incidence was in women receiving spinal anesthesia for deliveries. If the obstetric group is removed, the incidence dropped to 9.5%, and if the dural puncture was performed with a 22-gauge needle or smaller, the incidence dropped to 8.4%. In their series, 72% of post–lumbar puncture headaches lasted 1 week or less, and only 6% persisted 3 or more months. They also reported a 0.4%

incidence of occular complaints and a 0.4% incidence of auditory complaints. Although a patient who develops a post–lumbar puncture headache can be reassured that it will go away, it can be an extremely intense headache, unresponsive to usual remedies, and can delay recovery from the operation, because the best relief is obtained by maintaining recumbency. Treatment consists of bed rest, increasing fluid intake, and use of an abdominal binder.

Advantages of Regional Anesthesia

Regional anesthesia does offer significant advantages, the principal one being that the patient does not receive the myocardial depressant drugs that are used for general anesthesia. Regional anesthesia has a distinct advantage for the patient undergoing TURP in that the signs of water intoxication may be more readily recognized in the awake or semiawake patient. Patients usually feel less groggy and resume oral intake faster after regional.

There is increasing evidence that the use of epidural or intrathecal anesthesia with local anesthetics and/or narcotics postoperatively can decrease postoperative ventilatory dysfunction as well as provide long-acting pain relief with minimal respiratory depression. It has been shown that thoracic epidural block with local anesthetic partially reversed the decrease in forced vital capacity (FVC) caused by upper abdominal operations.[21] In a comparison of patients receiving continuous intravenous morphine with those having either intercostal or epidural local anesthetic after operation and having comparable levels of pain relief, more than half who received morphine had multiple episodes of oxygen desaturation, while none of the local anesthesia group did.[22]

Advantages of General Anesthesia

General anesthesia is the choice of many patients because they are afraid of spinal or they have been told to be afraid of it, or because they want to be asleep and "not know anything." General anesthesia does offer some real advantages in certain instances. Its main advantage is that it can be induced gradually and slowly, testing the patient's response at each step. It allows for controlled ventilation, which is necessary for some operations and patient positions. It is often believed that a regional technique is best for the patient with chronic obstructive pulmonary disease. However, in a patient who relies on his abdominal musculature for exhalation, a high spinal or epidural may not be best, and controlled ventilation under general anesthesia with attention to bronchial hygiene may be advantageous.

Thus, in the argument about regional vs. general anesthesia, the basic principle remains: the least anesthesia, carefully administered, is the best. Similarly, it is often held that for a minor procedure local is best. However, with a very anxious patient, an inadequate local or the stress of being wide-awake can produce symptoms such as angina or even precipitate cardiac decompensation. Other options, such as local anesthesia combined with intravenous sedation or regional or general anesthesia, should be considered.

Ambulatory Procedures

Many urologic procedures are now being done on an ambulatory basis and increasing numbers of surgical patients are not in the hospital the night before operation but are admitted on that morning. Obviously, if these patients are not as carefully evaluated and prepared for anesthesia and operation as are inpatients, an increased number of complications can be expected. However, with careful attention to evaluation standards and maintaining medical regimens and NPO status, handling patients this way is quite safe.

Many anesthesiologists would argue that there is no place for spinal or epidural anesthesia for outpatients because of the potential problem of a prolonged, subtle sensory and proprioceptive block which could lead to patient injuries. If one is dealing with a reasonable patient who understands the precautions when going home and discharge criteria are well established, regional anesthesia, using short-acting agents can be offered to outpatients. The fact that a post–lumbar puncture headache can occur after the patient has returned home is really not an issue, as it can be managed by telephone consultation, or, if necessary, by bringing the patient in for treatment. In one study of outpatients having significant headache after spinal anesthesia, the incidence was 11%.[23] There was a significantly greater incidence in females (16.6%) than in males (4%), and there were no headaches in patients over 55 years of age. For patients choosing regional anesthesia, epidural seems better for young women.

Complications of anesthesia that are considered to be minor in inpatients become greater problems in outpatients because they may require admission to the hospital. Protracted vomiting, fever, excessive sleepiness, bleeding, inability to void all can become significant. Overnight admission rates should be less than 2% if proper selection of patients and procedures is followed. Factors which have been shown to lead to higher admission rates are abdominal surgery, longer operating time, and higher ASA (American Society of Anesthesiologists) physical status.[24]

PROBLEMS WITH POSITIONING FOR OPERATION

In considering the risks of anesthesia, one usually thinks of problems caused by anesthetic agents and techniques. However, severe problems can be caused by positioning. Many urologic procedures utilize positions that can be physiologically compromising as well as having the potential for nerve damage. Any position change can lead to hemodynamic instability, due to shifts in intravascular volumes in the face of vasodilation with either regional or general anesthesia and the blunting of normal homeostatic mechanisms.

Kidney Position

Placing the patient into "kidney position" is potentially the most physiologically compromising. Not only is the patient's position shifted rapidly, but after that shift, the table is flexed and the kidney rest is raised. In addition to the shifts in blood volume, these maneuvers may cause impedance to venous return to the heart by compressing the vena cava. It is important that this position be achieved slowly, with frequent verification of blood pressure to assure adequate cardiac output.

Once the position has been achieved safely, there are other potential hazards. The down lung, because of the impaired descent of the diaphragm, often becomes atelectatic at the base, and although atelectasis is not a problem during the procedure because the patient's ventilation is controlled, it may lead to respiratory problems postoperatively. Additionally, the pleura may be entered on the side of the operation. If the air is not sufficiently evacuated at the end or if a chest tube is not placed, the patient is left with another potential for respiratory difficulty (pneumothorax) after a seemingly straightforward operation.

The potential for nerve damage in the kidney position is mainly in the down arm, with pressure on the brachial plexus at the axilla. This damage is prevented by the placement of an axillary roll slightly caudal to the axilla, to allow the vessels and nerves to be free from pressure. It is inadvisable to secure the up arm to the ether screen, as this may easily involve pressure to vulnerable points or stretching of the brachial plexus. Pillows or pads between the arms will allow adequate positioning. The most vulnerable point of the lower extremities is on the leg, where the common peroneal nerve comes around the head of the fibula. The leg should be checked for the necessity of extra padding, because pressure here can result in foot drop and sensory deficit along the lateral aspect of the leg.

Lithotomy Position

Placing a patient into the lithotomy position may actually be helpful in instances of hypotension caused by induction of regional or general anesthesia, since this elevation will cause a shift of blood from the legs back to the central circulation. However, the opposite effect may occur when the legs are put down at the end of the procedure. Thus, this move should be made slowly, while the anesthesiologist is checking the blood pressure, especially in patients whose cardiovascular status is precarious. The lithotomy position has been shown to reduce vital capacity, which can be of significance in the spontaneously breathing patient who is under regional anesthesia. However, the degree of compromise is not as great as in other positions.

Nerve damage to the lower extremities is associated with lithotomy position. If the patient is in ankle straps or hanging stirrups, care must be taken that the lateral aspect of the calf is not resting against the unpadded metal, causing pressure on the peroneal nerve. If the legs are supported behind the knees, these areas must be well padded. When putting the legs up, both legs should be moved together. The placement of the legs should always be symmetric. A patient with preexisting back or hip problems can be placed into position prior to the induction of general anesthesia to assure comfortable positioning.

Trendelenburg Position

Adding Trendelenburg to any position can cause aberrations in physiology proportional to the degree of head down-tilt. This position can mask uncompensated blood loss and lead to hypotension upon resuming a level position. If adequate ventilation is not maintained in this position, the weight of the abdominal contents will lead to hypoventilation and atelectasis. Head down-tilt can cause venous distention of the upper body, which can lead to facial edema if this position is maintained for long periods of time. More importantly, the increased venous pressure leads to decreased intracranial perfusion pressure. This is not a problem as long as other factors that can decrease perfusion pressure do not exist, such as the patient already having increased intracranial pressure or the arterial blood pressure not being adequately maintained. In theory, having the pelvis higher than the heart could lead to air entrainment through open veins and resulting air embolus; however, this complication does not seem to occur.

Lithotripsy

Water immersion lithotripsy presents an unusual situation where the anesthesiologist has very limited access to the patient. The procedure is usually done under either epidural or general anesthesia, and after induction the patient is placed in the semiseated position which can lead to hypotension because of the vasodilation caused by anesthesia. This may be partially overcome by the hydrostatic pressure of water immersion. Intrapleural infusion of local anesthetic[25] and intercostal block with local infiltration[26] are possible alternative anesthesia methods which can be used. It seems that local infiltration over the area of entry of the shock wave is necessary to prevent discomfort.[25]

The presence of a cardiac pacemaker can be a problem in any lithotripsy procedure because the shock wave can induce dysfunction. Certainly an abdominally placed generator is at great risk for induced arrhythmias. However, for generators in the chest wall, if a route for transvenous pacing is available and the pulse generator is checked before, during, and after the procedure for the stability of the programming, lithotripsy can be performed.[27]

Nerve Injury

In any position, care must be taken with arm position. The greatest incidence of peripheral nerve injuries following operations is to the nerves of the upper extremity. Overall, the incidence of peripheral nerve damage in two retrospective studies was less than 0.2%, but with upper extremity nerve damage comprising more than two thirds of the cases.[28, 29] The mechanisms of injury are several. The brachial plexus can be injured by stretching, which is caused by having the arm abducted greater than 90 degrees. For this reason it is important that arm boards on operating room tables lock into position, so that during the procedure the surgeon or his or her assistants cannot inadvertently force the arm into greater abduction. The ulnar nerve is most prone to injury, since it passes in the groove of the medial epicondyle of the humerus. If an arm is poorly tucked at the patient's side, or if the patient is too large to fit both arms safely on the table, the arm may loosen and rest on the metal side rail of the operating table. Even on an arm board, the ulnar nerve can be damaged, but if the arm is placed palm up, the elbow will be rotated so that the ulnar groove is free. The radial nerve is most vulnerable to pressure, since it winds around the lateral side of the midsection of the humerus. Median nerve damage is unusual, but it passes parallel and lateral to the basilic vein in the antecubital fossa so that it can be injured by venipuncture or extravasation of sclerosing solutions.

When any nerve damage is discovered following operation, the extremity should be protected to prevent further injury. Fortunately, a large percentage of the lesions resolve; however, it is important to obtain appropriate consultation so treatment can be started and any contributing conditions relieved.

POSTOPERATIVE RESPIRATORY COMPLICATIONS OF ANESTHESIA

Early Complications

Postoperative respiratory complications can be thought of as those occurring immediately after the operation and those occurring many hours later. Immediate respiratory difficulty or inadequate ventilation is caused by anesthetic drugs or an intraoperative event.

Residual Anesthetic Drugs.—Residual anesthetic drugs are the most common cause of respiratory insufficiency in the recovery room. Although almost any drug used in anesthesia or a combination of drugs can lead to respiratory depression, most often it is narcotics or muscle relaxants. Usually the presence of residual anesthetic drugs affecting respiration is recognized at the end of the case, and the patient is left with supplemental oxygen or intubated and on a ventilator. However, the signs of hypoventilation can be subtle, and a partially anesthetized patient will not complain of shortness of breath, and rising levels of carbon dioxide will make him more obtunded. Therefore, the less obvious signs, such as hypertension and tachycardia, must be considered as signs of respiratory problems before dismissing them as due to other causes.

Narcotic respiratory depression may not be immediately obvious, since the patient may seem fully awake while being transferred to the stretcher and the recovery room, only to become quite narcotized as soon as the stimulation ends. Even though narcotics were not given during the operation, a premedication of narcotics may be the problem if the operation itself was short. Although a narcotic antagonist, naloxone hydrochloride (Narcan), can be given, this agent should be used with great caution, for the sudden reversal it causes has been reported to result in extreme hypertension,[30] pulmonary edema,[31] and even sudden death.[32] Also, the reversal will often leave the patient in pain, which cannot be helped by narcotics until the antagonist has disappeared. If a narcotic antagonist is used, the ampule should be diluted and the drug titrated slowly until respiration improves, and the patient's heart rate and blood pressure need to be carefully monitored. Consequently, it is best to continue to stimulate and remind the patient to breathe or leave him on ventilatory support until the narcotic has worn off enough.

Muscle relaxants may be inadequately reversed after a procedure. Reversal consists of blocking the breakdown of acetylcholine, leading to its accumulation rather than a direct antagonism of a muscle relaxant. As a result, if there is too much muscle relaxant at the neuromuscular junctions, reversal will not work. Also, other factors lead to possible difficulty in reversal; for example, some antibiotics potentiate muscle relaxants. A patient who remains blocked after attempts at reversal needs to be ventilated until such time as reversal will work.

Intraoperative Events.—Many untoward events occurring during operation may lead to postoperative respiratory insufficiency. Sometimes these events are not recognized during the operation because the patient's ventilation has been controlled. They include pneumothorax, atelectasis, obstruction of a bronchus by a foreign body or mucous plug, pulmonary edema, aspiration, and bronchospasm. Other, less common, intraoperative "events" that can present as respiratory depression include hyponatremia, hypoadrenalism, or hypoglycemia.

Late Complications

Later respiratory complications (hours to days after operation) include events not related to anesthesia and operation. The late complications are mainly those of atelectasis, infection, and respiratory insufficiency in patients who had preexisting respiratory disease. These complications should be anticipated after operations affecting vital capacity, as discussed earlier. Postoperative management should include maneuvers to prevent atelectasis and promote clearing of secretions, such as deep breathing and incentive spirometry, as well as constant evaluation of pulmonary status. For patients with a high likelihood of respiratory failure as predicted by their pulmonary function tests, elective postoperative ventilation may be the best approach, with weaning from support after the maximum respiratory effects of the operation are over. Patients whose respiratory status is not bad enough to anticipate respiratory failure but who also have significant cardiac disease may also benefit from elective ventilatory support, because the additional stress of the work of breathing with reduced vital capacity can lead to cardiac dysfunction.

Aspiration

Aspiration remains a severe respiratory threat. The severity of the pneumonitis is relative to the amount and pH of the aspirate; more than 50 mL or a pH of less than 2.5 are indicative of a potentially serious aspiration.[33] Obviously, the presence of a full stomach greatly increases the possibility of aspiration despite the precautions of performing a "rapid sequence" induction. In one study of anesthetic and operative mortality, six of the 645 total deaths were due to aspiration.[1]

COMPLICATIONS OF INVASIVE MONITORING

As medical care has become more sophisticated, sicker patients are being brought to operation. Therefore, there has been a rapid escalation in invasive monitoring in anesthetic care. Of course, more invasive procedures lead to new complications. With all vascular catheters, infection, bleeding, and thrombosis are hazards. Reported rates of infection are 3% to 8%, rates of bleeding are 1% to 4%, and thrombosis probably occurs to some extent on all catheters.[34, 35]

The complications of obtaining central venous access varies with the route used; the external jugular route has minimal complications, the internal jugular has a 5% to 10% incidence of complications, and the subclavian, 10% to 15%.[36] The complications include inadvertent arterial puncture, sheared-off catheter segments, and misplaced catheters that send fluid into the pleural space or mediastinum. Reported unusual complications include thoracic duct damage, nerve damage, arrhythmias, neurologic deficits due to carotid manipulation, superior vena cava syndrome, creation of an atrioventricular fistula, and puncture of an endotracheal tube cuff.

The most frequent problem with the placement of pulmonary artery catheters is arrhythmias; however, only a small percentage are life-threatening. More serious complications include pulmonary artery rupture and pulmonary infarction. The unusual complications of catheter knotting and damage to tricuspid or pulmonic valves have also been reported.

COMPLICATIONS OF FLUID AND BLOOD ADMINISTRATION

Hazards of intraoperative fluid administration include those which can occur any time intravenous fluids are administered, such as infection, extravasation, and electrolyte imbalance. An infrequent problem that can lead to delayed awakening is nonketotic hyperglycemic hyperosmolar coma. This complication can happen even when the patient has received little dextrose-containing solutions. Predisposing factors include older age, adult-onset–type diabetes, hyperalimentation, uremia, and other drug therapy such as phenytoin (Dilantin) or steroids.

Mismatched blood is more of a problem in the patient under anesthesia because the early signs will be missed. The very first signs of a mismatch will be diffuse oozing in the operative field and "port wine" urine. Other hazards of blood transfusion include those of minor reaction and transmission of infection. With increasing levels of anxiety about blood bank products, autologous transfusion is becoming more frequent for elective operations. This practice eliminates all transfusion hazards, provided meticulous labeling practices prevail.

HYPOTHERMIA

In today's well air–conditioned operating suites, hypothermia is a too-common anesthetic operative complication. When a patient becomes too cold, he is slower to wake up, but what is more important, the oxygen demand of rewarming may be very high, and a sick, older patient may not have the respiratory and cardiac reserve to respond. Anesthesia suspends the normal mechanisms of temperature regulation, and with the added exposure of open body cavities, it is easy for patients' core temperatures to drop to around 31° to 33° C. Small children are more susceptible to a cold environment because their body surface–body mass ratio is much greater.

Several methods can be used to prevent hypothermia. The most effective one is to minimize loss by maintaining a higher room temperature, especially for small children and during longer operations on all patients. Warming lights and blankets work well on small children but are ineffective on adults. Heated humidification of respiratory gases is fairly effective, and fluids and blood can be warmed. Placing the head and extremities in plastic bags can greatly reduce convective heat loss.

COMPLICATIONS OF LARYNGOSCOPY AND INTUBATION

Complications of laryngoscopy and intubation include those caused by mechanical factors and reflex physiologic reactions. Minor trauma includes lacerations to lips, pharynx, and larynx, as well as dental trauma. Bleeding from trauma in these areas can be quite profuse. Potentially more serious, but much less frequent, is trauma to the vocal cords, which includes ulceration, formation of granulomas, polyps, or dislocation of an arytenoid. Fortunately, the most frequent sequela is a sore throat, which to some extent occurs after most intubations. There have been rare cases of more severe traumatic problems, such as tracheal rupture or perforation of the esophagus or pharynx.

Reflex reactions occur when manipulation of the airway is attempted in an insufficiently anesthetized patient. In the asthmatic patient or in children, a too-hasty intubation can precipitate severe bronchospasm. Any patient can get reflex arrhythmias, hypotension, or hypertension. These reflexes also can take place upon extubation.

Complications of the tube itself include bronchial intubation or occlusion by a foreign body, blood, secretions, or kinking. All can result in hypoventilation of the patient.

Postextubation edema that is sufficient to cause problems is more common in children, because their small airways have little tolerance for encroachment. Many children wake up after anesthesia sounding "croupy" due to edema. Most clear with time and the administration of humidity to the inspired gases, but occasionally reintubation and tracheostomy is required. Unfortunately, a few children and a lesser number of adults progress to tracheal stenosis, usually in cases where the tube was in place for more than 48 hours. However, with careful attention to technique, proper tube size, use of tubes with low-pressure cuffs, and minimization of tube motion, these complications can be kept to a minimum.

RARE COMPLICATIONS OF ANESTHESIA

There are a few conditions in which anesthesia can have devastating results in a patient who otherwise seems perfectly normal. These conditions should be suspected when the patient or a member of his family has had a serious problem while undergoing anesthesia. If the history is one of a relative dying solely because of anesthesia and not the disease or operation itself, this history needs to be explored.

Malignant Hyperthermia.—Malignant hyperthermia is a familial disease with an overall incidence of 1 in 15,000 in children and young adults and 1 in 50,000 or less in older adults.[37] This disease is triggered by many of the anesthetic agents. Once the reaction is started, the patient becomes extremely hypermetabolic, a high body temperature develops, and often brain damage and renal failure result. Mortality is as high as 50%. Therefore, if this entity is suspected in the family or the patient himself, the anesthesiologist needs to see this patient well before the operation so that special tests, such as a muscle biopsy, can be obtained.

Atypical Pseudocholinesterase.—If the history is one of a patient or his family member requiring ventilatory support after a minor operation, this condition may be suggestive of a pseudocholinesterase deficiency and an inability to metabolize succinylcholine. Again, the anesthesiologist needs to be involved, since levels of this enzyme can be obtained.

Halothane Hepatitis.—Halothane hepatitis is a rare complication with an incidence of 0.003% and a high mortality.[38] Many other factors can be confusing, such as viral hepatitis, drug toxicity, biliary disease, shock, or sepsis. It is felt that repeated exposures to halothane over short periods of time in adults increase the likelihood of this reaction. The exact cause is unknown, but it may be due to combinations of factors, such as preexisting liver disease, hypoxia, decreased blood flow to the liver, and the metabolic products of halothane. In general, halothane is avoided in adults with recent exposure to the drug or with known liver disease. Treatment is supportive.

EDITORIAL COMMENT

The greatest risk of surgery is usually related to anesthesia and respiratory complications. Increasingly, ill and older patients are undergoing extensive surgery and are being maintained with careful monitoring. We have performed thoracoabdominal surgery with removal of intracardiac tumor thrombus from renal cell carcinoma with cardiopulmonary bypass, hypothermia, and temporary cardiac arrest in three patients older than 76 years. They all survived the procedure.

Other important features worthy of emphasis include the severe reduction in respiratory function and vital capacity with abdominal surgery. For example, upper abdominal operations will cause a 60% to 75% reduction in vital capacity. The importance of preoperative assessment is, therefore, underscored. Many of the operative positions used in urology also require careful attention because of their effects on blood pressure and venous return.

Lumbar punctures are also performed now for outpatient procedures, although we have already had spinal headaches related to these procedures. On the other hand, these headaches were not severe as long as a very small needle was used. If multiple lumbar punctures have been made or if a larger needle has been used, admission overnight to keep the patient flat may be indicated, although such management remains controversial.

EDITORIAL COMMENT II

This chapter has been significantly revised to include discussion of anesthesia in the ambulatory patient, lithotripsy, and the increased use of regional anesthesia. Complications will be even more important in the ambulatory patient as there will be increased risk for the physician from both medical and legal exposure. Although some of the newer lithotriptors do not require anesthesia, the vast majority of patients are still being treated with original Dornier units which do require anesthesia. In our unit with more than 1,000 patients, 98% have been managed with epidural anesthesia and this technique has proved to be very satisfactory.

Increasingly sophisticated monitoring continues to reduce anesthetic morbidity and mortality. Pulse oximetry to monitor oxygen saturation has been a simple but exceedingly valuable addition to the monitoring of the anesthetic patient. It probably should be considered routinely.

REFERENCES

1. Marx GF, Mateo CV, Orkin LR: Computer analysis of postanesthetic deaths. *Anesthesiology* 1973; 39:54–58.
2. Farrow SC, Fowkes FGR, Lunn JN, et al: Epidemiology in anesthesia: II. Factors affecting mortality in hospital. *Br J Anaesth* 1982; 54:811–817.
3. Warner MA, Warner ME, Narr BJ: Perioperative mortality and major morbidity in ASA Physical Status I and II patients undergoing non-emergent procedures: 1985–87. *Anesthesiology* 1988; 69:A721.
4. National Center for Health Statistics: *Vital Statistics of the United States, 1985.* Vol 2-*Mortality, Part A.* US Department of Health and Human Services Publication No (PHS) 88-1101. Washington, DC, Public Health Service, Government Printing Office, 1988.
5. Tarhan S, Moffitt EA, Taylor WF, et al. Myocardial infarction after general anesthesia. *JAMA* 1972; 220:1451–1454.
6. Steen PA, Tinker JH, Tarhan S: Myocardial reinfarction after anesthesia and surgery. *JAMA* 1978; 239:2566–2570.
7. Rao TKL, Jacobs KH, El-Etr AA: Reinfarction following anesthesia in patients with myocardial infarction. *Anesthesiology* 1983; 59:499–505.
8. Ringsted C, Pedersen T, Eliasen K, et al: Estimated risk of postoperative pulmonary complications in relation to general and regional anesthesia. *Anesthesiology* 1988; 69:A715.
9. National Center for Devices and Radiological Health: *The Selection of Patients for X-Ray Examinations: Chest X-Ray Screening Examinations.* US Department of Health and Human Services Publication No. (FDA) 83-8204. Washington, DC, Public Health Service Government Printing Office, 1983.
10. Rucker L, Frye EB, Staten MA: Usefulness of screening chest roentgenograms in preoperative patients. *JAMA* 1983; 250:3209–3211.
11. Latimer RG, Dickman M, Day WC, et al: Ventilatory patterns and pulmonary complications after upper abdominal surgery determined by preoperative and postoperative computerized spirometry and blood gas analysis. *Am J Surg* 1971; 122:622–632.
12. Ali J, Weisel RD, Layug AB, et al: Consequences of postoperative alterations in respiratory mechanics. *Am J Surg* 1974; 128:376–382.
13. Pearce AC, Jones RM. Smoking and anesthesia: Preoperative abstinence and perioperative morbidity. *Anesthesiology* 1984; 61:576–584.
14. DeSoto H, Patel RI, Soliman IE, et al: Changes in oxygen saturation following general anesthesia in children with upper respiratory infection signs and symptoms undergoing otolaryngological procedures. *Anesthesiology* 1988; 68:276–279.
15. Tait AR, Knight PR: Intraoperative respiratory complications in patients with upper respiratory tract infections. *Can Anaesth Soc J* 1987; 34:300–303.
16. Hosking MP, Warner MA, Lobdell CM, et al: Regional versus general anesthesia for patients >90 years of age undergoing total hip arthroplasty or transurethral prostate resection: Perioperative morbidity and mortality and long-term outcome. *Anesthesiology* 1988; 69:A716.
17. Yeager MP, Glass DD, Neff RK, et al: Epi-

dural anesthesia and analgesia in high-risk surgical patients. *Anesthesiology* 1987; 66:729–736.

18. Beattie C, Christopherson R, Manolio T, et al: Myocardial ischemia may be more common with regional than with general anesthesia in high risk patients. *Anesthesiology* 1986; 65:A518.
19. Kane RE: Neurologic deficits following epidural or spinal anesthesia. *Anesth Analg* 1981; 60:150–161.
20. Vandam LD, Dripps RD: Long-term follow-up of patients who received 10,098 spinal anesthetics. III. Syndrome of decreased intracranial pressure (headache and ocular and auditory difficulties). *JAMA* 1956; 161:586–591.
21. Mankikian B, Cantineau JP, Bertrand M, et al: Improvement of diaphragmatic function by a thoracic extradural block after upper abdominal surgery. *Anesthesiology* 1988; 68:379–386.
22. Catley DM, Thornton C, Jordan C, et al: Pronounced episodic oxygen desaturation in the postoperative period: Its association with ventilatory pattern and analgesic regimen. *Anesthesiology* 1985; 63:20–28.
23. Perz RR, Johnson DL, Shinozaki T: Spinal anesthesia for outpatient surgery. *Anesth Analg* 1988; 67:S168.
24. Gold B, Kitz DS, Lecky JH, et al: Factors associated with unanticipated hospital admission following ambulatory surgery: A case-control study. *Anesthesiolgy* 1988; 69:A719.
25. Stromskag KE, Steen PA: Comparison of interpleural and epidural anesthesia for extracorporeal shock wave lithotripsy. *Anesth Analg* 1988; 67:1181–1183.
26. Malhotra V, Long CW, Meister MJ: Intercostal blocks with local infiltration anesthesia for extracorporeal shock wave lithotripsy. *Anesth Analg* 1987; 66:85–88.
27. Weber W, Bach P, Wildgans H, et al: Anesthetic considerations in patients with cardiac pacemakers undergoing extracorporeal shock wave lithotripsy. *Anesth Analg* 1988; 67:S251.
28. Dhuner KG: Nerve injuries following operations: Survey of cases occurring during 6-year period. *Anesthesiology* 1950; 11:289–293.
29. Parks BJ: Postoperative peripheral neuropathies. *Surgery* 1973; 74:348–351.
30. Azar I, Turndorf H: Severe hypertension and multiple atrial premature contractions following naloxone administration. *Anesth Analg* 1979; 58:524–525.
31. Prough DS, Roy R, Bumgarner J, et al: Acute pulmonary edema in healthy teenagers following conservative doses of intravenous naloxone. *Anesthesiology* 1984; 60:485–486.
32. Andree RA: Sudden death following naloxone administration. *Anesth Analg* 1980; 59:782–784.
33. Teabeaut JR II: Aspiration of gastric contents: An experimental study. *Am J Pathol* 1952; 28:51–63.
34. Sise MJ, Hollingsworth R, Brim JE, et al: Complications of the flow-directed pulmonary artery catheter: A prospective analysis in 219 patients. *Crit Care Med* 1981; 9:315–318.
35. Puri VK, Carlson RW, Bander JJ, et al: Complications of vascular catheterization in the critically ill: A prospective study. *Crit Care Med* 1980; 8:495–499.
36. Belani KG, Buckley JJ, Gordon JR, et al: Percutaneous cervical central venous line placement: A comparison of the internal and external jugular vein routes. *Anesth Analg* 1980; 59:40–44.
37. Gordon RA, Britt BA, Kalow W (eds.): *International Symposium on Malignant Hyperthermia.* Springfield, Ill, Charles C Thomas, 1973.
38. Bunker JP, Forrest WH, Mostellar F: *National Halothane Study.* Washington DC, Government Printing Office, 1969.

SECTION II

Surgical Complications

CHAPTER 9

Complications of Renal and Adrenal Surgery

C. Lee Jackson, M.D.
Thomas J. Maatman, D.O.
James E. Montie, M.D.

Operations on the kidney, ranging in magnitude from radical nephrectomy with cavectomy to open renal biopsy, are subject to the full spectrum of complications common to most surgical procedures and, in addition, present special problems unique to the excretory system. Operative mortality and morbidity can be minimized with thorough preoperative evaluation and patient selection, proper selection of incision, correct patient positioning, sound surgical technique, and postoperative care with emphasis on early detection of potential problems. In this chapter, the surgical procedure will be briefly described, with special emphasis on steps that may prevent operative complications. The recognition, diagnosis, and treatment of complications resulting from operations on the kidney will be discussed.

RENAL SURGERY

Radical Nephrectomy

Radical nephrectomy implies early control of the renal vasculature and excision of the kidney and adrenal gland extrafascially, with or without regional lymphadenectomy. It is considered the optimal form of therapy for patients with nonmetastatic renal cell carcinoma and is usually performed through a transabdominal-transperitoneal approach[1-4] or a thoracoabdominal approach.[5,6] The operative mortality for radical nephrectomy ranges from 2% to 5%.[7-10] Complications vary depending on the site of the tumor and will be discussed accordingly.

Right Radical Nephrectomy.—The transabdominal-transperitoneal approach offers maximum exposure, early access to the renal vasculature, and is our preferred method of radical nephrectomy in most cases. After entering the abdominal cavity and performing an exploratory laparotomy, the small bowel and ascending colon are retracted medially with a moist green towel. The posterior peritoneum is grasped with a forceps and a vertical incision is made lateral to the ascending colon over the white line of Toldt, extending from the aortic bifurcation inferiorly and around the hepatic flexure to the level of the right adrenal vein superiorly. The plane between the mesocolon and Gerota's fascia is then developed, either sharply or bluntly. Frequently, this can be done by applying gentle traction on the ascending colon with countertraction on the kidney. Occasionally, venous bleeding from the mesocolon occurs, but hemostasis can be achieved with coagulation or ligatures. A hematoma in the mesocolon is usually self-limiting, but if expanding, it should be opened and the actively bleeding vessels ligated. The colon should then be inspected for signs of ischemia, and if present, the ischemic portion of the bowel should be resected. Defects in the mesocolon are uncommon if the proper plane is developed but must be reapproximated with interrupted or running sutures to prevent possible internal herniation of small bowel. The duodenum is then encountered and Kocher's method is used to expose the inferior vena cava and aorta. Injury to the duodenum during the Kocher maneuver should be repaired in several layers. Intramural duodenal hematomas, if expanding, should be opened with expression of the hematoma, ligation of active bleeding vessels, and suture repair of the serosa. After exposing the great vessels, retraction can be maintained with a well-padded, self-retaining ring retractor. This type of retractor maintains, but does not and should not be used to develop, exposure. The bowel must be carefully padded with white lap pads and moist green towels. Throughout the case, the towels should be moistened with warm sterile saline, and the bowel should be inspected intermittently for evidence of vascular compromise. Improperly placed or padded retractor blades

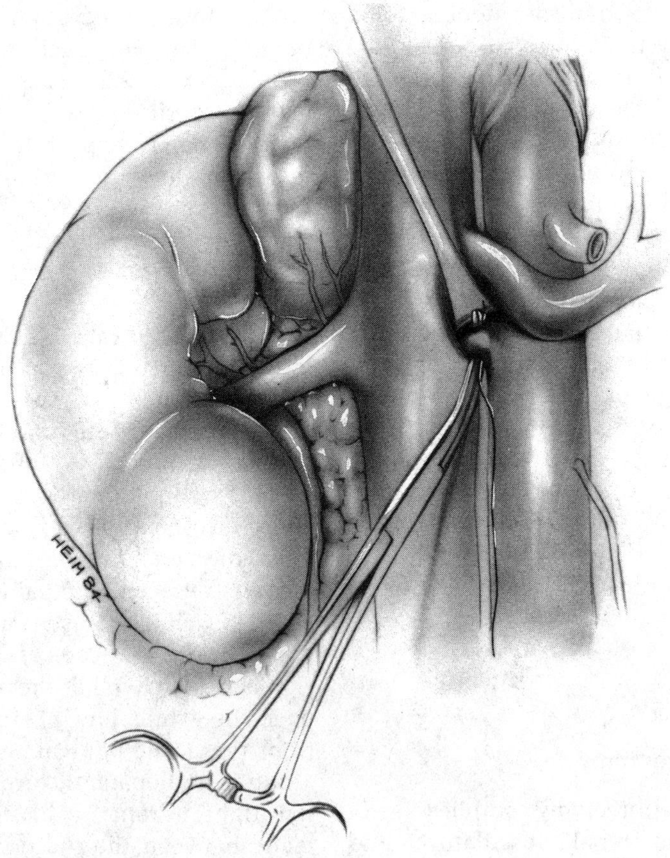

FIG 9–1.
Right renal artery is identified between the inferior vena cava and aorta.

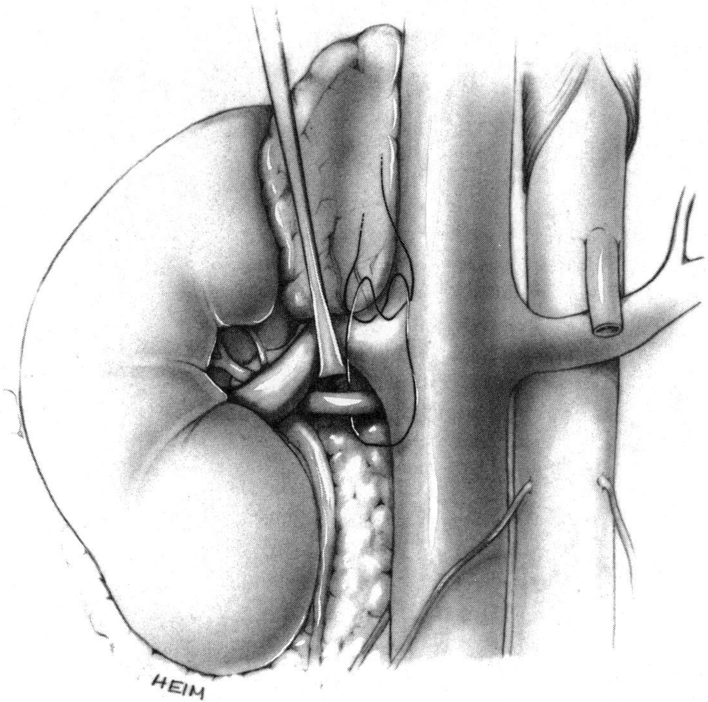

FIG 9–2.
Right renal artery is identified lateral to the inferior vena cava.

may cause vascular compromise to the bowel. Occasionally, ischemic bowel will have to be resected.

Next, the right renal artery is identified, either between the inferior vena cava and aorta (Fig 9–1), or just lateral to the inferior vena cava (Fig 9–2). The artery is dissected sharply and doubly ligated proximally. The right renal vein is then identified and gently palpated, and, if no thrombus is present, it is dissected and doubly ligated. An alternative approach that is used frequently is to singly ligate the renal artery but not divide it and then proceed with division of the renal vein (Fig 9–3). The renal artery can then be further dissected, ligated, and divided with better exposure. A plane is developed between the posterior sheath of Gerota's fascia and the anterior fascia or the psoas muscle. The ureter is then identified and ligated. Dissection proceeds cephalad toward the adrenal gland and is completed after securing the blood supply to the adrenal. The arterial supply to the adrenal gland is the same bilaterally. The inferior phrenic artery branches to form the superior adrenal artery, the middle adrenal artery branches from the aorta, and the inferior adrenal artery originates from the renal artery. The adrenal gland is drained by the central vein. The main right adrenal vein is short and enters directly into the posterior lateral aspect of the inferior vena cava. The vein can easily be avulsed, leading to major venous bleeding. If this occurs, Allis clamps should be carefully placed on the caval tear and the cava should be repaired with running 5-0 vascular sutures (Fig 9–4). Incomplete excision of the adrenal gland is another cause of venous bleeding. If there is no evidence of tumor, the adrenal gland may be oversewn with running 3-0 chromic sutures (Fig 9–5). An alternative method of managing bleeding from a partial adrenalectomy is to resect completely the remaining portion of the gland. Dur-

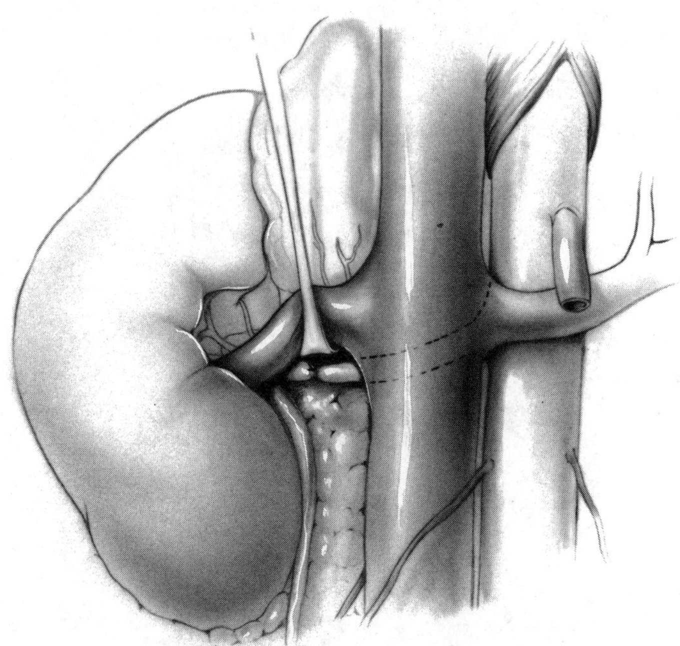

FIG 9–3.
Simple ligation of the right renal artery.

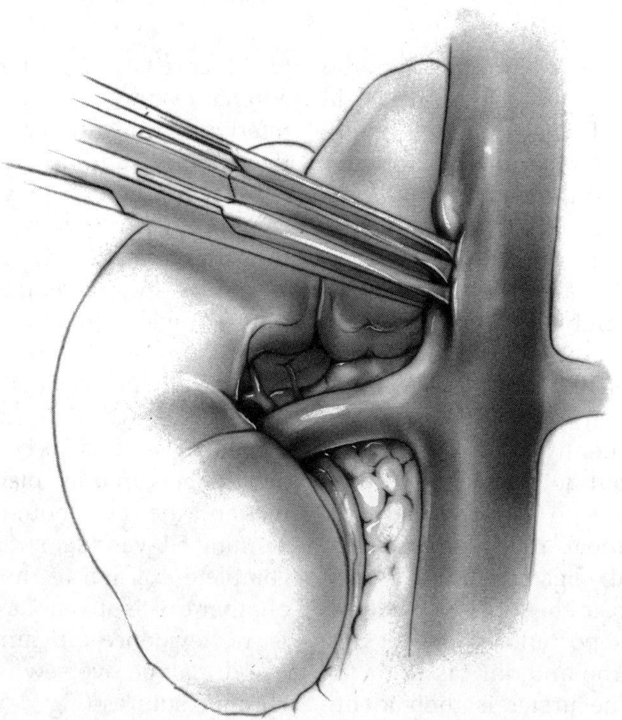

FIG 9–4.
Allis clamps applied to site of right adrenal vein avulsion.

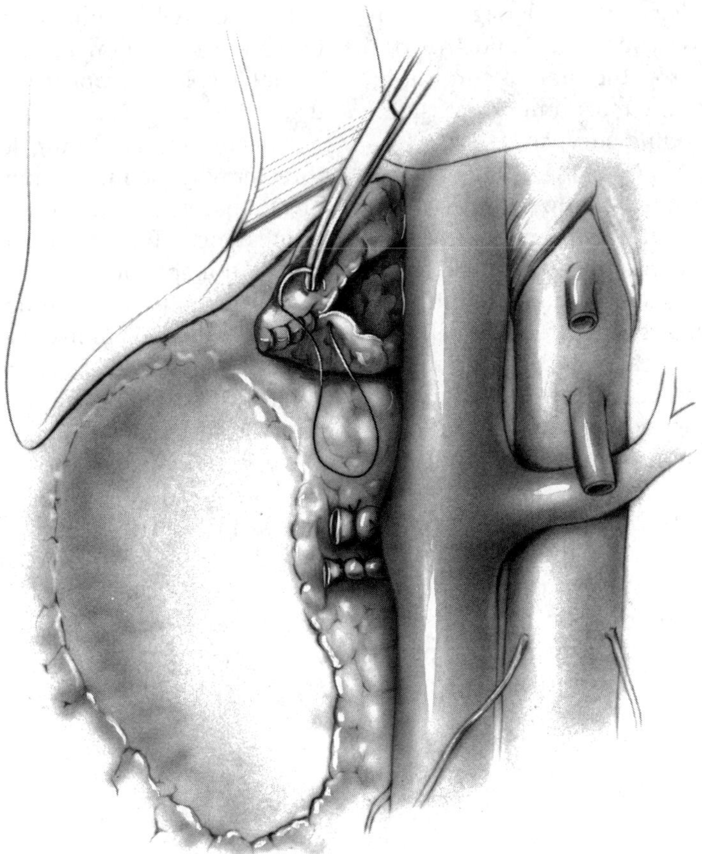

FIG 9–5.
Oversewing right adrenal for bleeding.

ing the course of dissection, all lymphatic tissue and lymphatic channels should be secured with ligatures or clips to prevent formation of a lymphocele or lymphatic fistula. The specimen is then removed and sent to the pathology laboratory for analysis. After making sure that the patient is normotensive, the renal fossa is inspected for active bleeding. At this time, the ligated pedicle can be inspected. If hemostasis is adequate, the fossa is then irrigated with warm saline. The colon may or may not be tacked back down to the posterior peritoneum with interrupted 3-0 sutures. The incision is closed in a single layer with the modified Tom Jones method.[11] No drains are used during this procedure.

Injury to the liver during right radical nephrectomy may occur if the liver retractor is not sufficiently padded. Liver lacerations may be repaired with interrupted horizontal mattress sutures. Direct involvement of the liver with renal cell carcinoma is unusual, despite the inability to see a plane between the two organs on computed tomography (CT) and the presence of neovascularity in the region of the liver on angiography. If, however, the liver is grossly involved with tumor, a decision must be made regarding the resectability of the mass, keeping in mind that major bleeding may be encountered, necessitating the Pringle maneuver (cross-clamping the porta hepatis with a vascular clamp) and/or partial hepatectomy. Injury to the biliary tree adds significantly to morbidity and mortality, and the local extent of tumor at the time of surgical intervention is the most important single variable in defining survival.[12]

Left Radical Nephrectomy.—After entering the peritoneum and performing exploratory laparotomy, the small bowel and descending colon are gently retracted medially with a moist green towel. The posterior peritoneal reflection is grasped with the forceps lateral to the colon, elevated, and incised, extending from the aortic bifurcation inferiorly, around the splenic flexure superiorly, to the level of the left adrenal vein. The descending colon can then be gently retracted medially to expose the aorta by developing the plane between mesocolon and the anterior sheath of Gerota's fascia. Incomplete transection of the peritoneal reflection and lienorenal ligament may result in unnecessary traction on the spleen and possibly splenic capsular tear or fracture.

Splenic injury during left radical nephrectomy is the most common intraoperative adjacent organ complication, with an incidence of 12.4% reported in a large series.[7] If a splenic injury is encountered, the spleen must be thoroughly inspected and the extent of injury assessed. Minor capsule tears and lacerations are best managed by packing with Avitene or Surgicel, protected with lap pads, and gently retracted cephalad out of the operative field. More severe bleeding may necessitate splenectomy. For immediate control of brisk splenic bleeding, the lesser sac may be opened and the tail of the pancreas grasped between the fingers and thumb, compressing the splenic artery and vein (Fig 9–6). This maneuver

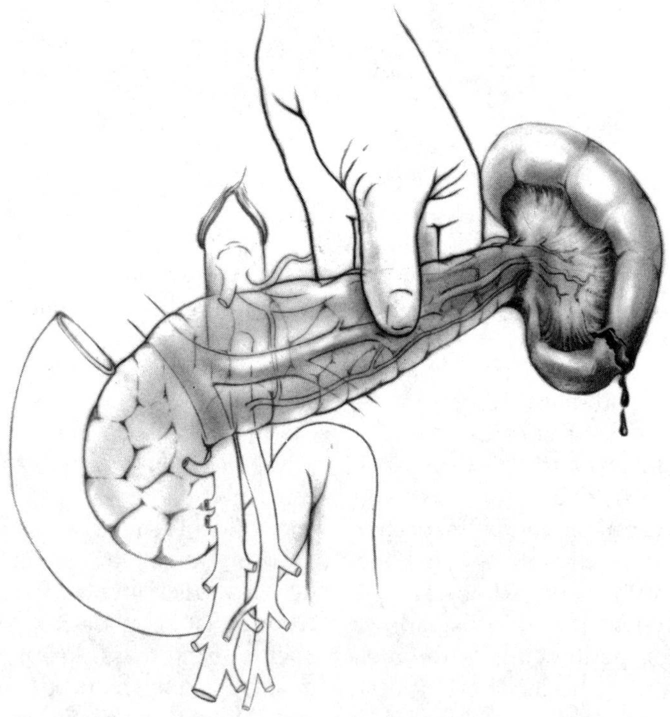

FIG 9–6.
The lesser sac is opened, and the splenic artery and vein are compressed along the tail of the pancreas to control splenic bleeding.

allows for rapid control of blood loss and a more relaxed inspection of the spleen.

If splenectomy is necessary, it should be performed at this time in the following manner: The spleen is mobilized by dividing the lateral peritoneal attachments from the colon and diaphragm. Adhesions to the diaphragm are sharply dissected. The spleen is then delivered into the wound by forward and medial rotation, and several dry lap pads are placed behind the spleen to prevent it from falling back into the splenic fossa. The short gastrics are then divided. The tail of the pancreas is then identified in the hilum of the spleen and the splenic artery and vein are identified, sharply dissected, ligated with silk suture, and then transected. The splenic bed is then inspected for bleeding and irrigated with 1% neomycin solution. It is not necessary to drain the splenic fossa after splenectomy. Postoperatively, the patient must be observed for left lower lobe atelectasis, which is common following splenectomy. If this occurs, it can be successfully managed with pulmonary physiotherapy.

It is generally accepted that patients who have undergone splenectomy are at greater risk for developing overwhelming infection (postsplenectomy sepsis) with bacterial organisms that produce polysaccharide capsules,[13] including *Streptococcus pneumoniae* and other streptococci, *Pseudomonas, Neisseria meningitidis, Escherichia coli, Haemophilus influenzae,* and *Staphylococcus aureus.*[14] For this reason, splenectomized patients should receive the 14-valent pneumococcal polysaccharide vaccine (Pneumovax) and prophylactic penicillin.[14–16]

It is rare for renal cell carcinoma to invade the spleen directly, but when confronted with this situation, the surgeon must assess the resectability of the tumor, keeping in mind once again the nature of metastatic renal cell carcinoma and the proximity of the pancreas and risk of pancreatic injury, which greatly increases morbidity and mortality.

After successfully reflecting the colon, attention should then be directed toward identifying, dissecting, ligating, and transecting the left renal artery. These procedures may be facilitated by dissecting the left renal vein first and gently retracting the vein cephalad with a vein retractor. Adequate exposure will require ligation of the adrenal vein, gonadal vein and lumbar vein which commonly enter into the left renal vein (Fig 9–7). Ligation of the left renal vein itself should follow ligation of the left renal artery to prevent blood loss into the kidney. Care must be taken to avoid injury to the adrenal vein and lumbar veins during dissection of the renal vein. Accidentally severed lumbar veins may retract into the paravertebral muscles. An Allis clamp may be placed over the area of active bleeding and, with gentle traction on the Allis clamp, the bleeding site can be secured with a figure-of-eight suture. The ureter is then identified and ligated. The plane between the posterior sheath of Gerota's fascia and the anterior psoas fascia is developed and dissected in a cephalad direction. The splenic hilum and pancreas are protected by developing the plane behind the posterior peritoneum superiorly (Fig 9–8). Collateral vessels are secured with clamps and ligatures. Dissection is completed with ligation and transection of the blood supply to the left adrenal gland. The main left adrenal vein is longer, enters into the superior aspect of the left renal vein, and is less likely to be avulsed. The specimen is sent to the pathology laboratory for analysis, and the renal fossa is irrigated with a warm saline solution. Once again, after one is certain that the patient is normotensive, the fossa and pedicle are inspected for active bleeding. Of great concern is the small vessel in spasm that retracts into the surrounding tissue and is missed during the inspection, only to cause significant bleeding later in the

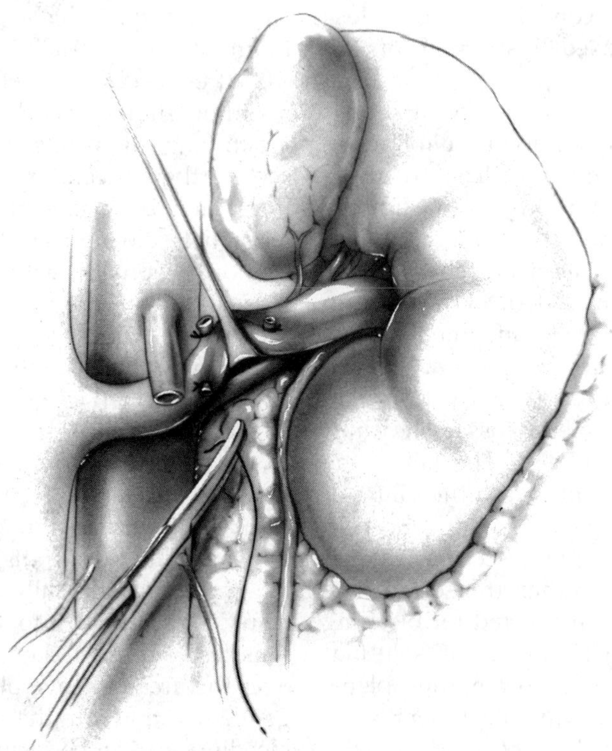

FIG 9–7.
The left renal artery is exposed after ligation of the adrenal, gonadal, and lumbar veins.

postoperative period. For this reason, a careful, controlled dissection, with clamping, transection, and suture ligation of the superior attachments of the kidney, is recommended.

The pancreas lies transversely in the retroperitoneum and extends from the descending portion of the duodenum across the midline to the hilum of the spleen (Fig 9–9). The gland is 10 to 20 cm in length and 3 to 5 cm in width. It has both an endocrine and an exocrine function and, when stimulated, is capable of producing 4.5 mL/min of an alkaline fluid with a pH ranging from 7.0 to 8.7. The pancreas is at greatest risk of injury during dissection of the superior attachments of the kidneys. It is the urologic surgeon's responsibility to be aware of this potentiality and to recognize pancreatic injuries when they occur. Intraoperative general surgical consultation is recommended once pancreatic injury is identified or suspected. Pancreatic injuries may be classified as (1) laceration of pancreatic parenchyma without major ductal injury, (2) laceration of pancreatic tissue and duct, (3) transection of the duct and tail of the pancreas, and (4) unrecognized pancreatic injury (Fig 9–10). Laceration of the pancreatic parenchyma without ductal involvement may be treated by simply closing the pancreatic capsule with interrupted 3-0 or 4-0 nonabsorbable permanent sutures and by sump drainage of the retroperitoneum. Others, however, would disagree with this treatment, since it may result in pseudocyst formation.[17] It is of utmost importance to inspect and ensure the integrity of the pancreatic duct in this type of injury, since unrecognized ductal injury will add significantly to morbidity

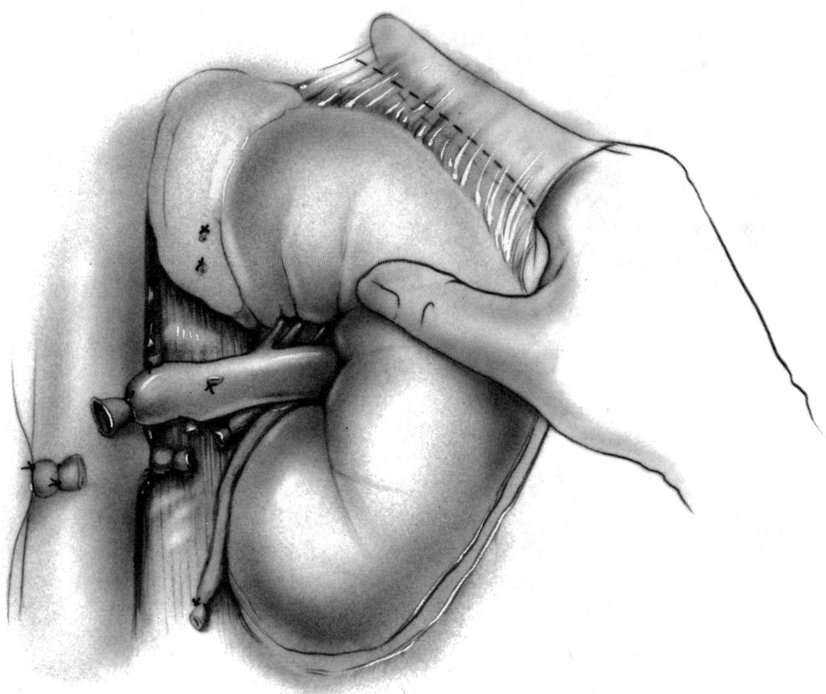

FIG 9–8.
The spleen and pancreas are protected by mobilizing the posterior peritoneum from Gerota's fascia.

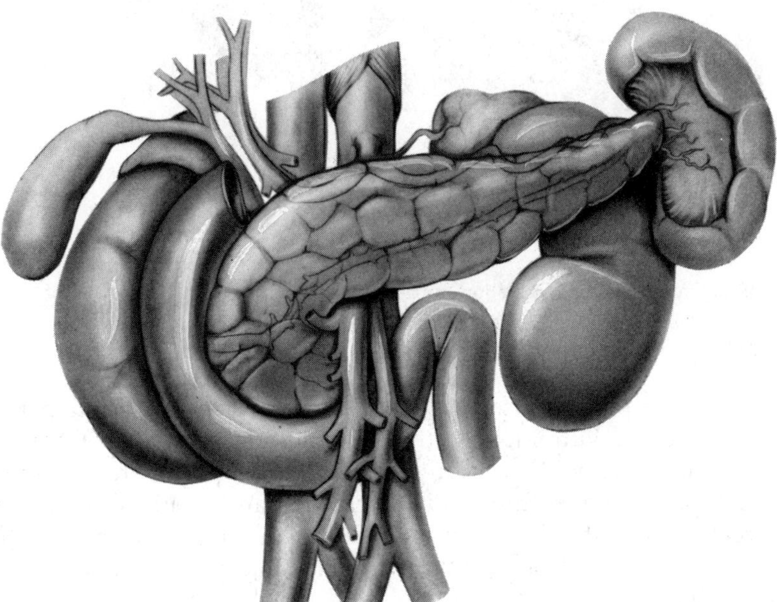

FIG 9–9.
The pancreas extends from the descending portion of the duodenum across the midline to the hilum of the spleen.

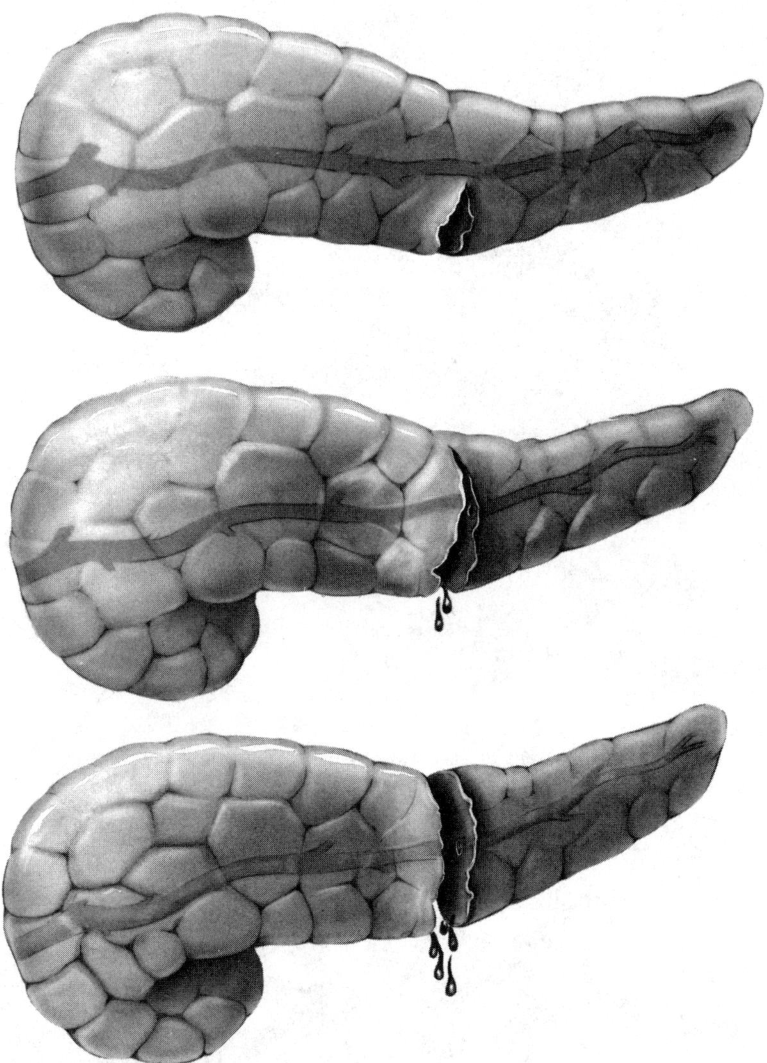

FIG 9–10.
Classification of pancreatic injuries: laceration of parenchyma without major ductal injury *(top)*; laceration of pancreatic tissue and duct *(center)*; and transection of the duct and tail of the pancreas *(bottom)*.

and mortality. Incomplete transection of the tail of the pancreas with injury to the duct should be managed with excision of the injured tail, permanent suture ligation of the pancreatic duct with closure of the capsule over the transected parenchyma, and sump drainage of the retroperitoneum. As much as 80% of the gland can be excised without producing pancreatic insufficiency.[18] Attempts to reanastomose the transected duct and parenchyma in this setting are not warranted and carry the risk of postoperative traumatic pancreatitis and death. Complete transection of the tail of the pancreas with coexistent ductal injury is treated with excision of the distal stump, permanent ligation of the duct, oversewing of the capsule, and sump drainage. A key factor in the successful management of pancreatic injury with ductal involvement is sump drainage of the retroperitoneum. The drain should be placed in the retroperitoneum near the site of injury but not touching the pancreas. Sump drainage is associated with a higher incidence of pancreatic fistula, but management of an isolated pancreatic fistula is not difficult.[19]

Perhaps the most distressing pancreatic injury is one not recognized at the time of surgery that manifests itself in the immediate postoperative period with signs and symptoms of acute pancreatitis with elevated serum amylase, fluid collection in the retroperitoneum, alkaline fluid draining from the incision, and/or sudden death. A CT scan of the abdomen will demonstrate a fluid collection in the retroperitoneum. Fluid draining from the incision should be analyzed for pH and the presence of amylase. Rarely, a sinogram is needed to make the diagnosis of pancreatic injury and fistula formation. The fluid must be drained either percutaneously or surgically with placement of sump drains, since pseudocysts and abscess formation are likely to occur if adequate drainage is not provided. Once drainage has been established, the majority of fistulas close spontaneously.[19–22] The patient should be supported with hyperalimentation, since the healing of a pancreatic fistula is often a slow process. Surgical closure by excising the fistulous tract and creating an anastomosis between the pancreas and the Roux-en-Y limb of the jejunum is only occasionally necessary in patients with prolonged pancreatic drainage.[23]

Radical Nephrectomy With Cavotomy or Cavectomy

Tumor thrombus extending from the renal vein into the vena cava occurs in 4% to 10% of patients with renal cell carcinoma[9, 24–28] and extension of the thrombus into the right atrium in as many as 14%-41% in this group of patients.[29–31] The diagnosis is suspected on the basis of intravenous pyelography (IVP), CT scan, or ultrasound, and is confirmed and the extent identified with magnetic resonance imaging (MRI) or inferior and superior vena cavography. In addition, the presence of caval involvement can be identified on occasion by recognizing arterialization of the tumor thrombus on renal angiography.[26, 32] Rarely, caval thrombus is unsuspected and found at the time of surgery by gentle palpation of the renal vein and inferior vena cava. Patients with vena cava extension (i.e., no other metastatic disease) have a cure rate, following radical nephrectomy and complete removal of the vena cava thrombus approaching that of patients with stage I or small stage II renal cell carcinoma.[33] For this reason, in properly selected patients, radical nephrectomy with cavotomy or cavectomy is recommended. The mortality rate for this procedure is 4% to 14%.[27, 28, 34, 35]

A transperitoneal approach (chevron or midline) is used in patients with a tumor thrombus extending into the inferior vena cava. For the more common right-sided tumors, a thoracoabdominal approach offers improved access to the uppermost portion of the inferior vena cava. For patients with upper vena cava and right atrial involvement, a chevron or midline incision with a median sternotomy is recommended. Coronary ligaments attaching the liver to the diaphragm may be incised to gain exposure to the intrahepatic cava. Short hepatic veins may be ligated, but two or more major hepatic veins should be preserved to prevent postoperative liver insufficiency. The majority of patients with caval thrombus have right-sided tumors because of the short right renal vein. In this setting, dissection begins with identifying, ligating, and transecting the right renal artery. The inferior vena cava and both renal veins are then gently dissected. Lumbar veins should be ligated and transected to prevent continued bleeding during cavotomy.

A Rumel tourniquet is placed below the renal veins and thrombus around the vena cava. The kidney is mobilized very carefully to avoid disrupting the thrombus until it is attached only by the involved renal vein and thrombus. The left renal vein is clamped with a bulldog clamp or Rumel tourniquet.

A Rumel tourniquet is placed around the vena cava above the upper limit of the thrombus. This can be associated with a profound drop in venous return to the heart and subsequently blood pressure; volume expansion may be adequate to compensate. If many collaterals have developed, hypotension is less of a problem. The cava is then incised over the thrombus with a scalpel, carrying the incision around the ostium of the right renal vein, and the tumor is gently extracted from the cava (Fig 9–11).

The cava is then closed with running 5-0 vascular sutures. Prior to closing the cava completely, the lower tourniquet is released, allowing blood to flow through the cava, forcing air out of the incompletely closed cavotomy site, and thereby preventing air embolism. When the cava is full of blood, the remaining portion of the cavotomy is closed and the bulldog clamp and upper tourniquets are released. The cava is then inspected for bleeding; occasionally, more interrupted silk sutures will be needed. If the tumor thrombus is small and friable, it is sometimes wiser to perform the extraction from

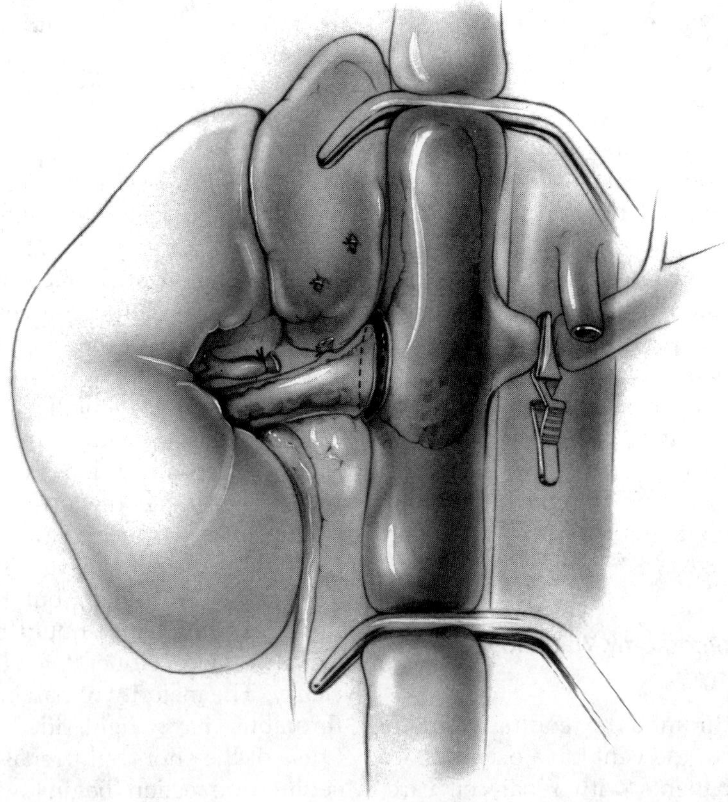

FIG 9–11.
Right vena caval tumor thrombus. Excision is made around the ostium of the right vein and thrombus is extracted.

the inferior vena cava prior to mobilization of the kidney. The disadvantage of this is the potential spill of cancer cells from the exposed thrombus during the rest of the dissection of the kidney. Sometimes, the inferior vena cava above the thrombus can be occluded completely during the mobilization of the kidney. Inferior vena cava clips or an umbrella above the thrombus have been used to trap tumor emboli but these can obstruct venous return as well and cause more backbleeding during the nephrectomy. Intraoperative tumor embolization is a devastating complication and even immediate pulmonary artery embolectomy may not prevent serious complications.

Intrahepatic tumor thrombi require other methods to insure vascular control. The upper inferior vena cava immediately above or below the diaphragm and the superior mesenteric and inferior mesenteric arteries is controlled and occluded. The porta hepatis is occluded to prevent engorgement of the liver and backbleeding from the hepatic veins. The liver can be reflected medially, thus exposing the intrahepatic inferior vena cava with complete vascular control. The porta hepatis can only be safely occluded for 20 to 30 minutes so this technique works well if the thrombus can be extracted easily. If there is extreme enlargement of the inferior vena cava with adhesion to the inferior vena caval wall, then use of cardiac bypass may allow more time to remove all the tumor fragments and reconstruct the inferior vena cava.

If the thrombus extends above the hepatic veins to the level of the diaphragm or into the atrium, or if it completely occludes or invades the inferior vena cava, cardiac bypass with or without circulatory arrest with deep hypothermia allows complete removal of the thrombus.[36–38]

The extent of caval involvement is determined by abdominal CT scan and MRI; inferior and superior venacavography and a cardiac echocardiogram may be needed in some cases. Good cardiac function is important to a successful recovery from circulatory arrest and deep hypothermia; therefore coronary angiography is also considered in the older patient to identify the rare individual who requires concurrent coronary revascularization to prevent a potentially lethal perioperative myocardial infarction. Patients with evidence of metastatic disease are not considered operative candidates.

The patient is explored through a transverse upper abdominal incision. After confirming resectability, a median sternotomy is made. Intraoperative monitoring is accomplished with an arterial line, a multiple-lumen central venous catheter, and a pulmonary artery catheter.

The kidney is mobilized entirely, leaving only the involved renal vein attached to the inferior vena cava. Venous collateral circulation is extensive making the dissection around the kidney more difficult and tedious. Precise hemostasis is particularly important prior to the initiation of bypass and heparinization. Ligation of the renal artery as early as possible in the dissection is beneficial. Control of the inferior vena cava below the tumor thrombus and to the contralateral renal vein is obtained. With the use of cardiac bypass, extensive dissection and mobilization of the upper involved inferior vena cava is not necessary. After heparinization, the aorta and right atrium are cannulated. Cannulation of the venous circulation from the lower half of the body is not required because the extensive collateral venous network ultimately drains into the superior vena cava. Cardiopulmonary bypass is begun immediately, and when the heart fibrillates the aorta is clamped and crystalloid cardioplegic solution is infused. A core temperature of 18 to 20 °C is achieved in approximately 15 to 30 minutes and the flow through the perfusion machine is stopped and 90% of the blood volume is drained into the pump.[39] The inferior vena cava is incised at the entrance of the ipsil teral renal vein and the ostium is circumscribed. If the tumor extends into the right atrium the atrium can be opened at the same time. An attempt is made to deliver the tumor extension intact into the inferior vena cava and to remove the kidney and inferior vena cava thrombus in one specimen. Frequently this is not possible because of adherence of the thrombus to the inferior vena cava wall and the extreme friability of the thrombus.

Occasionally it is necessary to remove part of the thrombus through the atriotomy and then the interior of the cava can be directly inspected for remaining fragments. The inferior vena cava is then closed with a running vascular suture and circulation is immediately reinstituted. Rewarming to a temperature of 35 °C is accomplished in approximately 30 to 40 minutes. After rewarming is done, cardiopulmonary bypass is terminated and the patient is transferred to a cardiac intensive care unit, intubated, and then extubated over the next 24 to 72 hours.

Between 1965 and 1987, 68 patients at the Cleveland Clinic have undergone radical nephrectomy with removal of an inferior vena caval thrombus. In 17 of these patients the use of circulatory arrest and deep hypothermia was carried out as just described. There is little argument that the use of cardiac bypass, especially with the use of circulatory arrest, makes the operative technique of removal of the thrombus easier. The unresolved issue is relative to the additional time and manpower used as well as the potential additional complications which may be seen with the addition of cardiac bypass with circulatory arrest.

A concern with the addition of cardiac bypass is the need for systemic heparinization. Because of the very large dissection needed with the radical nephrectomy, the potential exists for a significant degree of bleeding from exposed raw surfaces around the renal fossa. This can be minimized by ensuring precise hemostasis before initiating bypass and anticoagulation. The addition of circulatory arrest allows the thrombus to be removed in an entirely bloodless field. We have noted, however, a clinically significant coagulopathy after circulatory arrest in 15% to 20% of patients. Some patients require reexploration for bleeding and some resolve with time and blood-product replacement. Since circulatory arrest is a procedure which has not been widely used in adults in the past, there is a minimal amount of data to precisely quantitate the frequency with which this coagulopathy may be seen. Also, the mechanism that might cause this coagulopathy is as yet undetermined. The average blood loss in these 17 cases was approximately 2,000 cc and the duration of circulatory arrest ranged from 12 to 47 minutes. There have been no identifiable significant neurologic, hepatic, or renal consequences of circulatory arrest in deep hypothermia.[40]

Our clinical impression has been that the use of circulatory arrest in deep hypothermia has made the total operative technique easier. Difficult vena cava dissection is avoided and the potential for sudden massive bleeding is eliminated with a more precise removal of all tumor fragments and reconstruction of the inferior vena cava made possible with ideal exposure. The bloodless field reduces the risk of circulation of tumor cells during excision and the more serious potential complications of embolization of air, tumor, or blood clot.

Nephroureterectomy

Nephroureterectomy is indicated in patients with urothelial tumors of the renal collecting system and ureter. It can be performed through the following incisions: single anterior extraperitoneal,[41] paramedian extraperitoneal,[42] thoracoabdominal,[43] single midline, or through two separate incisions (flank or anterior subcostal with modified Pfannenstiel's incision).[44] A regional lymphadenectomy is not routinely performed. Nephrectomy is performed first through the upper incision, and the ureter is dissected as far distally as possible. The lower incision is then made, and the kidney and the ureter are passed downward and delivered through the lower incision. Dissection of the distal ureter continues to the ureterovesical junction. The bladder is then opened on the posterior lateral surface, and the incision is carried downward to, and circumscribes, the ureteral orifice. The specimen (including the kidney, ureter, and cuff of bladder) is then removed intact. An alternative method for excision of the distal ureter and cuff of bladder is to tent the bladder at the ureterovesical junction and excise the ureter and cuff of bladder extravesically. The bladder is closed in layers with chromic suture and the perivesicular space is drained with a Penrose. A Foley catheter is left indwelling for several days to allow the bladder to heal. Both incisions are then closed in layers.

Regardless of surgical approach and technique, it is important to inspect the distal ureter to ensure that an adequate bladder cuff has been excised, since failure to remove the distal ureter, ureteral orifice, and/or cuff of bladder has resulted in a 20% to 30%[45, 46] recurrence of cancer in the remaining portion of the ureter.

Simple Nephrectomy

Simple nephrectomy is performed when the function of a kidney has been irreparably destroyed due to disease processes, including calculi, obstruction, infection, trauma, uncontrolled renal vascular hypertension, and hemorrhage. The diseased kidney may be approached through a flank (subcostal, 11th rib, 12th rib, or modified), anterior transperitoneal (unilateral subcostal, bilateral subcostal, midline, or thoracoabdominal), or an anterior extraperitoneal incision, depending on the indication for surgery, the size and location of the kidney, the body habitus of the patient, and the experience of the surgeon. Operative mortality for simple nephrectomy is approximately 1% when done for reasons other than neoplasia.[47–50] The procedure, however, is associated with a significant number of operative and postoperative complications.[47]

The most alarming of these is intraoperative hemorrhage, which may be initially controlled by compressing the pedicle against the vertebral bodies. This maneuver allows for the addition of suction equipment, stabilization of the patient, and a more orderly approach to identifying the bleeding vessels. Arteriotomies and venotomies may be closed with 5-0 vascular silk sutures. Occasionally, the renal pedicle will be difficult to dissect because of the disease process and must be secured with a pedicle clamp. If a pedicle clamp is used, the duodenum must first be carefully reflected to prevent the inclusion of the retroperitoneal portion of the duodenum in the pedicle clamp, which leads to fistula formation. Another potential risk of using the pedicle clamp is the forming of an arteriovenous fistula when the vein and artery are ligated together. On rare occasions, an arteriovenous fistula may cause high-output cardiac failure.

Pneumothorax is a potential complication of any flank approach to the kidney and occurs when the pleura is inadvertently entered. Pleural injuries are usually recognized immediately by the presence of a sucking sound or bubbles in the operative field, but small rents may go unnoticed. The extent of the injury is identified, and running 3-0 or 4-0 chromic sutures are used to close the tear. Prior to complete closure, a red rubber catheter is inserted into the pleural cavity, and a pursestring suture is placed around the catheter. The anesthesiologist is then asked to hyperinflate the lungs. With hyperinflation and suction on the catheter, air and fluid in the hemithorax are forced out through the red rubber catheter, which is then removed, and the purse-string suture is secured. An alternative method is to place the distal end of the catheter in a basin of water. As the anesthesiologist hyperinflates the lung, air and fluid are forced out of the pleural cavity through the red rubber catheter, and bubbles will be seen in the basin of water. When bubbling stops, the catheter is removed, and a pursestring suture secured. When the pleura is entered, a chest roentgenogram should be obtained in the recovery room to ensure adequate reexpansion of the lung. A pneumothorax greater than 10%, tension pneumothorax, or one that is causing respiratory distress will require insertion of a chest tube.

Postoperative atelectasis is common in patients undergoing nephrectomy and is probably secondary to the positioning of the patient during the procedure. Atelectasis is a common cause of increased temperature postoperatively and may be effectively treated with pulmonary physiotherapy, including deep breathing, coughing, and incentive spirometry, but it may require chest physiotherapy.

An incisional hernia or bulge may occur postoperatively in patients when the surgeon uses a flank incision for exploration. The intracostal nerve lies immediately below the corresponding rib between the internal oblique and the transverse abdominal muscle. When this nerve is encountered, an effort should be made to spare it by dissecting both proximally and distally, enabling careful padding and retraction of the nerve out of the operative field, since transection may lead to muscle denervation. Postoperatively, muscle denervation with flank bulging must be differentiated from a flank incisional hernia, which is rare. In the latter, a fascial defect is usually palpable. Cosmetically, an asymmetric flank bulge may be very distressing.

Partial Nephrectomy

Partial nephrectomy implies removal of a portion of kidney with maintenance of functioning parenchyma in the remaining segment. This procedure may be indicated for calculus disease, renal trauma, segmental obstruction (in children with duplicated collecting systems and segmentally damaged parenchyma secondary to lower congenital anomalies), infections, vascular lesions and cancers in a solitary kidney, or bilateral tumors. The mortality rate for this procedure in most series is less than 1%. Essentially, there are five techniques for partial nephrectomy. Wedge resection with flaps of parenchyma reapproximated by deep mattress sutures has the disadvantage of leaving a devascularized margin of tissue and is associated with a high incidence of urinary fistula formation and ischemic tissue.[51] Transverse resection with individual ligation of blood vessels followed by closure of the capsule is applicable to almost all situations and is the preferred technique for polar segmental nephrectomy.[52, 53] Segmental resection with preliminary ligation of the appropriate renal artery branch is well suited for renal vascular lesions.[54] Segmental resection with intrarenal mass ligation with use of large sutures through the parenchyma has been advocated,[55] but it has the disadvantage of potentially compromising the blood supply of the tissue at the margin of resection. Mass ligation circumferentially around the polar segment,[56] which is used as a tightening noose to transect the renal parenchyma and ligate the major intrarenal blood vessels and collecting system, is not as precise as individual ligation of vessels and repair of the collecting system and may lead to bleeding problems and urinary fistula formation postoperatively.

Except in renal trauma, a flank incision is the preferred approach for partial nephrectomy. The kidney should be completely mobilized, and the renal artery should be identified and dissected free from the surrounding tissue.

Early control of the renal artery by vascular clamps and renal hypothermia with saline slush is usually necessary when performing partial nephrectomy for cancer. After mobilizing the kidney, the renal artery is identified, dissected free, and tagged with a vessel loop. Prior to clamping the renal artery, a 12.5-g dose of mannitol is given intravenously. Mannitol increases the osmolality of the glomerular filtrate, reduces the hazard of ice crystallization in renal tissue due to the cooling process, and ensures prompt diuresis once the renal artery clamp is removed.[57] The benefit of renal cooling with ice slush is well-established and lengthens the time that the renal artery can be safely clamped.[58] The goal of cooling is to achieve a renal core temperature of 15° C. To achieve this temperature, a rubber dam reservoir is needed, and icy physiologic salt solution must be continuously packed around the kidney during the procedure. The tumor is then identified and a circumscribing incision made in the parenchyma around the tumor.

The tumor is excised sharply with the back handle of the scalpel. If the collecting system is entered, it is closed with interrupted or running 3-0 or 4-0 chromic catgut sutures. Individual vessels are ligated with 4-0 chromic sutures. Hemostasis is checked by releasing the vascular clamp; if the bleeding is controlled, the capsule is then closed over the resection site with interrupted chromic sutures.

After completing a partial nephrectomy, the kidney is returned to Gerota's fascia, and the capsule and fascia are pexed to the posterior abdominal wall. Failure to do this may result in torsion of the kidney on the pedicle, with either infarction or venous congestion leading to ischemia or increased bleeding. The retroperitoneum should always be drained to prevent formation of a urinoma following partial nephrectomy.

Common complications of partial nephrectomy include hemorrhage, both immediate and delayed, urinary fistula formation, renal insufficiency, and infection. Significant intraoperative bleeding occurs frequently in patients undergoing partial nephrectomy and emphasizes the need for early control and easy access to the renal artery. For immediate control of significant bleeding, the pedicle can be compressed against the vertebral column to allow for the addition of suckers and a more controlled inspection of bleeding sites. In addition, manual compression of the parenchyma is frequently useful for immediate control of hemorrhage and placement of individual ligatures around active bleeding points. Postoperative hemorrhage may be confined to the retroperitoneum, in which case it is usually self-limiting, or it may be associated with gross hematuria. The initial management of postoperative hemorrhage is expectant and conservative, with absolute bed rest, serial hematocrit and hemoglobin determinations, and frequent monitoring of vital signs. Transfusions are administered when indicated. Angiography is useful in some patients to localize actively bleeding arteries that may be controlled via angioinfarction with Gelfoam or autologous blood clot. Life-threatening hemorrhage may necessitate reexploration with early control of the renal pedicle and individual ligation of active bleeding sites. If early control of the renal pedicle is achieved, nephrectomy is usually not needed.

The presence of urinary drainage after partial nephrectomy usually resolves as the collecting system closes with healing. Persistent drainage suggests the development of a urinary cutaneous fistula. The fluid should be collected in a bag and sent for a creatinine determination. If the creatinine level of the drainage fluid is greater than the patient's serum creatinine, it should be assumed that the fluid is urine. If the drainage creatinine level is the same as the serum creatinine, the fluid may be either serous or lymphatic in nature. Most urinary cutaneous fistulas will resolve spontaneously, provided adequate drainage of a nonobstructive unit is present. Poor drainage will result in the formation of a urinoma or abscess that will require formal drainage. Excretory urography or retrograde pyelography is important at this point to rule out obstruction of the collecting system distally. In an attempt to improve urinary drainage in patients with a persistent urinary leak, a ureteral catheter may be placed either in a retrograde fashion or percutaneously if there is evidence of hydronephrosis. Urinary fistulas that do not resolve will require formal re-exploration with excision of the tract, relief of obstruction, and closure of the collecting system. The repair should be reinforced with the addition of a layer of fat, peritoneum, or omentum to ensure adequate closure. Surgical closure of urinary fistulas, if needed, should be performed several months after the original surgery to allow for possible spontaneous closure and resolution of the surrounding tissue inflammation that is always associated with urinary leakage in the retroperitoneum.

Renal insufficiency postoperatively is expected in varying degrees when partial nephrectomy is performed in patients with solitary kidneys. It results from removal of some normal parenchyma along with the diseased portion of the kidneys and from ischemia secondary to occlusion of the renal artery. The degree of renal insufficiency is directly proportional to the duration of ischemia and severity of trauma to the kidney. Renal insufficiency postoperatively usually resolves spontaneously with proper fluid and electrolyte management. In addition, compensatory hypertrophy may occur over the long term in the remaining parenchyma. Severe renal insufficiency may require temporary hemodialysis and both the patient and hemodialysis team should be aware of this possibility preoperatively.

Postoperative infections are self-limiting if the operative site is well drained, but may be associated with a greater incidence of urinary fistula. For this reason, every effort should be made preoperatively to sterilize the urine with systemic antibiotics.

Unusual complications of partial nephrectomy include formation of aneurysm and arteriovenous fistulas in the remaining portion of the parenchyma.[59, 60]

Surgery for Renal Carbuncle and Perinephric Abscess

Modern antibiotic therapy has greatly reduced the incidence of renal carbuncle and perinephric abscess formation. Occasionally, this disease entity may be encountered and will require formal incision and drainage. Gram-negative abscesses are associated with ascending urinary tract infections, and causative genitourinary anomalies must be evaluated and treated if present. Gram-positive abscesses are associated with hematologically seeded infections. The patient presents with fever, chills, and flank pain, and the diagnosis is established via excretory urography, ultrasound, or CT, and needle aspiration of purulent material. Preoperative blood and urine cultures should be obtained, followed by institution of broad-spectrum antibiotics to control associated bacteremia that occurs both before and during surgery.[61] A flank approach is preferred, to confine the infection to the retroperitoneum. Dissection proceeds down to the abscess, which is opened, and purulent material is expressed and collected for aerobic and anaerobic cultures. Loculations are broken up with blunt dissection, and the wound is vigorously irrigated with saline and 1% neomycin solution. Several Penrose drains or sump drains are placed to ensure continuous drainage. Muscle and fascia may be packed open with povidone-iodine (Betadine)–soaked gauze or closed in layers with absorbable sutures. The skin and subcutaneous tissue are left open to heal by secondary intention. Closure of the skin is associated with a high incidence of wound infection. The drains are sutured securely to the skin with permanent sutures. The number of drains used and location of each should be carefully documented on the patient's chart.

Postoperatively, the amount of drainage from each drain is recorded. The cultures are checked, and antibiotic therapy is modified as indicated. The dressing is changed on a daily basis and the wound cleansed with half-strength povidone-iodine diluted with either hydrogen peroxide or saline. When drainage subsides, the drains are advanced and subsequently removed. Documentation of each drain removed is important. Persistent drainage indicates obstruction, retained foreign body, calculus, fistula tract (urinary), or persistent abscess collection. A retained Penrose drain that has slipped beneath the surface of the skin may be retrieved with alligator forceps and a cystoscope inserted into the fistula tract.

An abscess associated with a nonfunctioning kidney should generally be managed with incision and drainage only as the initial step in therapy. Postoperative function can be reevaluated and frequently will return if the unit is not obstructed.[62] The mortality rate for primary nephrectomy with perinephric abscess is significantly higher than for simple incision and drainage alone.[63]

Surgery for Renal Cysts

With improved diagnostic modalities, including selective angiography, ultrasound, CT, and cyst puncture, the need to explore renal cysts has greatly diminished. Infected, hemorrhagic, calcified, and certain peripelvic cysts may require surgery. In addition, when the diagnosis of cyst is uncertain, surgical exploration may be needed as both a diagnostic and therapeutic procedure. When indicated, renal exploration of a cystic mass can be done with no mortality and minimal morbidity.[64] The kidney may be explored through a flank, anterior-extraperitoneal, or transperitoneal approach. Gerota's fascia is opened over the cyst. Simple renal cysts have a blue dome. A needle may be inserted into the cyst and fluid collected for cytologic study. If the fluid is clear, the cyst should be incised and unroofed. The back wall is then inspected for the presence of tumor or communication with the collecting system. Suspicious areas should be biopsied. Any communication with the collecting system should be closed in a watertight fashion with 4-0 chromic catgut sutures. The incised edges of the cysts are then sutured with running interlocking 3-0 chromic catgut sutures. Drains are used only if the cyst is infected or communicates with the collecting system.

Exploration of peripelvic cysts requires a more thorough dissection of the proximal ureter, pelvis, and kidney. In addition, the renal artery must be identified and tagged with a vessel loop for easy access, in case major bleeding is encountered when dissecting in the hilum near the segmental vessels.

Cystic lesions within the parenchyma of the kidney are the most difficult to explore. By clamping the renal artery and cooling the kidney, the mass may become easier to palpate as the parenchyma softens. If the mass is cystic, needle aspiration may proceed. A small nephrotomy over the cyst may be necessary to gain access for unroofing.

Caliceal cutaneous fistulas occur when a communication between the unroofed cyst and collecting system goes unrecognized or when closure of the collecting system is not watertight. With adequate drainage, the fistula resolves as the collecting system closes, assuming there is no obstruction distally. Without adequate drainage, a urinoma or abscess will form requiring formal drainage.

Surgery on Kidneys With Fusion Anomalies and Ectopia

Patients with fusion anomalies and renal ectopia are susceptible to the same disease processes that affect normally formed and placed kidneys, including hydronephrosis, calculus formation, infections, tumor, and trauma. During surgery, the danger of vascular injury increases because of the associated anomalous blood supply. For this reason, it is essential to obtain preoperative renal angiograms when major renal operations are contemplated in patients with fusion anomalies and renal ectopia.

Open Renal Biopsy

Open renal biopsy is performed in patients with solitary, small, malformed, or ectopic kidneys, severe renal insufficiency, or coagulation disorders, and in patients who are not likely to cooperate during percutaneous needle biopsy. The kidneys may be approached through a traditional flank incision or through a posterior lumbotomy incision. The posterior approach offers diminished morbidity, minimal postoperative pain and recovery time, and a cosmetic advantage. The patient is placed in the prone position and the operating room table is flexed. A laminectomy frame may be used to accentuate this position. A vertical incision is made along the lateral margin of the sacrospinalis muscle, extending from the 12th rib superiorly to the iliac crest inferiorly. The lumbodorsal fascia is incised laterally to the sacrospinalis and quadratus lumborum muscles, which are retracted medially to allow access to the renal fossa. Gerota's fascia is opened, usually over the inferior pole of the kidney. The perirenal fat is swept off the capsule to expose the biopsy site. An eliptic incision (3×1×1 cm) is made in the capsule and parenchyma of the kidney with a scalpel, and the tissue is removed with sharp scissors. Unnecessary handling of the tissue with forceps should be avoided. Tissue is immediately sent to the pathology laboratory and inspected with the dissecting microscope to ensure that there are enough glomeruli for complete analysis, which includes light microscopy, electron microscopy, and immunofluorescence studies. The incision should not be closed until the pathologist confirms receipt of adequate tissue. The surgeon closes the biopsy site by placing three or four 3-0 chromic catgut sutures on a tapered needle, being careful not to tear through the diseased parenchyma. The sutures are tied over oxidized cellulose with surgeon's knots. Pressure is then applied to the biopsy site, and the wound is irrigated with 1% neomycin solution. Gerota's fascia is reapproximated with 3-0 chromic sutures. The lumbodorsal fascia is closed with 1-0 or 2-0 chromic sutures. The subcutaneous tissue may be reapproximated, and the skin is closed with running subcuticular sutures and reinforced with Steristrips. No drains are required for this procedure.

There was no mortality, and only a single superficial wound infection occurred when this approach was used for open renal biopsy in a large series of patients.[65] The most serious potential complication is postbiopsy hemorrhage in patients who are typically hypertensive, uremic, and have minor coagulation disorders. Bleeding is typically confined to the retroperitoneum, and the majority of patients can be managed conservatively, with bed rest, frequent monitoring of vital signs, serial hemoglobin or hematocrits, and blood transfusions when indicated. Severe or prolonged bleeding may require exploration, but rarely nephrectomy. The retroperitoneal hematoma from a postbiopsy hemorrhage may become infected with subsequent abscess formation and should be drained, either percutaneously or through a small incision posteriorly.

The urologic surgeon may also be called upon to manage complications following percutaneous needle biopsy of the kidney. Postbiopsy retroperitoneal hemorrhage is managed conservatively as mentioned above. A deep needle biopsy may produce gross hematuria if the needle penetrates into the collecting system. Most patients with gross hematuria can be managed conservatively. Occasionally, life-threatening hematuria may occur, requiring angioinfarction or nephrectomy. Late hematuria may occur 7 to 10 days after needle biopsy, and patients should be instructed to limit activity for 2 weeks. Arteriovenous fistula formation has been reported and is probably a result of the needle having penetrated a large artery. The fistula is usually self-limiting, but, rarely, high-output cardiac failure may develop. Percutaneous biopsy of bowel, spleen, liver, pancreas, adrenal gland, and diaphragm has been performed with no associated sequelae reported.

Nephrostomy

Nephrostomy drainage of the kidney is used to provide supravesical urinary diversion in selected patients. Nephrostomy tubes may be placed percutaneously under fluoroscopic, ultrasonic, or CT guidance, or through a formal flank incision. If the tube is to be placed surgically, the proximal ureter, pelvis, and kidney are mobilized, and a small pyelotomy is made. A curved clamp, Randall forceps, or nephrostomy hook is placed through the pyelotomy and into a dependent calix. A small nephrostomy incision is made over the tip of the instrument, which is then pushed through the parenchyma. A Foley or Malecot catheter may then be grasped with the instrument and delivered into the pelvis of the kidney. Bleeding is usually controlled by the tube's tamponading of the tract. Occasionally, mattress sutures are placed into the parenchyma to control brisk bleeding. The tube is then secured in the parenchyma with 3-0 chromic figure-of-eight sutures, and the balloon is inflated with 2 to 3 mL of sterile water or contrast material. The pyelotomy is repaired with a running 4-0 chromic suture or interrupted sutures to ensure a watertight closure. The tube is brought out through a separate stab incision that provides dependent drainage. The retroperitoneum is drained, and the incision is closed in layers. The nephrostomy tube should be securely fastened to the skin with permanent suture material to ensure proper placement until a tract is well established.

Postoperative hemorrhage is usually self-limiting, but if significant hematuria occurs, the tube should be clamped. By clamping the tube, the pelvis fills with blood, forming a clot that acts as a tamponade. When active bleeding has ceased, the tube is unclamped and left to gravity drainage. In several days, the clot will be completely autolyzed.

A nephrostomy tube that fails to drain should be carefully inspected for kinks and straightened if necessary. If no kinks are found, the tube should be gently irrigated with sterile water or saline. If the tube cannot be irrigated freely, a gentle-gravity antegrade nephrostogram should be promptly obtained to ensure proper placement of the tube. If the tube is in the collecting system, it may be assumed that the kidney is not producing a normal amount of urine, and the patient should be managed with appropriate fluid and electrolyte therapy. If the tube is not in the collecting system, it may be repositioned percutaneously via the established tract.

Chronic urinary infection associated with nephrostomy tube drainage is common and not usually significant if drainage is adequate. If the patient becomes symptomatic, appropriate antibiotic therapy is indicated. The use of long-term, low-dose suppressive antimicrobial therapy is of questionable benefit in this setting.

Stone formation associated with

nephrostomy tube drainage may occur, especially if the urine is chronically alkaline or infected with urea-splitting organisms. This may be treated with urinary acidification or gentle irrigation of the nephrostomy tube periodically with an acidic solution. The use of Silastic catheters and frequent nephrostomy tube changes (every 6 to 8 weeks, or more frequently if needed) after the tract has been established will minimize stone formation.

Persistent urinary tract drainage after removal of the nephrostomy tube indicates fistula formation, is usually associated with distal obstruction of the collecting system, and will persist until the obstruction is relieved.

Conclusion

A small but significant rate of mortality and morbidity accompanies renal surgery. Prompt recognition and swift action to reverse both surgical and postoperative complications cannot be overemphasized in the successful management of these urologic patients.

ADRENAL SURGERY

Adrenal disease may pose a neoplastic as well as a metabolic threat to the patient. Preoperative complications associated with adrenal disease may be physiologic in addition to those typically seen in general surgical and renal procedures. Physiologic complications may result from preoperative excess production, and postoperative absence of glucocorticoids in Cushing's disease and adrenal neoplasm; mineralocorticoids in primary aldosteronism; and norepinephrine and epinephrine in pheochromocytoma. These adrenal hormones have a profound effect upon fluids, electrolytes, and hemodynamic homeostasis. Understanding these effects and appropriate preoperative preparation and postoperative management will allow adrenal surgery to be performed with a low morbidity and mortality.

Preoperative Preparation

Hyperocortisolism and Adrenocortical Insufficiency.—Patients with Cushing's syndrome or disease or cortisol-producing adrenal carcinomas are subject to a variety of physiologic effects. The excess cortisol produced in these conditions causes sodium and fluid retention with consequent volume-dependent hypertension. The excess cortisol production also promotes protein catabolism and abnormal collagen synthesis with subsequent derangements in wound healing and bone mineralization. It promotes peptic ulcer disease and thromboembolism, and has a well-recognized immunosuppressive effect, placing patients at increased risk for wound infection and sepsis.

In view of these risks, preoperative preparation of patients with adrenal disease should include antihistamine blockade, miniheparin or pneumatic stockings, care in positioning of the patient to avoid fractures, meticulous wound care, and perioperative antibiotics.

If the excess cortisol is produced by a unilateral adrenal tumor, suppression of adrenocorticotropic (ACTH) secretion by the pituitary will produce atrophy of the contralateral adrenal cortex. The atrophied adrenal may not be sufficient to respond to perioperative stresses and will permit adrenocortical insufficiency when the cortisol-producing tumor is removed. Perioperative preparation requires adequate steroid replacement. This may be done by administering 100 mg of hydrocortisone prior to surgery followed by an additional 100 mg of hydrocortisone every 6 hours for the next 24 to 48 hours postoperatively. A gradual steroid taper to maintenance levels is then provided until the hypothalamic pituitary adrenal axis recovers. Patients undergoing total bilateral adrenalectomy will require lifelong steroid replacement.[66]

Primary Aldosteronism.—Primary aldosteronism is most commonly caused by unilateral aldosterone-producing adrenal cortical adenoma. It is characterized by hypertension, elevated aldosterone levels, low plasma renin, and hypokalemic metabolic alkalosis. Preoperative preparation consists of sodium restriction, potassium-sparing diuretics, and attention to serum electrolytes. The most effective and commonly used diuretic is spironolactone. Given over a 2-month period preoperatively, it helps to improve hypertension. It also allows total body potassium reserves to be replenished and reduces the risk of perioperative cardiac arrhythmia. The medication is typically continued up until the time of surgery.[67]

Pheochromocytoma.—Pheochromocytoma is a catecholamine-secreting tumor of chromaffin tissue, most commonly occurring in the adrenal medulla. The excess catecholamines produced by these tumors can cause severe sustained or paroxysmal hypertension with subsequent end organ damage, including cardiomyopathy and cardiac arrhythmias. Intraoperative manipulation of the tumor can cause further catecholamine release with rapid and dangerous hemodynamic shifts. Preoperative preparation for these hemodynamic shifts includes preoperative fluid replacement, adequate anesthetic monitoring, and adrenergic blockade.[68]

The goal of adrenergic blockade is preoperative and perioperative blood pressure control. This is most commonly done with Phenoxybenzamine started 14 days prior to surgery.[69, 70] Adrenergic blockade also causes preoperative vasodilation and allows for reexpansion of a contracted plasma volume. Instead of adrenergic blockade, plasma volume may be reexpanded with the transfusion of 2 units of whole blood.[71] This was the preferred method prior to the development of sophisticated imaging equipment, including CT scanning and indobenzylguanidine (MIBG) scanning. It was preferred because it allowed for the intraoperative detection of extra-adrenal tumors by intraoperative palpation and exploration. However, in view of modern infectious risks associated with transfusion and increasingly reliable preoperative detection with scanning techniques, adrenergic blockade may be preferred to transfusion in the future.

Immediate preoperative preparation by the anesthesia team with ample central venous peripheral arterial and cardiopulmonary access for monitoring is critical. Central venous access is important for the immediate intraoperative delivery of labetalol and sodium nitroprusside (Nipride), which are required to respond to the rapidly changing hemodynamic situation.

Surgical Options.—The surgical approach to adrenal disease depends upon the size and character of the lesion.

Cortisol-secreting carcinomas should be approached transabdominally to allow wide en bloc dissection including the ipsilateral kidney. Large carcinomas are best approached thoracoabdominally for adequate exposure.

Bilateral, hyperplastic, pituitary-dependent adrenals uncommonly require removal. Instead, the pituitary adenoma responsible for the adrenal hyperplasia should be resected by transphenoidal exploration or irradiated. This produces a 80% to 90% success rate.[72] Those hyperplastic adrenals that do not respond to pituitary ablation, however, are best approached through a posterior retroperitoneal incision. These patients frequently have truncal obesity, which can make an anterior transabdominal approach very difficult. By placing such patients in a prone position and making separate bilateral posterior incisions, carried directly through the diaphragm, the hyperplastic adrenals are easily exposed at skin level.

The posterior approach is also useful for surgical management of primary aldosteronism. The preoperatively identified adenoma is easily approached through a unilateral posterior incision. However, those patients with primary aldosteronism suspected to be secondary to bilateral nodular hyperplasia should be managed with a bilateral adrenalectomy through separate posterior incisions as described above.

Pheochromocytoma is best approached transabdominally to allow for early ligation of the main adrenal vein prior to tumor manipulation to limit intraoperative catecholamine release and facilitate hemodynamic control. Large pheochromocytomas, like adrenocortical carcinomas, are best approached thoracoabdominally.

Postoperative Complications

Adrenocortical Insufficiency.—Adrenocortical insufficiency will occur in all patients following bilateral adrenalectomy and will probably occur in patients following unilateral removal of a hypercortisol-secreting tumor that caused atrophy of the remaining contralateral gland. Symptoms may appear gradually or rapidly with physiologic stresses. Rapid onset may be seen in the immediate postoperative period or delayed until after discharge when symptoms are precipitated by the onset of infection or some other stress. Patients presenting with delayed adrenocortical insufficiency may have sufficient adrenal function for routine metabolic function but lack the adrenal reserve for physiologic stresses such as sepsis.

Symptoms are characterized by fever, abdominal pain, nausea, vomiting, and diarrhea. The decreased ability to retain sodium, intravascular volume, and to excrete potassium leads to hypotension and cardiovascular collapse. Serum laboratory values are remarkable for hyponatremia, hyperkalemia, and azotemia in these patients. Hypoglycemia may also be present secondary to imparied hepatic gluconeogenesis. Therapy depends upon rapid diagnosis, volume replacement, and steroid supplementation.[73]

Aldosteronism.—Following adrenalectomy for an aldosterone-producing adenoma, aldosterone secretion is reduced and may not respond to sodium depletion or angiotensin. Antihypertensive medications are therefore discontinued and serum electrolytes are followed closely. There is typically sufficient mineralocorticoid activity to prevent hypokalemia if sodium intake is adequate, and potassium supplementation is rarely required. If given, however, serum potassium levels should be closely monitored. Aldosterone secretion typically recovers quickly, but may take up to 3 to 12 months.[71]

Pheochromocytoma.—The most common hemodynamic response to removing a pheochromocytoma is hypotension. Catecholamine levels fall rapidly following resection leading to increased vascular compliance and hypotension. This typically responds to volume replacement and may require large volumes of fluid administration in the immediate postoperative period.[74, 75]

Lethargy and slow emergence from anesthesia may be secondary to hypoglycemia and should be diagnosed and corrected immediately to avoid encephalopathy and prolonged neurologic damage. Hypoglycemia occurs postoperatively in response to falling catecholamine levels.[76, 77] Preoperatively, high circulating catecholamine levels inhibit insulin release, stimulate glycogenolysis and lipolysis, and decrease glucose uptake in peripheral tissues, thus promoting hyperglycemia. The preoperative hyperglycemia depletes glycogen reserves which cannot respond to hyperinsulinism that results from the sudden release of insulin inhibition following removal of the pheochromocytoma.[78, 79] Intravenous glucose replacement accompanied by vigorous hydration is required.

The rapid fall in catecholamine levels may also precipitate postoperative bronchospasm. Epinephrine is a potent bronchial smooth muscle dilator that when rapidly reduced by removing a pheochromocytoma may cause a rebound spasm and require subcutaneous supplementation to reverse.[80]

Summary

The adrenal gland governs much of the body's physiology. Disease of the adrenal gland and its treatment may therefore produce a wide variety of physiologic disturbances. A thorough understanding of normal adrenal gland function and the consequences of adrenal disease is fundamentally helpful in preoperative preparation and postoperative management of patients with surgical adrenal disease. Thoughtful preoperative preparation and postoperative management often require cooperation among the endocrinologist, anesthesiologist, and surgeon.

EDITORIAL COMMENT

A new section in this chapter covers the technique of cardiopulmonary bypass, hypothermia, and temporary cardiac arrest in the treatment of patients with intracaval neoplastic extension from renal cell carcinoma.* Magnetic resonance imaging is increasingly utilized as a modality to investigate the vena cava. It is particularly helpful when there is total occlusion of the cava. On the other hand, it may not perfectly delineate the tumor thrombus if there is movement of the distal end of the tumor thrombus. We have utilized transesophageal ultrasonography in five patients and have found this to be a valuable additional diagnostic test. It has identified greater extension of the tumor thrombus in several patients when it was not expected. The necessity for complete dissection of the renal tumor in these patients before initiation of cardiopulmonary bypass, hypothermia, and arrest is very important. The potential for a coagulopathy and extensive bleeding will be enhanced if long bypass and arrest times are utilized. We have also been less inclined to perform coronary angiography or consider coronary revascularization at the same time, especially in patients who have no significant symptoms.

A new section on adrenal surgery has been added. I think most physicians now feel that in patients with a pheochromocytoma α-adrenergic blockade preoperatively is preferable to a blood transfusion.

*1. Marshall FF, Reitz BA: Technique for removal of renal cell carcinoma with suprahepatic vena caval tumor thrombus. *Urol Clin North Am* 1986; 13:551.

2. Marshall FF, Dietrick DD, Baumgartner WA, et al: Surgical management of renal cell carcinoma with intracaval neoplastic extension above the hepatic veins. *J Urol* 1988; 139:1166.

REFERENCES

1. Chute R., Baron JA Jr, Olsson CA: The transverse upper abdominal 'chevron' incision in urological surgery. *J Urol* 1968; 99:528.
2. Montie JE: Management of stage I, II, and III renal adenocarcinoma, in Javadpour N (ed): *Principles and Management of Urologic Cancer.* Baltimore, Williams & Wilkins Co, 1984, pp 492–521.
3. Poutasse EF: Anterior approach to upper urinary tract surgery. *J Urol* 1961; 85:199.
4. Stewart BH, Hewitt CB, Kiser WS, et al: Anterior transperitoneal operative approach to the kidney. *Cleve Clin Q* 1969; 36:123.
5. Chute R, Soutter L, Kerr WS Jr: Value of thoracoabdominal incision in removal of

kidney tumors. *N Engl J Med* 1949; 241:951.
6. Robson CJ: Radical nephrectomy for renal cell carcinoma. *J Urol* 1963; 89:37.
7. Swanson DA, Borges PM: Complications of transabdominal radical nephrectomy for renal cell carcinoma. *J Urol* 1983; 129:704.
8. Skinner DG, Colvin RB, Vermillion CD, et al: Diagnosis and management of renal cell carcinoma. A clinical and pathologic study of 309 cases. *Cancer* 1971; 28:1165.
9. Waters WB, Richie JP: Aggressive surgical approach to renal cell carcinoma: Review of 130 cases. *J Urol* 1979; 122:306.
10. Middleton RG, Presto AJ III.: Radical thoracoabdominal nephrectomy for renal cell carcinoma. *J Urol* 1973; 110:36.
11. Hermann RE: Abdominal wound closure using a new polypropylene monofilament suture. *Surg Gynecol Obstet* 1974; 138:84.
12. Selli C, Hinshaw WM, Woodard BH, et al: Stratification of risk factors in renal cell carcinoma. *Cancer* 1983; 52:899.
13. Ammann AJ, Addiego J, Wara DW, et al: Polyvalent pneumococcal-polysaccharide immunization of patients with sickle-cell anemia and patients with splenectomy. *N Engl J Med* 1977; 297:897.
14. Dickerman JD: Splenectomy and sepsis: A warning. *Pediatrics* 1979; 63:938.
15. Gopal V, Bisno AL: Fulminant pneumococcal infections in 'normal' asplenic hosts. *Arch Intern Med* 1977; 137:1526.
16. Stollerman GH: Pneumococcal vaccine (letter). *JAMA* 1982; 247:1809.
17. Lucas CE: Diagnosis and treatment of pancreatic and duodenal injury. *Surg Clin North Am* 1977; 57:49.
18. Child CG III, Frey CF, Fry WJ: A reappraisal of removal of ninety-five percent of the distal portion of the pancreas. *Surg Gynecol Obstet* 1969; 129:49.
19. Zinner MJ, Baker RR, Cameron JL: Pancreatic cutaneous fistulas. *Surg Gynecol Obstet* 1974; 138:710.
20. Werschky LR, Jordan GL Jr: Surgical management of traumatic injuries to the pancreas. *Am J Surg* 1968; 116:768.
21. Northrup WF III, Simmons RL: Pancreatic trauma: A review. *Surgery* 1972; 71:27.
22. Jordan GL Jr: Complications of pancreatic and splenic surgery, in Artz CP, Haag JD (eds): *Management of Surgical Complications*. Philadelphia, WB Saunders Co, 1975, pp 534–572.
23. Spirnak JP, Resnick MI, Persky L: Cutaneous pancreatic fistula as a complication of left nephrectomy. *J Urol* 1984; 132:329.
24. Marshall VF, Middleton RG, Holswade GR, et al: Surgery for renal cell carcinoma in the vena cava. *J Urol* 1970; 103:414.
25. Siminovitch JMP, Montie JE, Straffon RA: Inferior vena cavography in the preoperative assessment of renal adenocarcinoma. *J Urol* 1982; 128:908.
26. Skinner DG, Pfister RF, Colvin R: Extension of renal cell carcinoma into the vena cava: The rationale for aggressive surgical management. *J Urol* 1972; 107:711.
27. Scheftt P, Novick AC, Straffon RA: et al: Surgery for renal cell carcinoma extending into the inferior vena cava. *J Urol* 1978; 120:28.
28. Clayman RV, Gonzales R, Fraley EE: Renal cell cancer invading the inferior vena cava: Clinical review and anatomical approach. *J Urol* 1980; 123:157.
29. Ney C: Thrombus of the inferior vena cava associated with malignant renal tumors. *J Urol* 1946; 55:583.
30. Svane S: Tumor thrombus of the inferior vena cava resulting from renal carcinoma: A report of 12 autopsied cases. *Scand J Urol Nephrol* 1969; 3:245.
31. Arkless R: Renal carcinoma: How it metastasizes. *Radiology* 1965; 84:496.
32. Kahn PC: The epinephrine effect in selective renal angiography. *Radiology* 1965; 85:301.
33. Cherrie RJ, Goldman DG, Lindner A, et al: Prognostic implications of vena caval extension of renal cell carcinoma. *J Urol* 1982; 128:910.
34. Abdelsayed MA, Bissada NK, Finkbeiner AE, et al: Renal tumors involving the inferior vena cava: Plan for management. *J Urol* 1978; 120:153.
35. Kearney GP, Waters WB, Klein LA, et al: Results of inferior vena cava resection for renal cell carcinoma. *J Urol* 1981; 125:769.
36. Montie JE, Jackson CL, Cosgrove DM, et al: Resection of large inferior vena caval thrombi from renal cell carcinoma with the use of circulatory arrest. *J Urol* 1988; 139:25.

37. Krane RJ, White R, Davis Z, et al: Removal of renal cell carcinoma extending into the right atrium using cardiopulmonary bypass, profound hypothermia and circulatory arrest. *J Urol* 1984; 131:945.
38. Marshall FF, Reitz BA, Diamond DA: A new technique for management of renal cell carcinoma involving the right atrium: Hypothermia and cardiac arrest. *J Urol* 1984; 131:103.
39. Klein FA, Smith MJV, Greenfield LJ: Extracorporeal circulation for renal cell carcinoma with supradiaphragmatic vena caval thrombi. *J Urol* 1984; 131:880.
40. Montie JE, Pontis JE, Novick AC, et al: Intratrial extension of renal cell carcinoma: Results of surgical management. Second International Symposium on Advances in Urologic Oncology. ed. *Acta Urol* 1989;
41. Culp OS: Anterior nephro-ureterectomy: Advantages and limitations of a single incision. *J Urol* 1961; 85:193.
42. Tessler AN, Yuvienco F, Farcon E: Paramedian extraperitoneal incision for total nephroureterectomy. *Urology* 1975; 5:397.
43. Skinner DG: Considerations for management of large retroperitoneal tumors: Use of the modified thoracoabdominal approach. *J Urol* 1977; 117:605.
44. Montague DK, Straffon RA: Complications of renal surgery, in Smith RB, Skinner DG (eds): *Complications of Urologic Surgery*. Philadelphia, WB Saunders Co, 1976, pp 54–86.
45. Bloom NA, Vidone RA, Lytton B: Primary carcinoma of the ureter: A report of 102 new cases. *J Urol* 1970; 103:590.
46. Strong DW, Pearse HD: Recurrent urothelial tumors following surgery for transitional cell carcinoma of the upper urinary tract. *Cancer* 1976; 38:2178.
47. Scott RF Jr, Selzman HM: Complications of nephrectomy: Review of 450 patients and a description of a modification of the transperitoneal approach. *J Urol* 1966; 95:307.
48. Pearlman CK, Kobashigawa L: Nephrectomy: Review of 200 cases. *Am Surg* 1968; 34:438.
49. Sakati IA, Marshall VF: Postoperative fatalities in urology. *J Urol* 1966; 95:412.
50. Schiff M Jr, Glazier WB: Nephrectomy: Indications and complications in 347 patients. *J Urol* 1977; 118:930.
51. Goldstein AE, Abeshouse BS: Partial resections of the kidney. Report of 6 cases and review of the literature. *J Urol* 1937; 38:15.
52. Semb C: Partial resection of the kidney: Operative technique. *Acta Chir Scand* 1955; 109:360.
53. Wein AJ, Carpiniello VL, Murphy JJ: A simple technique for partial nephrectomy. *Surg Gynecol Obstet* 1978; 146:621.
54. Poutasse EF: Partial nephrectomy: New techniques, approach, operative indications and review of 51 cases. *J Urol* 1962; 88:153.
55. Kim SK: New techniques of partial nephrectomy. *J Urol* 1969; 102:165.
56. Williams DF, Schapiro AE, Arconti JS, et al: A new technique of partial nephrectomy. *J Urol* 1967; 97:955.
57. Straffon RA, Novick AC (eds): *Vascular Problems in Urologic Surgeries.* Philadelphia, WB Saunders Co, 1982, pp 101–102.
58. Wilson GSM: Clinical experience in renal hypothermia. *J Urol* 1963; 89:666.
59. Rezvani A, Ward JN, Lavengood RW Jr: Intrarenal aneurysm following partial nephrectomy. *Urology* 1973; 2:286.
60. Snodgrass WT, Robinson MJ: Intrarenal arteriovenous fistula: A complication of partial nephrectomy. *J Urol* 1964; 91:135.
61. Thorley JD, Jones SR, Sanford JP: Perinephric abscess. *Medicine* 1974; 53:441.
62. Malgieri JJ, Kursh ED, Persky L: The changing clinicopathological pattern of abscesses in or adjacent to the kidney. *J Urol* 1977; 118:230.
63. Gonzalez-Serva L, Weinerth JL, Glenn JF: Minimal mortality of renal surgery. *Urology* 1977; 9:253.
64. Stanisic TH, Babcock JR, Grayhack JT: Morbidity and mortality of renal exploration for cyst. *Surg Gynecol Obstet* 1977; 145:733.
65. Novick AC: Posterior surgical approach to the kidney and ureter. *J Urol* 1980; 124:192.
66. Dluhy RG, Gittes RF: The adrenals, in Walsh PC, Gittes RF, Perlmutter AD, et al (eds): *Campbell's Urology.* Philadelphia, WB Saunders Co, 1986, pp 2999–3007.
67. Bravo EL, Dustan HP, Tanae RC: Spirino-

lactone as a nonspecific treatment for primary aldosteronism. *Circulation* 1973; 48:491.

68. Cullen ML, Staren ED, Strans AK, et al: Pheochromocytoma: Operative strategy. *Surgery* 1985; 98:927.
69. Temple WD, Voitk AK, Thomson AE, et al: Phenoxybenzamine blockade in surgery of pheochromocytoma. *J Surg Res* 1977; 22:59.
70. Wheeler MH, Chanz MJB, Austin TR, et al: The management of the patient with catecholamine excess. *World J Surg* 1982; 6:735.
71. DeOreo GA, Stewart BH, Tarazi RC, et al: Preoperative blood transfusion in the safe surgical management of pheochromocytoma: A review of 46 cases. *J Urol* 1974; 111:715.
72. Tyrell B, Brooks RM, Fitzgerald PA, et al: Cushing's disease: Selective transsphenoidal resection of pituitary microadenomas. *N Engl J Med* 1978; 298:753.
73. Bell NH: The glucocorticoid withdrawal syndrome, in Avioli JV, Genvani C, Imbimbo B (eds): *Glucocorticoid Effects and Their Biological Consequences.* New York, Plenum Press, 1984; pp 293–299.
74. Ross EJ, Pritchard BNC, Kaufman L, et al: Preoperative and operative management of patients with pheochromocytoma. *Br Med J* 1967; 1:191.
75. Bergman SM, Sean HF, Jaadpour N, et al: Postoperative management of patients with pheochromocytoma. *J Urol* 1978; 120:109.
76. Costello GT, Moorthy SS, Vane DW, et al: Hypoglycemia following bilateral adrenalectomy for pheochromocytoma. *Crit Care Med* 1988; 16:562.
77. Channa AB, Mofti AB, Atylor GW, et al: Hypoglycemic encephalopathy following surgery on pheochromocytoma. *Anesthesia* 1987; 42:1298.
78. Sagalowski A, Donohue JP: Possible mechanism of hypoglycemia following removal of pheochromocytoma. *J Urol* 1980; 124:422.
79. Ellis S: The metabolic effects of epinephrine and related amines. *Pharmacol Rev* 1956; 8:485.
80. Nishikawa T, Dolzi S, Auzai Y: Recurrence of bronchial asthma after adrenalectomy for pheochromocytoma. *Can Anaesth Soc J* 1986; 33:109.

CHAPTER 10

Complications of Renal, Vesical, and Urethral Trauma

Jack W. McAninch, M.D.

Complications of injury to the urinary system can result in high morbidity and, at times, mortality. This chapter will focus on the most significant complications in each area and detail their diagnosis and management as well as appropriate preventive measures.

COMPLICATIONS OF RENAL TRAUMA

Early Complications

Delayed Renal Bleeding

Delayed bleeding after major injury to the urinary system may be seen as retroperitoneal bleeding or gross blood in the urine. This bleeding occurs most often 5 to 20 days after injury and can be massive. Excessive activity, lifting heavy objects, or prolonged Valsalva maneuvers tend to increase the likelihood of delayed bleeding. Patients may become abruptly hypotensive and present in frank hypovolemic shock. More often the process is slower, with the patient complaining of flank pain and gross hematuria.

Patients with retroperitoneal bleeding will have flank and upper quadrant abdominal tenderness on the involved side. With gross hematuria, obstructive clots in the ureter may cause symptoms typical of colic, mild irritative bladder symptoms, and dysuria. Excessive blood loss will result in a drop in blood pressure; massive bleeding may cause severe shock.

Occasionally, heavy retroperitoneal bleeding may not be accompanied by gross hematuria, but in most circumstances microhematuria will be noted on urinalysis. Significant blood loss will cause serial hematocrit readings to decrease significantly over a few hours' time.

Computed tomography (CT) is the single best diagnostic study for retroperitoneal bleeding. With contrast enhancement, CT can demonstrate the area of renal injury as well as the size and extent of the retroperitoneal hematoma.[1] Excretory urography (intravenous pyelogram [IVP]) may be used, but it is nonspecific and provides very little diagnostic information.

Massive renal bleeding causing hypovolemic shock that does not respond to immediate fluid therapy will require immediate surgical intervention. The operation is best done through a midline transabdominal incision, with immediate isolation of the renal artery and vein on the involved side before renal exposure. Vascular clamps should be placed on the renal artery at the time of isolation to prevent additional blood loss and allow for deliberate renal exposure and inspection. When renal exploration is required for delayed bleeding, the incidence of complete nephrectomy is very high.[2, 3] When blood loss occurs more slowly, intravenous infusion of Ringer's lactate will often correct any developing hypotension, and transfusion with packed red blood cells will permit observation and delay operative intervention. Several units of blood may be used to stabilize the patient, and, on many occasions, the bleeding will subside spontaneously. When bleeding persists, angiography may be done (time permitting) and bleeding arteries embolized for control.[4]

In most patients, clot formation develops immediately after injury, and clot breakdown by the natural enzymatic process and wound healing begin as early as 5 days later. This enzymatic process may occur over a period of up to 20 days after injury, and it is during this time that delayed bleeding is most likely. Renal lacerations that extend through the cortex and into the deep medulla are more subject to delayed bleeding than are superficial lacerations, because the larger vessels coursing within the renal parenchyma lie more medial and central to the renal vascular pedicle. This anatomical arrangement is true of both arteries and veins.

Prevention of delayed bleeding hinges on the appropriate selection of patients for operation. Fewer than 10% of patients with blunt renal trauma will have major injuries, and not all of these will require operation, but patients with deep lacerations through the cortex and into the medulla are more prone to delayed bleeding. Patients with deep lacerations and minimal retroperitoneal hematoma at presentation may be less prone. Patients with major blunt injuries should be cautioned against excessive physical activity and allowed to return to their habitual state of activity only progressively.

Prolonged Urinary Extravasation

Prolonged urinary extravasation occurs after major blunt or penetrating injuries. These patients are often asymptomatic, unless the urine or retroperitoneal urinoma becomes infected. When the extravasation is extensive and prolonged, the patient may complain of increasing abdominal discomfort and distention, lethargy, poor appetite, and weight loss.

Large urinomas in the retroperitoneum may cause low-grade fevers. On palpation, an abdominal mass may be noted; tenderness is usually minimal unless infection is present. Ileus and abdominal distention are common.

On IVP, the involved kidney, particularly the area of injury, will be poorly visualized. Delayed films will usually demonstrate opacified urine in the retroperitoneum and in the urinoma. Computed tomography will provide more sensitive definition of the area of injury and the extent of extravasation (Fig 10–1).[1]

Small degrees of urinary extravasation after trauma are probably insignificant. In most circumstances, extravasation confined to the renal capsule appears to cease within a short time and does not interfere with wound healing. Extravasation beyond the capsule may be more significant and early operative intervention should be considered. If it continues and a large urinoma develops, fluid drainage is indicated. Percutaneous measures should be tried; if unsuccessful, open operation via flank approach with the placement of drains usually corrects the problem. It is seldom necessary to explore the kidney formally and close the opening in the collecting system. Extensive tissue reaction in the retroperitoneum often prevents clear identification of the precise area of injury and hampers closure under direct vision. Drainage alone is adequate in most cases.

The pathogenesis of urinomas and prolonged extravasation can be traced to deep lacerations extending into the urinary collecting system. Minor lacerations usually close promptly and heal without difficulty, but extensive injury to a calix

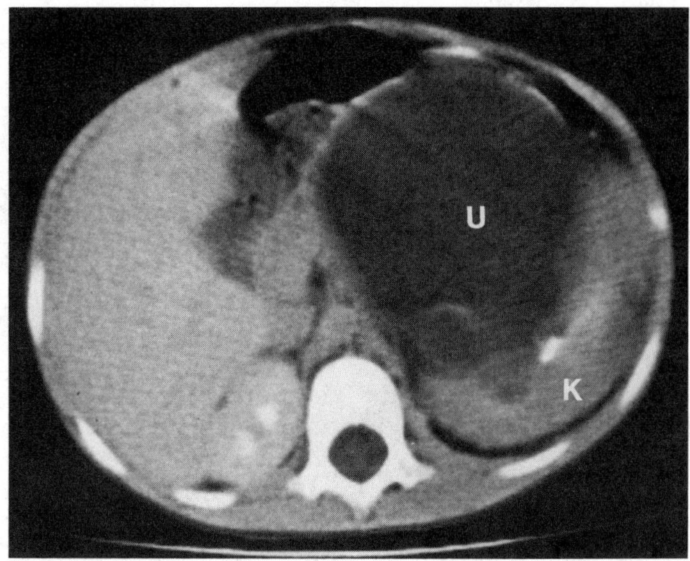

FIG 10–1.
Computed tomography in a 6-year-old child a few weeks after blunt abdominal trauma. The child had a deep left renal laceration managed nonoperatively. Chronic urinary extravasation resulted in a large urinoma *(U)*. The kidney *(K)* is posterior and lateral. Surgical drainage corrected the problem.

may cause prolonged extravasation. Any obstruction distal to the area of injury will decrease the chances of spontaneous closure, and any surrounding nonviable tissue may, through chemolysis and tissue breakdown, allow an avenue for continued extravasation.

Extensive extravasation beyond the renal capsule on initial evaluation is often predictive of the development of a urinoma. These injuries are frequently associated with massive retroperitoneal bleeding and large amounts of nonviable tissue and require immediate surgical correction. Proper selection of these patients for operation is the best preventive. Should the ureter or renal pelvis be obstructed by clot, congenital abnormalities, or calculi, prompt drainage from an area above the obstruction will allow the injured site to heal spontaneously.

Retroperitoneal Abscess

Abscess formation within the retroperitoneum is usually secondary to infection of the accumulated hematoma or the existing urinoma, and it is suspected if the patient has chills, fever, and increasing abdominal and flank pain. The abscess may develop within 5 to 7 days of injury; the patient usually has had operative exploration, which is the source of the infection, or infected urine that seeds the retroperitoneal space. Chronic abscess will result in lethargy, appetite suppression, and weight loss. Generalized sepsis may occasionally develop.

Most patients have high spiking temperatures with marked tenderness of the abdomen and flank. Extensive abscess may cause overlying skin erythema and "pointing" in the area of Petit's triangle.

The urine should be carefully inspected for infectious organisms and a culture obtained. The IVP will often suggest an abscess by the displacement of bowel from a retroperitoneal mass; the kidney may also be displaced. Sonography will demonstrate a hypoechogenic mass; in some cases, gas may be present in it. Ultrasonography may at times be diagnostic. Computed tomography of the retroperitoneum is more often diagnostic: a large mass with a density of 10 to 60 Hounsfield units is typical, and gas produced by bacteria within the abscess cavities is often detected.

Drainage is the best management and may be accomplished by percutaneous insertion of a small catheter to evacuate the pus, followed by intermittent irrigation with small volumes of antibiotic solution to allow sterilization and contraction of the abscess cavity. Large loculated abscesses may require open surgical drainage, which is best done by a retroperitoneal approach.

Bacteria may reach the retroperitoneal hematoma by implantation during a surgical procedure (this is uncommon), by tracking along drains left in place, by seeding of the hematoma from the vascular system, or by extravasated infected urine. Prolonged urinary extravasation increases the potential of infection.

Careful, early assessment of the patient is the best prevention. Antibiotics providing broad-spectrum coverage for gram-negative and gram-positive organisms should be initiated promptly. Retroperitoneal drains left in place should be monitored carefully, since they represent an external source by which bacteria can enter the retroperitoneal space and propagate abscess formation. Early removal is indicated when drainage has subsided. All patients with accumulated retroperitoneal blood or urine should be carefully followed; any suspicion of infection should prompt immediate diagnostic procedures.

Delayed Complications

Hypertension

Although the literature suggests that the incidence of hypertension after renal injury is 5% or less, the true rate is difficult to determine. Patients tend not to return for follow-up, and the time of onset can vary from months to years after injury.

Patients who have severe hypertension present with headaches and blurred vision. However, they may very often be asymptomatic, and hypertension will be detected only by routine blood pressure measurement. They will report a history of renal trauma, which at the time may have appeared to be of no clinical significance. Other clinical clues suggestive of renal vascular hypertension related to trauma include absence of family history of hypertensive disease, abrupt onset of moderate to severe hypertension, development of malignant hypertension, and unresponsiveness to standard diuretic therapy or antihypertensive medications.

In adults, diastolic blood pressure will be over 90 mm Hg; in children, it will vary according to age. With malignant hypertension, examination of the eyegrounds will often demonstrate hemorrhage, exudate, and papilledema. Occasionally, an abdominal or flank bruit will be heard; this usually indicates severe arterial stenosis or an aneurysm of the main renal artery.

Mild microscopic hematuria may be present. Serum electrolytes may demonstrate some degree of metabolic acidosis and hypokalemia.[5] A rapid-sequence IVP should be obtained (Fig 10–2). Delayed excretion of contrast in the calices on the involved side is typical of main renal artery stenosis; segmental renal artery lesions will be more difficult to diagnose by IVP. Renal arteriography is the best method to demonstrate anatomical arterial lesions likely to cause hypertension. Renal vein renin levels should be measured; in some cases, the segmental renal veins will require sampling. The renal vein renin ratio is calculated by dividing the plasma renin activity of the stenotic side by that of the normal side. Values above 1.5 are considered typical of renal vascular hypertension.[5]

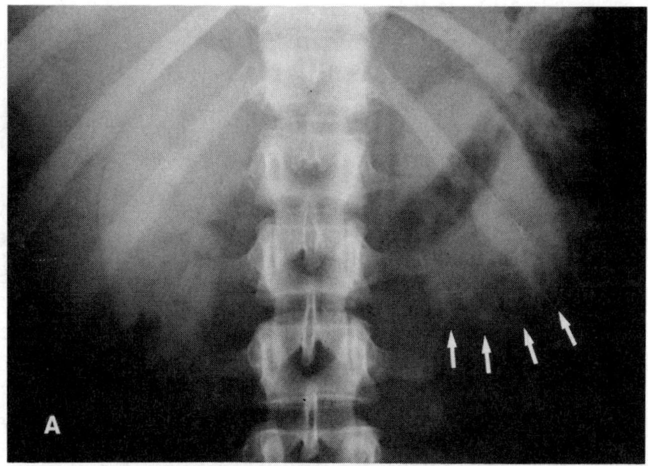

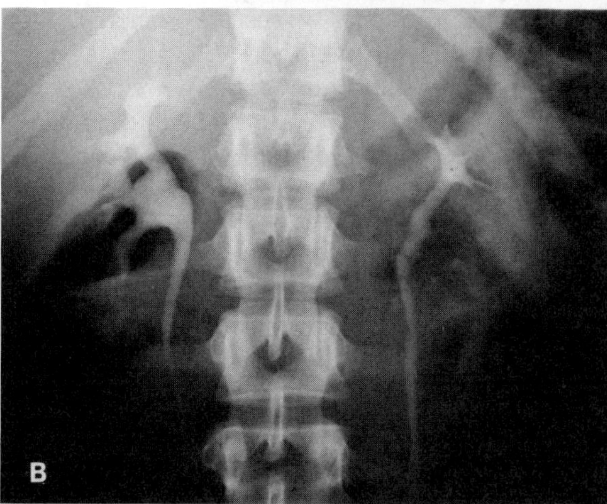

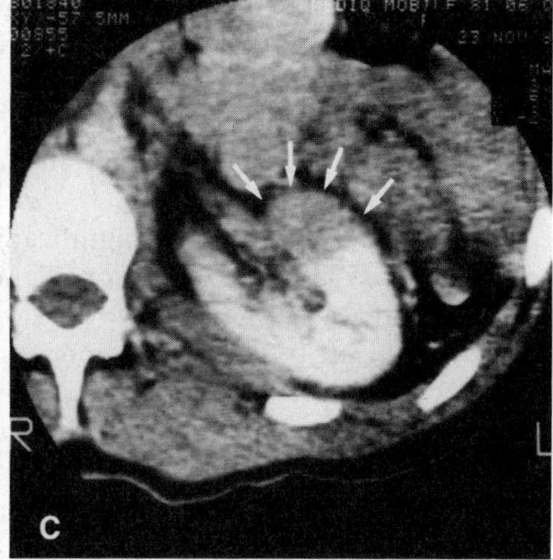

FIG 10–2.
A, a rapid-sequence IVP in a 30-year-old woman 6 months after a blunt injury to the left kidney was managed nonoperatively. The nephrotomogram shows nonvisualization of the left lower pole *(arrows)*. **B,** the lack of contrast excretion from the left lower pole indicates that the area of injury is large. **C,** computed tomography at the level of injury demonstrates poor perfusion of the injured segment *(arrows)*. The patient is at risk of developing hypertension and should have frequent blood pressure checks.

The initial management approach should be medical. If this treatment fails, surgical exploration is indicated, with partial nephrectomy of any localized area of previous injury that excretes excessive renin. Should the cause of the hypertension be main renal artery stenosis consequent to trauma, nephrectomy is usually required.

The pathogenesis of hypertension after renal injury is that of relative ischemia to the renal parenchyma, which causes excessive renin secretion. The ischemia may result from main or segmental renal artery injury or parenchymal lacerations. The last-named may be associated with large intrarenal hematomas, which cause relative compression of the parenchymal margins and thus ischemia and hypertension. This form of hypertension may occur shortly after injury and last for a few weeks before spontaneous resolution.

Hypertension after trauma can be prevented with prompt initial management of main and segmental renal artery lesions.

Page Kidney.—In 1939, Page[6] described arterial hypertension caused by cellophane perinephritis consequent to renal injuries. The presentation is similar to hypertension; indeed, most patients are hypertensive on examination. Headache, blurred vision, and facial flushing are common. Palpitations and tachycardia accompanied by shortness of breath may be other suggestive symptoms. Many patients may be totally asymptomatic; however, a careful history will invariably elicit trauma to the flank or a kidney in previous years.

Examination will reveal significant diastolic and systolic hypertension. Patients with severe cases may have retinopathy as well as left ventricular hypertrophy. Cardiac murmurs will be heard occasionally. The abdomen should be carefully palpated, but invariably no masses or renal abnormalities will be detected. Bruits of the renal vessels will not be present.

Patients with Page kidney have been reported to have polycythemia, but this is not a typical laboratory finding. A plain roentgenogram of the abdomen will usually demonstrate an absent psoas shadow on the involved side with evidence of an enlarged renal shadow; a small percentage will show calcification in the area of the kidney. Arteriography will demonstrate a patent arterial tree and delayed contrast medium perfusion on the involved side. The segmental and interlobar arteries are often splayed and stretched, and the kidney appears to be diffusely enlarged. Computed tomography[7] can be useful: characteristically, there is minimal contrast enhancement of the renal tissue with surrounding bandlike tissue engulfing the kidney; renal scans demonstrate decreased uptake and poor function.

Therapy involves the release of surrounding fibrosis constricting the renal parenchyma. If this cannot be accomplished, a nephrectomy should be performed. Medical therapy appears to be of limited benefit.

Arterial hypertension caused by cellophane perinephritis[6] is the result of constrictive trauma to the kidney and retroperitoneum that constantly compresses the parenchyma, activating the renin-angiotensin system. The traumatic cause appears to be a subcapsular hematoma, which produces excessive scarring beneath the capsule and subsequent severe parenchymal compression within a confined space. Renins localized to the involved kidney are uniformly elevated.

The incidence of Page kidney is extremely low, much less than 1%. Patients at high risk are those with a significant subcapsular hematoma that has not been drained. Patients with kidneys that show decreased function on nucleotide scans and that have large subcapsular hematomas should have the hematoma drained as a preventive measure.

Arteriovenous Fistula

Arteriovenous fistula is a troublesome problem. These patients present many years after renal trauma with evidence of hypertension or renal bleeding. The exact incidence is unknown but is reportedly no more than 1% of patients sustaining renal injury.[8]

Hematuria is the most common presenting symptom, usually gross and intermittent. Patients may occasionally complain of flank pain if clot obstruction within the ureter occurs. Headache and other symptoms of hypertension may be the initial presenting symptom in a small percentage. A past history of an abdominal stab wound or gunshot wound is typical, although blunt traumatic injuries can also cause arteriovenous fistulas.

The finding of massive gross hematuria together with a past history of abdominal trauma should make one immediately suspicious. Hypertension with diastolic blood pressure in excess of 90 mm Hg may also be present; when severe, papilledema, retinal changes, and headaches will be noted. Careful auscultation of the abdomen often reveals a bruit.

Digital subtraction renal angiography or selective renal arteriography will clearly establish the diagnosis. Characteristically, the involved kidney is smaller than its counterpart, and contrast material will be rapidly shunted from the arterial to the venous system (Fig 10–3).

Management is controversial. Complete nephrectomy is the simplest answer

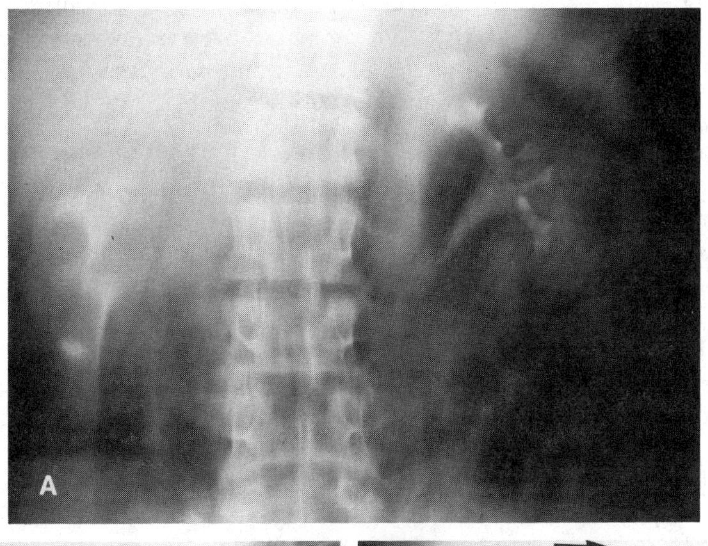

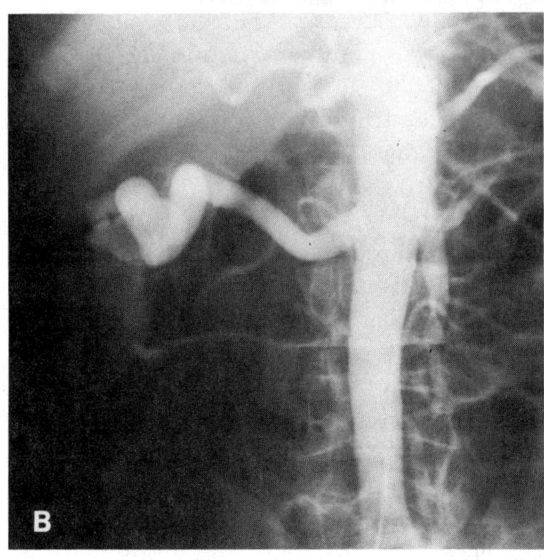

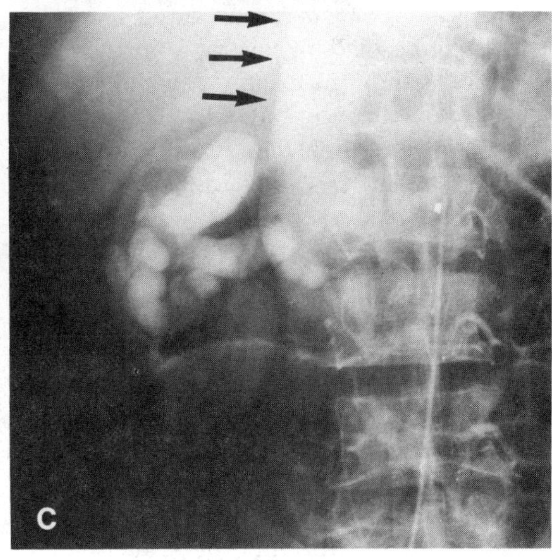

FIG 10–3.
A, excretory urogram in a man with gross hematuria who had blunt right renal trauma 20 years previously. The film shows a small right kidney with severe caliceal distortion. **B,** renal arteriogram shows a large tortuous right renal artery. **C,** immediate contrast filling of the right renal vein is seen during arteriography, confirming the diagnosis of arteriovenous fistula. The vena cava is promptly visualized *(arrows)*. A right nephrectomy was performed.

for large fistulas. When the upper or lower pole of the kidney is involved, partial nephrectomy can be done. Very often severe surrounding fibrosis will make any operation difficult. In general, the fistula should not be embolized, because of potential shunting into the venous system. Cosgrove and associates have used segmental ligation of the renal vessels in the fistula with some success.[9]

Stab wounds appear to be the most common cause of arteriovenous fistulas, gunshot wounds and blunt trauma less so. The exact mechanism by which fistulas form is unclear, nor can their development be predicted.

Prevention requires careful reconstruction of the injured area at initial operation, including meticulous hemostasis and individual suture ligation of bleeding points. The parenchymal defect should be covered with an omental pedicle graft or other existing tissue in the area, such as free peritoneal grafts or perirenal fat.

Hydronephrosis

Ureteral obstruction is a recognized complication of renal trauma and most often becomes evident several months later.

The symptoms usually develop slowly over weeks or months and include, most notably, increasing flank pain. Although the pain is usually constant, it is not debilitating initially. However, as the obstruction progresses, more and more pain will develop; some patients report varying intensity, but they are never totally pain-free. The pain may be localized to the flank or the upper abdominal quadrant on the involved side. Pyelonephritis may be a complicating factor of the obstructive process.

Palpation will usually elicit flank or upper abdominal tenderness; occasionally, a mass may be noted. Urinalysis is usually normal. The IVP will demonstrate delayed contrast excretion on the involved side; delayed films will show columning of contrast material in the upper ureter or renal pelvis to the site of obstruction. The most common area involved is the upper ureter along the lower renal pole or at the ureteropelvic junction. Sonography will establish the presence of hydronephrosis but will not localize the point of obstruction, and retrograde ureteropyelography may be necessary.

The pathogenesis involves periluminal fibrosis of the ureter or renal pelvis, producing extrinsic obstruction. Extrarenal urinary extravasation, urinomas surrounding the kidney, and infected perirenal hematomas appear to increase the risk.

Management is difficult. The existing perirenal scar makes ureterolysis and excision of fibrotic tissue surrounding the renal pelvis difficult.

Ideally, the ureter and renal pelvis should be totally freed of the scar tissue, and omentum or viable adipose tissue should be placed in the area to prevent recurrence of the scar formation. Nephrectomy may be necessary when extensive renal damage has occurred from the obstruction or when adequate reconstruction of the area cannot be accomplished.[10]

Upper ureteral obstruction can be prevented at the time of initial operative repair by assuring that the ureter is free from the lower pole of the renal capsule, since in this area the ureter often adheres to the capsule and becomes engulfed in the perinephric fibrosis. Maintaining the ureter in a separate plane is best accomplished by placing a small amount of viable fatty tissue between the kidney and the upper ureter at the completion of any reconstructive procedure.

COMPLICATIONS OF BLADDER TRAUMA

Persistent Pelvic Bleeding

Major traumatic injuries to the bony pelvis and pelvic vessels cause persistent pelvic bleeding. Because patients usually have numerous associated injuries, including long-bone fractures and abdominal injuries, they can be in great discomfort or unconscious, and the diagnosis is not aided by specific patient complaints. The hematomas may accumulate slowly over several hours and be reflected by increasing lower abdominal distention and tenderness, and bladder injuries are common.

Catheterization of the bladder typically reveals gross hematuria. Cystography demonstrates extravesical extravasation of contrast and will also depict the deformity on the bladder caused by the large developing pelvic hematoma. With continued bleeding, pelvic angiography can be done (time permitting) to localize any arterial bleeding (Fig 10–4). Embolization provides successful control.[11] An IVP or abdominal CT scan should be done to be certain that the kidneys and ureters are free of injury.

Surgical therapy is the primary treatment for bladder ruptures. Exploration through a lower abdominal midline incision allows an easy approach to the bladder and provides access to the abdominal cavity for further exploration. A peritoneotomy should be done to determine if free blood is in the abdomen; if so, full exploration should be performed. Once the lower abdominal fascia has been opened, the bladder should be approached by avoiding the large retroperitoneal hematomas that may have accumulated on either side of the midline. The bladder is opened in the midline and repaired from inside with 2-0 chromic sutures in a single layer.

To maintain the natural tamponade, avoid opening the lateral hematomas. Heavy bleeding will be encountered in some cases, most often from disruption of pelvic veins, and one should avoid excessive pelvic dissection to find venous bleeding sites. Little benefit is obtained from ligation of the hypogastric arteries. In such cases, the best management is surgical packing of the pelvis with laparotomy tapes and closure of the abdomen. Reexploration in 24 hours with removal of the tapes usually provides control of these difficult bleeding problems. Fresh frozen plasma should be given to provide the patient with appropriate clotting factors during the process of resuscitation with packed red blood cells and electrolyte solutions.

These large hematomas develop both from pelvic fractures and from the disruption of arteries and veins within the deep pelvic floor upon massive traumatic insult. Arterial bleeding can be identified and controlled, but venous bleeding is much more difficult to define and localize. The development of large pelvic hematomas is often insidious and their significance often underestimated. Mortality may be as high as 20%.[12]

Prevention is not always possible. However, certain points in management should be noted. At surgical exploration, lateral dissection along the bladder wall should be avoided to maintain the tamponade effect. When the patient is stable, angiography should be done early to determine if arterial bleeding is the source and to allow embolization to control the problem. Should heavy bleeding be encountered during exploration, packing of the area with laparotomy packs and closure of the abdomen with planned removal in 24 hours offers an excellent method of preventing further bleeding and hematoma development.

Pelvic Abscess

Patients presenting with pelvic abscess after trauma usually have had bladder rupture managed by catheter drainage alone or by surgical exploration that promoted an infection of the pelvic hematoma. The patients ordinarily have not been discharged from the hospital and develop increasing lower abdominal discomfort 7 to 10 days after the initial injury. Night sweats, fever (spiking tempera-

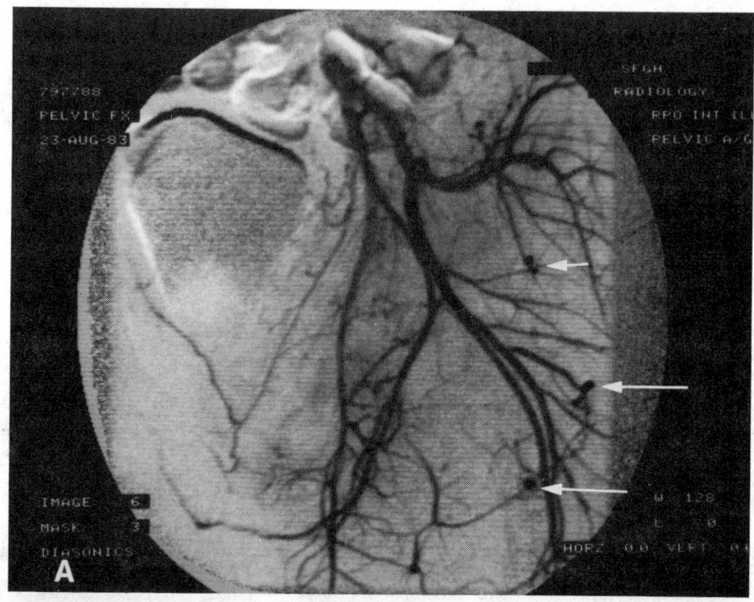

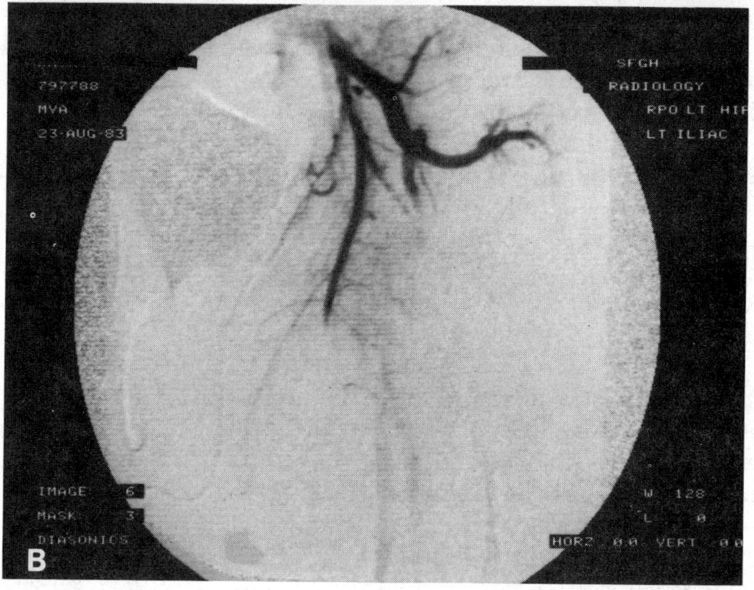

FIG 10–4.
A, digital subtraction arteriogram of the hypogastric artery in a patient with pelvic fracture and persistent retroperitoneal bleeding. *Arrows* indicate points of arterial rupture and site of bleeding. **B,** repeated arteriogram after embolization with Gelfoam shows complete occlusion of the ruptured areas. Bleeding was controlled and the patient became hemodynamically stabilized.

tures), and evidence of systemic sepsis may be present. Abdominal ileus is common, but other findings will be minimal on examination. Lower abdominal tenderness is often absent.

Hematocrit levels are often low because of chronic blood loss and hemolysis from infection. White blood cell counts are elevated, in many cases above 20,000/mm^3 with a marked left shift. Ultrasonography and CT of the pelvic area may demonstrate these abscesses, but distinguishing hematoma from abscess is often difficult. Diagnosis is best based on the accumulated facts of the patient's condition.

Surgical drainage is the recommended management. In isolated cases, percutaneous drainage may be acceptable, but the hematomas are often multiple and loculated, and surgical drainage offers the most complete and safest form of therapy. A lower or midline abdominal incision provides access to the abscess; multiple drains should be placed in the area to provide complete evacuation. Antibiotics should be instituted before surgery and maintained postoperatively. These antibiotics should provide broad-spectrum coverage to include anaerobes, aerobes, and gram-positive and gram-negative organisms. The urinary bladder should be decompressed with catheter drainage during the healing process.

The pathogenesis of pelvic abscess development originates with infection of the pelvic hematoma. This infection may be initiated at the time of surgery to correct bladder rupture, but more commonly occurs at the drain site. Catheter drainage only of extraperitoneal ruptures is another source of pelvic hematoma infection (Fig 10–5). Bladder colonization occurs approximately 72 hours after placement of the catheter, allowing bacteria to migrate into the surrounding hematoma through the existing rupture site.

Prevention is crucial. The high morbidity (20%) of pelvic hematomas results largely from abscess formation. Drains should be avoided at the initial surgery and at bladder repair. Catheter drainage of the bladder for urinary diversion is sufficient to prevent urinary extravasation; thus, drains to the pelvis are seldom indicated to remove accumulated blood. The drain sites represent the major source of infection in the pelvic hematoma. If drains are left in place, they should be removed as soon as possible.

Because pelvic abscess can develop secondary to using catheter drainage alone as a form of managing bladder rupture, one must select patients judiciously

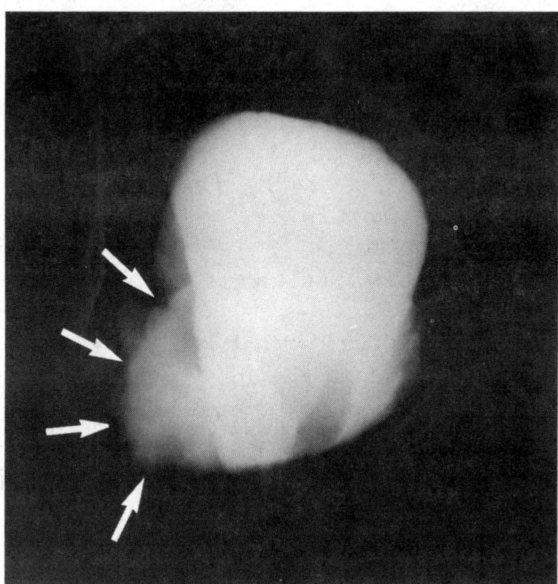

FIG 10–5.
Cystogram in a patient 10 days after an extraperitoneal bladder rupture was managed by urethral catheter drainage. The film shows persistent extravasation *(arrows)*, which leads to pelvic hematoma infection. Surgical drainage of the abscess and bladder closure were successful.

for such therapy. Hayes and associates[13] have recently reported 16 patients thus managed in whom no complications developed, but Cass et al.[14] found significant complications in a similar group. Our own experience has indicated that the extent of extravasation seen on cystography does not correlate with the size or number of bladder lacerations.[15] For this reason, all patients at our institution continue to have formal surgical repair. Should one choose catheter drainage alone, we recommend cystography with a limited volume of contrast material at approximately 8 to 10 days after injury, at which time patients should receive systemic antibiotics. When no extravasation is present, the catheter may be removed and the patient followed carefully. Should evidence of pelvic abscess begin to develop, complete diagnostic studies should be performed to establish an accurate diagnosis. With sonography, CT, and cystography, the size and location of the abscess can be determined.

Incontinence

Incontinence may develop after major bladder trauma in a select number of patients. During the early postoperative period after catheter removal, patients often note intermittent urgency and urge incontinence, but total incontinence is rare. Stress incontinence is common in women during the first few weeks; in most cases, it will subside slowly and disappear. Total incontinence leaves the patient with constant wetness and no sensation of voiding. This is more common in women and occurs primarily because of injuries to the bladder neck. Catheterization reveals no evidence of stricture or bladder neck contraction, and the bladder has a normal capacity.

Results of cystometrography will be normal, but urodynamic studies of the bladder neck and urethra will demonstrate an inability to close and very low resistance.

Careful diagnostic evaluation with urodynamic studies should be done before any type of repair. Procedures to correct total incontinence after trauma have had limited success; however, Tanagho's tube flap[16] offers perhaps the best overall rates. Of endoscopic urethral suspension techniques, limited information is available, but some encouraging results have been obtained.[17]

The mechanism by which incontinence occurs after major bladder trauma depends upon the type of injury. Lacerations along the trigone extending down through the bladder neck appear to be the major source of the problem. These injuries largely result from massive pelvic fracture after severe blows to the bony pelvis and cause extensive damage to the smooth muscle and skeletal muscle of the bladder neck and the urethra in women.

Incontinence is best prevented by refined surgical technique at the initial repair. Lacerations extending into the bladder neck should be meticulously repaired with fine chromic sutures of 3-0 and 4-0 placed in an interrupted fashion. This careful reconstruction reassembles the injured tissue anatomically, such that healing can occur under optimal circumstances.

Fistulas

Vesicocutaneous or vesicovaginal fistulas are uncommon but may develop after major bladder ruptures and massive pelvic injuries. Patients with vesicovaginal fistulas often have had penetrating injuries through the vagina and bladder and present with vaginal urinary leakage 10 to 20 days later. Vesicocutaneous fistulas may occur at suprapubic cystostomy sites after catheter removal and generally develop with impaired wound healing or distal bladder outlet obstruction.

Cystoscopy and cystography will often establish the diagnosis and localize the site of the fistula. Occasionally, methylene blue cystography is necessary to establish the presence of a vesicovaginal fistula and localize its site. This will also aid in excluding ureterovaginal fistulas, as will the IVP.

Surgical correction of vesicovaginal fistulas can be done by a transabdominal or vaginal approach. The technique is beyond the scope of this discussion, but numerous types of repair have been successful. Management of vesicocutaneous fistulas should begin with the elimination of any bladder outlet obstruction. Spontaneous closure of the fistulous tract may occur. Should no obstruction be apparent on diagnostic studies, urethral catheter drainage alone is often successful. The last resort should be surgical excision of the fistula and closure of the bladder and skin.

The pathogenesis of fistula formation is generally connected to poor wound healing and incomplete reconstruction at initial injury. Prevention requires meticulous multilayered repair of coexisting injuries to the bladder and vagina. Hyperalimentation in patients with massive injuries will maintain high-quality wound healing. Once the bladder and vagina have been closed, a silicone urethral catheter should be left in place and a suprapubic cystostomy tube inserted to maintain urinary diversion for 10 days to 2 weeks.

COMPLICATIONS OF URETHRAL TRAUMA

Urethral Stricture

Stricture disease is a common complication of urethral trauma and is influenced by the location and mechanism of injury as well as the method of management. It will develop in patients with complete transection of the urethra managed by suprapubic cystostomy alone and, in most cases, will require operative correction. This type of stricture results from the initial therapy and does not truly represent a complication of injury. Patients with prostatomembranous urethral disruption managed by initial primary realignment have approximately a 30% to 40% incidence of stricture formation, with a high percentage requiring dilatation, endoscopic urethrotomy, or formal urethroplasty.[18, 19] Trauma to the anterior urethra commonly occurs from straddle injuries or from endoscopic procedures and leaves residual stricture disease in the bulbar and pendulous urethra.

Patients who have traumatic injury to the urethra and develop stricture disease will complain of slowing of the urinary stream, spraying, and a prolongation of micturition. They may at times have urinary tract infection. Long-standing obstructive stricture disease may cause urinary frequency, hesitancy, and nocturia. Patients usually have complete bladder emptying with insignificant residual urine. Small amounts of urethral discharge and occasional dysuria are common.

Physical findings are unremarkable, unless the patient has developed urethrocutaneous fistulas proximal to the stricture area. In these cases, deep subcutaneous infection may be present, with purulent discharge through the fistulous tract. The patient will also have urinary leakage when voiding. With significant stricture disease, flow rates will be diminished to below 10 mL/sec.

Urinalysis commonly reveals small degrees of pyuria without evidence of urinary tract infection. Retrograde urethrography is the best study to evaluate the location and extent of the stricture. In patients with prostatomembranous disruption initially managed by cystostomy alone, urethrography should be performed simultaneously with cystography. In these patients, it is important to visualize the prostatic urethra. To fill this area with contrast, the patient is asked to void, which will allow the bladder neck to open and fill the proximal urethra. Patients with partial urethral disruption of the prostatomembranous junction or anterior urethra should have voiding cystourethrography performed through the cystostomy catheter approximately 3 weeks after injury to evaluate the status of healing and extravasation.

Numerous methods of management are available. Stricture disease of the prostatomembranous junction can be managed by direct-vision urethrotomy if there is continuity of the urethral mucosa. Formal urethroplasty by perineal or transpubic route can also be done.[20, 21] Endoscopic reestablishment of urethral continuity after traumatic disruption of the prostatomembranous urethra is another option.[22] This procedure is done by placing a lighted cystoscope through the suprapubic cystostomy tube into the prostatic urethra and, with a direct-vision urethrotome coming from the anterior urethral position, lysing the stricture by cutting toward the visualized lighted unit. This approach seems simple and can be done successfully in some cases. However, difficulties arise when the urethra has been subluxated at initial injury so that the opposing ends are not in apposition. Skin graft urethroplasty can be used in both the anterior and posterior urethra.

The pathogenesis of stricture disease after traumatic injury derives from partial or complete urethral transection that heals with significant scar tissue. Devitalization of tissue in the area of injury may significantly influence the development of this scarring. Initial repairs of the injury may be difficult because of excessive bleeding and hematoma. Posterior urethral strictures create major difficulties in visualization during corrective surgery under the best of circumstances; in traumatic injury, the problem is even worse. The ability to prevent stricture disease after trauma is highly unpredictable. Careful preoperative assessment will allow one to select an initial operative procedure that is best indicated for a given injury. The surgeon must be familiar with the anatomy, experienced in traumatic injury management, and possess meticulous surgical technique to prevent stricture formation.

Incontinence

Incontinence after urethral injury is uncommon and occurs when the injury involves the posterior urethra. Patients with crushing injuries to the bladder neck, prostate, and prostatomembranous junction are at risk: the incidence of incontinence has been reported to be as high as 33%. However, recent reports indicate that the incidence of incontinence should be less than 5%.[23]

Complete incontinence would be noted when urethral continuity has been established and the patient has continuous leakage of urine and does not void. This finding is extremely rare and occurs in only the most severe injuries. Stress incontinence is fairly common and may be seen in up to 10% of patients immediately after repair, but generally will improve slowly and disappear with time. A careful history should be taken after traumatic urethral injuries to elicit complaints of small amounts of dribbling, which results from urethral pooling of urine after voiding. This is particularly true in patients who have had anterior urethral injury and corrective surgery. It can easily be managed by having the patient gently palpate the length of the urethra after voiding to express any residual drops within the lumen.

The objective findings will be constant dribbling when standing and small amounts of urine lost when coughing or straining. Urodynamic and urethral pressure profile studies are the best methods to establish the location of poor sphincteric activity and the site of major damage.

The cause for incontinence in these major injuries to the posterior urethra is damage to the voluntary and involuntary sphincteric mechanisms during either the initial trauma or the initial management. Extensive traumatic damage may destroy the sphincteric mechanism. Primary urethral realignment with a urethral catheter left in place on prolonged extensive traction may cause sphincteric damage sufficient to result in incontinence.

Total incontinence after trauma presents an extremely difficult management problem. Pharmacologic manipulation is of little benefit. Surgical repair by a Tanagho tube flap[16] or other procedures will be successful in no more than 50% of patients. The artificial sphincter may be required and offers a reasonable solution. In addition, newer techniques of neural stimulation are promising and may prove beneficial in selected patients.

Incontinence can generally be prevented. When primary realignment is the initial treatment, the surgeon should avoid prolonged excessive catheter traction. Any operative procedures involving the posterior urethra require meticulous surgical technique. With massive injury to the prostate, bladder neck, or the prostatomembranous junction, the best initial approach is suprapubic cystostomy drainage without any attempt at surgical reconstruction. Later reconstruction will often then be performed in a continent patient free of stricture disease.

Impotence

Impotence consequent to prostatomembranous disruption is perhaps the single most severe complication of urethral trauma. There appears to be a difference in the impotence rate relative to the initial method of management. In 1953, Johanson[21] described a method that included only simple cystostomy drainage and then delayed repair of the subsequent urethral stricture. With this approach, the incidence was less than 10%—a dramatic improvement over other methods. Since that time, numerous authors have reported impotence rates of less than 15% with this technique.[20, 23] In 1970, Gibson[24] reviewed the literature and found the mean incidence of impotence after primary urethral realignment to be approximately 50%, improving slowly over time to a permanent rate of approximately 30%. Since then, Patterson et al.[18] have reported a 15% incidence of impotence in 27 patients treated with primary urethral realignment. This improvement may be the result of careful surgical technique and follow-up. Virtually all patients are impotent immediately after injury. Within 1 year, most patients who will recover have done so, although return of erectile function can be delayed up to 3 years. The general trend is slow and gradual improvement in the first few months. The work of Lue et al.[25] and Walsh and Donker[26] has demonstrated the importance of the erectile nerves and has identified their location in the 4- and 8-o'clock positions adjacent to the prostatomembranous junction. This knowledge should allow the attentive surgeon to avoid secondary injury during repairs in this area. Some patients will have vasculogenic impotence because of injury to pelvic vessels and the internal pudendal artery within Alcock's canal.

During the weeks immediately following prostatomembranous disruption, when virtually all patients are impotent, they will need a great deal of emotional support. As erectile function returns, the patient will note small degrees of partial erections, which will improve with time. Those who have been managed by initial cystostomy drainage should have delayed stricture repair within 3 months; this should not interfere with the recovery of erectile function.

Patients who complain of impotence after injury usually have a normal physical examination. The sensation to the penile skin and glans penis will be normal, as will rectal sphincteric tone and sensation. Arteriogenic erectile dysfunction can be detected with an injection of 60 mg of papaverine in 20 mL of saline directly into the corpus cavernosum. The patient should experience a near-normal erection within 5 minutes; if arterial blood is impeded, normal erection may not develop for 20 to 30 minutes.[27] Patients with neurogenic impotence will have a normal response to the papaverine test. Nocturnal penile tumescence monitoring may also be done to evaluate erections, but false-negatives are often encountered, and the conditions under which the study must be performed are difficult.

Patients with prostatomembranous disruption and impotence have associated pelvic fractures. These fractures may damage the internal pudendal vessels along Alcock's canal as it crosses near the posterior pubic rami. The massive trauma that occurs when the urethra is transected may well transect the nearby erectile nerves. Prevention of additional injury to these nerves should be the surgeon's objective, irrespective of the type of repair. Knowledge of neuroanatomy and the arterial blood supply to the erectile bodies will allow the surgeon to manage these patients confidently with a minimal incidence of impotence.

Abscess and Fistula

Abscesses may be seen soon after urethral rupture (more commonly at the prostatomembranous junction), and fistulas will most often appear several weeks later. Manifestations of abscess are chills, fever, lower abdominal pain, lethargy, and poor appetite. These symptoms reflect a deep abscess within the pelvic floor, which usually involves the pelvic hematoma. Fistulas develop as small sinus tracts leading from the area of injury to the retropubic space. They may be secondary to previous abscesses and are very often asymptomatic; however, should they become infected, frank abscess development will be noted along with associated systemic symptoms. Early indications of fistulas are low-grade fever and pelvic pain of undetermined origin.

Deep pelvic abscess is typified by high spiking fevers over a 24-hour period, lower abdominal tenderness, and induration of the overlying lower abdominal skin. Careful examination of the perineum may reveal tenderness and swelling. The diagnosis can be made by history, physical examination, and the patient's current clinical state. Useful diagnostic studies include cystography, sonography, pelvic CT, and (with suspected urinary extravasation from a ureteral injury) IVP.

The diagnosis of fistula after urethral rupture is best made by a combination of cystography and urethrography. After bladder filling with contrast material, the patient is asked to void; as the bladder neck opens and contrast reaches the apex of the prostate, the fistulous tract will usually be demonstrated (Fig 10–6). Very often multiple tracts will be present, and their number and extent should be carefully noted. Retrograde urethrography may also be useful.

The therapeutic approach to pelvic abscess is surgical drainage, either with multiple Penrose drains in the retropubic space or with other, more closed drainage systems. Gram-negative organisms are usually the cause (rarely staphylococci or streptococci), and the patient should be placed on systemic broad-spectrum antibiotic coverage.

Fistulas occur near the apex of the prostate or in the area of the urogenital diaphragm, and their location creates difficulties in management. Proper treatment is complete and total excision of the fistulous tract, which requires careful definition preoperatively. A transpubic approach combined with a perineal incision will allow complete access and total excision of the tracts. This approach also permits total reconstruction of the stricture that has developed in the area of injury.

Pelvic abscess usually develops within the first 2 weeks of injury and is caused by gram-negative or gram-positive organ-

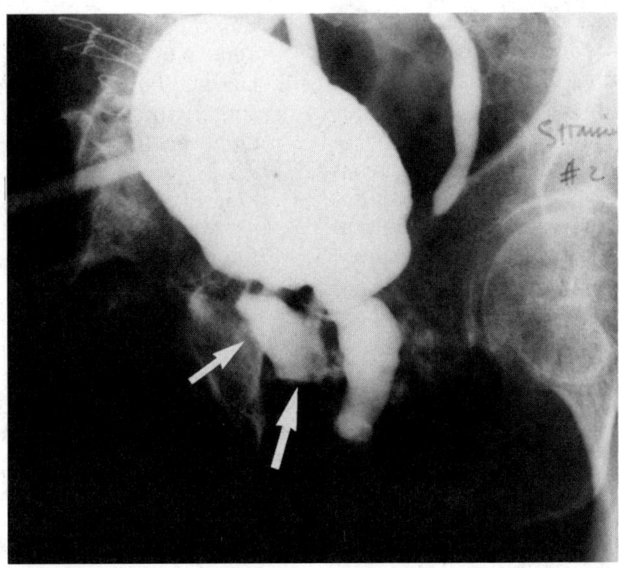

FIG 10–6.
Cystogram in a patient 3 months after massive pelvic fracture and prostatomembranous disruption shows a large fistulous tract *(arrows)*. A combined transpubic perineal surgical approach was used to remove the fistula and perform a urethroplasty.

isms from associated bowel injury or from contamination at the time of surgical exploration, which infect the hematoma. Fistulas develop because of small microabscesses and small amounts of urinary extravasation persisting within the area. Their development may be enhanced by the nonviable tissue that results from the injury.

Abscess formation can often be prevented by avoiding extensive dissection in the deep pelvic and lateral hematomas at initial surgical exploration. When the bladder is well drained, there is little reason to leave Penrose drains or others in the retropubic space. Bacteria tracking along these external drains may often lead to hematoma infection. In addition, the rectosigmoid area should be carefully investigated to be certain that rectal injury has not resulted in perforation that would cause hematoma infection. Should rectal or sigmoid injury be noted, proximal diverting colostomy should be done.

Prevention of fistula formation may be difficult, but it is important to have adequate bladder drainage to prevent urinary extravasation in the area of the prostatic apex. Appropriate early management, as described above for abscess formation, will also help prevent fistula formation.

EDITORIAL COMMENT

Complications of renal, vesical, and urethral trauma are outlined in detail in this chapter. It is clear that computed tomography has greatly aided the management of the trauma patient, although CT scanning may not be available on emergent basis in many hospitals. Complications occur most commonly with kidneys that have a rupture through the corticomedullary junction, devitalized tissue, major urinary extravasation, or a possible pedicle injury. It also should be remembered that any kidney that is abnormal in location (pelvic kidney, horseshoe kidney) or abnormal in size (ureteral pelvic junction obstruction) is much more prone to trauma. For this reason, patients presenting with lesser amounts of trauma and hematuria should still be investigated at the time of injury.

Although the management of renal arteriovenous fistula remains controversial, we have found that detachable silicone balloons are very helpful in the management of this difficult problem and may also preserve more renal parenchyma than most operative procedures.*

*Marshall FF, White RI, Kaufman SC, et al: Treatment of traumatic renal arteriovenous fistulas by detachable silicone balloon embolization. *J Urol* 1979; 122:237.

REFERENCES

1. McAninch JW, Federle MP: Evaluation of renal injuries with computerized tomography. *J Urol* 1982; 128:456–460.
2. Holcroft JW, Trunkey DD, Minagi H, et al: Renal trauma and retroperitoneal hematomas—indications for exploration. *J Trauma* 1975; 15:1045–1052.
3. McAninch JW, Carroll PR: Renal trauma: Kidney preservation through improved vascular control—a refined approach. *J Trauma* 1982; 22:285–290.
4. McAninch JW, Spring DB: Autologous clot embolization to control renal hemorrhage from trauma. Relationship of clot volume to renal infarction. *Invest Urol* 1980; 17:499–502.
5. Vaughan ED Jr, Case DB, Pickering TG, et al: Clinical evaluation of renovascular hypertension and therapeutic decisions. *Urol Clin North Am* 1984; 11:393–407.
6. Page IH: The production of persistent arterial hypertension by cellophane perinephritis. *JAMA* 1939; 113:2046–2048.
7. Takahashi M, Tamakawa Y, Shibata A, et al: Computed tomography of "Page" kidney. *J Comput Assist Tomogr* 1977; 1:344–348.
8. Cosgrove MD, Mendez R, Morrow JW: Traumatic renal arteriovenous fistula: Report of 12 cases. *J Urol* 1973; 110:627–631.
9. Cosgrove MD, Mendez R, Morrow JW: Branch artery ligation for renal arteriovenous fistula. *J Urol* 1973; 110:632–638.
10. Jakse G, Putz A, Gassner I, et al: Early surgery in the management of pediatric blunt renal trauma. *J Urol* 1984; 131:920–924.
11. Ring EJ, Athanasoulis C, Waltman AC, et al: Arteriographic management of hemorrhage following pelvic fracture. *Radiology* 1973; 109:65–70.
12. Carroll PR, McAninch JW: Major bladder trauma: Mechanisms of injury and a unified method of diagnosis and repair. *J Urol* 1984; 132:254–257.
13. Hayes EE, Sandler CM, Corriere JN Jr: Management of the ruptured bladder secondary to blunt abdominal trauma. *J Urol* 1983; 129:946–948.
14. Cass AS, Johnson CF, Kahn AU, et al: Nonoperative management of bladder rupture from external trauma. *Urology* 1983; 22:27–29.
15. Carroll PR, McAninch JW: Major bladder trauma: The accuracy of cystography. *J Urol* 1983; 130:887–888.
16. Tanagho EA, Smith DR: Clinical evaluation of a surgical technique for the correction of complete urinary incontinence. *J Urol* 1972; 107:402–411.
17. Stamey TA: Endoscopic suspension of the vesical neck for urinary incontinence. *Surg Gynecol Obstet* 1973; 136:547–554.
18. Patterson DE, Barrett DM, Myers RP, et al: Primary realignment of posterior urethral injuries. *J Urol* 1983; 129:513–516.
19. Crassweller PO, Farrow GA, Robson CJ, et al: Traumatic rupture of the supramembranous urethra. *J Urol* 1977; 118:770–771.
20. McAninch JW: Traumatic injuries to the urethra. *J Trauma* 1981; 21:291–297.
21. Johanson B: Reconstruction of the male urethra in strictures. *Acta Chir Scand [Suppl]* 1953; 176:1–103.
22. Gonzalez R, Chiou R-K, Hekmat K, et al: Endoscopic re-establishment of urethral continuity after traumatic disruption of the membranous urethra. *J Urol* 1983; 130:785–787.
23. Morehouse DD, MacKinnon KJ: Management of prostatomembranous urethral disruption: 13-year experience. *J Urol* 1980; 123:173–174.
24. Gibson GR: Impotence following fractured

pelvis and ruptured urethra. *Br J Urol* 1970; 42:86–88.

25. Lue TF, Zeineh SJ, Schmidt RA, et al: Neuroanatomy of penile erection: Its relevance to iatrogenic impotence. *J Urol* 1984; 131:273–280.
26. Walsh PC, Donker PJ: Impotence following radical prostatectomy: Insight into etiology and prevention. *J Urol* 1982; 128:492–497.
27. Lue TF, Hricak H, Marich KW, et al: Evaluation of arteriogenic impotence with intracorporeal injection of papaverine and the duplex ultrasound scanner. *Semin Urol* 1985; 3:43–48.

CHAPTER 11

Complications of Surgery for Removal of Renal and Ureteral Stones

Donald R. Bodner, M.D.,
Martin I. Resnick, M.D.

The management of renal and ureteral stones has changed greatly over the past few years with the majority of stones being treated today with extracorporeal shock wave lithotripsy and some with percutaneous nephrostolithotomy. Due to the popularity of these new techniques, fewer open surgical procedures are being performed and there has been a tendency to forget the great improvements that have been made in open renal surgical techniques. While the role of open surgical procedures for the removal of stones from the kidney and ureter will be less frequent in the future, it is clear that open procedures will be required for the more complex stones and it is therefore necessary for urologists to maintain their proficiency in open surgical techniques.

The complications encountered with open surgical procedures on the kidney and ureter will remain directly related to the actual procedure performed and the amount of intraoperative dissection and manipulation required. Appropriate preoperative and postoperative management can help to minimize morbidity. The objective of stone management remains—to preserve renal function and remove all the stone fragments in an expeditious manner.

PREOPERATIVE CARE OF URINARY INFECTION

To prevent the postoperative complication of sepsis, wound infection, and abscess formation, preoperative treatment of urinary tract infections is necessary based upon culture and sensitivity testing and preferably the urine should be sterile at the time of open renal surgery. Approximately 15% to 20% of urinary calculi are struvite in composition and their formation is directly related to the presence of a urinary tract infection. They are found twice as frequently in females as in males. Neurogenic bladder dysfunction, as well as chronic indwelling catheters, stents, and urinary diversion, places a patient at higher risk for the development of these stones.

Infection stones are caused by urinary tract infections secondary to urea-splitting bacteria, most notably *Proteus mirabilis, Klebsiella, Providencia,* and occasional strains of *Pseudomonas*. The *Pseudomonas* infections are often the most difficult to eradicate and are associated with the highest stone recurrence rate.[1] Of note, *Escherichia coli* is not a urea-splitting bacterium and infections caused by this organism in association with urolithiasis usually represent a superinfection.

Documented urinary tract infections should be treated for a minimum of 24 to 48 hours prior to the surgical procedure, and the choice of antibiotics should be based upon in vitro culture and sensitivity studies. Ideally, the antibiotic should attain high urine and serum levels and be non-nephrotoxic. The preferred agents include semisynthetic penicillins, cephalosporins, and some of the newer quinolones. Aminoglycosides should be reserved for those infections sensitive only to them. In these instances, renal function should be monitored closely and peak and trough levels should be routinely obtained. The drug must be discontinued if deleterious side effects are noted. Whenever possible the urine should be sterile at the time of open renal or ureteral procedures.

RENAL ANATOMY

To understand the complications from open procedures on the kidney and ureter, the renal and intrarenal anatomy must first be briefly reviewed. In approximately 70% to 80% of kidneys, the main renal artery divides in its distal third prior to entering the renal hilum into a larger anterior and smaller posterior segment, each of which is an end artery (Fig 11–1). The posterior segment is the first branch from the main renal artery in 50% of cases while the segmental branch to the inferior pole comes off first in 30%.

Further branching continues in an orderly manner to form eight to 12 interlobar arteries, which in turn branch to form transmedullary arteries, and some continue as arcuate arteries. The kidney is thus divided into four surgical segments (superior, inferior, anterior, and posterior) by the division of the renal artery (Fig 11–2). The anterior division, which is the direct continuation of the main renal artery, supplies the superior, inferior, and anterior segments. The posterior segment continues without further branching to supply the posterior surface of the kidney. It is important to remember that the

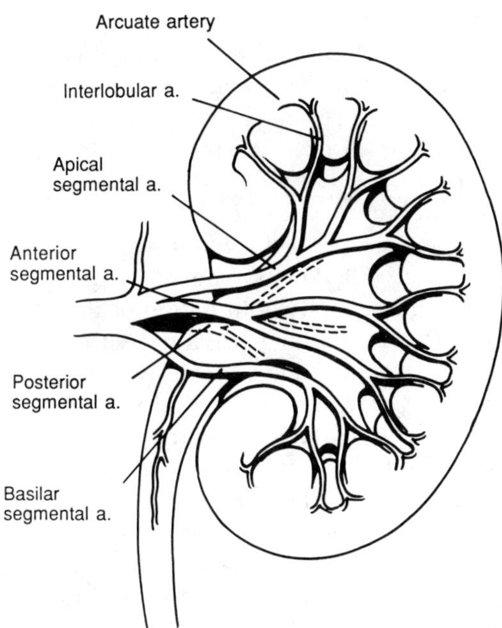

FIG 11–1.
The distribution of the main renal artery with its sequential branches is shown.

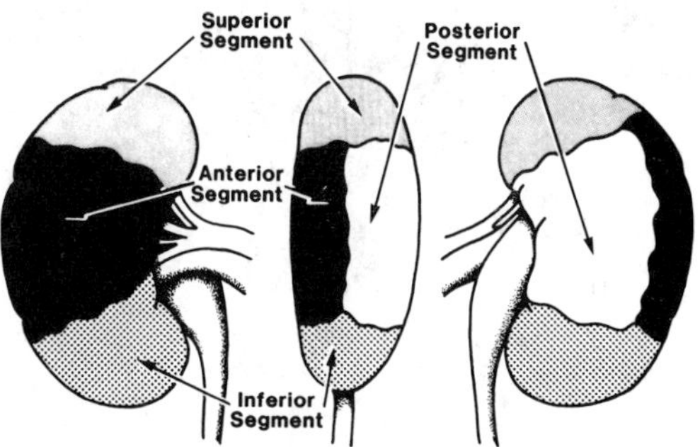

FIG 11–2.
The superior, inferior, anterior, and posterior surgical segments of the kidney are formed by the branching of the renal artery.

artery to the inferior segment of the kidney enters the renal hilum and then descends obliquely to its lower border where it crosses the renal pelvis and divides into an anterior and posterior segment.

The most variable portion of renal anatomy is the distribution and number of calices (Fig 11–3). The renal pelvis is generally a direct continuation of the ureter. The pelvis then divides within the substance of the kidney into two or three main divisions known as major calices or infundibula, which in turn divide into secondary and tertiary divisions known as minor calices. The calices can be simple and drain one papilla or they may be complex and drain multiple papillae. Polar calices are the most variable and are frequently complex. The total number of calices ranges from four to 12 and averages eight. The calix from the most superior division is frequently complex. The remainder of the calices are paired anterior and posterior to an imaginary line that divides the kidney longitudinally. The anterior calices are irregularly arranged at an angle of 70 to 75 degrees from the frontal plane while the posterior calices are more regularly arranged at a 20-degree angle from the frontal plane.

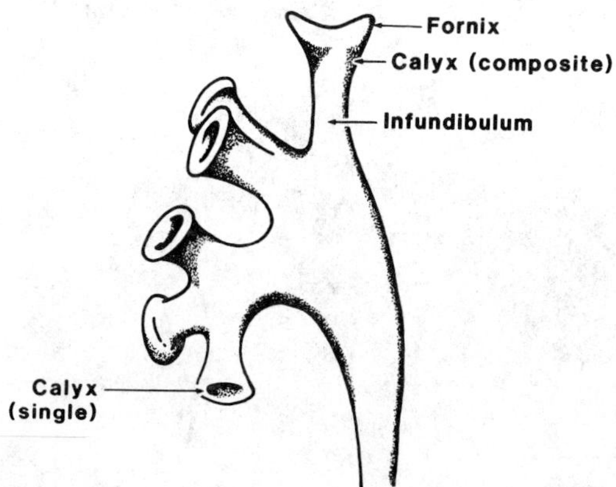

FIG 11–3.
The number and distribution of the calices is the most variable part of renal anatomy.

INTRAOPERATIVE AND POSTOPERATIVE COMPLICATIONS

Infections

Boyce and Harrison reported that damaged kidneys containing renal calculi, stenosed or obstructed calices, and patchy pyelonephritis may retain bacteria after administration of seemingly adequate doses of antibiotics, and even though initial bladder urine may be sterile, optimal microbiologic assessment of the patient is achieved only by frequent urine cultures obtained during the postoperative period.[2] Intraoperatively, any mucinous material and portions of the removed stone should be sent for cultures. Fowler stressed the importance of stone culture in the management of patients with infection stones.[3] In only two of 16 patients was the stone bacteriology precisely predicted by urine cultures alone. The value of stone culture is in the guidance of postoperative antibiotic selection, which may be markedly different from preoperative therapy. If the infected stone is completely removed from the collecting system and the urine is carefully monitored postoperatively to detect recurrent urinary tract infections early so that appropriate therapy can be administered, the incidence of recurrent urinary calculi associated with infections can be markedly diminished.[4] In the presence of adequate urinary levels of appropriate antibiotics, only the surface of an infection stone will be sterile and deeper layers will continue to harbor bacteria below the surface.[5, 6] It is therefore important that all of the infection stone fragments be removed at surgery, and frequent urine cultures are required during the postoperative follow-up period.

Pulmonary Complications

Postoperative pulmonary dysfunction is perhaps the most frequent morbidity noted with open renal surgery.[5] Birch and

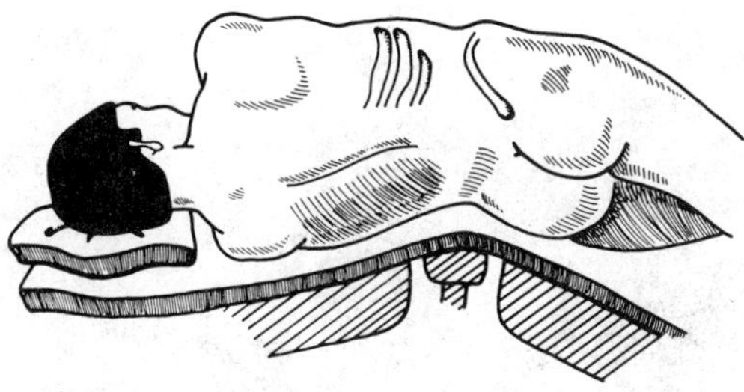

FIG 11–4.
The lateral or flank position provides excellent exposure to the kidney and is optimal when hypothermia is required.

Nims found a 37% incidence of pulmonary complications when they reviewed their experience with patients undergoing anatrophic nephrolithotomy.[7] This is in part explained by the fact that most surgery on the kidney to remove the stone is performed through a lateral or flank approach (Fig 11–4). In this position, lateral flexion is used to maximize the distance between the iliac crest and the costal margin to make exposure of the kidney optimal. The patient's head is in the Trendelenburg position and the feet are down. This position creates such stress on the skeletal and respiratory systems that most unanesthetized subjects cannot tolerate it. Case and Stiles reported that this position caused a 14.5% decrease in vital capacity in conscious subjects.[8] Comparable reductions in vital capacity have been reported in anesthetized patients and these reductions are felt to be secondary to restriction in chest wall excursion in all directions.[9, 10]

Atelectasis.—There has been concern that the down lung is at increased risk for developing pulmonary complications because of its decreased ability to fully expand and because of venous congestion, but this has not been shown clinically to be true. Atelectasis occurs with equal frequency in both lung fields.[7] Postoperative atelectasis can be reduced by having the patient perform deep breathing and coughing exercises. The routine use of incentive spirometry appears to be of benefit in reducing pulmonary complications. Pulmonary physiotherapy should be instituted in the preoperative period and continued well into the postoperative period.

Pneumothorax.—Pneumothorax occurs in less than 5% of operative procedures performed on the kidney for removal of stone. A history of prior surgery on the kidney or pyelonephritis places a patient at higher risk for developing this complication. Pneumothorax occurs because of adherence of the upper pole of the kidney to the diaphragm and attached pleura making inadvertent entry more possible. Because of the attachment of the pleura to the ribs, pleural injury is more common when an 11th or 12th interspace incision is used rather than a 12th rib or subcostal incision. When a small opening of the pleura is recognized at surgery, it can be closed with a running chromic catgut suture after the lung is hyperinflated to ensure that no air remains. If there is concern that the pleural opening is not adequately repaired, a small chest tube can be left in place for 24 to 48 hours postoperatively. A chest x-ray should be performed in the recovery room if a pleural repair has been performed or a pneumothorax is suspected (Fig 11–5). Depending on the size of the pneumothorax, a chest tube may be required and follow-up chest films are essential.

Thrombophlebitis, Pulmonary Emboli, and Cardiovascular Complications.—These serious complications are addressed elsewhere in this book. Tables 11–1 and 11–2 depict the low morbidity and mortality that Boyce reported in his large series[11] of anatrophic nephrolithotomies. The incidence of pulmonary emboli and myocardial infarctions is also quite low.

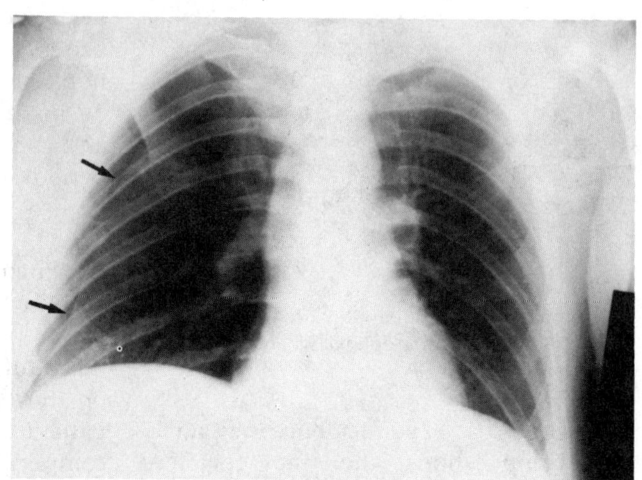

FIG 11–5.
A 30% pneumothorax is noted by the *arrows*.

Hemorrhage

The surgeon's ability to perform bloodless renal surgery while preserving renal function is directly related to his knowledge of the intrarenal arterial anatomy and the vascular surgical segments[12] (see Figs 11–1 and 11–2). Careful placement of intersegmental nephrostomy incisions should present little problem with bleeding since no vessel of significant size should be disrupted. These procedures are best performed after isolation and control of the main renal artery and occlusion of the vessel in association with cooling the kidney to prevent ischemic injury. When an anatrophic nephrolithotomy is to be performed, the avascular plane between the distribution of the anterior and posterior branches of the renal artery can be defined by giving methylene blue after placing a nontraumatizing vascular clamp about the posterior segment of the renal artery (Fig 11–6). The avascular plane is found posterior to Brödel's white line (Fig 11–7). The nephrostomy incision is made through the avascular plane with minimal risk of bleeding or loss of renal parenchyma (Fig 11–8). Precise closure of the collecting system and renal capsule will result in compression of the small intrarenal vessels and will help to prevent subsequent hemorrhage. Boyce reported 778 cc as the average blood loss for anatrophic nephrolithotomies and noted that 6.8% had greater than 1,000 cc of blood loss, which he considered to represent hemorrhage.[11]

When bleeding occurs postoperatively, it is frequently intrapelvic and oc-

TABLE 11–1.
Anatrophic Nephrolithotomy 1963–1982: Complications With Recovery in 951 Patients*†

Complications	No. of Patients (%)
Hemorrhage >1000 mL (reoperation 3)	65(6.8)
Arteriovenous fistulas, reoperated	4(0.4)
Atelectasis, any degree by x-ray	232(24.2)
Pneumothorax	36(3.8)
Pulmonary embolus	9(0.9)
All others including temperature >100° F, gastrointestinal, etc.	153(16.1)

*From Boyce WH: *Urol Clin North Am* 1983; 10:538. Used by permission.
†Average stay in hospital: 9.6 days (mean 11.6, maximum 68).

TABLE 11–2.
Anatrophic Nephrolithotomy 1963–1982: Mortality (0.42%) in Under 3 Months*

Cause of Death	No. of Patients
Myocardial infarction	1
Pulmonary embolus	3

*From Boyce WH: *Urol Clin North Am* 1983; 10:585. Used by permission.

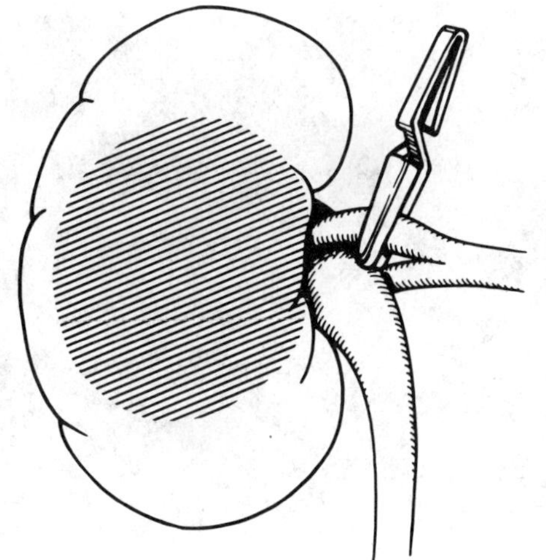

FIG 11–6.
A vascular clamp is placed about the posterior branch of the renal artery to define the avascular plane.

curs 7 to 14 days after surgery. Bleeding generally results from inadequately closed intrarenal vessels. Expectant therapy with bed rest, fluids, and blood replacement will often suffice.

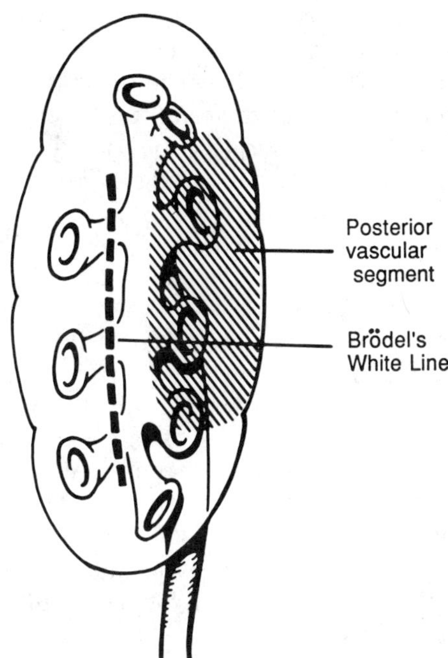

FIG 11–7.
The avascular plane is found to be posterior to Brödel's white line.

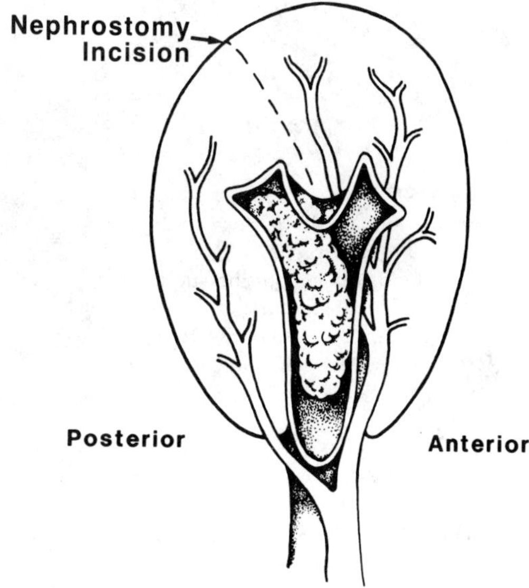

FIG 11–8.
The nephrostomy incision for anatrophic nephrolithotomy is made through the avascular plane, which minimizes the risk for hemorrhage.

If bleeding persists, the use of aminocaproic acid (EACA, Amicar) is of controversial value in controlling intrarenal hemorrhage.[13] The agent is administered intravenously and then maintained by the oral route for several days once bleeding is controlled. EACA can make the clot more dense in the absence of fibrinolysis activity and result in ureteral obstruction and subsequent colic. Consequently, EACA should be used selectively.

When bleeding is of such significance that control cannot be obtained with these measures, or if significant hypotension is present, arteriography should be performed to further define the cause and site of bleeding (Fig 11–9). If open vessels or arteriovenous fistulas are identified, they can usually be managed by an experienced angiographer who is familiar with embolic techniques (Fig 11–10). Only when all these methods fail to control active bleeding should open surgical techniques be considered for the direct repair of the damaged vessel.

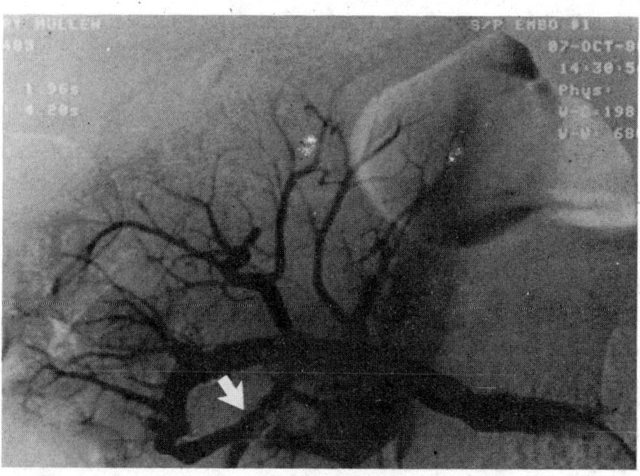

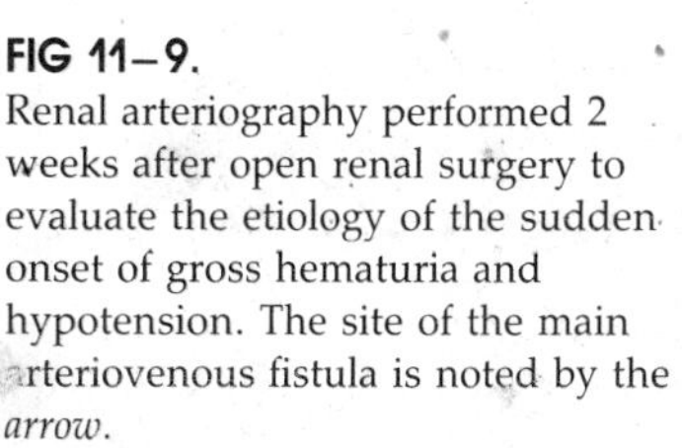

FIG 11–9.
Renal arteriography performed 2 weeks after open renal surgery to evaluate the etiology of the sudden onset of gross hematuria and hypotension. The site of the main arteriovenous fistula is noted by the *arrow*.

Complications of Vascular Manipulation

Ischemic Injury.—When extensive nephrotomies and intrarenal reconstructive procedures are required, it is advisable to temporarily occlude the renal artery. This maneuver not only decreases the magnitude of intraoperative hemorrhage, but by reducing renal tissue turgor it facilitates improved access to the intrarenal collecting system. Care should be taken in dissecting the renal artery to prevent inadvertent damage. The adventitia and small vessels about the renal artery should be preserved. Atraumatic vascular clamps should be applied precisely. Prior to occluding the renal artery, the patient should be well hydrated and the intraoperative blood pressure should be sufficient to ensure constant renal plasma flow.[14] The intraoperative administration of mannitol (25 g IV) prior to clamping of the renal artery will increase renal plasma flow and decrease intrarenal vascular resistance.[15, 16] It is also believed that mannitol will increase the osmolality of the tubular fluid and protect the kidney from hypothermic damage during the period of renal ischemia and cooling.

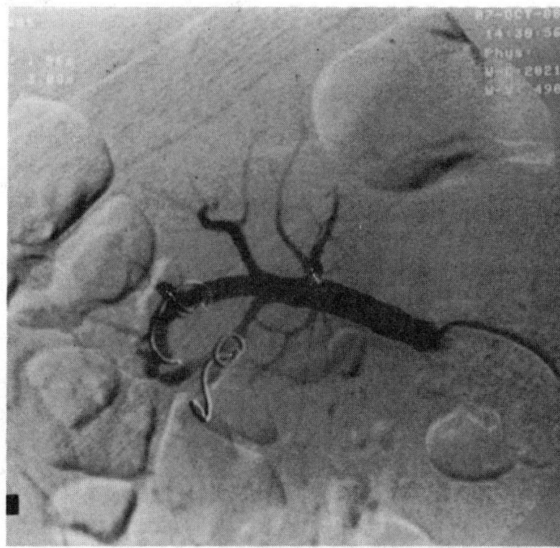

FIG 11–10.
Renal bleeding was controlled by angioinfarction of the arteriovenous malformations. Coils are noted in the small branches of the renal artery where the fistulas were located.

Postischemic renal failure can be avoided by cooling the kidney by a multitude of equally effective techniques.[17–20] Direct surface cooling with an ice slush solution placed within a rubber dam about the kidney after occlusion of the renal artery is as effective as other methods (Fig 11–11). Warm ischemia beyond 30 minutes is generally poorly tolerated in paired kidneys, but evidence suggests that solitary kidneys may be able to withstand slightly longer ischemic insults.[21] Renal cooling reduces cellular metabolic activity so that the parenchymal cells, particularly those of the proximal convoluted tubule, are able to tolerate a period of

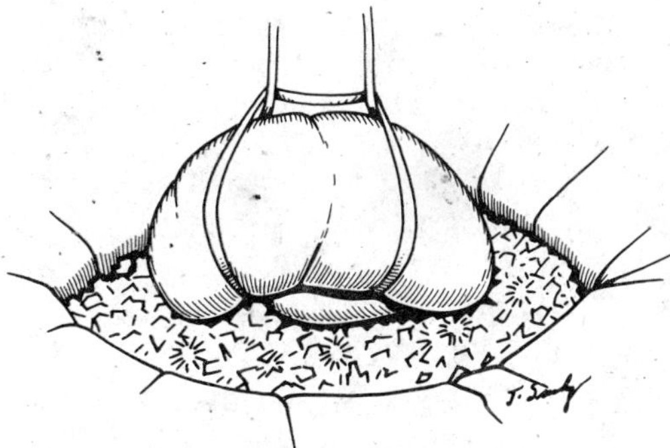

FIG 11–11.
Surface cooling of the kidney is performed by placing an ice slush solution within a rubber dam in direct contact with the kidney. The renal artery is occluded immediately prior to cooling.

ischemia. The optimal temperature needed to prevent ischemic changes has been a matter of controversy, but experimental studies and clinical experience indicate that the kidney maintained at approximately 15 to 20° C will be optimally protected from injury. Temperatures of 0° C may in fact be damaging to the kidney.[22]

In Boyce's experience in performing 951 anatrophic nephrolithotomies, no instance of renal artery injury, either acute or delayed, was reported.[11] Renal vein injuries are very uncommon because the renal vein is typically not occluded during the hilar dissection. Occluding the renal artery and not the renal vein reduces the chance of venous thrombosis and subsequent renal infarction. Care should also be exercised that not too much traction be placed on the kidney during intraoperative manipulation with tapes placed about the kidney as this may lead to intimal arterial injuries.

During surgery in which the renal artery is temporarily occluded, an injury of a segmental artery will result in no visible alteration of the color or turgor of the kidney. When the occluding vascular clamp is removed, the vascular injury will become apparent and an attempt should be made at that time to repair it.

Renal Failure

Despite following all the principles described above to preserve renal function, some patients will suffer loss of renal parenchyma and note diminished renal function postoperatively. Studies in patients with solitary kidneys indicate that removal of the stone, with subsequent relief of obstruction and resolution of infection, will result in an overall improvement in total renal function.[19] As previously mentioned, ischemic injury to the kidney can be minimized by carefully clamping the renal artery and cooling the kidney. Incisions through avascular segments of the kidney and careful closure of the small vessels that are opened and of the renal capsule will help to preserve renal function. Although some renal damage has been reported to occur with extensive intrarenal procedures as documented by changes on postoperative compared to preoperative radionuclide studies, the benefits of the procedure consistently appear to outweigh the deleterious effects. In the extensive experience of Boyce and colleagues, although some patients with solitary kidneys experienced transient elevations in serum creatinine, in no instance did patients experience frank episodes of acute renal failure.[2, 11, 19]

Retained Calculi

The presence of retained stone fragments is a major concern after an open surgical procedure for stone. The immediate danger is of a stone fragment passing into the ureter and causing acute ureteral obstruction, prolonged postoperative pain, and urine leakage. If the acute ureteral obstruction is associated with infection, the patient may become septic and emergent intervention with stent or percutaneous nephrostomy tube placement is required. At the time of anatrophic nephrolithotomy or when other procedures are performed for the removal of a large stone burden from the kidney, consideration should be given to placement of a Silastic stent or double-J catheter from the renal pelvis into the bladder. These stents can be removed endoscopically if they do not pass spontaneously (Fig 11–12). On rare occasions, the stent can actually migrate up the ureter and not be present in the bladder at the time for removal. Ureteroscopy or distal ureteral basketing under fluoroscopy will nearly always retrieve the stent.

Retained stone fragments also present a nidus for further calculus formation and are reported to have an incidence of 5% to 30% after open surgical techniques.[11, 23, 24] Residual stone fragments are perhaps of less concern when the composition of the stone is calcium oxalate, uric acid, or cystine. These stones can grow in size but are influenced by the concentration of the active products in the urine and the formation product of these substances and not by the mere presence of a retained fragment.[23] Retained fragments are of more concern when the composition of the stone is struvite since bacteria are incorporated within the body of the stone and thus remain a source of infection. The bacteria will continually alkalinize the urine and form an environment that encourages further stone formation and growth.[5] Sleight and Wickham reported that 70% of retained infected stones increased in size while only 30% of the retained nonstruvite stone fragments enlarged.[24]

To ensure that all of the stone fragments have been removed from the kidney, intraoperative renal x-rays are critical (Figs 11–13, 11–14). Initial x-rays localize all of the stone fragments and subsequent films confirm that all of the fragments have been removed. Once the bulk of the stone burden is removed, further films should be obtained to identify the location of any remaining stone fragments. A variety of techniques have been described to help localize stone fragments in the kidney and generally radiopaque stones larger that 2 mm in diameter can be consistently detected intraoperatively.[25–29] Keith needles can be placed in the kidney to help localize the stone, and final films should reveal no stone fragments.

Nephroscopy can help to localize stone fragments when intraoperative x-rays reveal their presence but is not very helpful in determining their exact location.[30] Intraoperative ultrasonography, another technique that is widely available, utilizes high-frequency tranducers to assist in localizing the retained fragments.[31–34] Both superficial and deep parenchymal stones can usually be localized

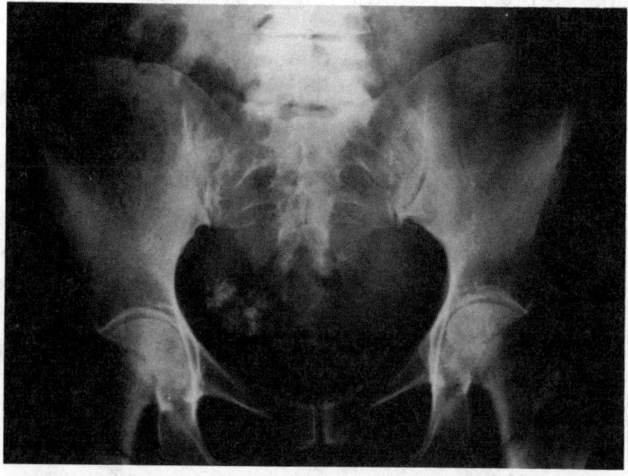

FIG 11–12.
The double-J stent placed at the time of nephrolithotomy was found on routine follow-up to have migrated into the bladder.

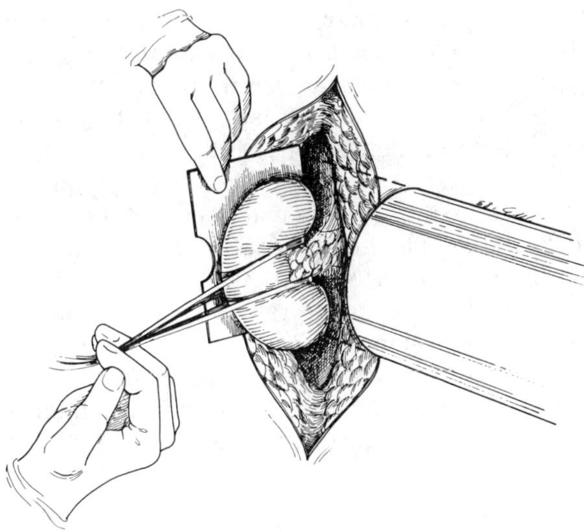

FIG 11–13.
Intraoperative x-rays of the kidney are essential to ensure that all of the stone fragments are removed.

with this technique. Also of significance, ultrasound offers the advantage of being able to localize radiolucent stones that otherwise may not have been identified using conventional techniques. If tiny fragments are believed to remain, consideration should be given to leaving a nephrostomy tube and planning chemolysis in the postoperative period. The tract should be as straight as possible if later percutaneous procedures are considered.

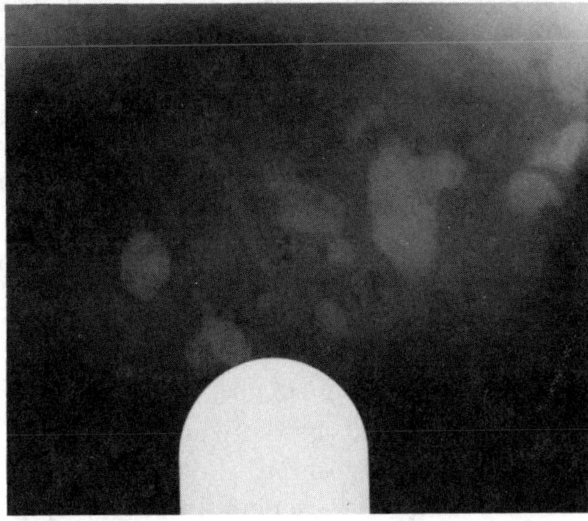

FIG 11–14.
This intraoperative film was obtained prior to removing any of the stone. The film helps to localize all the stone fragments and subsequent films confirm that the kidney is stone-free.

Chemolysis.—Chemolysis can be used as secondary therapy when small stone fragments remain in the kidney. The most appropriate approach is dependent on the location and type of stone remaining as determined by stone analysis. Systemic alkalinization is the initial form of therapy for treating both cystine and uric acid stones. Open surgical procedures are rarely required for uric acid stones as uric acid is a weak organic acid with a pK_a of 5.35 in urine at 37° C. Stone formation occurs when uric acid is in the nondissociated form. When the pH of the urine approaches 7.0, more than half of the uric acid is in the dissociated form and dissolution occurs.[35, 36] Oral sodium bicarbonate, potassium citrate, and intravenous 0.166M lactate have all been used successfully in dissolving these stones.[37] A variety of solutions have also been used to directly dissolve retained stones.[38] Highly alkaline solutions such as sodium bicarbonate and tris(hydroxymethyl)-aminomethane (THAM) have been used to dissolve cystine and uric acid stones.[39–42] Acetylcystine has been used successfully in conjunction with alkaline solutions to dissolve cystine stones.

Struvite stones are soluble in acid and are susceptible to dissolution with local therapy. Hemiacidrin (Renacidin) is an irrigant that is composed of a 10% solution of citric acid, D-gluconic acid, magnesium hydroxycarbonate, magnesium acid citrate, calcium carbonate, and water at a pH of 4.0. Local irrigation with this solution results in complete chemolysis in 73% to 100% of patients, and the incidence of recurrent urolithiasis has been reported to vary form 0% to 25%.[43–46] When irrigation solutions are used to dissolve stones, it is essential that the urine remain sterile. Daily urine cultures should be obtained from the nephrostomy tube and the patient should be kept on appropriate antibiotics. In addition, the irrigation must be immediately discontinued in the presence of urinary obstruction. During irrigation, a system should be developed to provide continuous intrapelvic pressure monitoring (Fig 11–15). When intrapelvic pressures exceed 20 to 25 cm of water, the patient becomes at greater risk for the development of toxicity secondary to the systemic infusion of the irrigating solution and possible sepsis.[47] A nephrostogram should confirm that there is no leakage prior to beginning the irrigation. The irrigation can be run at a rate not to exceed 120 mL/hr and it must be immediately stopped if the patient experiences pain, fever, or increased intrapelvic pressures. Serum magnesium and calcium should be monitored. Several early deaths were reported with the use of hemiacidrin irrigation and profound absorption of magnesium can occur in the presence of higher intrapelvic pressures.[48–50] For these reasons, the principles of administration discussed above must be closely followed.

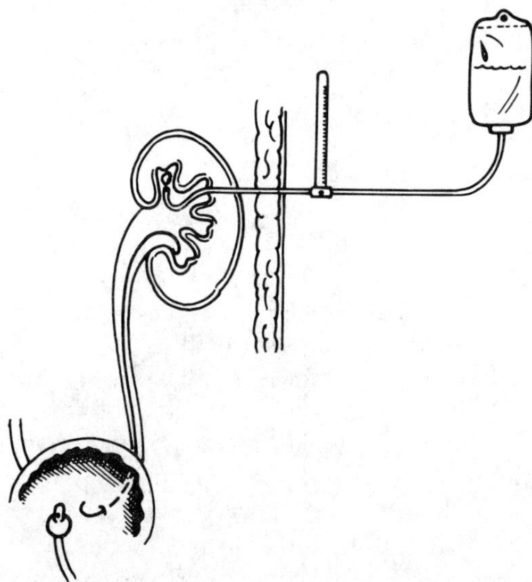

FIG 11–15.
Hemiacidrin irrigation is run through a nephrostomy tube connected to a monometer to continuously monitor intrapelvic pressure. A double-J stent is also noted in the ureter.

Hypertension

The potential for developing or aggravating preexisting hypertension would seem a concern following any open surgery on the kidney. Yet, the complication appears to be unusual.[51, 52] Boyce and Elkins[51] noted only two patients out of their early series of 100 undergoing anatrophic nephrolithotomy that became mildly hypertensive postoperatively. Both patients were easily controlled with oral medications. By meticulous dissection about the renal artery, careful mapping of the avascular plane, and the use of hypothermia, the incidence of hypertension should remain negligible.

Stone Recurrence

After eradication of all stone fragments, recurrent stone formation remains a potential problem for all patients (Fig 11–16). The stone recurrence rate has been reported to be between 20% and 30% over a period of 6 to 10 years.[53, 54] As noted, postoperative chemolysis has been reported to decrease the rate of recurrent disease. Better control of infections and full metabolic evaluation to determine an etiology for the stone formation will help to lower the rate of stone recurrence.

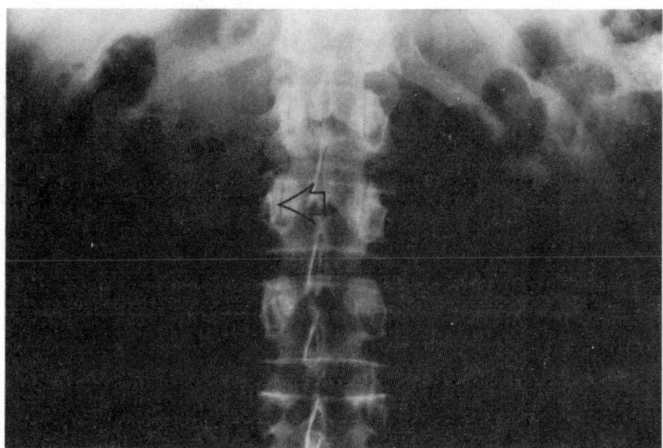

FIG 11–16.
The *arrow* points to a small stone recurrence in a quadriplegic patient 2 years after anatrophic nephrolithotomy for a full staghorn calculus.

Complications of Ureteral Stone Surgery

The frequency of open surgery on the ureter for stone has drastically decreased as extracorporeal shock wave lithotripsy and new endourologic techniques have been popularized. The main problems encountered after surgery on the ureter involve ureteral strictures and persistent ureteral fistulas. If the blood supply to the ureter is disrupted by the inadvertent removal or extensive dissection of periureteral tissue, there will be a delay in the healing of the ureterotomy, and a ureteral stricture may form (Fig 11–17). An attempt should be made to place a ureteral stent and consider endoscopically dilating the stricture under fluoroscopic control. If these techniques fail, treatment will be determined by the location of the ureteral stricture.

Ureteral Reimplantation.—Distal ureteral strictures can best be managed with ureteral reimplantation. In adults, reimplantation into the dome by direct end-to-side ureteroneocystostomy without concern for an antirefluxing tunnel is sufficient. Only distal lesions are suitable for this form of correction. Adequate length of the ureter must be present to create an anastomosis without tension. A low midline incision is best for this procedure. The distal third of the ureter must be exposed. The ureter is transected proximal to the lesion where it is felt that the blood supply is adequate. The ureter is mobilized from the peritoneum to gain adequate length such that the entry site of the ureter is extraperitoneal. The ureter is spatulated and then anastomosed to the bladder dome in an end-to-side manner.

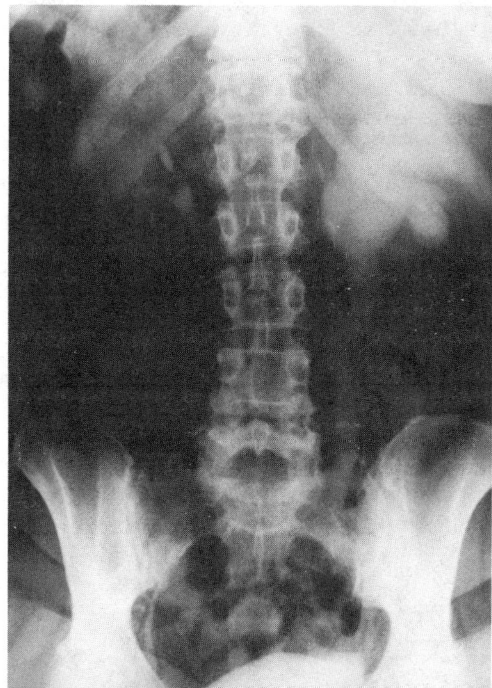

FIG 11–17.
This patient presented with flank pain 1 month after uneventful removal of distal left ureteral stone without reimplantation. She subsequently required ureteral reimplantation.

The sutures should be of 4-0 or 5-0 chromic catgut and be full thickness of the ureter and mucosal layer of the bladder. A stent and drain should be left. If additional length is needed, a psoas hitch can be performed by mobilizing the bladder and taking down the contralateral vascular pedicle. The serosa of the bladder can then be tacked to the psoas muscle with 2-0 chromic catgut sutures gaining several centimeters in length (Fig 11–18).

Boari Bladder Flap.—When the stricture of the ureter is higher, added length can be obtained by making a Boari bladder flap.[55, 56] As much as 15 cm of length can be created with a Boari flap and the ureter can be reimplanted into the flap in a submucosal manner to prevent reflux if this is desired (Fig 11–19). The Boari flap is ideal for replacing the lower third of the ureter. A Gibson incision provides good exposure to the distal ureter and bladder. The ureter is isolated and the amount of ureteral injury is noted. The bladder flap should be 2 to 4 cm longer than the ureteral defect. The base of the flap is created at the cephalad portion of the bladder and should be 2 to 5 cm in length. The distal portion of the flap gradually narrows and can be angulated across the bladder to gain length. The bladder is closed with interrupted 0 chromic sutures and the flap can be tublarized with the same suture. Equally good results are obtained if the ureter is anastomosed in a refluxing or an-

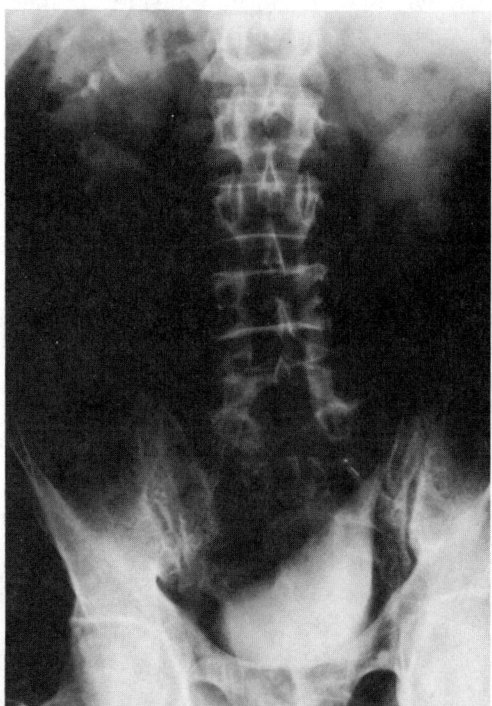

FIG 11–18.
A left psoas hitch was performed on this patient at the time of ureteral reimplantation for repair of distal left ureteral obstruction. The x-ray was taken in the early postoperative period and the chronic calicectasis had not yet resolved.

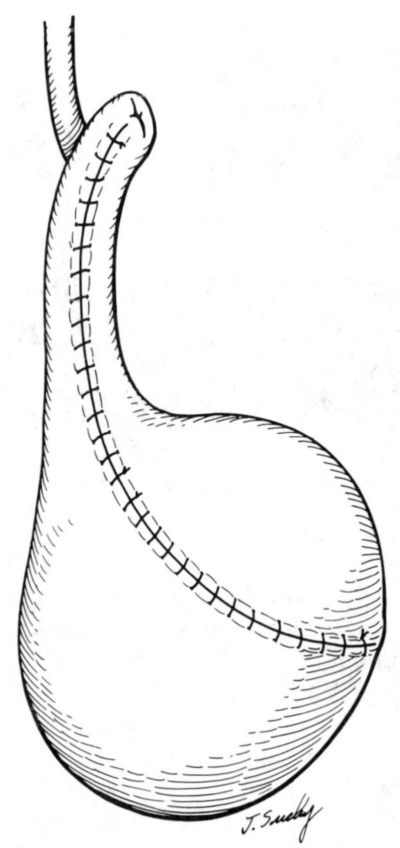

FIG 11–19.
The Boari-Ockerblad bladder flap for replacement of the distal ureter is shown. The ureter can be reimplanted into a submucosal tunnel to prevent reflux if this is desired. The bladder and the flap are closed with a running absorbable suture.

tirefluxing manner. A ureteral stent should be considered and the wound drained.

Transureteroureterostomy.—If the strictured or diseased ureter involves the lower half of the ureter, transuretero-ureterostomy has been considered. The length of the proximal ureter must be sufficient to cross the midline to join the other ureter (Fig 11–20). Unfortunately this technique is contraindicated in the presence of stone disease. Should a stone pass down the ureter, it could effectively obstruct both renal units and result in anuria.

Ileal Ureter.—When the injury occurs to the proximal ureter, or when the entire ureter is lost, replacement of the ureter can be achieved with an ileal ureter. The replacement of damaged ureter with small bowel was first reported at the turn of the century.[57] It creates a wider conduit in patients with recurrent stone disease. The serum creatinine should be less than 2 mg/dL (Figs 11–21 through 11–23).

Adequate exposure is key to performing this procedure. A midline transabdominal incision is ideal. A segment of distal ileum of adequate length on a well-vascularized pedicle is isolated and transected. Continuity of the divided bowel is reestablished. Generally, the entire ureter is destroyed and the intent is to create a proximal ileopyelostomy and a distal ileovesicostomy. The ileal segment is retroperitonealized or brought through a segment of mesocolon. A single-layer ileopyelostomy and a single-layer ileovesicostomy are performed with absorbable suture. The distal anastomosis with the bladder need not be antirefluxing at the discretion of the surgeon. Any redundant bowel is resected distally. Drains are left extraperitoneally and brought out through a separate stab incision.

The production of mucus from the en-

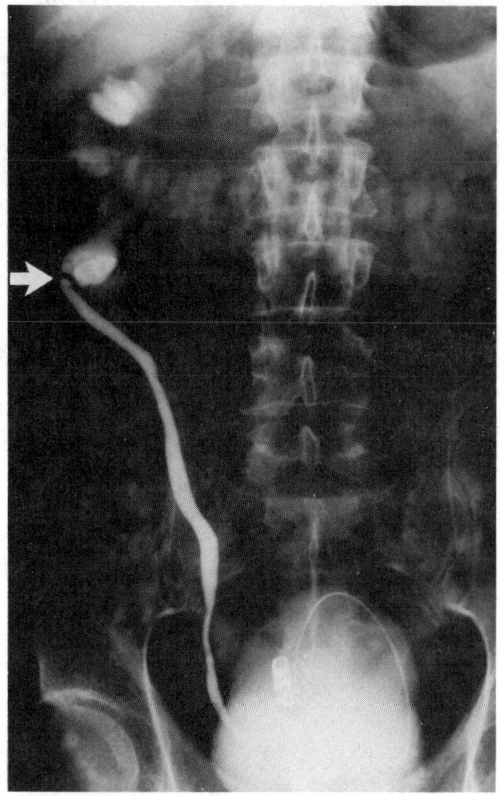

FIG 11–21.
This dense stricture *(arrow)* occurred after two prior pyelolithotomies. The patient has formed multiple stones and the stricture failed endoscopic dilatation.

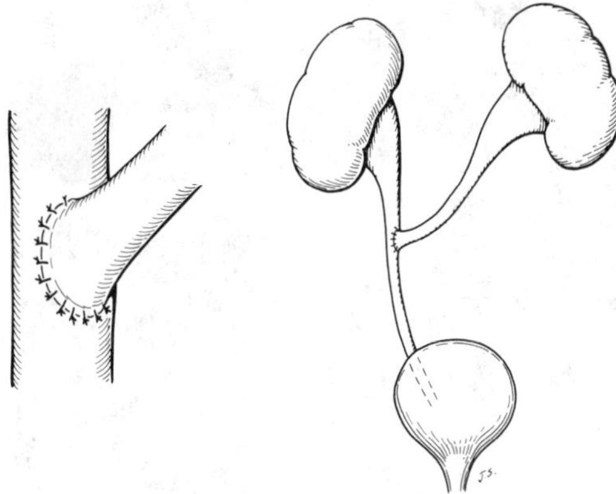

FIG 11–20.
Schema of a transureteroureterostomy to restore ureteral integrity when there is injury or loss of the distal half of the ureter. This technique should be used as a last resort in patients with a history of stone disease as passage of a stone could effectively result in anuric renal failure.

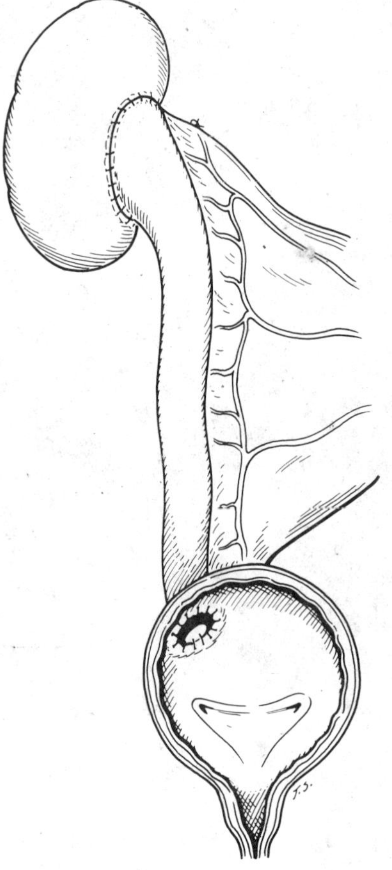

FIG 11–22.
The ileal ureter is shown. The ileum is anastomosed to the renal pelvis proximally and to the bladder distally. The entire ileal segment can be passed through a window in the mesocolon.

teric mucosa can be a problem postoperatively and can be minimized by having the patient maintain adequate fluid intake. Reabsorption of filtered renal solutes can create electrolyte problems and must be monitored carefully postoperatively.

Autotransplantation.—When the entire ureter must be replaced, autotransplantation is an alternative to creation of an ileal ureter. This technique can change the position of the kidney to the pelvis by reestablishing the blood supply to the hypogastric vessels. The advantages of this procedure include the fact that there is no mucus production or electrolyte abnormalities because the bowel is not used. The ureter can be reimplanted into the bladder in an antirefluxing manner if so desired. If the entire length of the ureter has been lost, a vesicopyelostomy can be created. Minimal long-term follow-up is available, but early reports indicate that little damage to the kidney occurs and this appears to be a viable option.

Ureterocutaneous Fistulas.—Ureterocutaneous fistulas are the other complication of ureteral surgery (Figs 11–24, 11–25). Distal ureteral obstruction, infection, or the presence of a foreign body are the usual causes, and correction will lead to healing of the fistula.[58] In addition, if extensive ureteral dissection is performed, with resultant compromise of the periureteral vasculature, prolonged urinary extravasation through the ureterotomy is not infrequent. Most cases of prolonged urinary extravasation will resolve within 2

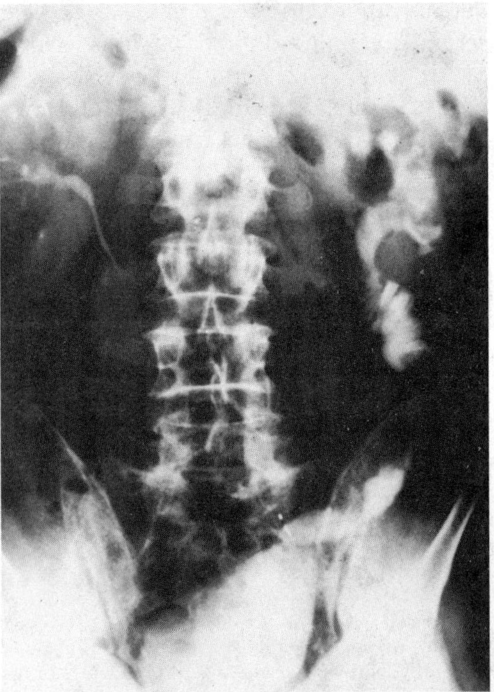

FIG 11–23.
A postoperative excretory pyelogram revealing a left ileal ureter. There is prompt excretion bilaterally.

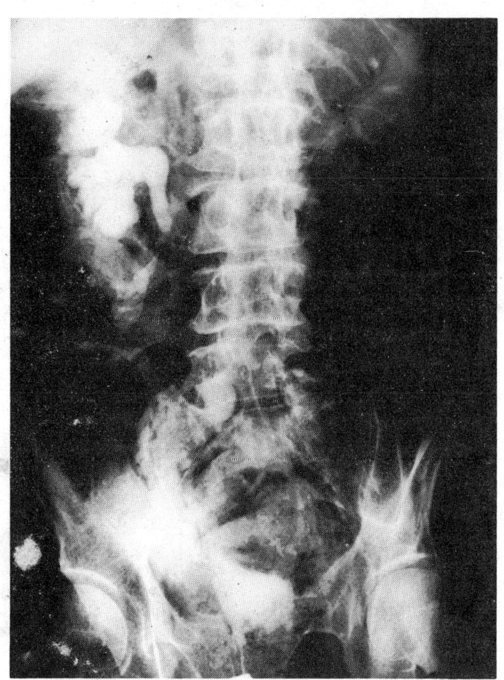

FIG 11–24.
The excretory pyelogram demonstrates persistent extravasation from the ureterolithotomy incision in the proximal right ureter.

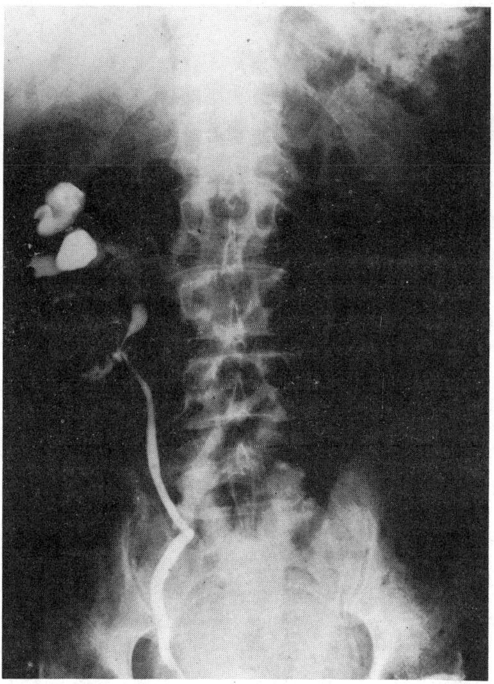

FIG 11–25.
A retrograde pyelogram confirms the presence and location of the persistent fistula. The fistula resolved spontaneously after a double-J stent was placed.

to 3 weeks postoperatively. Early surgical intervention should be avoided. When drainage persists, insertion of a double-J stent is useful. Open surgical repair will occasionally be required but is often necessitated by the development of strictures that are likely due to the extensive scarring associated with the ureteral injury and the associated prolonged urinary extravasation.

Urinoma formation is a rare complication of open ureteral surgery when the drains have been removed prematurely. If the urine becomes infected, antibiotics and drainage of the urinoma are required. Often, placement of a ureteral stent will help to correct prolonged extravasation.

EDITORIAL COMMENT

Extracorporeal shock wave lithotripsy remains effective for most renal calculi so that renal surgery for renal calculi is becoming increasingly rare. The surgical anatomy is carefully defined in this chapter. Use of intraoperative ultrasound can be very helpful in the localization of these calculi.

REFERENCES

1. Resnick MI, Boyce WH: Bilateral staghorn calculi: Patient evaluation and management. *J Urol* 1980; 123:338–341.
2. Boyce WH, Harrison LH: Complications of renal stone surgery, in Smith RM, Skinner DG (eds): *Complications of Urologic Surgery: Prevention and Management.* Philadelphia, WB Saunders Co, 1976, pp 87–105.
3. Fowler JE: Bacteriology of branched renal calculi and accompanying urinary tract infection. *J Urol* 1984; 131:213–215.
4. Silverman DE, Stamey TA: Management of infection stones: The Stanford experience. *Medicine* 1983; 62:44–51.

5. Nemoy NJ, Stamey TA: Surgical, bacteriological and biochemical management of infection stones. *JAMA* 1971; 215:1470–1476.
6. Stamey TA: Infection stones, in Stamey TA (ed): *Pathogenesis and Treatment of Urinary Tract Infections.* Baltimore, Williams & Wilkins Co, 1980, pp 430–474.
7. Birch AA, Nims GR: Anesthesia considerations during nephrolithotomy with slush. *J Urol* 1975; 113:433–435.
8. Case EW, Stiles JA: The effect of various surgical positions on vital capacity. *Anesthesiology* 1946; 7:29–31.
9. Jones JR, Jacoby J: The effect of surgical positions on respiration. *Surg Forum* 1955; 5:686–691.
10. Wellborn SG: Anesthesiologic considerations: Urology, in Martin JT (ed): *Positioning in Anesthesia and Surgery.* Philadelphia, WB Saunders Co, 1978, pp 170–174.
11. Boyce WH: Surgery of urinary calculi in perspective. *Urol Clin North Am* 1983; 10:585–594.
12. Resnick MI, Elkins IB: Applications of renal anatomy to intrarenal surgery, in Resnick MI, Parker MP (eds): *Surgical Anatomy of the Kidney.* Mt Kisco, NY, Futura Publishing Co, 1982, pp 165–176.
13. Juengst KN, Kursh ED: Pyelolithotomy. *Urol Clin North Am* 1983; 10:649–658.
14. Novick AC: Renal hypothermia: In vivo and ex vivo. *Urol Clin North Am* 1983; 10:637–644.
15. Collins GM, Green RD, Boyer P, et al: Protection of the kidneys from warm ischemic injury: Dosage and timing of mannitol administration. *Transplantation* 1980; 29:83–84.
16. Nosowsky EE, Kaufman JJ: The protective action of mannitol in renal artery occlusion. *J Urol* 1963; 89:295–299.
17. Wickham JEA, Coe N, Ward JP: One hundred cases of nephrolithotomy under hypothermia. *J Urol* 1974; 112:702–705.
18. Marberger M, Eisenberger F: Regional hypothermia of the kidney: Surface or transarterial perfusion cooling? A functional study. *J Urol* 1980; 124:179–183.
19. Stubbs AJ, Resnick MI, Boyce WH: Anatrophic nephrolithotomy in the solitary kidney. *J Urol* 1978; 119:457–460.
20. Resnick MI: Anatrophic nephrolithotomy. *Mod Techniques Urol Surg* 1982; 25:1–13.
21. Askeri A, Novick AC, Stewart BH, et al: Surgical treatment of renovascular disease in the solitary kidney: Results of 43 cases. *J Urol* 1982; 127:20–22.
22. Ward JP: Determination of the optimum temperature for regional renal hypothermia during temporary renal ischemia. *Br J Urol* 1975; 47:17–24.
23. Roth RA: Residual stones, in Roth RA, Finlayson B (eds): *Stones: Clinical Management of Urolithiasis.* Baltimore, Williams & Wilkins Co, 1983; pp 422–439.
24. Sleight MW, Wickham JEA: Long-term followup of 100 cases of renal calculi. *Br J Urol* 1977; 49:601–604.
25. Marshall FF: Intraoperative localization of renal calculi. *Urol Clin North Am* 1983; 10:629–636.
26. Beck AD: Intraoperative radiography in conservative surgery for renal calculi. *J Urol* 1973; 110:494–497.
27. Boyce WH: The localization of intrarenal calculi during surgery. *J Urol* 1977; 118:152–157.
28. Feldman RA, Shearer JK, Shield DE, et al: Sensitive method for intraoperative roentgenograms. *Urology* 1977; 9:695–697.
29. Singh M, Marshall V, Blandy J: The residual renal stone. *Br J Urol* 1975; 47:125–129.
30. Zingg ES, Futterlieb A: Nephroscopy in stone surgery. *Br J Urol* 1980; 52:333–337.
31. Cook JH III, Lytton B: Intraoperative localization of renal calculi during nephrolithotomy by ultrasound scanning. *J Urol* 1979; 117:543–546.
32. Resnick MI, Saunders R: *Ultrasound in Urology.* Baltimore, Williams & Wilkins Co, 1979.
33. Sigel B, Coelho JCU, Shariti R, et al: Ultrasonic scanning during operation for renal calculi. *J Urol* 1982; 127:421–424.
34. Spirnak JP, Resnick MI: Anatrophic nephrolithotomy. *Urol Clin North Am* 1983; 10:665–676.
35. Fried FA, Vermuelen CW: Artificial uric acid concretion and observations on uric acid solubility and supersaturation. *Invest Urol* 1964; 2:131.
36. Burns JR, Ganthier JF, Finlayson B: Disso-

lution kinetics of uric acid calculi. *J Urol* 1984; 131:708.

37. Kursh ED, Resnick MI: Dissolution of uric acid calculi with systemic alkalinization. *J Urol* 1984; 132:286–287.
38. Sheldon CA, Smith AD: Chemolysis of calculi. *Urol Clin North Am* 1982; 9:121–130.
39. Crissey MM, Gittes RF: Dissolution of cystine ureteral calculus by irrigation with tromethamine. *J Urol* 1979; 121:811–812.
40. Hardy B, Klein LA: In situ dissolution of ureteral calculus. *Urology* 1976; 8:444–446.
41. Gordon MR, Carrion HM, Politano VA: Dissolution of uric acid calculi with THAM irrigation. *Urology* 1978; 12:393–397.
42. Rodman JS, Williams JJ, Peterson CM: Dissolution of uric acid calculi. *J Urol* 1984; 131:1039–1043.
43. Fam B, Rossier AB, Yalla S, et al: The role of hemiacidrin in the management of renal stones in spinal cord injury patients. *J Urol* 1976; 116:696.
44. Blaivas JG, Pais VM, Spellman RM: Chemolysis of residual stone fragments after extensive surgery for staghorn calculi. *Urology* 1975; 6:686.
45. Royle G, Smith JC: Recurrence of infected calculi following postoperative renal irrigation with stone solvent. *Br J Urol* 1976; 48:531–537.
46. Sant GR, Blaivas JG, Meares EM: Hemiacidrin irrigation in the management of struvite calculi: Long-term results. *J Urol* 1983; 130:1048–1050.
47. Mulvaney WP: The hydrodynamics of renal irrigations: with reference to calculus solvents. *J Urol* 1963; 89:765.
48. Kohley FP: Renacidin and tissue reaction. *J Urol* 1962; 87:102.
49. Fostvedt GA, Barnes RW: Complications during lavage therapy for renal calculi. *J Urol* 1963; 89:329.
50. Cato AR, Tulloch AGS: Hypermagnesemia in a uremic patient during renal pelvis irrigation with renacidin. *J Urol* 1974; 300:341–343.
51. Boyce WH, Elkins IB: Reconstructive renal surgery following anatrophic nephrolithotomy: Follow-up of 100 consecutive cases. *J Urol* 1974; 111:307–312.
52. Gil-Vernet JM: Pyelolithotomy, in Roth RA, Finlayson B (eds): *Stones: Clinical Management of Urolithiasis.* Baltimore, Williams & Wilkins Co, 1983, pp 297–331.
53. Griffith DP: Infection induced stones, in Coe FL (ed): *Nephrolithiasis, Pathogenesis and Treatment.* Chicago, Year Book Medical Publishers, 1978.
54. Russell JM, Webb RT, Harrison LH, et al: Long-term followup of 100 anatrophic nephrolithotomies. Presented at International Urinary Stone Conference, Perth, Australia, Aug 4–8, 1979.
55. Boari A: Chirurgia dell'uretere con prefazione del Dott. I. Albarran, 1900. Contributo sperimentale alla plastica delle uretere. Quoted by Spies JW, Johnson CW, Wilson CS: Reconstruction of the ureter by a bladder flap. *Proc Soc Exp Biol Med* 1932; 30:425.
56. Williams JL, Porter RW: The Boari bladder flap in lower ureteral injuries. *Br J Urol* 1966; 38:528–533.
57. Boxer RJ, Fritzsche P, Skinner DG, et al: Replacement of the ureter by small intestine: Clinical application and results of the ileal ureter in 89 patients. *Trans Am Assoc Genitourin Surg* 1979; 70:99–102.
58. Cohen JD, Persky L: Ureteral stones. *Urol Clin North Am* 1983; 10:699–708.

CHAPTER 12

Complications of Endourology

Joseph W. Segura, M.D.

COMPLICATIONS OF PERCUTANEOUS STONE REMOVAL

While percutaneous procedures for stone removal are considerably less invasive than standard surgical techniques, a variety of complications may ensue at any point in the percutaneous nephrolithotomy. As in other surgical procedures, recognizing the problems that *can* occur will help prevent them, and recognizing *when* such problems have occurred will minimize their impact.

The three essential steps in percutaneous stone removal are nephrostomy tube insertion, tract dilatation, and removal of the stone. The temporal relationship of these three steps to one another varies from institution to institution, and has no bearing on the overall stone removal success. These three steps provide a convenient framework within which to consider the incidence and nature of complications related to endourologic stone removal.

Complications Related to Access

While nephrostomy tube placement may be done under fluoroscopic or ultrasonic control, we feel that optimum results are achieved with the precision available with fluoroscopy.[1] Despite this precision, initial placement of the nephrostomy tube may be suboptimal for subsequent stone removal. In large measure, the complication rate and, indeed, the ultimate success of the final procedure is a function of accurate tract placement. The first step toward minimizing the risk of complications is an accurate assessment of one's ability to obtain proper access in a given situation.

Trauma

Successful percutaneous access depends upon the fact that the kidney is a retroperitoneal organ and that it may be approached posterolaterally without compromise to adjacent structures (Fig 12–1). Review of the pertinent anatomy reveals a "window" through which access may be safely achieved. Variations in normal anatomy and/or errors in technique may result in trauma to adjacent organs.

Spleen.—When the spleen is of normal size and in normal position, it is unlikely to be traumatized by nephrostomy tube placement through a typical sub-12th rib approach. Splenomegaly may be present to such a degree that safe nephrostomy tube placement is impossible. Often, splenomegaly is obvious on the plain x-ray film, and review of such films will reveal the marginal case wherein the risk of injury is increased. If there is any doubt about the position of the spleen relative to the kidney, a computed tomographic (CT) scan should be obtained to accurately delineate the anatomical relationship. The CT guidance of nephrostomy placement in these cases may be

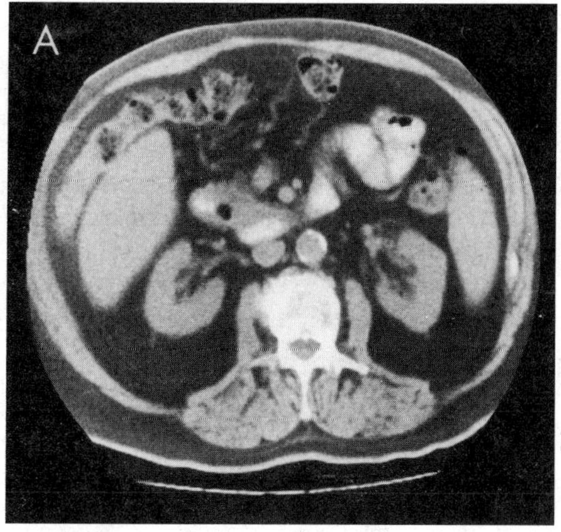

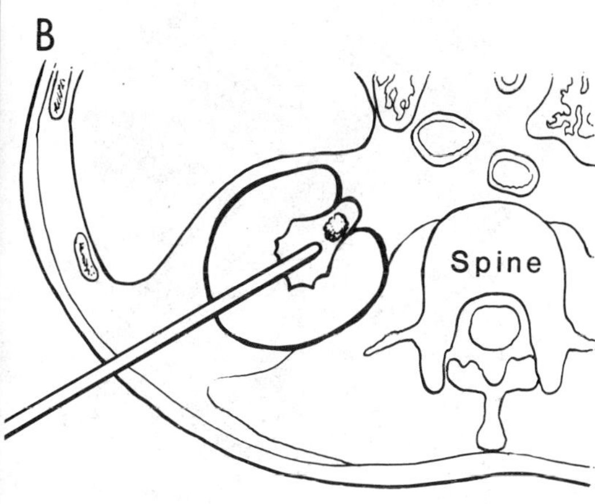

FIG 12–1.
A, CT scan through lower half of kidneys. **B,** access on right side should miss liver and adjacent organs. A posterolateral approach optimally accesses the posterior calices of the collecting system and spares the colon, liver/spleen, and the paraspinal muscles, as well as the perineal cavity. Normal anatomical variations as well as pathologic changes in adjacent organs may result in injury despite an appropriate approach.

helpful. Trauma to the spleen will certainly result in acute blood loss with the necessity for emergency splenectomy.

Liver.—Injury to the normal liver is very unlikely in a typical approach. Some patients may have hepatomegaly, and a rare patient will have a liver configuration that may prohibit a percutaneous approach. Hepatomegaly of such a degree to compromise the procedure is usually apparent on the plain film, and doubtful cases may be evaluated by CT scan.

Duodenum.—Because of its proximity to the right kidney, the duodenum is occasionally injured. Ordinarily this injury will occur when needles, trocars, or guide wires that have already been inserted as far as the kidney are inserted too far, with perforation of the medial pelvis and subsequent perforation of the duodenum. If careful fluoroscopic control is employed during nephrostomy insertion and during tract dilatation, the risk of this complication is minimal. Treatment is conservative: the patient should receive nothing by mouth, with nasogastric tube drainage for several days, until the surgeon is certain that the hole in the duodenum has sealed.[2]

Colon.—The kidneys lie posterior to the colon, although the colon may extend to the lateral aspect of the kidney. If the colon is enlarged, this lateral extension may project posteriorly and seem to wrap around the kidney. This extension is more likely in the region of the splenic flexure and descending colon. It is not possible to predict who will have a colon of such size and position that nephrostomy tube placement is unsafe. In an occasional individual, a normal colon seems to be positioned posterolateral to the kidney in a position of distinct risk. Patients who have had a jejunal-ileal bypass for chronic morbid obesity have enlarged colons, presumably due to the increased volume of material presented to the colon, and are at increased risk for this complication. In one such patient, percutaneous tract

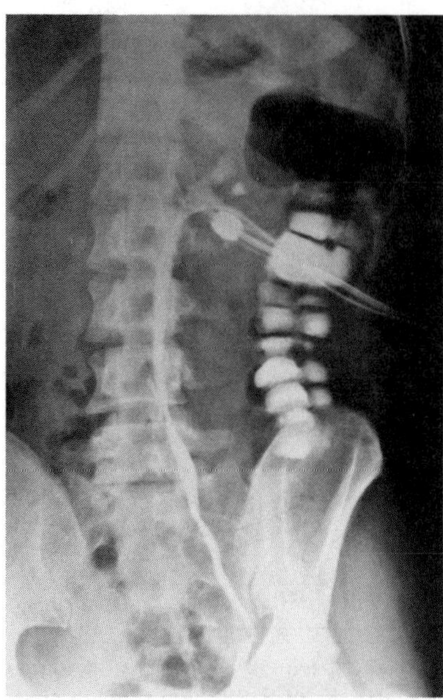

FIG 12–2.
A nephrostogram done 48 hours after percutaneous ultrasonic lithotripsy. Contrast medium is in the collecting system, as well as the descending colon. The patient was asymptomatic.

placement nicked the descending colon (Fig 12–2). Almost all of the stone was removed at the time of percutaneous ultrasonic lithotripsy, although the procedure was terminated before all of the stone was removed because of a discrepancy in input and output irrigation fluid levels. A nephrostogram 48 hours after the procedure revealed contrast medium in the colon. The patient had no systemic signs and was otherwise well.

The problem was managed by inserting a double-J stent from bladder to kidney in order to obtain internal diversion of the urine. The nephrostomy tube was withdrawn out of the kidney into the colon in order to provide maintenance of the tract without risk of uncontrolled fecal leakage into the retroperitoneum as well as to decompress the colon. After several days, contrast media injected through the nephrostomy tube entered the colon but not the kidney. After a few more days, the "colostomy" tube was then removed and the tract closed spontaneously. A diverting colostomy was not necessary. This and a similar case are described in detail by LeRoy et al.[3] Neustein et al. reported a similar case, which was also managed conservatively but complicated by a small pelvic tear and difficulty obtaining internal diversion.[4] The colonic fistula responded to conservative measures, but surgery was required to remove the stone.

It appears difficult to predict in which patient this complication is likely to occur, other than in the above-mentioned specific situation. If there is any doubt, CT scan might precisely delineate the relationship of the colon to the kidney. While the trauma in these cases was manageable conservatively, more significant trauma to the colon or damage to a significant colonic vessel with significant bleeding would probably require surgical repair.

Pleura.—The risk of injury to the pleura is a function of several variables: how far inferior the pleural cavity extends, how cephalad the kidney is, and whether the percutaneous access was created above the 12th rib. In general, if the kidney is in relatively normal position and access to the collecting system is below the 12th rib, the risk of pleural damage is very slight. If access routes above the 12th or 11th ribs are chosen, the risk of pleural injury becomes greater. We have had one proven case. While treatment could well require chest tube insertion, our case was asymptomatic, with approximately a 15% pneumothorax, and did not require a chest tube. In a case managed at the University of Minnesota, a hematothorax was present, but this responded to chest tube placement and was otherwise conservatively treated.[5] It is likely that other asymptomatic pleural injuries have occurred but, because they were not clinically significant, have not been diagnosed.

Kidney.—Less than optimal tract placement may result in renal damage separate from what might occur at the time of stone removal. A too-lateral or too-medial placement of a nephrostomy tract through a portion of the kidney, with insufficient parenchyma, may predispose to tearing or laceration of the parenchyma as the dilatation progresses. This problem is not evident while the nephrostomy tube is in place but becomes obvious as bleeding ensues during the dilatation. Renal vascular pedicle injury may also occur. If the pedicle is injured by anything larger than a skinny needle, significant bleeding may occur. Whether this bleeding would require surgical intervention would largely depend on the situation.

A bleeding diathesis is the only absolute contraindication to percutaneous nephrostomy placement. Any such bleeding diathesis should be corrected before nephrostomy tube placement. Drugs that affect bleeding and clotting time, such as dipyridamole (Persantine), warfarin (Coumadin), and aspirin or aspirin-containing drugs, should be stopped prior to the procedure. The effect of dipyridamole is usually over after 24 hours, but that of warfarin and aspirin may last considerably longer. We have not routinely measured bleeding or clotting parameters, unless patients are taking one of these medicines or there is some suspicion, based on the patient's history, of a bleeding diathesis.

Larger renal arteries and veins are located near the central portion of the kidney, and the smallest are at the tips of calices. Proper placement of the nephrostomy tract through a calix, through the infundibulum, and thence into the renal pelvis will minimize the risk of significant large vessel injury. Variations in renal anatomy and limitations in the fluoroscopic guidance systems are such that occasionally a significant vessel may be injured. Despite this risk, the chance of causing bleeding that is sufficient to require transfusion appears to be small. In about 1,400 nephrostomy tube placements prior to percutaneous stone removal, no patient has bled to the extent that transfusion has been required (although transfusion was subsequently necessary in 3% of patients because of bleeding associated with the stone removal portion). We believe that the bleeding, when it occurs, is probably venous in origin and in no case has the bleeding been such that we suspected significant arterial injury. In general, when significant bleeding occurs in association with percutaneous stone removal, it accompanies the tract dilatation and the lithotripsy itself.

Sepsis

A rise in temperature associated with percutaneous access may often occur, but such a temperature spike is usually not high or associated with overt signs of sepsis unless acute infection is present at the time of access or if an infected stone is present. If the stone removal follows closely upon percutaneous access, it may not be possible to separate temporally fever that is secondary to the access from fever that is a result of the percutaneous manipulation and stone removal. The chances of sepsis are minimized if the patient is receiving prophylactic antibiotics. We prefer cephalosporins for this purpose unless an overt infection is present and sensitivities dictate another antibiotic. If an infected stone is present, the patient should receive the appropriate antibiotics for 1 or 2 days prior to the percutaneous access. Sepsis is also less likely if catheter manipulation is minimized and external urinary drainage is provided at the time of nephrostomy placement.

Complications Related to Tract Dilatation

When tract dilatation and stone removal are done as one procedure, the relationship of a given complication to a particular phase of the procedure may be obscured. In general, if the tract has been correctly placed, the risk of a complication associated with dilatation is small.

The most troublesome complication to occur during dilatation is inadvertent removal of the guide wire. At best, the operator must return to "square one" and reestablish access; at worst, the situation will be complicated by a bleeding tract with no ready access to the collecting system. The risk of tract loss is minimized if the guide wire is placed down the ureter and coiled in the bladder, so that unintentional loss of a few inches of wire would not result in loss of the tract. Placement of a second or reserve guide wire through the tract is essential to avoid these problems.

Some tracts may be so long that dilators cannot pass over the wire without buckling the wire in the retroperitoneum. Such long tracts may be more likely in patients with high-riding kidneys or in obese patients with marked amounts of retroperitoneal fat. The buckling is most prominent with flexible fascial dilators and less likely with the Amplatz dilators or metal concentric dilators. Kinking of the guide wire is a frequent problem, and usually the guide wire should be replaced if this happens, since the kink simply makes every subsequent step in the procedure more difficult. The dilators should be placed no further than the renal pelvis, since pushing the dilators in too far may tear the renal pelvis or avulse or tear the ureteropelvic junction, as the large caliber dilators are forced through a small ureteropelvic junction and upper ureter. Consistent use of fluoroscopic control while the dilators are passed will reduce the risk of such an occurrence. In situations in which the stone fills most of the available space in the renal pelvis, the dilator should proceed only as far as the stone, since there may not be enough room in the pelvis for both stone and dilator. If advanced too far, a tear in the pelvis may occur.

Bleeding

Tract dilatation always causes bleeding. Occasionally, this bleeding is forceful, with blood running profusely out of the tract. This bleeding is renal in origin but also can result from damage to the intercostal vessels. In our experience, this bleeding is always tamponaded by the presence of the dilator and/or the nephroscope sheath. Such bleeding should not be a cause for flank exploration.

Complications Related to Stone Removal

While all aspects of percutaneous stone removal are interrelated, some complications seem related to the stone removal itself.

Bleeding

All of these patients bleed to a greater or lesser extent, much like a patient undergoing a transurethral resection of the prostate. The average patient, in fact, loses 1.2 g of hemoglobin during a typical case. Most bleeding is parenchymal in origin and is controlled by tract tamponade and continuous irrigation. Over the operating time of the typical case (average 48 minutes), the degree of bleeding is usually not important. Sometimes the bleeding gradually increases during a case so that stone removal is compromised; the rate of stone removal decreases and it becomes difficult to visualize endoscopically the renal pelvis and stone. Usually, it is then best to stop the procedure, insert a large-caliber nephrostomy tube, and reinsert the nephroscope 48 hours later. Intraoperative bleeding may be aggravated by an up-and-down, side-to-side movement of the nephroscope. Indeed, such movements, which may be necessary to access difficult stones, are best undertaken after the simpler stones have been removed. For example, if the prime reason for the procedure was a pelvic stone and the secondary reason was some smaller caliceal stones, the pelvic stone, which requires minimal nephroscopic manipulation, should be done first, and then the caliceal stones.

Occasionally, at the end of the stone removal procedure, large quantities of venous blood will come out the nephrostomy tube, making it seem as if there were a direct connection between the collecting system and the renal vein. Injection of contrast into the nephrostomy tube will often demonstrate contrast medium entering into the renal venous system through the parenchymal veins along the acute tract (Fig 12–3). A clue during the procedure that this is happening is when the operator notices that the suctioned irrigating fluid is quite bloody but that the pelvis readily clears when the irrigating fluid is turned on. Also, discrepancies between fluid input and output may sometimes be accounted for by intravenous extravasation.

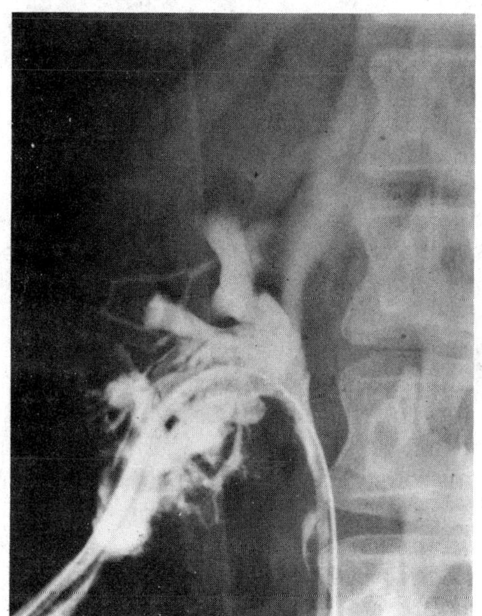

FIG 12–3.
Operative nephrostogram. The nephrostomy tube has been placed, and a guide wire and stent are down the ureter. Contrast injected through the nephrostomy tube goes through the renal venous system and clearly outlines the renal vein and inferior vena cava. Bleeding from such a fistulous connection will cease after clamping of the nephrostomy tube and tamponade of the renal pelvis.

We treat this bleeding by clamping the nephrostomy tube, which results in tamponade of the venous bleeders. Concurrently, the patient receives mannitol, 22.5 mg intravenously. After 30 to 60 minutes, the nephrostomy tube is opened and urine output ensues after 1 to 3 hours. The renal pelvic blood clots will lyse over the next 1 to 3 days. We have performed this maneuver many times without compromise of the clinical situation or long-term complication.

The most serious complication of percutaneous stone removal is arteriovenous fistula or pseudoaneurysm formation. We have six definite cases in about 1,400 patients who underwent percutaneous stone removal (0.5%). Other centers have also reported incidences of less than 1%.[6]

These patients all presented with marked amounts of postoperative bleeding. Indeed, the brisk bleeding was noted through the nephrostomy tube and around the nephrostomy tube when present, and this blood also went down the ureter and into the bladder. The degree of bleeding demands immediate transfusion and treatment. Arteriography with embolization of the peripheral bleeding vessel is the preferred method of treatment and is immediately curative (Fig 12–4). Flank exploration should be avoided if possible, since the emergent nature of the surgery may make nephrectomy necessary or, at best, result in partial nephrectomy.

Patterson et al. have reviewed our cases in detail.[7] In four patients, the bleeding was clearly associated with traumatic intraoperative maneuvers or postoperative trauma. One of these patients was hypertensive. In two patients, the ultrasonic probe was pushed blindly into the renal parenchyma in an attempt to access the stone, and one patient pulled his Foley catheter nephrostomy tube out through the kidney with the balloon in-

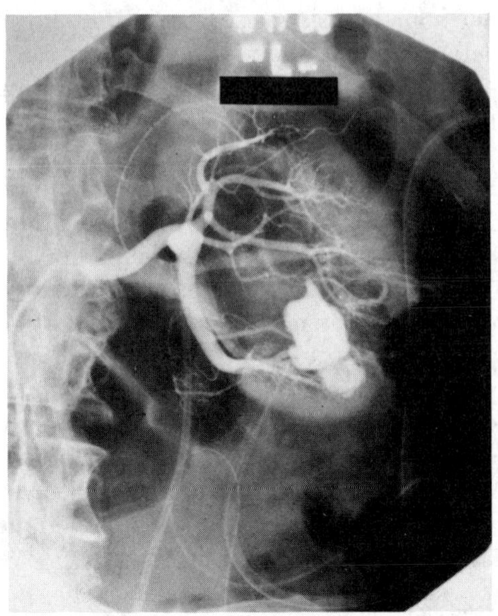

FIG 12–4.
Left selective arteriogram. A pseudoaneurysm was present at the lower pole at the site of percutaneous access. This was a difficult percutaneous stone removal and required subsequent ureterolithotomy. The peripheral vessel is selectively embolized, immediately stopping the bleeding with successful results.

tact. Two patients had no history of traumatic procedures and bled spontaneously 7 to 10 days after the surgery. The exact cause of arteriovenous fistula formation is not known, and it is difficult to predict in which case arteriovenous fistula formation might develop. Marberger believes that the incidence of fistula formation may be related to the use of large (22 –26 French) nephrostomy tubes, since there is a very low fistula rate in his own practice and he consistently uses a 14F nephrostomy tube.[8] The exact incidence is, in fact, unknown, since subclinical cases may spontaneously resolve.

Extravasation

The preferred irrigating solution is 0.9% sodium chloride, so that if and when extravasation occurs, its consequences will be manageable. Water should never be used, nor should glycine. Schultz and his colleagues reported a case of ammonium toxicity in a patient who absorbed considerable quantities of glycine during a percutaneous procedure.[9] Extravasation of contrast medium at the time of access is common and of no significance if adequate drainage is provided. Whether extravasation is important depends largely on how much fluid is absorbed, where it goes, and the patient's ability to tolerate this. The risk of extravasation is greater in a sealed system (such as with a nephroscope or Ruttner cannula) and is less if an Amplatz sheath is used, since the fluid leaks out around the sheath. Generally, the best treatment of extravasation is prevention. It should be standard practice in the operating room for the circulating nurse to measure the volume of fluid in the suction, urethral catheter, and other fluid outputs and compare these to the quantity of irrigating fluid used. If the discrepancy cannot be accounted for by leakage or by fluid in the bladder, extravasation must be assumed to have occurred.

How much extravasation is significant? This depends on where the fluid is going and the condition of the patient. As a general rule, we think that if the discrepancy reaches 500 mL, and this difference cannot be accounted for by spillage or other loss, the surgeon should seriously consider stopping the procedure. While any individual in reasonable health can absorb 1,000 mL of normal saline intravenously with little difficulty, the quantity absorbed may mount up rapidly and become dangerous. When absorption, particularly intravenous absorption, has occurred, intravenous furosemide (Lasix) is useful for inducing as rapid a diuresis as practical.

Retroperitoneal extravasation is not uncommon and is usually related to a tear or hole in the collecting system. This hole may be obvious, and while the rate of extravasation is not as fast as that in intravenous extravasation, it will often be necessary to terminate the case unless it can be quickly completed. If the hole is made, our practice is to monitor closely the input and output and proceed with the case as long as it can be completed expeditiously and as long as there is no discrepancy in the input and output. The most common spot for a tear to occur is in the inferior border of the renal pelvis, just above the ureteropelvic junction. This is because the dilators and nephroscopes are constantly passing over this area, presumably weakening it and making it more susceptible to tear. Also, maneuvering the nephroscope to visualize the ureteropelvic junction will sometimes put considerable stress on this area. The recognition that a tear has occurred (here or elsewhere) is the most important factor. The tear may dissect down to the ureteropelvic junction, and the procedure should be stopped before this happens. Intraperitoneal extravasation is not common. We have had two cases in our experience and Carson and Nesbitt reported two cases from Duke University.[10]

In our cases (done before we monitored input and output), 5,000 mL or more of 0.9% saline were absorbed. These patients were managed with diuretics, and fluid was mobilized over the next 2 to 3 days. Carson and Nesbitt treated their patients with peritoneal taps, which resulted in immediate relief of abdominal distention. Whichever method is chosen, the use of diuretics and careful monitoring of electrolytes are important.

The treatment of extravasation is straightforward. The procedure should be stopped and a nephrostomy tube placed indwelling. There will often be no x-ray evidence of extravasation whatsoever after 12 hours and almost never at 48 hours. Indeed, we will routinely re-treat these patients at 48 hours, at which time there will be no visual evidence of extravasation regardless of whether the extravasation was intravenous or retroperitoneal. The site of the tear is usually visible, but it will be sealed and appear as if it were, for example, a diverticulum. An exception to these rules is if a large amount of retroperitoneal fluid has leaked; in that case the patient may require longer for the defects to seal. In such a patient, the large amount of fluid that has extravasated has the effect of creating significant retroperitoneal space, which is not present in other patients with relatively minor leakage. Perinephric abscess or urinoma formation may rarely arise in this situation.

Retained Fragments

The incidence of retained fragments in our practice has varied from 3% in our best selected series of patients to about 9% or 10% overall. While not a complication, strictly speaking, we would prefer to have removed these residual stones if possible. These stones become a complication if their size is such that spontaneous passage could not reasonably be expected, or if they are residual infected stones. In the former case, another procedure may be required should the stones move; in the latter, stone regrowth may result. The presence of such stones should be identified before the nephrostomy tube is removed, so that the nephroscope may be reinserted if necessary. The decision as to whether the nephroscope should be reinserted depends largely on whether removal of the residual stones is thought to be worth the extra time, expense, and discomfort occasioned by the repeat procedure. There is no evidence that such residual stones contribute to recurrent stone formation (unless they are infected). The incidence of recurrent stone formation appears to be a function of the underlying metabolic abnormality rather than a function of the type of procedure used to remove the stone. Marberger et al.[11] and Segura et al.[12] have found no increased incidence of stone formations in patients whose recoveries were followed for 1 to 4 years after percutaneous stone removal. Fragments sometimes exit through holes or tears in the collecting system. If these fragments are not infected, it is usually not a significant problem, and it is not our practice to operate on these patients to remove the fragments. Tiny fragments are sometimes also visible in the percutaneous tract, and we believe that repeat surgical procedures to remove these fragments are also not indicated.

Sepsis

Sepsis may occur immediately after percutaneous stone removal irrespective of when the initial nephrostomy tube was placed. We have had two patients develop acute septic shock immediately postprocedure in the recovery room. These patients had infected stones and were covered with the appropriate antibiotic. It seems likely that the immune systems in these two elderly people were overwhelmed because of the absorption of irrigating fluid containing a suspension of infected stone from the center of the stone. Both patients were treated immediately and vigorously, with successful result.

Sepsis is occasionally obvious after the procedure, when the temperature may climb to high levels, but adequate and appropriate antibiotic treatment and supportive measures should reduce the fever levels to normal after 1 or 2 days.

Miscellaneous Complications

We have performed these procedures on patients with a wide variety of general medical problems—on patients who have been in general good health and patients who have been distinctly ill. It has been consistently observed that the general medical complications in this group of patients have been minimal. Only one patient developed a postoperative thrombophlebitis and he subsequently turned out to have a hypercoagulable state secondary to carcinoma of the pancreas. A second patient developed thrombophlebitis 3 weeks after the procedure. One 65-year-old woman died after undergoing bilateral removal of staghorn calculi on two separate operating days a week apart. The procedure on the first side went well, as did the second, with an operating time of 53 minutes in the second procedure. Twenty-four hours after the second procedure, she developed an arrhythmia secondary to probable myocardial infarction.

The general lack of significant medical complications may relate to the fact that, for the typical patient, the clinical course is parallel to that of a patient undergoing transurethral resection of the prostate—most patients are up and eating 12 to 24 hours after the procedure and out of the hospital after just a few days.

Long-Term Complications

The long-term results of endourologic stone removal are unknown. Marberger et al. carefully studied 82 patients 1 to 4 years after the original procedure and were able to find no abnormality or untoward result.[11] We have noted no special incidence of unusual problems with follow-ups of nearly 4 years in some patients. We have identified one patient with mild postoperative ureteropelvic junction stricture, which has not required treatment. The exact incidence of this complication is not known, but all other urograms in patients who have had postprocedure urograms have been normal.

Intuitively, one would expect little in the way of long-term problems in the typical case. Urologists have been putting nephrostomy tubes in kidneys for two generations without any evidence of long-term problems relative to the nephrostomy tube. To a great extent, this procedure simulates what happens when a percutaneous nephrostomy tube is inserted. The risk of significant long-term complications in those who have had some short-term problem remains unknown.

COMPLICATIONS OF ENDOPYELOTOMY

In recent years percutaneous management of ureteropelvic junction (UPJ) strictures has become a practical method of managing obstruction at the ureteropelvic junction.[14, 15] Most patients who are candidates for this procedure have had a previous failed pyeloplasty or have an unoperated "typical" UPJ obstruction.

Bleeding

There may be enough bleeding with the freshly dilated access tract to compromise vision and prevent an accurate incision at the UPJ. If so, a nephrostomy tube should be placed and the procedure continued 2 to 3 days later. Some bleeding at the site of incision is inevitable, but large amounts of blood should not result, unless the aberrant vessel which frequently passes adjacent to most UPJs is injured. Because the anatomical relation of these vessels to the UPJ is determined embryologically, damage can be avoided by making the incision laterally and posteriorly.[16]

Whether damage to these vessels requires exploration or management by arteriography depends on the clinical situation.

Extravasation

Some extravasation is desirable as an indication that the incision has gone completely through the ureter and pelvis. Excessive operating time spent after this point in the procedure could result in undesirable levels of extravasated fluid. This problem will be uncommon if the quantity of irrigating fluid is routinely compared with the suction output as noted above.

Long-Term Complication

There is not enough experience with this procedure to know if any specific long-term problems will occur. Except for the risk that the procedure might fail to produce the desired result, there would seem to be no reason to suspect that long-term problems would be any different from those attendant on any other percutaneous procedure.

The risk of recurrent stricture is about 10% to 20%, and is probably minimized by the use of stents for 6 to 8 weeks postprocedure.[17, 18]

COMPLICATIONS OF ENDOSCOPY OF THE UPPER URINARY TRACT

Ureteroscopy

Considerable evolution has occurred in the technique of ureteroscopy in the last few years since a variety of instruments have become available for the routine direct endoscopic examination of the ureter and renal pelvis.[19, 20] This improvement in instrumentation has facilitated the whole procedure, increased the range of indications for ureteroscopy, and reduced the chance of complication. While the principles of endoscopic examination extant elsewhere in the urinary tract remain the same in the ureter, the size of these instruments relative to the small size of the ureter and the smaller margin for error given these geometric and anatomical facts all conspire such that ureteroscopy has a greater risk of complication than any other urologic endoscopic procedure.

Ureteroscopy may be regarded as a two-part procedure: (1) dilatation of the intramural ureter and manipulation of the ureteroscope to the area of interest, and (2) operative ureteroscopy. Ureteroscopy should always be performed under fluoroscopic control. Complications may occur at any point in the procedure and recognition of situations where the risk of complication is increased will help avoid problems. Also, the surgeon must learn to recognize defeat and accept that he may need to temporize and return another day to deal with the situation.

Complications Related to Access

Except when the smallest ureteroscopes are being used, the intramural ureter must be dilated to a size which will permit easy passage of the ureteroscope to the area of interest. We have preferred balloon dilatation for this purpose as it is rapid and effective and it traumatizes the anatomy only once instead of multiple times, as with the other kinds of dilators.

False Passage

The operator should be entirely certain of the anatomy and course of the ureter. Unusual tortuosity may be suspected on excretory urography and confirmed with immediate retrograde urography. Such tortuosity may compromise guide wire placement prior to dilatation and if there is any doubt that the placement of the wire is correct, dilatation should not proceed. In doubtful cases I will often use an 8.5F direct-vision ureteroscope without dilatation to identify the true lumen so that a guide wire may be accurately placed. Perforation of the ureteral wall by the wire is usually obvious on fluoroscopy, but a submucosal false passage of the wire may not be so apparent. On fluoroscopy, the wire appears as if it is passing in the course of the ureter, but the urologist will notice somewhat more resistance than normal as he passes the wire. Recognition that this has happened is important because if the ureteroscope is passed submucosally up to the kidney, destruction of the ureter may ensue. Submucosal ureteroscopy can also be suspected after inspection of the ureteral "mucosa" when the ureteroscope is in the distal ureter. This will reveal circular striations which resemble the prostatic capsule after transurethral prostatic resection (TURP). Gradual retreat with the ureteroscope will then identify the true channel and the operation can then proceed.

Occasionally, a stone is impacted in the intramural ureter such that a wire cannot bypass it despite efforts at manipulation. If perforation seems inevitable, the stone should be approached under direct vision with a small ureteroscope to identify the passage around the stone or to consider destruction in situ. A false passage per se is not a contraindication to ureteroscopy, as long as the true channel can be identified and the instrument manipulated easily into the channel (Fig 12–5). If there is any doubt whether the contemplated procedure is safe, a double-J stent should be left in place for a few days before the procedure is repeated.

Inadequate Dilatation

The intramural ureter should be dilated to a size such that the ureteroscope which is to be used may be accommodated. For example, if one anticipates that the 11.5F unit will be employed, dilatation should proceed to 15F or so. Inadequate dilatation commonly is revealed by a "waist" effect or narrow area revealed in the balloon by fluoroscopy (Fig 12–6).

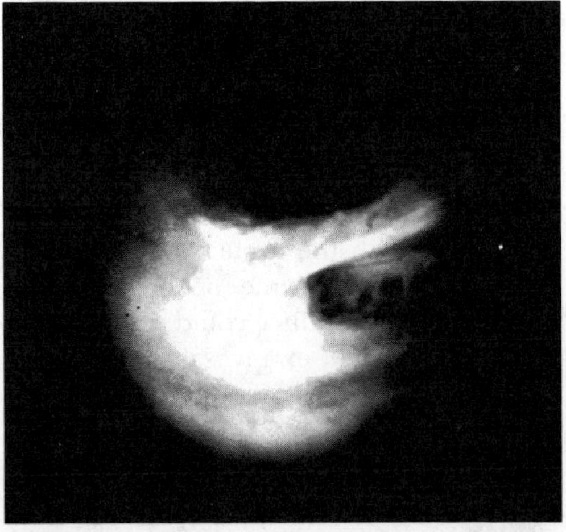

FIG 12–5.
A false passage in the left pelvic ureter. The location is at the 5-o'clock position, the usual position where catheters and guide wires inadvertently perforate.

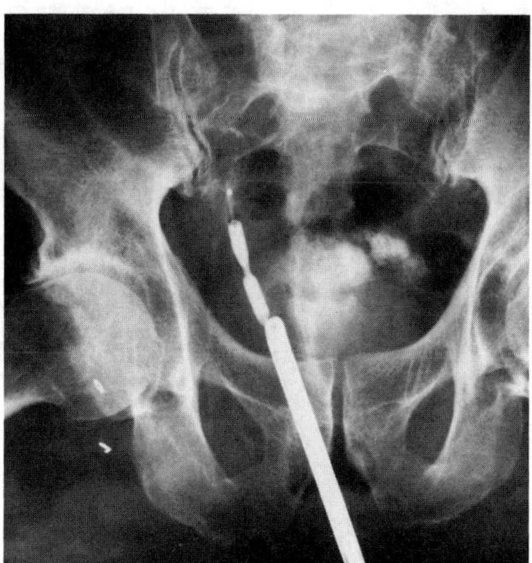

FIG 12–6.
Inadequate dilatation of the intramural ureter. A stronger balloon should be tried. If the "waist" does not disappear, the size of instrument that can be inserted will be limited.

The balloon should be changed so that greater pressures can be accommodated. Most ureters will yield to a 21-atm balloon, although occasionally the narrowing will persist. It is best not to try to force the area with the ureteroscope. A double-J stent left indwelling for a few days will often dilate the ureter such that ureteroscopy is then possible.

Passage of the instrument up to the area of interest may be compromised by several factors. First, the ureter may simply be too small for the chosen instrument. Usually, this is obvious because the ureter seems to "grip" the instrument and the ureter appears to telescope ahead in the visual field. Attempts to force the instrument can result in ureteral avulsion. The problem can be avoided by switching to a smaller instrument or, if a shorter segment of ureter seems to be the problem, by balloon-dilating the segment.

The normal course of the ureter describes several curves which must straighten out for successful rigid ureteroscopy. Postoperative scar tissue may prevent the mobility of the ureter necessary to permit passage of the ureteroscope. Also, the smaller instruments are less rigid and may bend to the point that the operator cannot see the lumen.

Perforation by a large ureteroscope in the process of passage, or at any other time during the procedure, will usually produce a hole large enough that the operation should be stopped. The main reason for stopping is that further manipulation may cause the hole to get worse and become a tear. Insertion of a double-J stent for several days will cause the hole to seal and permit further manipulation. If the operator is unable to get a stent past the hole from below, then a stent should be placed percutaneously. If this is not done, a urinoma will likely form.

Complications Related to Ureteroscopic Surgery

Operative complications are a function of the particular procedure, although certain problems, such as the risk of perforation, attend all procedures.

Ureteral and Renal Stones

The most vexing complications happen in managing stones: small stones may be washed up to the renal pelvis by the irrigating fluid, thereby converting an easy case into a difficult one. Limiting the force of irrigating fluid will minimize this problem; also, passage of a basket beyond the stone may entrap it before it escapes. A stone that is fixed in the ureter should be loosened before attempting to engage it with the basket because of the risk of perforation. Power lithotripsy will accomplish this and will also break into pieces small enough to manipulate a stone too big to basket. Small fragments of stone are occasionally pushed through the ureteral wall. These are significant only in that they may cause confusion on plain films in the future. Attempts to retrieve the stones are unnecessary and only serve to make the hole larger.[21, 22]

Some complications may be related to the method of lithotripsy employed. The most common problem we have observed with the ultrasonic probe is inadvertent perforation of the ureter in the edematous tissues adjacent to a stone. The electrohydraulic probe, particularly the new small 3F and 2F probes, can easily be used under direct vision and are safe. Still, firing the probes adjacent to the ureteral wall will damage the ureter and can easily result in perforation. Laser lithotripsy involves no particular unusual risk. Perforation with the fiber is quite common and not important.

Ureteroscopic Ureterostomy

Perforation is a routine consequence of this operation and becomes a complication only if the anatomy is such that the ureteral lumen above the point of incision cannot be accessed for stent insertion. Also, bleeding may totally obscure the visual field, effectively ending the procedure. Such endoscopic surgery is best performed with a reserve guide wire in place to ensure adequate stent placement.

Ureteral Tumors

Biopsy of suspicious lesions on the ureteral mucosa has become a standard procedure. Such biopsies should be conservative owing to the chance that a perforation may result in spillage of tumor cells into the retroperitoneum. Careful fulguration of such lesions appears to be safe in the short term, but the risk of subsequent stricture at the site of fulguration remains unknown.[23]

Complications Related to Renoscopy

The rigid ureteroscope can be inserted as far as the renal pelvis in about two thirds of patients. In many patients, flexible renoscopy is possible. Except for the risk of perforation at the time of access, there are no particular risks associated with inspection of the collecting system per se. Most of the endoscopic surgical options possible in the ureter are also, at least theoretically, practical in the kidney, but are usually limited by shortcomings of the rigid instruments.

The greatest possible problem of renoscopy is that one might not be able to reinsert the instrument back into the renal pelvis. In other words, if the instrument must be removed for whatever reason, one runs the risk of leaving the job only half done, because the instrument cannot be maneuvered back into the pelvis of the kidney.

Post-ureteroscopic Complications

Blute et al.[21] reviewed the complications that we identified in 346 patients who underwent ureteroscopy. The most common problem was a postoperative fever of greater than 38°C, despite the fact that nearly all patients were receiving perioperative anibiotics. Sepsis was uncommon, occurring in only one patient (Fig 12–7).

We routinely leave a stent in place for 48 hours afterward and believe that the stent has kept the risk of immediate postoperative obstruction to a minimum. Many patients will experience pain or colic after stent removal owing to passage of clots and an occasional small residual stone fragment.

Long-Term Complications

The incidence of long-term postoperative complications is unknown. Only a handful of patients have had ureteral strictures identified, although not every patient has had a postoperative urogram.

Clayman[24] noted an incidence of reflux of 14% in a group of patients dilated to 24F. The incidence in patients dilated to the more usual 16F to 18F is not known, but clinically has not appeared to be a problem. Lyon[25] has followed a small group of patients with upper tract tumors who have had multiple ureteroscopies for surveillance and has noted no strictures

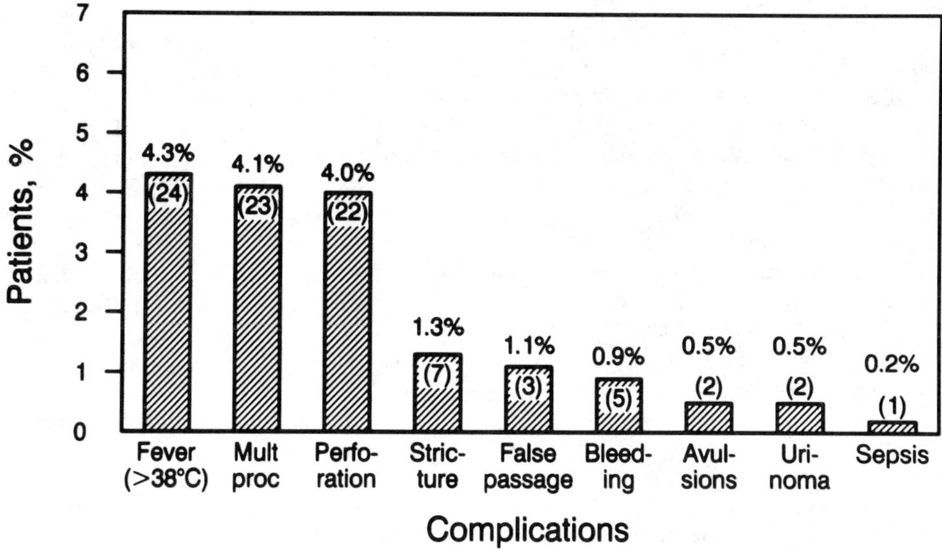

FIG 12–7.
Complications of ureteroscopy in 89 patients. Those with temperature greater than 38° C were not in frank sepsis.

or reflux. The "controlled trauma" that ureteroscopy inflicts upon the ureter may actually be less damaging than that resulting from the blind basketing we did routinely prior to the era of ureteroscopy.

EDITORIAL COMMENT

This chapter on the complications of percutaneous stone removal reflects the extensive experience of the author. We have performed several hundred percutaneous procedures and our incidence of bleeding may be slightly higher. It is surprising there is not a somewhat higher incidence of postoperative traumatic ureteropelvic junction obstruction. This complication does not appear to be common. We have already seen more problems following ureteroscopy with ureteral perforation or ureteral obstruction than with percutaneous renal manipulation.

We have also investigated x-ray exposure to both the patient and personnel. In general, the x-ray exposure to personnel has been in the millirad range and well within the acceptable guidelines for medical personnel. All our procedures have been done with an x-ray beam originating under the patient or with a C-arm in the operating room, which has an under-the-table beam. If an above-the-table radiographic machine is used, x-ray exposure is far greater. If there is careful attention to detail, it is apparent that percutaneous stone manipulation can be done with a low morbidity and mortality.

EDITORIAL COMMENT II

Ureteroscopy has greater potential for injury and complications than endoscopy of the urethra or bladder. If the ureteral injury or stricture is short, sometimes balloon dilatation of a stricture will suffice with stenting for a month. In other cases, if there is a longer stricture, additional surgical reconstruction may be necessary.*

*Chang R, Marshall FF: Management of ureteroscopic injuries. *J Urol* 1987; 137:1132.

REFERENCES

1. LeRoy AJ, May GR, Bender CE, et al: Percutaneous nephrostomy for stone removal. *Radiology* 1984; 151:607.
2. White EC, Smith AD: Percutaneous stone extraction from 200 patients. *J Urol* 1984; 132:437.
3. LeRoy AJ, Williams HJ Jr, Bender CE, et al: Colon perforation following percutaneous nephrostomy and renal calculus removal. *Radiology* 1985; 155:83.
4. Neustein P, Barbaric ZL, Kaufman J: Nephrocolic fistula: A complication of percutaneous nephrostolithotomy. *J Urol* (in press).
5. Lange P: Personal communication.
6. Clayman RV, Surya V, Miller RP, et al: Percutaneous nephrolithotomy: Extraction of renal and ureteral calculi from 100 patients. *J Urol* 1984; 131:868.
7. Patterson DE, Segura JW, LeRoy AJ, et al: The etiology and treatment of delayed bleeding following percutaneous lithotripsy. *J Urol* 1985; 133:447.
8. Marberger M: Personal communication.
9. Schultz RE, Hanno PM, Wein AJ, et al: Percutaneous ultrasonic lithotripsy: Choice of irrigant. *J Urol* 1983; 130:858.
10. Carson CC, Nesbitt JA: Peritoneal extravasation during percutaneous lithotripsy. *J Urol* (in press).
11. Marberger M, Staekel W, Hruby W, et al: Late sequela of ultrasonic lithotripsy of renal calculi. *Urology* 1984; 133:170–173.
12. Segura JW, Patterson DE, LeRoy AJ, et al: Percutaneous removal of kidney stones: Review of 1,000 Cases. *J Urol* 1985; 134:1077.
13. Segura JW, Patterson DE, Leroy AJ, et al: Percutaneous removal of kidney and ureteral stones (abstract 579). *J Urol* 1984; 131:248.
14. King LR, Coughlin PW, Ford KK, et al: Initial experience with percutaneous and transureteral ablation of postoperative ureteral strictures in children. *J Urol* 1984; 131:1167.
15. Karlin GS, Badlani GH, Smith AD: Endopyelotomy versus open pyeloplasty: comparison in 88 patients. *J Urol* 1988; 140:476.
16. Badlani GH, Karlin G, Smith AD: Complications of endopyelotomy. *J Urol* 1988; 146:473.
17. Badlani GH, Smith AD: Stent for endopyelotomy. *Urol Clin North Am* 1988; 15:445.
18. Amer M, Abdel H: Endopyelotomy for ureteropelvic junction obstruction—Is long-term stenting mandatory? *J Endourol* 1987; 1:265.
19. Pérez-Castro Ellendt E, Martínez-Pinẽiro JA: Transurethral ureteroscopy: a current urological procedure. *Arch Esp Urol* 1980; 33:445.
20. Huffman JL, Bagley DH, Lyon ES: Treatment of distal ureteral calculi using rigid ureteroscope. *Urology* 1982; 20:574.
21. Blute ML, Segura JW, Patterson DE: Ureteroscopy. *J Urol* 1988; 139:510.
22. Lingeman JE, Sonda LP, Kahnoski RJ, et al: Ureteral stone management: Emerging concepts. *J Urol* 1986; 135:1172.
23. Huffman JL, Bagley DH, Lyon ES: Endoscopic diagnosis and treatment of upper-tract urothelial tumors. A preliminary report. *Cancer* 1985; 55:1422.
24. Clayman RV: Personal communication.
25. Lyon ES: Personal communication.

CHAPTER 13

Complications of Shock Wave Lithotripsy

Joseph W. Segura, M.D.

Extracorporeal shock wave lithotripsy (ESWL) has become one of the most common procedures urologists perform. This widespread experience has also established that it is also one of the safest procedures, at least in the short term. The American Urological Association Lithotripsy Committee surveyed a number of centers 3 years ago asking for reports of complications.[1] The rate of complications reported was quite small, considerably less than 1.0%, and many of these were the same cardiovascular problems found after other procedures. This relative safety and ease of use should not blind the urologist to the fact that complications can occur and that some of them may be avoidable.

Most procedures performed to date in this country have been with the Dornier HM-3. It remains to be seen whether or not the complications of shock wave lithotripsy will vary significantly from machine to machine.

COMPLICATIONS RELATED TO STONE FRACTURE

Inadequate breakup is probably the most common complication of ESWL. Plain films taken after the procedure may reveal a residual fragment which is obviously too large to pass, or a large piece may have already dropped down into the ureter with resulting pain and obstruction. Recognition that cystine stones are unlikely to fracture completely and that large stones, particularly those made of calcium oxalate monohydrate, will not break up easily with only one treatment, will help keep the problems generated by such fragments from reaching the level of complications. Preliminary insertion of stents will often keep these large fragments out of the ureteropelvic junction (UPJ) and ureter.

Immediate Postoperative Complications

Hematoma.—A significant subcapsular hematoma will form in a small group of patients (approx. 0.5%) (Fig 13–1). This complication may be suspected if the patient complains of an unusual amount of pain after the treatment or if there is a greater-than-usual drop in serum hemoglobin. The diagnosis is confirmed by ultrasound examination or, preferably, computed tomography (CT) scan. No treatment is usually necessary as these eventually resolve spontaneously. Bleeding requiring transfusion is rare. We saw one patient treated with ESWL elsewhere who had hemorrhaged into his collecting sys-

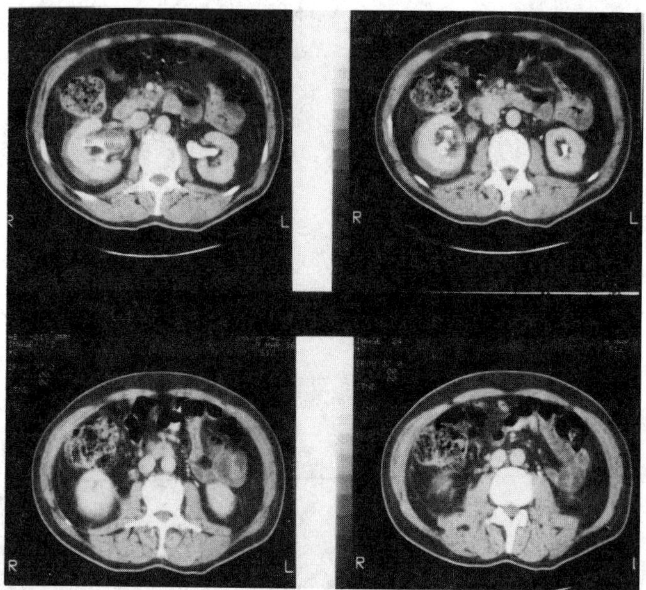

FIG 13–1.
Subcapsular hematoma of the right kidney noted 2 days after extracorporeal shock wave lithotripsy. The hematoma resolved spontaneously.

tem and required several units of blood.

He stopped bleeding spontaneously, and we later performed a percutaneous stone removal without difficulty. Magnetic resonance imaging studies have demonstrated a much higher incidence of small hematomas and interstitial bleeding, but the large majority of these have been without clinical significance.

Sepsis.—Extracorporeal shock wave lithotripsy in the presence of an uncontrolled urinary tract infection may result in sepsis. The risk is less if appropriate preoperative antibiotics are used, although such use may not prevent sepsis if a large-volume struvite stone is treated when adequate drainage is not provided, either by the percutaneous or ureteroscopic route.

Petechiae.—Petechiae are occasionally seen on the skin at the entry site of the shock wave and also sometimes at the exit point and are associated with a certain amount of cutaneous soft tissue swelling. These are most likely to be found in thin people. They disappear readily, and are of little significance.

Posttreatment Complications

Pain.—Ten percent of patients will have significant colic which will require narcotics and usually hospitalization. While this is more common during the immediate posttreatment period, colic may start days later as a stone begins to make its way down the ureter. Such colic occurs with a fragment of any size but is more common with larger fragments. If the fragment is 5.0 mm or greater, spontaneous passage is unlikely and the fragment should be removed ureteroscopically or possibly re-treated with ESWL.

Some patients may have ureteral obstruction and a nonfunctioning kidney secondary to stone fragments in the ureter. Intravenous pyelography (IVP) should be performed if a postprocedure kidney-ureter-bladder (KUB) follow-up at 1 month shows fragments in the course of the ureter. Unfortunately, many patients have the idea that once they are treated with the machine, their problems are over. Every effort should be made to emphasize the importance of follow-up care.

After treatment, many patients complain of flank pain, which they describe as a severe ache. This pain usually disappears after a few days, although a number of patients complain that the ache persists for months after treatment.

Steinstrasse.—The quantity of broken-up fragments may be such as to exceed the capacity of the ureter to pass expeditiously. The fragments collect in the ureter and form a column of stone referred to as a "steinstrasse" or "stone street" (Fig 13–2). Surprisingly, many patients who have such large quantities of stone have little pain, although others may be markedly symptomatic. While many steinstrassen will pass spontaneously, many will not, and it is my feeling that all of these should be removed when diagnosed. This is easily done ureteroscopically by loosening the distal portion of the stony column. It should not be necessary to insert a guide wire or dilate the orifice. Ordinarily, the ureteroscope may be inserted directly into the orifice. There is often a "keystone," which when displaced will be followed by a rush of smaller particles.

This problem can be avoided by placing a stent before lithotripsy in patients with large stones. This will prevent the formation of a steinstrasse, although it will not increase the stone-free rate and will itself cause significant discomfort. One may also avoid this complication by treating large stones percutaneously, a course of action we have found preferable.

Compromises of Renal Function.—It has been known that renal function in the treated kidney will decrease after treatment but will return to normal after 2 to 3 months. Thomas[2] has recently shown that bilateral lithotripsy will cause permanent suppression of renal plasma flow. Studies by Williams et al.[3] demonstrate decreased renal plasma flow to the treated area of the kidney. The long-term significance of these findings is uncertain, but it would seem prudent to avoid concurrent bilateral lithotripsy.

Long-Term Complications

This topic is an area of considerable interest at the present time, fueled largely by worries concerning whether or not hypertension might result from shock wave lithotripsy. It is fair to state that as of this writing, there is no evidence that this is a major problem, at least in a time frame of a few years after treatment. A careful retrospective study by Lingeman and colleagues[4] has demonstrated no general increase in the incidence of hypertension in nearly 1,000 patients. A statistically significant increase in diastolic blood pressure of 0.78 mm Hg at 1 year was documented, however. At the present time, the risk of hypertension after ESWL does not seem great, but a final opinion must await longer follow-up of treated patients.

Stone Recurrence Rate

There are some data to suggest that the rate of new stone formation and the size of preexisting stones may be increased after ESWL. Lingeman et al.[5] reported a rate of 22% in a group of post-ESWL patients followed for 2 years, a rate about double what one would expect and about double what has been reported after percutaneous lithotripsy.[6] Whether this is in fact related to ESWL is not known.

SUMMARY

There have been few short-term problems and complications related to shock

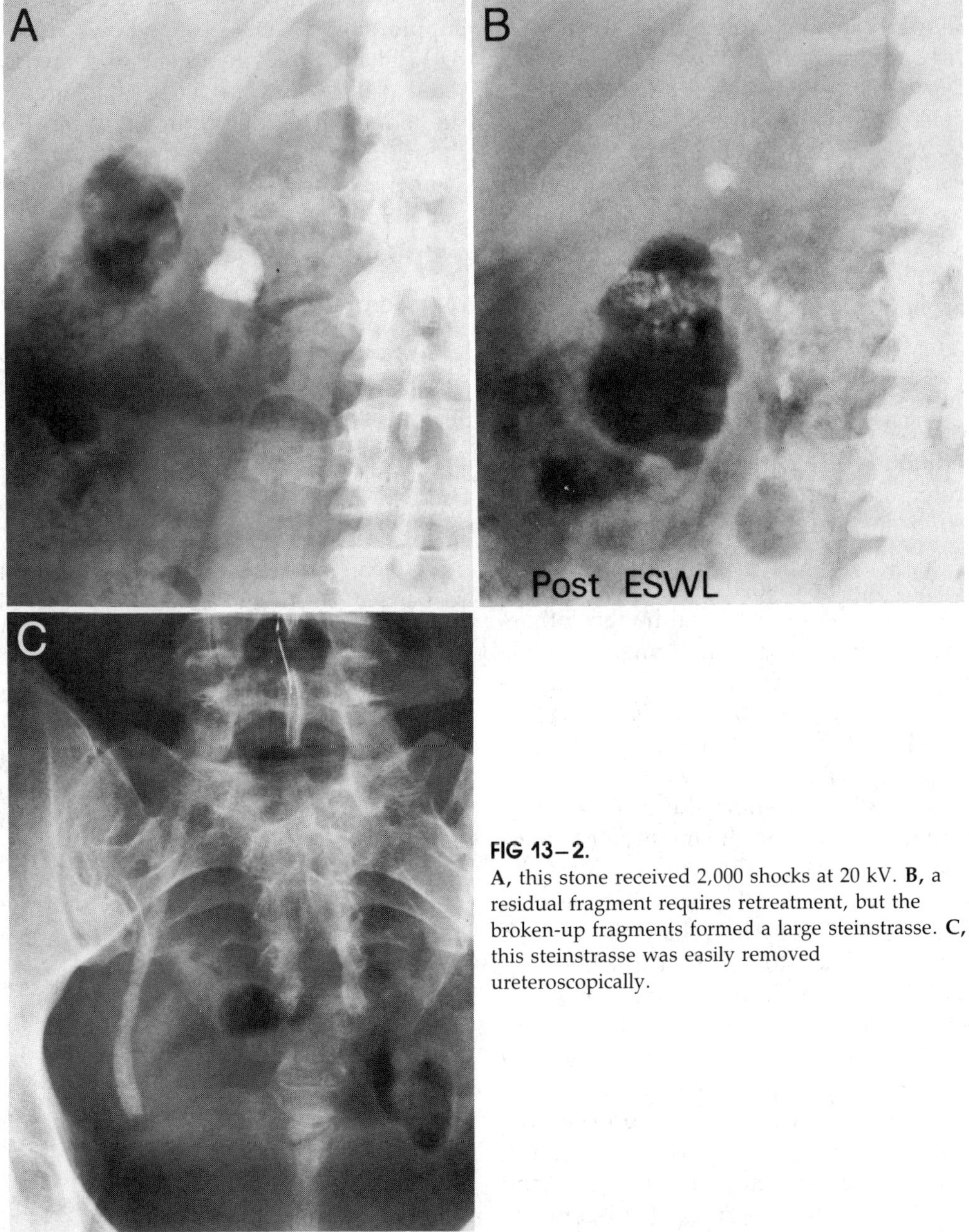

FIG 13–2.
A, this stone received 2,000 shocks at 20 kV. **B,** a residual fragment requires retreatment, but the broken-up fragments formed a large steinstrasse. **C,** this steinstrasse was easily removed ureteroscopically.

wave lithotripsy except for problems concerned with incomplete breakup of stones and the need for re-treatment of patients who have pain associated with the passage of fragments.

It should be remembered that ESWL has only been performed in large numbers of patients for a little over 5 years and that a precise definition of long-term risk at this point cannot be expected.

EDITORIAL COMMENT

Shock wave lithotripsy has revolutionized the management of the stone patient. Not only has it been very effective therapy, it has also been a very safe procedure. It should be added that calcifications in the area of the kidney, either vascular or pancreatic, should be viewed with caution. Pancreatitis has been reported and I did not perform ESWL on one patient with renal calculi because of extensive pancreatic calcification.

REFERENCES

1. Report of American Urological Association Ad Hoc Committee to Study the Safety and Clinical Efficacy of Current Technology of Percutaneous Lithotripsy and Noninvasive Lithotripsy, May, 1987.
2. Thomas A: Personal communication.
3. Williams CM, Kaude JV, Newman RC, et al: Extracorporeal shock-wave lithotripsy: Long-term complications. *AJR* 1988; 150:311–315.
4. Lingeman JE, Kulb TB: Hypertension following extracorporeal shock-wave lithotripsy (abstract). *J Urol* 1987; 137:142A.
5. Lingeman JE, McAteer JA, Kempson SA, et al: Bioeffects of extracorporeal shock-wave lithotripsy. *Urol Clin North Am* 1988; 8.
6. Knoll LD, Segura JW, Patterson DE, et al: Long-term followup in patients with cystine urinary calculi treated by percutaneous ultrasonic lithotripsy. *J Urol* 1988; 140:246–248.

CHAPTER 14

Complications of Renal Vascular Surgery and Percutaneous Transluminal Angioplasty

Andrew C. Novick, M.D.

Renal arterial occlusive disease is most often due to atherosclerosis or one of the fibrous dysplasias. Intervention for these disorders is indicated either in the presence of severe associated hypertension or when renal function is threatened by progressive vascular disease.[1] Renal artery aneurysms are relatively uncommon but may require treatment when they are the cause of significant hypertension or to obviate the risk of rupture associated with certain clinical features.[2] Other rare renal vascular lesions include an arteriovenous fistula, renal artery thrombosis or embolism, neurofibromatosis, and the middle aortic syndrome.[1] The diagnosis of these conditions is also characteristically made during an evaluation for hypertension.

There are currently two forms of nonmedical or intervention therapy for patients with renal artery disease, namely surgery and percutaneous transluminal angioplasty (PTA). Surgical treatment generally comprises renal vascular reconstruction, and the long-term efficacy of this approach is well established. Percutaneous transluminal angioplasty is a newer method that has yielded promising early results, particularly in patients with fibrous dysplasia. In this chapter, the various complications of renal vascular surgery and PTA are reviewed with emphasis on etiologic factors and appropriate management.

RENAL VASCULAR SURGERY

Currently, renal vascular reconstruction is possible in most patients with renal artery disease who require surgical treatment, and total or partial nephrectomy is infrequently performed. (Complications of the latter operations are reviewed in another chapter of this book and will not be dealt with here.) Of the various available revascularization techniques, aortorenal bypass with an autogenous or synthetic vascular graft is the preferred approach in most centers.[3–6] Transrenal endarterectomy, which was formerly a popular method for atherosclerotic lesions, has now largely been abandoned. In patients with severe aortic disease that precludes safe performance of an aortorenal bypass, alternate techniques are currently employed, such as hepatorenal bypass,[7,8] splenorenal bypass,[9,10] iliorenal bypass,[11] or mesenterorenal bypass.[12] In patients with complex branch renal artery disease, extracorporeal microvascular reconstruction and autotransplantation are indicated.[13] There are several previous publications which describe the performance of each of these operations in detail.

All renal revascularization operations are performed transabdominally, through either a bilateral subcostal or midline incision. As such, general complications associated with any type of major intraabdominal surgery can develop postoperatively. These include wound infection, atelectasis, pneumonia, paralytic ileus, mechanical bowel obstruction, pulmonary embolism, myocardial infarction, or cerebrovascular accident. Complications that relate specifically to the performance of renal vascular surgery are outlined below.

Hypertension

Patients undergoing renal revascularization often experience hypertension postoperatively, even with a technically satisfactory vascular repair. This hypertension may be due to hypervolemia, vasoconstriction from total body hypothermia, poorly controlled incisional pain, or renal ischemia sustained intraoperatively. Such blood pressure elevation may be quite severe immediately after surgery and, if not properly controlled, can promote hemorrhage from the fresh vascular anastomoses. Therefore, these patients are initially placed in an intensive care unit for monitoring the central venous pressure, blood pressure, urine output, pulse rate, and serum levels of hemoglobin and creatinine. During this time, the diastolic blood pressure is maintained at 90 to 100 mm Hg to ensure satisfactory renal perfusion. We prefer to manage postoperative hypertension with a continuous intravenous infusion of sodium nitroprusside for the first 24 to 36 hours. At this time, if hypertension persists, maintenance therapy with agents such as methyldopa and/or hydralazine (Apresoline) is initiated, and the nitroprusside infusion is gradually discontinued.

Approximately 50% of patients who are ultimately cured of hypertension by renal revascularization will experience blood pressure elevation for a period of time postoperatively. In fact, it is not uncommon for such hypertension to persist for several weeks following surgery before gradually resolving. Of course, when this occurs, patency of the reconstructed renal artery must be confirmed with isotope renography and/or digital subtraction angiography.[14]

Hemorrhage

Early hemorrhage following renal revascularization is generally a consequence of poor surgical technique. Bleeding from a vascular anastomotic site can occur if this is under tension, if one or both of the anastomosed vessels are diseased, or if the vascular sutures have not been placed sufficiently close together. Eversion of intima through the anastomosis may also predispose to hemorrhage and should be avoided.

Early hemorrhage may also be due to poor surgical hemostasis. This complication is most likely to occur because of unsecured collateral vessels in the renal hilum, because of damage to the left adrenal gland, which is often closely apposed to the left renal artery, or because of inadequately secured lumbar arteries that have been divided during aortic mobilization. When a saphenous vein bypass graft has been used, bleeding can occur from avulsion of a ligature applied to one of the branches of the vein graft; this can be avoided by suture ligation of all such branches.

Factors that predispose to early postoperative hemorrhage include incomplete reversal of systemic heparinization, an episode of hypertension, or unrecognized coagulopathy. Mild bleeding that ceases spontaneously in an asymptomatic patient does not require reoperation. Such small hematomas generally undergo complete reabsorption without sequelae, although, occasionally, extrinsic cicatrical stenosis of the repaired renal artery may result. With severe or uncontrolled bleeding, immediate reoperation is indicated to evacuate the accumulated blood and secure hemostasis.

In unusual cases, late hemorrhage can occur weeks, months, or even years following renal revascularization. This may be due to infection involving the vascular suture line,[15, 16] rupture of a noninfected false aneurysm at the anastomotic site into the retroperitoneum or gastrointestinal tract,[17] or erosion of a prosthetic bypass graft into the duodenum.[18] All present as sudden catastrophic hemorrhage that requires immediate operation. Prosthetic graft erosion can be avoided at the original operation by interposing peritoneum or omentum between such grafts and the duodenum or by placing the graft retrocaval on the right side. It is also appropriate to state that prosthetic renal artery bypass grafts should be used only when an autogenous vascular graft is not available.

Renal Artery Thrombosis

Thrombosis of the repaired renal artery is an uncommon complication that occurs in less than 5% of patients undergoing revascularization, generally within the first few days of surgery. Postoperative hypotension, a hypercoagulable state, and hypovolemia are factors that predispose to this problem. Significant intrarenal arteriolar nephrosclerosis causes poor run-off, which can also lead to arterial thrombosis, particularly with synthetic Dacron grafts.[19] Nevertheless, arterial thrombosis is usually due to poor technical performance of revascularization and, in this regard, several points deserve emphasis.

All of the vessels used for anastomosis should be free of disease that may cause subsequent occlusion. Complete excision of all renal artery disease is necessary. Occasionally, a local aortic endarterectomy is performed when an aortorenal bypass is done. All vascular anastomoses must be done precisely, to avoid intraluminal intrusion of adventitia and trauma to the intima. The latter may result from improperly applied surgical forceps or vascular clamps and is known to promote intraluminal platelet aggregation, fibrin deposition, and the development of a thrombus. When an endarterectomy is done, the resulting traumatized arterial surface can also predispose to thrombus formation.

If an intimal flap is present in the distal renal artery at revascularization, this must be tacked down with interrupted sutures to avoid intramural dissection and occlusion following restoration of blood flow. End-to-end anastomosis of vessels that are more than 50% disparate in diameter should also be avoided. This invariably leads to bunching of the smaller vessel and unfavorable hemodynamics that can eventuate in thrombus formation and vascular occlusion.

When performing a renal artery bypass procedure, the bypass graft must be properly placed to avoid angulation, kinking, or malalignment with the renal artery. Figures 14–1 and 14–2 illustrate the most common errors in the positioning of an aortorenal bypass graft that can lead to thrombosis or stenosis. These same considerations apply to all renal revascularization operations, especially extracorporeal branch repairs. In the last-named, multiple renal arterial branch anastomoses are commonly done, and it is important to anticipate the position that the various branches will assume in relation to one another upon completion of the repair and following autotransplantation.

Embolization of an atheroma from a

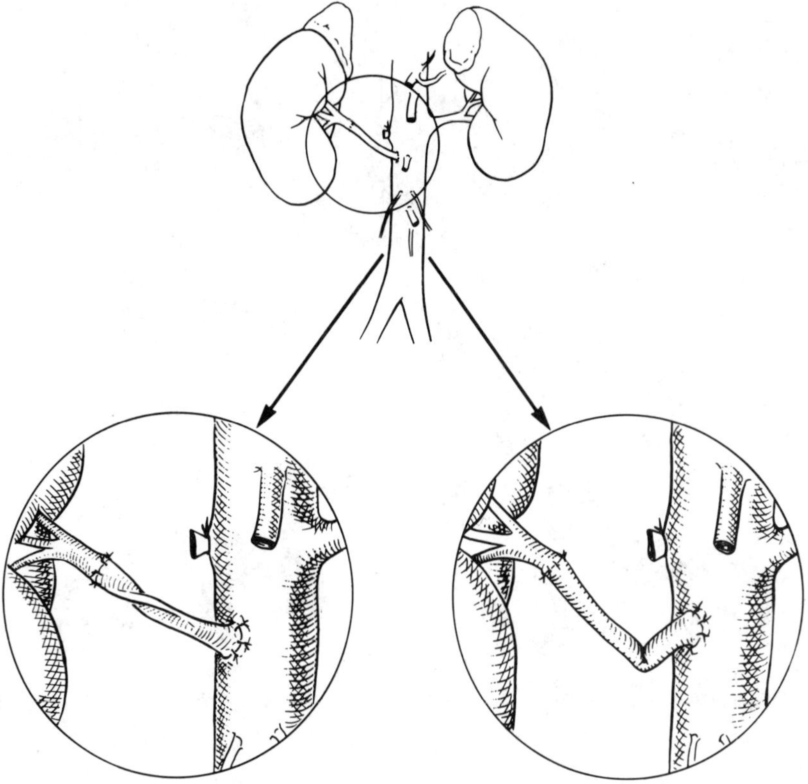

FIG 14–1.
Sketch illustrating improper placement of an aortorenal bypass graft with longitudinal torsion *(left)* or angulation *(right)* that can lead to postoperative thrombosis or stenosis.

traumatized aorta into the kidney and external compression of the repaired renal artery by a retroperitoneal fluid collection are additional causes of postoperative thrombosis. Finally, although thrombosis is typically an early event, occlusion of an aortorenal bypass graft can occur months or years later from progressive aortic atherosclerosis at the origin of the graft.

The diagnosis of renal artery thrombosis must be established almost immediately in order for salvage of the kidney to be possible. In some cases, a subtotally occlusive thrombus and/or extensive collateral renal arterial supply allow additional time to undertake successful intervention. The most helpful clinical clues to postoperative thrombosis are persistent or sudden hypertension and an elevated serum creatinine level. However, both of these findings may initially be present with a patent vascular repair. Therefore, a radiographic renal imaging study should be routinely done within the first 24 hours of surgery, and, in this regard, we have found isotope renography with technetium to be an excellent noninvasive method. Since we always perform direct end-to-end anastomosis of the bypass graft to the distal renal artery, renal uptake of isotope assures patency of the vascular repair. This study is less reliable if an end-to-side anastomosis of the bypass graft to the distal renal artery has been done. If isotope renographic findings are equivocal and/or clinical suspicion for arterial thrombosis remains high, then angiography should be done immediately.

The traditional treatment for postoperative renal arterial thrombosis has been emergency surgical reexploration with thrombectomy and/or graft revision if the

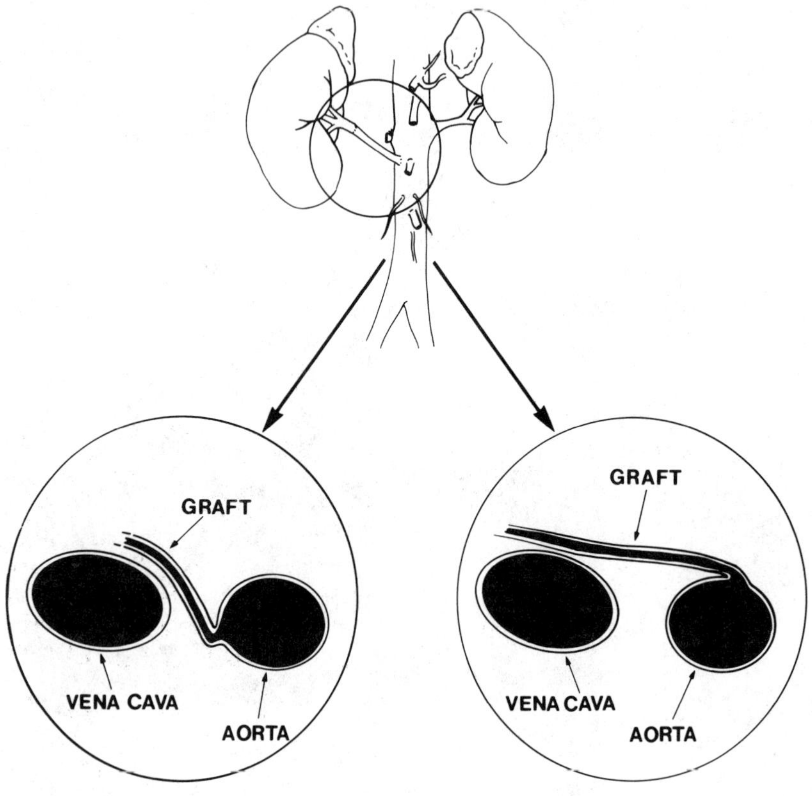

FIG 14–2.
In performing aortorenal bypass, it is important for the graft to be brought off the anterolateral aspect of the aorta. If the graft originates too far posteriorly *(left)* or anteriorly *(right)*, this can predispose to postoperative thrombosis or stenosis at the origin of the graft.

kidney is found to be viable. More commonly, the kidney is no longer viable, in which case a nephrectomy is done. Percutaneous low-dose intraarterial infusion of streptokinase is a new method that may be undertaken as an alternative to surgery.[20–22] Although successful clot lysis has been reported with this technique, there also appears to be an increased risk of bleeding from hypofibrinogenemia. Percutaneous transcatheter thrombectomy has also been described as treatment for acute renal artery thrombosis or embolism; however, this technique cannot be safely done in the presence of a fresh vascular anastomosis.[23] Systemic anticoagulation with heparin is not effective as primary therapy for postoperative arterial thrombosis but is a useful adjunctive measure following surgical thrombectomy or intraarterial streptokinase infusion.

Renal Artery Stenosis

The incidence of stenosis of a surgically reconstructed renal artery is less than 10% with current techniques, and this complication typically occurs weeks, months, or even years following revascularization.[1] Many of the causes are similar to those outlined for postoperative thrombosis, such as faulty suture technique, intimal trauma, incomplete excision of primary vascular disease, wide disparity in vessel size, dissection of a distal intimal flap created at surgery, and torsion, angulation, or kinking of the vessels. When performing an end-to-end vascular anastomosis, the likelihood of subsequent stenosis can be minimized by spatulating the ends of the two vessels to fashion a suture line that is wider than the normal circumference of the renal artery. Tension on the vascular suture line can also cause narrowing in this area and should be avoided. Finally, during procurement of a saphenous vein graft, care should be taken not to overdistend the vein or injudiciously dissect periadventitial tissue, both of which may cause devascularization of the graft that leads to subsequent stenosis.

Other causes of late postoperative renal artery stenosis include diffuse subendothelial fibroplastic proliferation in saphenous vein grafts, neointimal proliferation at the suture line of synthetic grafts, recurrent primary vascular disease, and obstruction from a valve in a segment of saphenous vein.[6] Concerning the last, these grafts should always be reversed so that blood flow is directed toward the cephalic end, which allows venous valves to assume a neutral position. However, even when this is done, such valves may undergo fibrotic contracture to produce a weblike stenosis of the vein graft (Fig 14–3). This occurrence, although rare, suggests that a valveless segment of vein should be used, if possible.

All patients undergoing renal revascularization should be followed at yearly intervals with blood pressure measurements, determination of renal function, and isotope renography with technetium. Postoperative renal artery stenosis that is more than 70% occlusive is invariably accompanied by an elevation in the blood pressure and, not uncommonly, evidence of deteriorating renal function. When either of these conditions is present, or if there is isotope renographic evidence of

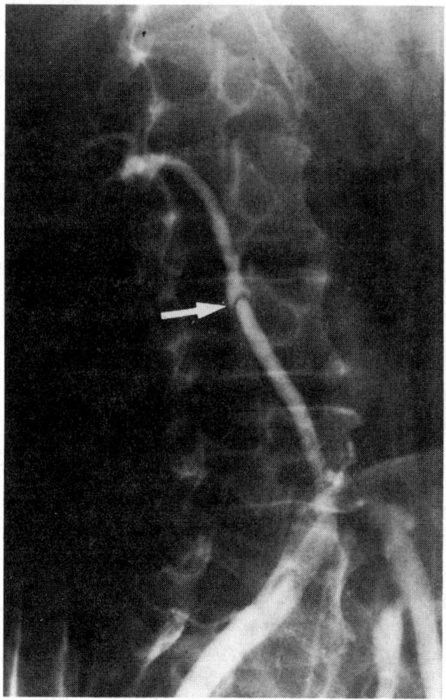

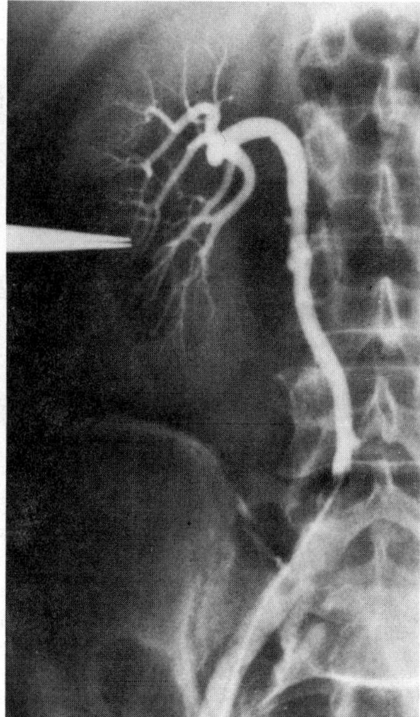

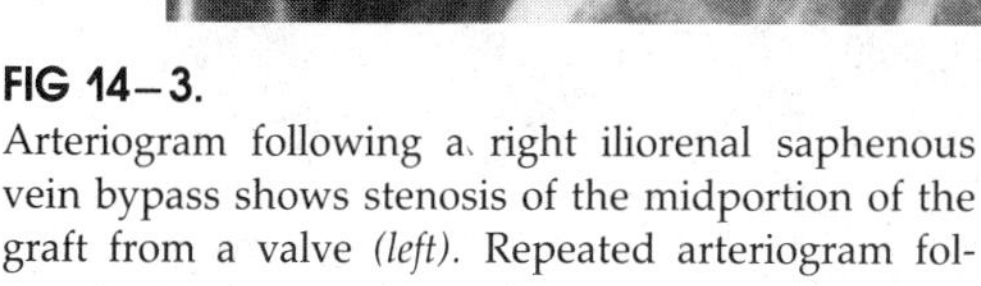

FIG 14–3.
Arteriogram following a right iliorenal saphenous vein bypass shows stenosis of the midportion of the graft from a valve *(left)*. Repeated arteriogram following percutaneous transluminal dilatation of the stenotic area shows improved blood flow through the graft *(right)*.

diminished renal perfusion, digital subtraction or conventional angiography should be done. Recurrent arterial stenosis is most often located at a vascular suture line (Fig 14–4) but may present anywhere along the course of the reconstructed renal arterial supply (Fig 14–5). The therapeutic options are surgical reoperation or PTA. Since secondary revascularization in such cases is quite difficult and may eventuate in nephrectomy, PTA is a reasonable initial approach to therapy, if it is technically feasible.

Renal Artery Aneurysm

Long-term angiographic studies of patients who have undergone aortorenal saphenous vein bypass have revealed graft dilatation in 25% to 52% of patients and frank aneurysm formation in 5% to 8% of patients.[24, 25] These findings have been observed more often in children than in adults. The clinical significance of these abnormal-appearing vein grafts remains uncertain, since most of these patients continue to be normotensive with excellent renal function. In some cases, graft dilatation has been associated with a distal anastomotic stenosis, suggesting the latter as a possible inciting factor (Fig 14–6). However, in other cases, similar dilatation has been found with no evidence of stenosis (Fig 14–7). This problem has only rarely been encountered with autogenous arterial grafts. It may be possible to prevent saphenous vein graft dilatation by more careful procurement and storage of the graft in chilled heparinized Ringer's lactate or autologous blood

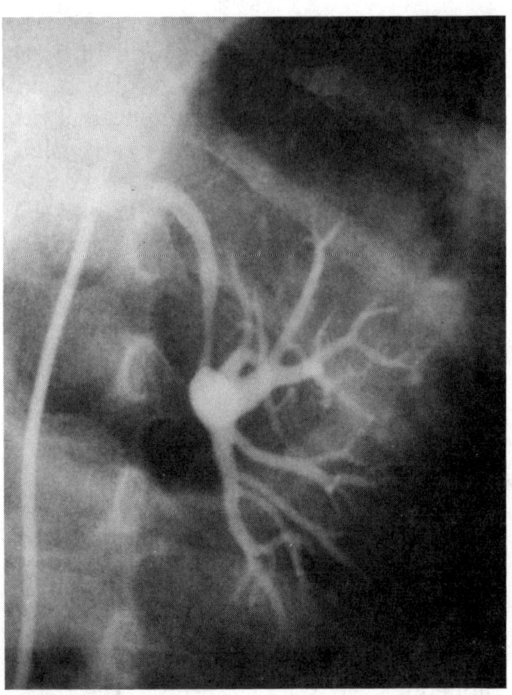

FIG 14–5.
Postoperative selective celiac arteriogram after splenorenal bypass shows a long stenotic segment of the splenic artery proximal to the anastomosis with the left renal artery. (From Novick AC, Banowsky LH, Stewart BH, et al: *Surg Gynecol Obstet* 1977; 144:891. Used by permission.)

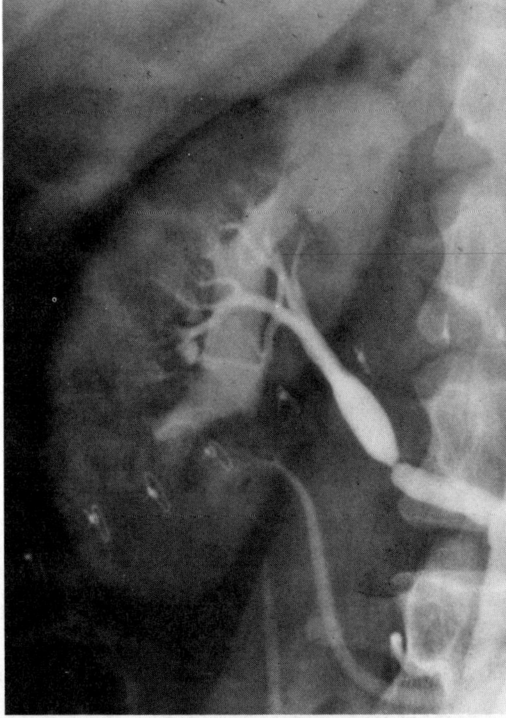

FIG 14–4.
Selective right renal arteriogram following an aortorenal bypass operation demonstrates high-grade stenosis at the distal anastomosis of the graft to the renal artery. (From Novick AC: *AUA Update Series,* lesson 40, vol 2, 1983. Used by permission.)

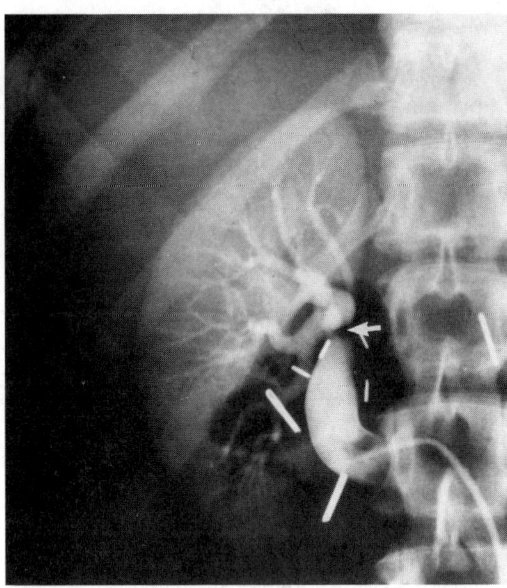

FIG 14–6.
Right renal arteriogram following aortorenal saphenous vein bypass demonstrates dilatation of the graft with a distal anastomotic stenosis *(arrow)*. (From Jordan ML, Novick AC, et al: *J Vasc Surg* 1985; 2:385. Used by permission.)

to prevent transmural ischemia. When severe aneurysmal dilatation is present, or if graft expansion is associated with recurrent hypertension, reoperation and attempted secondary revascularization are indicated.

Postoperative aneurysm formation has also been associated with use of the spermatic or ovarian veins for renal artery bypass surgery. These veins are extremely friable, cannot withstand the stress of arterial pressure, and undergo severe dilatation or frank rupture (Fig 14–8). Therefore, their use as bypass grafts in arterial reconstruction is absolutely contraindicated.

Following renal revascularization, a false aneurysm may develop at a vascular anastomotic site months or years later. Mycotic false aneurysms are caused by deep wound infection involving the vascular suture line.[16] Contrary to a widely held impression, there is no increased risk of infection with vascular silk sutures

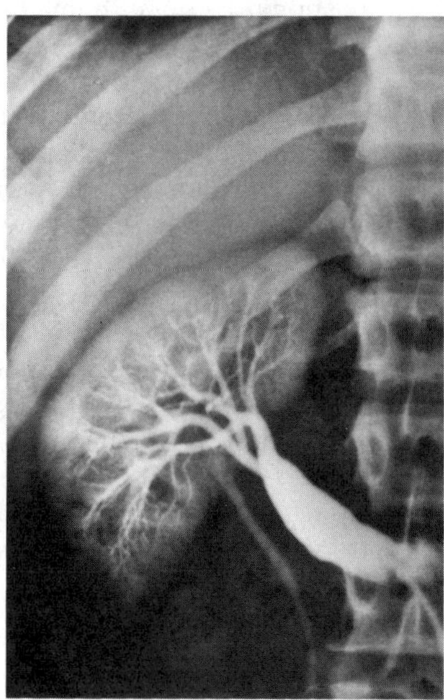

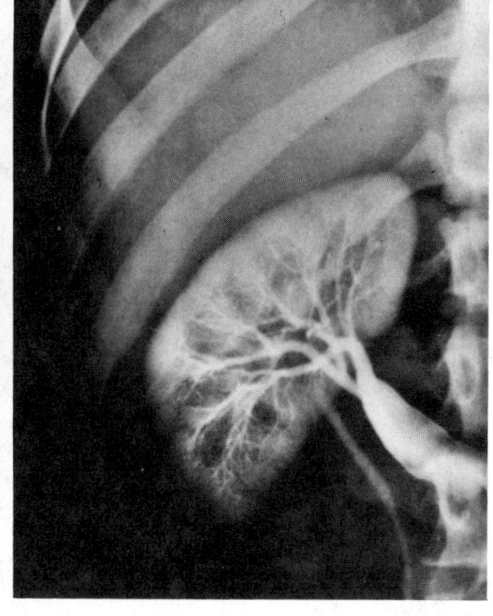

FIG 14–7.
Right renal arteriogram following aortorenal saphenous vein bypass demonstrates aneurysmal dilatation of the bypass graft with no evidence of stenosis. (From Novick AC, et al: *J Urol* 1978; 119:794. Used by permission.)

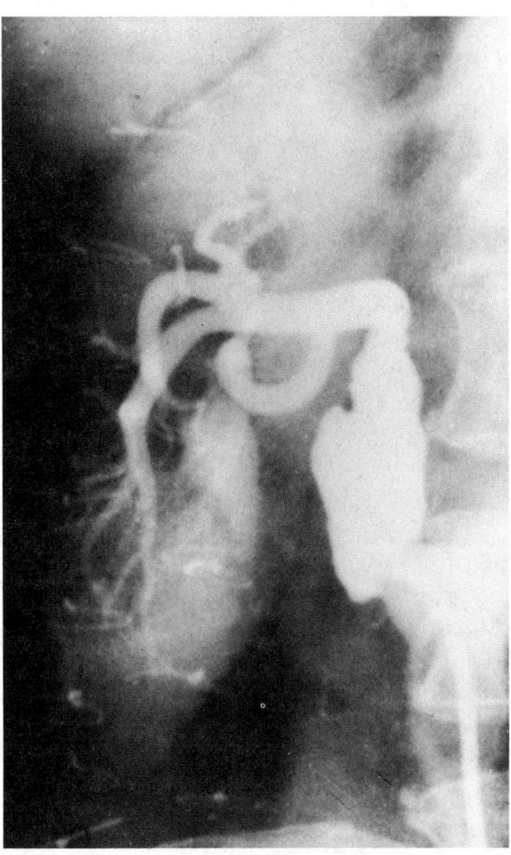

FIG 14–8.
Right renal arteriogram following aortorenal bypass with a segment of the gonadal vein demonstrates aneurysmal dilatation and irregularity of the venous bypass graft. (From Novick AC: *AUA Update Series,* lesson 40, vol 2, 1983. Used by permission.)

when these are used for anastomosis of autogenous vessels. Noninfected false aneurysms have most often been associated with synthetic bypass grafts, since anastomoses of native vessels with these grafts never acquire significant strength other than that determined by the suture line.[17] For this reason, synthetic graft anastomoses should always be done with a nonreabsorbable suture, such as polypropylene, rather than with silk, which loses its tensile strength over time. Infected or uninfected false anastomotic aneurysms can rupture spontaneously and should be repaired as soon as the diagnosis is established.

Aortic Complications

During an aortorenal bypass operation, clamping and unclamping of the abdominal aorta is performed. When the aorta is involved with atherosclerosis, this maneuver can cause dislodgment of plaque, resulting in aortic thrombosis and/or distal embolization. This occurrence can be minimized by selecting the healthiest portion of the abdominal aorta for use in such operations. Intraoperative systemic heparinization also helps to prevent this problem. Ultimately, the most effective prevention is to avoid operation on the extensively diseased aorta by using alternate techniques, such as hepatorenal or splenorenal bypass.

Whenever aortic surgery is undertaken, the peripheral pulses and lower extremities should always be examined before and immediately after revascularization. If there is evidence of compromised peripheral circulation postoperatively, emergency transbrachial abdominal aortography should be done. Immediate surgical thromboembolectomy is indicated to relieve aortic or major peripheral vascular occlusion. Minor discoloration of the toes from cholesterol microemboli can be observed easily when good peripheral pulses are present. This problem will generally resolve spontaneously, and digital amputation is rarely necessary.

Clamping and unclamping of the aorta may also produce an intraluminal aortic dissection, especially if a local endarterectomy has been done. This can be prevented by suturing down distal flaps of intima within the aorta when the lumen is exposed. This type of aortic dissection can cause peripheral ischemia or may be entirely asymptomatic, in which case simple observation is sufficient (Fig 14–9).

Visceral Complications

Visceral-renal arterial bypass operations are indicated in patients with severe

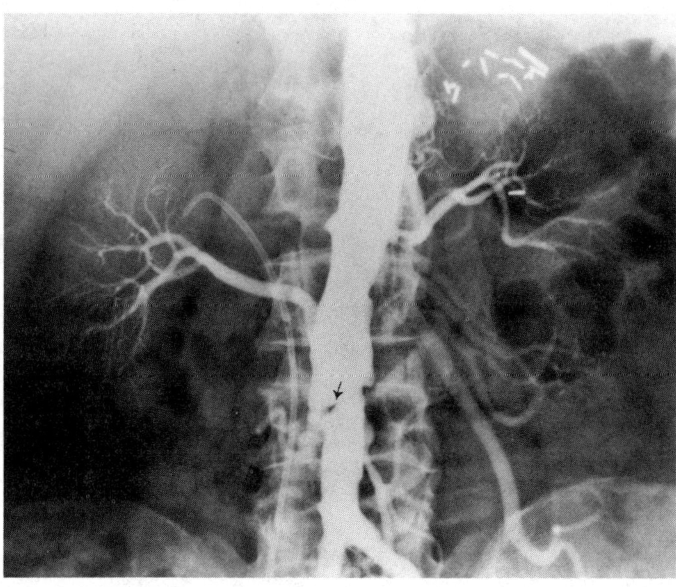

FIG 14–9.
Aortogram following a right aortorenal bypass demonstrates intraluminal aortic dissection from a flap of intima *(arrow)*, which was not present preoperatively. In this case, there is good flow through the aorta, the patient is asymptomatic, and no further intervention is indicated.

aortic disease and may be associated with specific complications. When splenorenal bypass is done, splenic viability is maintained by collateral vascular supply from the short gastric and gastroepiploic arteries. Nevertheless, a retractor-induced splenic laceration may be sustained during mobilization of the splenic artery, which necessitates performance of an incidental splenectomy. In our initial series of splenorenal bypasses, this complication occurred in five of 32 cases (16%).[9] During mobilization of the splenic artery, the splenic vein, which is thin-walled and directly adjacent to the artery, may be inadvertently damaged. Lacerations of the splenic vein are repaired with interrupted 5-0 vascular sutures. Injury to the pancreas, with resulting pancreatitis or pseudocyst formation, is a potential complication of splenorenal bypass which we have not thus far encountered in our experience with this operation.[10]

When performing hepatorenal bypass, the common hepatic artery and its major branches can be mobilized quite readily without damaging the portal vein or common bile duct. Hepatorenal bypass is usually done by end-to-side anastomosis of a saphenous vein graft to the common hepatic artery, which allows preservation of distal hepatic arterial flow.[7] However, in some cases, a direct end-to-end anastomosis of the hepatic and right renal arteries is done, which produces complete hepatic dearterialization.[8] This is well tolerated by the liver due to the increased extraction of oxygen from portal venous blood and the fairly rapid development of collateral hepatic arterial flow. Thus, although transient abnormalities in liver function parameters may occur, permanent hepatic damage has not yet been observed. However, the gallbladder is more susceptible to ischemic damage and may undergo postoperative necrosis when its blood supply from the right hepatic artery is interrupted. This problem can be avoided by performing an adjunctive cholecystectomy in patients whose blood flow through the common hepatic artery is totally diverted to the kidney.

A bypass from the superior mesenteric artery to the kidney is occasionally an option in patients with severe aortic atherosclerosis.[12] Since the superior mesenteric artery (SMA) is the only source of blood supply to a large portion of the bowel, this operation may produce postoperative intestinal ischemia. Such ischemia can be avoided by limiting this approach to patients with infrarenal aortic occlusion, in whom a significantly enlarged SMA is invariably present.

Acute Renal Failure

Acute renal failure induced by ischemia is a potential complication of surgical revascularization that, fortunately, can be prevented in most cases. Since all revascularization operations require temporary occlusion of the renal artery, it is important to understand renal responses to warm ischemia. If the period of arterial occlusion exceeds that which may be safely tolerated, then specific renal preservative measures are indicated.

In general, 30 minutes is the maximum period of arterial occlusion that the kidney can withstand before permanent damage is sustained.[26] In some clinical situations, this time may not apply and a longer period of ischemia may be safely tolerated. It is acknowledged that the solitary kidney is more resistant to ischemic damage than the paired kidney, although precise limits have not been defined. We reviewed the outcome of renal revascularization in 43 patients with a solitary kidney in whom warm ischemic intervals ranged from 14 to 59 minutes and where no specific renal protective measures were employed. In this series, there were no cases of acute renal failure postoperatively, indicating, in many of these patients, the ability of the solitary kidney to safely withstand periods of warm ischemia longer than 30 minutes.[27] Another situation that may enhance renal tolerance to temporary arterial occlusion is the presence of an extensive collateral vascular supply, which is often observed in patients with renal arterial occlusive disease.

There are several general measures that can help to limit the occurrence of postoperative acute renal failure in patients undergoing renal revascularization. These include generous preoperative and intraoperative hydration, intraoperative administration of mannitol,[28] avoidance of unnecessary manipulation or traction on the renal artery, continuous rather than intermittent clamping of the renal artery,[26] and prevention of hypotension during induction of anesthesia and/or aortic declamping. These measures help to limit postischemic renal injury by ensuring both optimal perfusion with absence of cortical vasospasm at the time of arterial occlusion and uniform restoration of blood flow throughout the kidney when the renal artery is unclamped. Mannitol is most effective when given 5 to 15 minutes prior to arterial occlusion; its benefits include increasing renal plasma flow, decreasing intrarenal vascular resistance, minimizing intracellular edema, and promoting an osmotic diuresis when the renal circulation is restored. Systemic or regional heparinization is also necessary prior to renal arterial occlusion to prevent intrarenal vascular clotting during the period of ischemia.

When in situ renal revascularization is done, it is generally possible to design the operation so that the kidney is only ischemic during the performance of a single vascular anastomosis, which should be done in well under 30 minutes. For operations involving placement of a bypass graft to the kidney from the aorta, hepatic, iliac, or mesenteric arteries, the renal circulation is not interrupted during the proximal anastomosis of the bypass graft to one of these vessels; therefore, the kidney is ischemic only during the distal anastomosis of the bypass graft to the renal artery. Splenorenal bypass also involves only a single vascular anastomosis of the splenic and renal arteries. When in situ revascularization is done in patients with branch renal arterial disease, the use of a prefashioned branched saphenous vein graft to achieve aortorenal bypass can help to limit renal ischemia.[5] In this approach, following anastomosis of the bypass graft to the aorta, each graft branch is anastomosed end-to-end to a branch of the renal artery and the ischemic interval to each supplied renal segment is thus limited to the time needed to perform a single end-to-end anastomosis. In this manner, in situ repair of branch renal artery disease may be done with no need for additional specific measures to protect the kidney from ischemia.

If the anticipated period of renal arterial occlusion exceeds 30 minutes, or if extracorporeal revascularization and/or autotransplantation are done, additional protection from postischemic renal injury is necessary. For in situ revascularization, the most useful techniques are external surface cooling of the kidney with ice slush[29] or renal flushing with a single intraarterial injection of 200 mL of chilled Collins solution[30]; when the latter method is used, since the Collins solution has a high potassium content, the renal vein is temporarily clamped and the effluent is drained through a short proximal venotomy. Both of these adjunctive techniques are effective in preventing acute renal failure following up to 2 hours of ischemia in situ. When extracorporeal revascularization and/or autotransplantation are done, renal preservation is achieved by immediate intraarterial flushing of the removed kidney with 500 mL of chilled Collins solution. The removed flushed kidney is then protected by immersion in ice slush to maintain hypothermia until the extracorporeal repair is completed. This method of simple cold storage provides safe and effective extracorporeal renal preservation for at least 24 hours.[31]

When postoperative acute renal failure occurs, it is generally manifested by a fall in urine output and a rise in the serum creatinine level. Alternatively, nonoliguric renal insufficiency may be observed. The cornerstone of therapy for such acute renal failure is judicious fluid management to ensure normal extracellular volume and sodium content. In older patients, the central venous pressure is not reliable for monitoring fluid replacement and the pulmonary artery wedge pressure provides a more accurate measurement of the left ventricular filling pressure. This information allows precise control of the volume and rate of fluid infusion, so that maximum cardiac output can be achieved without inducing left ventricular decompensation. The role of diuretic and vasoactive drug therapy to improve renal perfusion after ischemic injury is controversial. Furosemide administration appears to be of value, since this is known to increase renal blood flow by stimulating the release of intrarenal prostaglandin E, a potent dilator of the afferent renal arterioles.[32]

PERCUTANEOUS TRANSLUMINAL ANGIOPLASTY

Since 1980, percutaneous transluminal angioplasty has been evaluated extensively as a method of treatment for occlusive renovascular disorders. PTA offers the advantages of avoiding general anesthesia, reduced cost, ability to be repeated, and a shorter period of hospitalization. Also, in most cases, surgery is not precluded if PTA is unsuccessful.

The therapeutic results with PTA for renovascular hypertension have varied according to the pathologic diagnosis and the extent of vascular disease. In patients with fibrous lesions of the main renal artery, the technical and clinical success of PTA has been 85% to 90% and these results are comparable to those that can be obtained with surgical revascularization. The incidence of recurrent stenosis following successful PTA in this group has been approximately 5% and successful redilatation has been possible in some patients. Therefore, PTA presently represents the treatment of choice for patients with main renal arterial fibrous dysplasia. However, up to 30% of patients with fibrous disease have involvement of one or more renal artery branches. In such cases, PTA is technically more difficult and often impossible to perform. Therefore, for most patients with branch renal artery disease, surgical revascularization currently remains the treatment of choice.

In patients with atherosclerotic renal artery disease, the success rate with PTA has been excellent (80%–90%) for nonostial plaques located exclusively within the renal artery. However, atherosclerotic renal artery plaques that originate within the aorta (i.e., ostial) have responded poorly to PTA with only 25% to 30% success rate. In many of these lesions, PTA is not technically possible to perform; in other cases, following balloon dilatation of ostial lesions, the aortic plaque often returns to its original position, causing recurrent renal artery stenosis. Such ostial lesions are very common in patients with atherosclerotic renal artery disease, particularly in those with generalized atherosclerosis and bilateral disease, and surgical revascularization currently provides the most effective form of treatment.

In the original description of PTA for atherosclerotic lesions, the mechanism of action was attributed to compression and redistribution of atheromasa within the vessel wall. Subsequent experimental and autopsy studies on the pathophysiology of PTA showed that atherosclerotic plaques are not compressed. Rather, the caliber of the vessel is increased by the splitting of the plaque, with disruption of the intima and overstretching of the media.[33, 34] It is postulated that healing of the separated arterial layers occurs by the formation of a new layer of neointima and fibrous tissue. However, in some cases, PTA leads to intrusion of intimal plaque into the lumen, which creates a local flap and the opportunity for complicating dissection and/or thrombosis. In fibrous dysplasia of the renal artery, it is believed that rupture and stretching of the collagenous bundles in the arterial wall is the mechanism for successful dilatation. The specific technique for performing renal PTA is described in detail elsewhere.[35]

Based on the above description, it is obvious that PTA is an invasive technique wherein the internal structure of the renal artery is manipulated in the hope of fashioning a wider lumen. As such, complications may develop relative to percutaneous arterial puncture to introduce the catheter, passage of the catheter through the aorta, manipulation of the renal artery, or the use of contrast material and adjunctive systemic anticoagulation. Initially, major complications following renal PTA were reported in up to 33% of patients.[36] Currently, technical advances in angiographic guide wires and balloon catheters along with increasing experience have reduced the incidence of complications to 5% to 10% in the hands of a skilled radiologist. It is also apparent that complications following PTA are more likely to occur in patients with generalized atherosclerosis and ostial renal artery stenosis, compared to patients with focal nonostial atherosclerosis or fibrous dysplasia.

The following is a list of major complications that have been reported following PTA of the renal arteries.

1. Thrombosis (Fig 14–10) and/or severe intramural dissection (Fig 14–11) of the main renal artery caused by trauma to the intima.[35, 37–41] (In some cases, renal salvage has been accomplished through emergency surgical revascularization, whereas in others nephrectomy has been necessary.)

2. Segmental renal infarction caused by thrombosis and/or dissection of a renal artery branch[37, 41] (Fig 14–12).

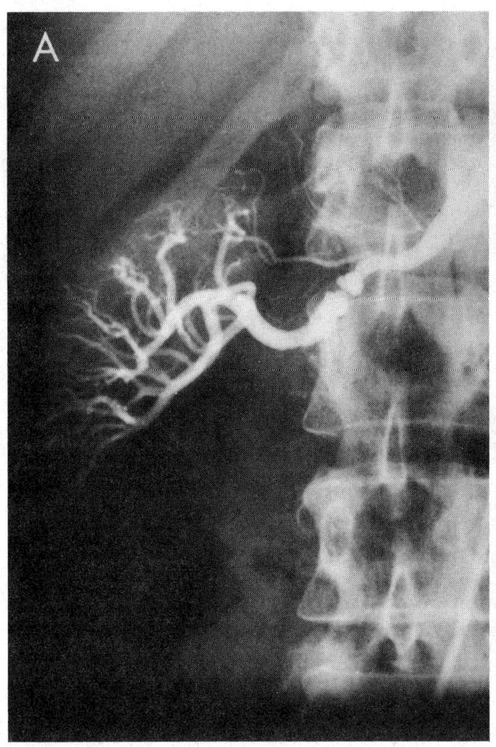

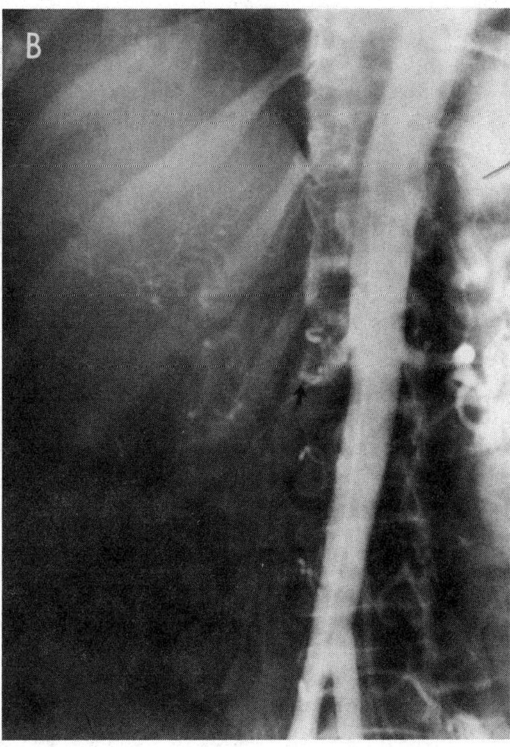

FIG 14–10.
A, right renal arteriogram shows stenosis of the midportion of the main renal artery from fibrous dysplasia. **B,** aortogram obtained immediately following attempted percutaneous transluminal dilatation shows thrombosis of the right renal artery at the site of attempted dilatation. (From Novick AC: *AUA Update Series,* lesson 40, vol 2, 1983. Used by permission.)

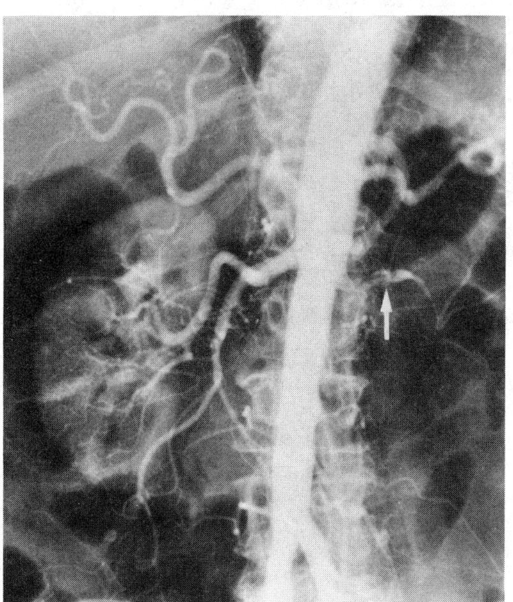

FIG 14–11.
Aortogram following percutaneous transluminal angioplasty of atherosclerotic left renal artery stenosis shows intramural dissection extending from proximal third of left renal artery into distal intrarenal branches *(arrow).* (From Flechner S, Novick AC, Vidt D, et al: *J Urol* 1982; 127:1072. Used by permission.)

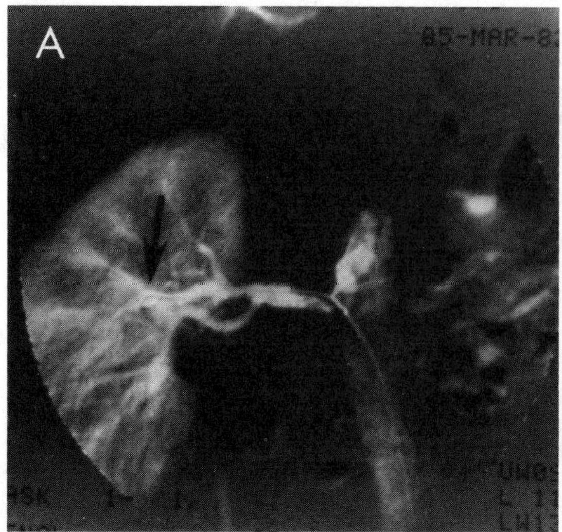

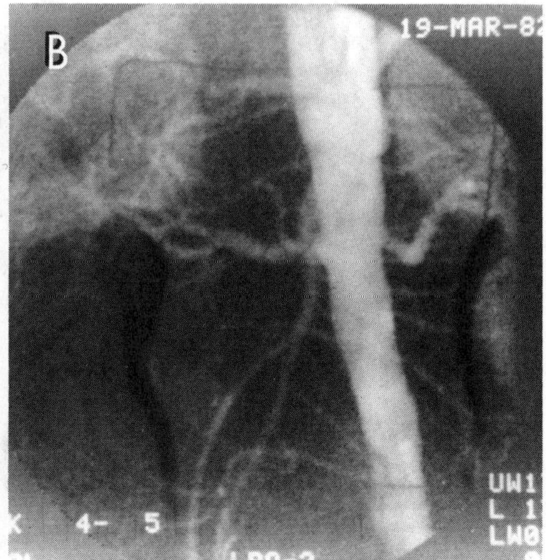

FIG 14–12.
A, right renal digital subtraction angiogram in patient with proximal main arterial stenosis undergoing percutaneous transluminal dilatation. The guide wire extends far beyond the area of stenosis into the kidney *(arrow).* **B,** digital subtraction angiogram following attempted percutaneous transluminal dilatation shows absent vascularity to the lower half of the kidney due to traumatic thrombosis of major segmental artery.

3. Development of a renal arteriovenous fistula.[42, 43]

4. Perforation of the renal artery during manipulation with resulting retroperitoneal hemorrhage.[40, 44, 45]

5. Acute renal failure related to the use of iodinated contrast material.[39, 41, 44, 46–48] In most cases, this has been reversible; however, permanent renal failure has been reported in some patients.

6. Cholesterol microembolization peripherally into the kidney caused by manipulation of atherosclerotic plaque within the aorta and/or renal artery.[39]

7. Catheter-induced trauma to the aorta with resulting local aortic thrombosis (Fig 14–13), distal embolization to lower extremities, or embolization to the mesenteric circulation.[35, 37, 45, 46, 49] The sequelae of such embolization have included emergency embolectomy, amputation, and death.

8. Hemorrhage from percutaneous puncture of the femoral or axillary artery, requiring transfusion and/or surgical repair for hemostasis[38, 41, 44, 50–52] (Fig 14–14).

9. Spontaneous retroperitoneal or gluteal hemorrhage occurring 2 to 4 weeks after PTA as a result of systemic oral anticoagulation.[45]

10. Rupture of the catheter balloon leading to distal embolization of balloon fragments or inability to remove the dilating catheter, necessitating a femoral arteriotomy.[44, 53]

11. Paraplegia caused by spinal cord vascular insufficiency.[48]

Every attempt should be made to minimize these complications and to deal with them promptly, should they occur. Repeated unsuccessful attempts to pass the guide wire across a severely obstructed artery enhance the likelihood of vascular trauma and should be avoided. The PTA should be undertaken only after consultation with a vascular surgeon and with an operating room available in the event that emergency surgical intervention is necessary. The risk of contrast-

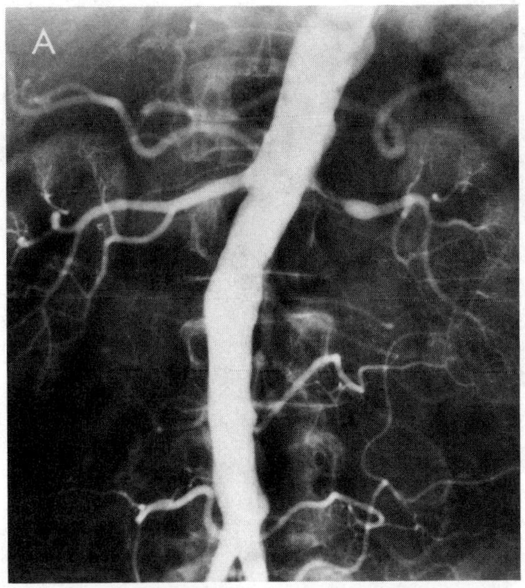

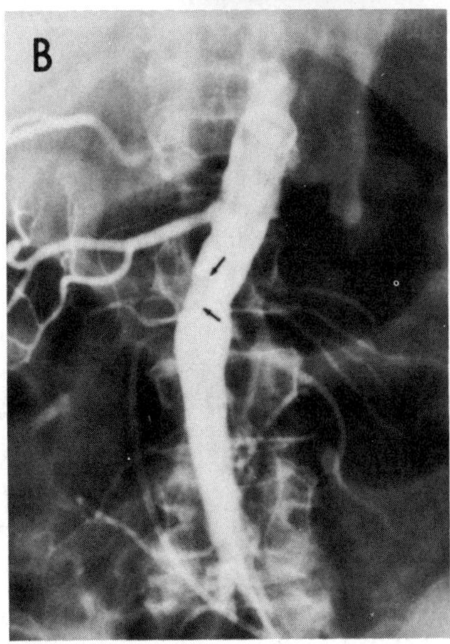

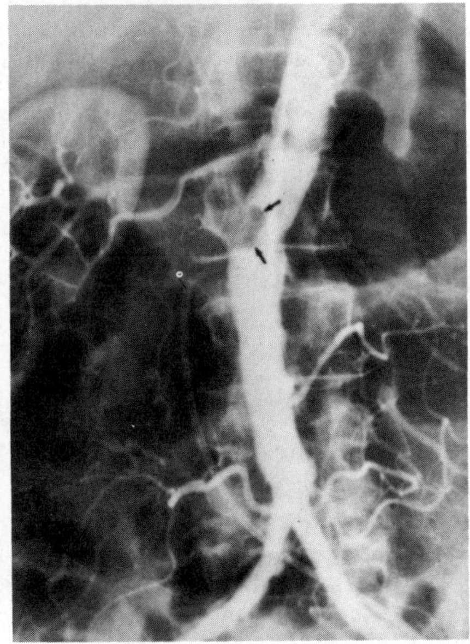

FIG 14–13.
A, aortogram shows atherosclerotic stenosis of the left renal artery. **B,** repeated aortography after percutaneous transluminal dilatation of the left renal artery shows thrombosis with complete occlusion. Note the aortic filling defect *(arrows),* which proved to be clot formation on traumatized aortic surface. (From Flechner S, Novick AC, Vidt D, et al: *J Urol* 1982; 127:1072. Used by permission.)

induced renal failure can be reduced by ensuring that the patient is well hydrated, by preliminary administration of mannitol, and by minimizing the contrast dose. Similarly, the risk of hemorrhage can be reduced by avoiding PTA in patients with poorly controlled hypertension or a recent history of anticoagulant use.

Immediately after dilatation of the renal artery, before removing the catheter from the patient, an aortogram should be done to assess the initial result and to rule

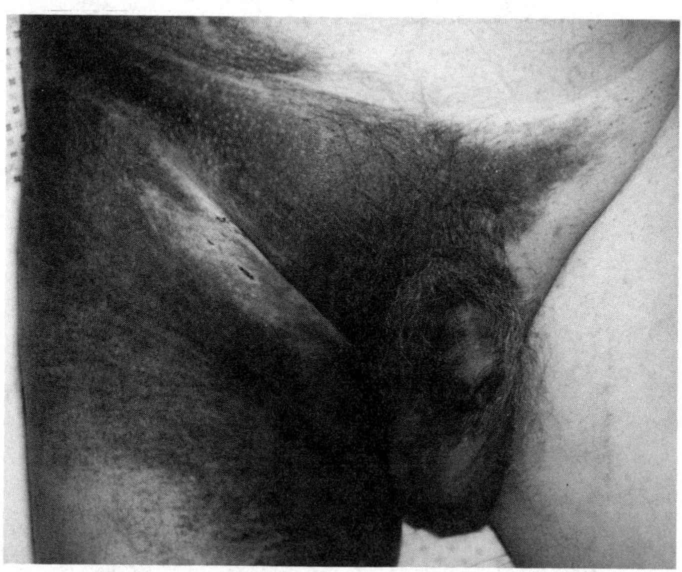

FIG 14–14.
Photograph of large groin hematoma following percutaneous femoral arterial puncture for transluminal renal angioplasty. (From Flechner SM: *Urol Clin North Am* 1984; 11:515. Used by permission.)

out significant vessel trauma. During the first few days following PTA, it is important to monitor the blood pressure, urine output, hematocrit, and serum creatinine level, particularly in patients with a solitary functioning kidney. The presence of acute flank pain, an unstable blood pressure, a rising serum creatinine level, or a falling hematocrit is an indication for emergency repeat angiography. The long-term follow-up of patients undergoing renal PTA is similar to that described earlier in this chapter for patients treated with surgical revascularization.

EDITORIAL COMMENT

This chapter covers in detail the complications of renal vascular surgery and percutaneous transluminal angioplasty. It is well illustrated by an author with extensive experience. Microvascular experience is also quite helpful, especially if small tertiary renal arterial branches are anastomosed. We have found that the use of detachable silicone balloons within the kidney has provided excellent control of arteriovenous fistulas or hemorrhage.[1, 2] Occasionally, these techniques are probably more effective than surgery, since the precise vessels can be easily identified angiographically and can be hard to locate surgically.

Percutaneous transluminal angioplasty has become more commonplace since the first edition and Dr. Novick has expanded discussion of this treatment. As indicated, single fibrous lesions in the main renal artery may respond very well to PTA but atherosclerotic lesions of the renal arterial ostium with involvement of the aorta are much less likely to respond. The many complications associated with this procedure are summarized.

1. Marshall FF, White RI, Kaufman SL, et al: Treatment of traumatic renal arteriovenous fistulas by detachable silicone balloon embolization. *J Urol* 1979; 122:237.

2. Kadir S, Marshall FF, White RI, et al: Therapeutic embolization of the kidney with detachable silicone balloons. *J Urol* 1983; 129:11.

REFERENCES

1. Novick AC: Renovascular hypertension, in Kendall R, Karaffin L (eds): *Practice of Surgery*. New York, Harper & Row, 1983.
2. Poutasse EF: Renal artery aneurysms. *J Urol* 1975; 113:443.
3. Novick AC, Stewart BH, Straffon RA: Autogenous arterial grafts in the treatment of renal artery stenosis. *J Urol* 1977; 118:919.
4. Straffon RA, Siegel DF: Saphenous vein bypass graft in the treatment of renovascular hypertension. *Urol Clin North Am* 1975; 2:337.
5. Streem SB, Novick AC: Aortorenal bypass with a branched saphenous vein graft for in situ repair of multiple segmental renal arteries. *Surg Gynecol Obstet* 1982; 155:885.
6. Dean RH: Late results of aortorenal bypass. *Urol Clin North Am* 1984; 11:425.
7. Chibaro EA, Libertino JA, Novick AC: Use of the hepatic circulation for renal revascularization. *Ann Surg* 1984; 199:406.
8. McElroy J, Novick AC: Renal revascularization by end-to-end anastomosis of the hepatic and renal arteries. *J Urol* 1985; 134:1089.
9. Novick AC, Banowsky LH, Stewart BH, et al: Splenorenal bypass in the treatment of stenosis of the renal artery. *Surg Gynecol Obstet* 1977; 144:891.
10. Khauli R, Novick AC, Ziegelbaum W: Splenorenal bypass in the treatment of renal artery stenosis: Experience with 69 cases. *J Vasc Surg* 1985; 2:547.
11. Novick AC, Banowsky LH: Ilial-renal saphenous vein bypass: Alternative for renal revascularization in patients with surgically difficult aorta. *J Urol* 1979; 122:243.
12. Khauli R, Novick AC, Coseriu G: Superior mesenterorenal bypass for renal revascularization in patients with infrarenal aortic occlusion. *J Urol* 1985; 133:188.
13. Novick AC: Management of intrarenal branch arterial lesions with extracorporeal microvascular reconstruction and autotransplantation. *J Urol* 1981; 126:150.
14. Zabbo A, Novick AC: Digital subtraction angiography for non-invasive imaging of the renal artery. *Urol Clin North Am* 1984; 11:409.
15. Szilagy DE, Smith RF, Elliot JP, et al: Infection in arterial reconstruction with synthetic grafts. *Ann Surg* 1972; 176:321.
16. Nerstrom B, Engell HC: Operative treatment of renovascular hypertension: A study of 60 consecutive patients with follow-up findings between 1 and 7 years postoperatively. *Ann Surg* 1972; 176:590.
17. Moore WS, Hall DD: Late suture failure in the pathogenesis of anastomotic false aneurysms. *Ann Surg* 1970; 172:1064.
18. Cerny JC, Fry WJ, Gambee J, et al: Aortoduodenal fistula. *J Urol* 1972; 107:12.
19. Kaufman JJ: Dacron grafts and splenorenal bypass in the surgical treatment of stenosing lesions of the renal artery. *Urol Clin North Am* 1975; 2:365.
20. Cronan JJ, Dorfman GS: Low-dose thrombolysis: A nonoperative approach to renal artery occlusion. *J Urol* 1983; 130:757.
21. Dardik H, Sussman BC, Kahn M, et al: Lysis of arterial clot by intravenous or intra-arterial administration of streptokinase. *Surg Gynecol Obstet* 1984; 158:137.
22. Berni GA, Bandyk DF, Zierler RE, et al: Streptokinase treatment of acute arterial occlusion. *Ann Surg* 1983; 198:185.
23. Milan VG, Sher MH, Deterling RA, et al: Transcatheter thromboembolectomy of acute renal artery occlusion. *Arch Surg* 1978; 113:1086.
24. Dean RH, Wilson JP, Burko H, et al: Saphenous vein aortorenal bypass grafts: Serial arteriographic study. *Ann Surg* 1974; 180:469.
25. Stanley JC, Ernst CB, Fry WJ: Fate of 100 aortorenal vein grafts: Characteristics of late graft expansion, aneurysmal dilatation and stenosis. *Surgery* 1973; 74:931.
26. Novick AC: Renal hypothermia: in vivo and ex vivo. *Urol Clin North Am* 1983; 10:637.
27. Askari A, Novick AC, Stewart BH, et al: Surgical treatment of renovascular disease in the solitary kidney: Results in 43 cases. *J Urol* 1982; 127:20.
28. Collins GM, Green RD, Boyer D, et al: Protection of kidneys from warm ischemic injury: Dosage and timing of mannitol administration. *Transplantation* 1980; 29:83.
29. Metzner PJ, Boyce WH: Simplified renal hypothermia: An adjunct to conservative renal surgery. *Br J Urol* 1972; 44:76.
30. Abele RP, Novick AC, Ishigami N, et al: Comparison of flushing solutions for in situ renal preservation. *Urology* 1981; 18:485.

31. Novick AC, Magnusson MO: Extracorporeal and in situ renal preservation, in Novick AC, Straffon RA (eds): *Vascular Problems in Urologic Surgery.* Philadelphia, WB Saunders Co, 1982.
32. Patak RV, et al: Antagonism of the effects of furosemide by indomethacin in normal and hypertensive men. *Prostaglandins* 1975; 10:649.
33. Block PC, Fallon JT, Elmer D: Experimental angioplasty: Lessons from the laboratory. *Am J Radiol* 1980; 135:907.
34. Castaneda-Zuniga WR, Formanek A, Tadavarthy M, et al: The mechanism of balloon angioplasty. *Radiology* 1980; 135:565.
35. Flechner SM, Novick AC, Vidt D, et al: The use of percutaneous transluminal angioplasty for renal artery stenosis in patients with generalized atherosclerosis, *J Urol* 1982; 127:1072.
36. Flechner SM: Percutaneous transluminal dilatation: A realistic appraisal in patients with stenosing lesions of the renal artery. *Urol Clin North Am* 1984; 11:515.
37. Connolly JE, Kwaan JH, McCar PM: Complications after percutaneous transluminal angioplasty. *Am J Surg* 1981; 142:60.
38. Flechner SM, Sandler CM, Childs T, et al: Screening for transplant renal artery stenosis in hypertensive recipients using digital subtraction angiography. *J Urol* 1983; 130:440.
39. Grim CE, Luft FC, Yune HY, et al: Percutaneous transluminal dilatation in the treatment of renovascular hypertension. *Ann Intern Med* 1981; 95:439.
40. Guzzetta PC, Potter BM, Kapur S, et al: Reconstruction of the renal artery after unsuccessful percutaneous transluminal angioplasty in children. *Am J Surg* 1983; 145:647.
41. Sos TA, Pickering PG, Sniderman KW, et al: Percutaneous transluminal renal angioplasty in renovascular hypertension due to fibromuscular dysplasia. *N Engl J Med* 1983; 309:274.
42. Mills SR, Wertman DE, Grossman SH: Renal cortical arteriovenous fistula complicating percutaneous renal angioplasty. *Am J Radiol* 1981; 137:1251.
43. Oleaga JA, Grossman RA, McLean GK, et al: Arteriovenous fistula of a segmental renal artery branch as a complication of percutaneous angioplasty. *Am J Radiol* 1981; 136:988.
44. Schwarten EE, Yune HY, Klatte E, et al: Clinical experience with percutaneous transluminal angioplasty of stenotic renal arteries. *Radiology* 1980; 135:601.
45. Tegtmeyer CJ, Dyer R, Teates CD, et al: Percutaneous transluminal dilatation of renal arteries. *Radiology* 1980; 135:589.
46. Katzen BT, Chang J, Lukowsky GH, et al: Percutaneous transluminal angioplasty for treatment of renovascular hypertension. *Radiology* 1979; 131:53.
47. Katzen BT, Chang J, Know WG: Percutaneous transluminal angioplasty with a Gruntzig balloon catheter. *Arch Surg* 1979; 113:1389.
48. Luft FC, Grim CE, Weinberger MH: Intervention in patients with renovascular hypertension and renal insufficiency. *J Urol* 1983; 130:654.
49. Tegtmeyer CJ, Teates CD, Crigler N, et al: Percutaneous transluminal angioplasty in patients with renal artery stenosis. *Radiology* 1981; 140:323.
50. Mahler F, Probst P, Haertel M, et al: Lasting improvement of renovascular hypertension by transluminal dilatation of atherosclerotic and non-atherosclerotic renal artery stenosis. *Circulation* 1982; 65:611.
51. Martin EC, Mattern RF, Baer L, et al: Renal angioplasty for hypertension: Predictive factors for long-term success. *Am J Radiol* 1981; 127:951.
52. Paolini RM, Marcondes M, Wideman A, et al: Percutaneous transluminal angioplasty of renal artery stenosis. *Acta Radiol [Diagn] (Stockh)* 22:571, 1981.
53. Grim CE, Yune HY, Weinberger M, et al: Balloon dilatation for renal artery stenosis causing hypertension: Criteria, concerns, and cautions. *Ann Intern Med* 1980; 92:117.

CHAPTER 15

Complications of Renal Transplantation

James F. Burdick, M.D.

This chapter will consider the anatomy and surgical technique that are important for avoiding—and managing—complications after renal transplantation. Isolation of this aspect of the management of transplants is somewhat arbitrary. However, several general texts on transplantation[1-3] provide excellent treatment of the many other aspects of patient care important in this field. It is recognized that bacterial and nonbacterial infection, steroid-connected and other immunosuppression-related metabolic changes, duodenal ulcer, cecal erosion, pancreatitis, hepatitis, hematologic pathology, psychiatric problems, cosmetic changes, tumors, recurrence of original disease, and poor compliance all threaten the transplant. These possibilities must be remembered in any assessment of possible complications.

The importance of the diagnosis of rejection and the use of immunosuppression cannot be overemphasized in the care of the transplant patient. The diagnosis of allograft rejection is far from a reliable science. We have shown that interpretation of renal allograft biopsies is complicated by the presence of a marked inflammatory infiltrate even in patients who are doing well but have a biopsy performed on routine protocol.[4] The exact nature of allograft rejection is not totally understood. The prospect for the success of a transplant has recently improved, due to the improved safety and effectiveness of immunosuppression.[5] The remarkable value of cyclosporine has become apparent over the 5 years since it became generally available.[6] Cadaver donor graft survival at 1 year has increased approximately 20%. However, immunologic issues are impossible to deal with successfully in a routine way unless patient care is based upon a firm foundation of excellent technical practice. That foundation is the subject of this chapter.

PERIOPERATIVE COMPLICATIONS

Selected points to consider before, during, and after the transplant procedure are summarized and depicted anatomically in Figure 15–1.

Inadequate Preoperative Assessment

The renal transplant patient should have undergone appropriate evaluation well before the time of the final arrangements for the specific transplant procedure. Possible infection, serious heart disease, and urologic abnormalities, such as congenital problems or benign prostatic hypertrophy, should be evaluated appropriately prior to transplantation. The de-

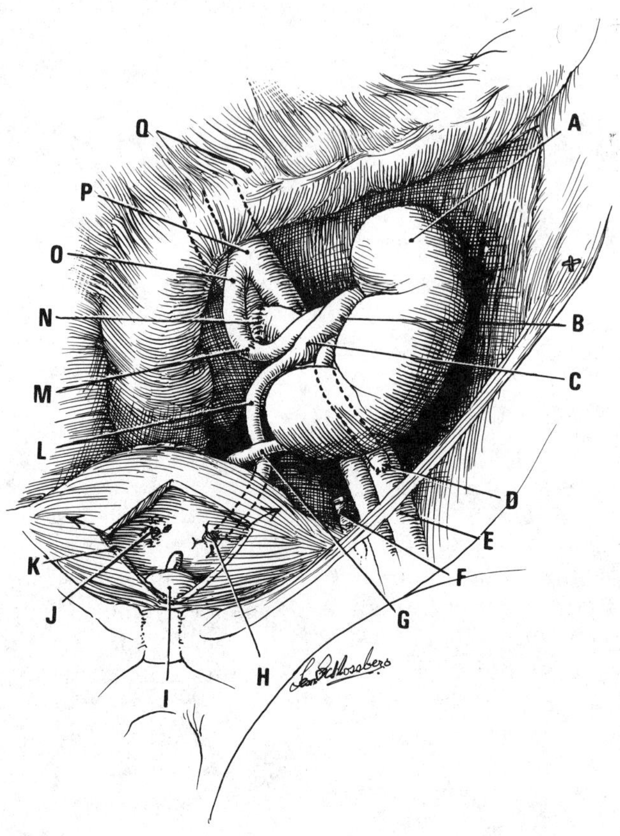

FIG 15–1.
Possible trouble spots to remember and evaluate during the transplant procedure. *A-Q:* Structures (and their potential complications). *A,* parenchyma (hyperacute rejection, perfusion injury); *B,* hilum (unligated bleeder); *C,* ureter and pelvis (electrocautery or other operative damage); *D,* accessory artery (occlusion producing ureteropelvic necrosis); *E,* distal external iliac artery (embolus, clamp injury, flap of atheroma); *F,* ligated lymphatic (leak producing lymphocele); *G,* spermatic cord (ureteral obstruction); *H,* ureteroneocystostomy (leak, stenosis); *I,* Foley (balloon puncture, clot occlusion); *J,* bladder mucosa (hemorrhage from abrasion); *K,* cystotomy (leak at closing suture line); *L,* ureter (obstruction, twist, leak, devascularization); *M,* arterial anastomosis (stenosis, leak); *N,* venous anastomosis (leak); *O,* internal iliac artery (twist, clamp trauma); *P,* iliac bifurcation (atherosclerotic disease); and *Q,* peritoneum (hole with gastrointestinal tract damage or leakage and peritoneal dialysis fluid).

gree to which other factors, such as underlying abnormalities of the patient's teeth, mental state, and gastrointestinal tract, are investigated will vary from center to center. Specific note should be made of previous surgery in the lower abdomen and groins, the presence of iliac bruits in older or diabetic patients at risk for atherosclerosis, and, in patients with a history of a previous transplant, the status of the graft and vessels. It is currently the practice to perform bilateral autologous nephrectomies in cases presenting a risk of infection or severe hypertension but not otherwise to do routine nephrectomy, since this does not improve results.[7–9] It is our routine practice to perform bilateral nephrectomy on patients with polycystic renal disease, since the problems of infection and bleeding are such a great threat and the nephrectomy procedure posttransplantation is a major undertaking in this disease. However, other centers have found bilateral nephrectomy not to be necessary in the asymptomatic patient with polycystic kidneys,[10] and we have begun to reconsider our policy of routine polycystic nephrectomy since cyclosporine became available.

Potential Problems With the Shared Cadaver Donor Kidney

Major factors in the success of modern renal transplantation are the comparative uniformity of excellent harvesting technique by surgeons trained specifically in the en bloc approach and the openness and honesty with which organs are shared between centers. We feel that early flushing followed by dissection after the kidneys are cold and bloodless[11] improves flushing. However, the surgeon performing implantation of the organ must always be prepared to encounter a graft that is somewhat different from what was expected. The kidney may mistakenly be from the opposite side, which can necessitate a rearrangement of the arterial anastomosis that had been planned. The kidney should be examined very carefully for small additional arteries which may have been unwittingly divided during the retrieval procedure. This may not be important if a small upper pole vessel is affected, but revascularization of lower pole arteries is critically important, since they supply the pelvis and ureter of the kidney, which have no collateral supply in the transplant setting. The vein should be inspected carefully for major lacerations and unligated branches, since massive bleeding after opening the venous anastomosis may be troublesome or catastrophic, and this can be avoided by tying or sewing the defects while the kidney is still on ice. The arteries should be inspected to make sure that traction has not produced defects or intimal injury. Subcapsular hematomas, although esthetically displeasing, do not seem to be of any functional or prognostic significance. Finally, once the renal blood supply has been restored, the ureter and pelvis should be inspected to ensure that they are well perfused. If adequate tissue has not been left with the ureter and it is without appropriate blood flow, then anastomosis of the ureteropelvic junction to the recipient ureter is usually advisable, instead of the usual ureteroneocystostomy.

Bleeding

The particular predisposition that renal transplant patients have to bleeding is caused by the interference with platelet function caused by toxic metabolites not cleared during dialysis. Heparin is not routinely used during the performance of an end-to-end anastomosis between the renal artery and the internal iliac artery, since this artery is clamped at the iliac bifurcation and thrombosis is therefore avoided. However, if the external iliac is to be employed for an end-to-side anastomosis, which is indicated in situations in which several renal vessels are to be anastomosed on a renal pedicle, or in a man with a previous transplant on the opposite side (see later in the chapter), or in a patient with significant atherosclerosis at the iliac artery bifurcation, then we think that the patient should be heparinized prior to clamping this artery to prevent thrombosis and embolization from this occluded arterial segment.

Although the patient will have an increased tendency to bleed if heparin is used, careful hemostasis must be obtained in all patients with renal failure at the end of any procedure because of their azotemic coagulopathy. Prior to closure, the areas of blunt retroperitoneal dissection should be inspected for small areas that are bleeding, and the anastomoses should be examined carefully, since a small needle hole may continue to leak and produce a prolonged hemorrhage that necessitates reoperation. Additionally, the hilum of the kidney should be carefully inspected for bleeding points that were overlooked during the donor nephrectomy; the inspection should be done initially when the anastomoses are first opened up, and again just before closure of the wound. Initial spasm of a small vessel may give way, and, without an appropriate platelet plug, bleeding may arise minutes or hours after the initial restoration of flow to the transplant.

Compromise of Renal Allograft Vasculature

Since the renal artery is posterior to the renal vein, the kidney sits most comfortably when the (medial) internal iliac artery and (lateral) iliac vein of the contralateral side are used for anastomosis. Conversely, if the external iliac artery is to be used, the transplant is best placed in the ipsilateral iliac fossa, because the artery lies lateral to the vein. If the renal artery is of sufficient length, this rule may be violated, but the course of the vessels should then be carefully evaluated at the end of the procedure. After reestablishing flow through the artery and vein, flow through the kidney may be tested by very briefly occluding the renal vein and noting the swelling of the transplant, which will then be relieved by releasing the renal vein occlusion. This maneuver provides reassurance that actual flow is present in addition to pulsation in the renal artery. Not uncommonly, the kidney may have parenchymal vasospasm, which may cause the flow to be very poor. The most common technical cause for impaired flow is probably obstruction of an end-to-end anastomosis between the internal iliac artery and the renal artery. This obstruction can be caused by excessive tension on a running suture, by a flap of vessel edge if the anastomosis is uneven, or by a fine film of adventitia on the donor artery that may extend over its end and partially occlude the lumen. These problems may go unnoticed unless the surgeon is looking specifically for them during creation of the anastomosis. A noticeable thrill will often be palpable in the renal artery just distal to the anastomosis if the flow through the kidney is very high immediately after establishment of the anastomosis, even if no technical problem exists. If the thrill is prominent, or if it appears that the pulsation is weaker in the renal artery than in the internal iliac artery proximal to the anastomosis, the anastomosis should be reexplored, preferably employing about 200 mL of ice-cold Ringer's lactate, containing 18 g mannitol and 2,000 units of heparin per liter, to perfuse the kidney after opening the suture line, before recreating the anastomosis. Another site that may produce interference with the arterial flow is kinking or a periadventitial restricting band at the iliac artery bifurcation. Also, if the iliac artery is found to be quite atherosclerotic and an endarterectomy of the internal iliac artery is attempted, there may be a flap left that will interfere with perfusion. Anticipation of this problem with the planned use of the external iliac (rather than the contralateral internal iliac) is advisable. Important venous obstruction is uncommon unless most of the opposite wall of the venous anastomosis becomes incorporated in a suture line or unless multiple stitches are required to reinforce leaking areas after completion of the suture line, with resultant narrowing of the outflow. Slight "ballooning" of the vein above the anastomosis is not an indication for revision. Of course, care must be taken during retraction and manipulation of the kidney as the arterial and venous anastomoses are formed, to ensure that neither vessel becomes twisted and then anastomosed in an improper orientation.

Vascular and Neurologic Compromise of the Leg

The use of an end-to-side renal artery-to-external iliac artery anastomosis threatens the distal vasculature of the leg because of the possibilities of embolus and creation of a distal intimal flap if the iliac artery is diseased. Care must be taken to use heparinization, avoid clamp injuries of the vessel, and carefully flush the vessel, first proximally and then by backbleeding distally, before tying down the suture and releasing the vascular occlusions permanently. The peripheral pulse status should be known preoperatively in all cases, and it should be checked carefully while the patient is still on the operating table after an external iliac artery anastomosis is performed. If an embolus occurs, balloon catheter embolectomy should be done through a separate transverse incision on the iliac artery distal to the renal artery anastomosis, to preserve flow through the kidney during this time. An important avoidable operative complication is femoral neuropathy due to compression by a self-retaining retractor blade.[12–14]

Hyperacute Rejection

This disaster will be nearly nonexistent if an appropriate cross-match has been performed by the tissue-typing laboratory. However in rare cases, the transplant may become extremely plethoric and swollen within minutes after flow is reestablished. A biopsy provides the evidence that hyperacute rejection has occurred.[15] In such cases, it may be appropriate to remove the transplant immediately since systemic toxicity, particularly leukopenia and thrombocytopenia, may present a serious threat to the patient if the hyperacute rejection is allowed to progress. In many other instances, the turgor and color of the transplant may fluctuate considerably, often changing from firm and pink to a softer and more purple color, without an apparent technical problem with the vasculature or other underlying cause. Unless definite evidence for hyperacute rejection is found, the transplant should be left in place, under the presumption that this represents a more common reversible change that may accompany acute tubular necrosis but is consistent with eventual good function. Occasionally, if vigilance in washing powder off operating gloves is relaxed, enough starch-particle emboli may be flushed into the kidney to cause dysfunction.

The First Postoperative Day

The most important problems facing the transplant patient in the hours following the procedure are hyperkalemia, bleeding, and fluid shifts. Unless the patient is hypertensive and has severe salt overload, intravenous fluid replacement and intravascular volume support should be maintained with normal saline or its equivalent in sodium chloride content. Salt restriction should be achieved as part of overall fluid restriction, as necessary. A particular metabolic danger is represented by the diabetic who has severe postoperative hyperglycemia. Replacement with hyponatremic solutions in the presence of hyperglycemia will result in severe hyponatremia (in spite of normal or elevated osmolarity) which, typically accompanied by hyperkalemia, produces life-threatening cardiovascular instability on occasion.

It is our practice to leave a drain in the retroperitoneal space for 24 to 48 hours to monitor for postoperative bleeding. We have not found the increased risk of wound infection due to a drain which has been reported by others.[16] Hemodialysis should be considered even during the first few postoperative hours if hyperkalemia or fluid overload is a serious problem and the transplant is not functioning well. The heparinization required for dialysis may result in additional bleeding, and it is appropriate to leave the wound drain in place until after the first dialysis if dialysis is required within 24 to 36 hours posttransplant. Attention should also be directed to the Foley catheter if there is poor urine output, since the catheter may become occluded with blood clot. Careful sterile flushing of the Foley should be performed once or twice during the first day if urine output is not profuse.

The routine use of a central venous pressure line is advocated by some. This allows excellent maintenance of appropriate filling pressure and may assist in ameliorating the degree of acute tubular necrosis that develops posttransplant.

Hyperkalemia is slightly less of a threat in the chronic dialysis patient, who has a chronic tendency toward this state. However, potassium may still achieve critical levels and produce cardiac arrhythmias rather quickly posttransplantation in the dialysis patient. Initial management includes the administration of glucose, insulin, bicarbonate, and calcium. Sodium polystyrene sulfonate (Kayexalate) may be employed, but there is a serious question about its safety. Colonic necrosis in the absence of gross vascular obstruction is not uncommon in patients following renal transplantation,[17, 18] and there is evidence that this complication may be due to synergism between immunosuppression and Kayexalate.[19] If used, Kayexalate must be cleansed from the colon with follow-up saline enemas. Posttransplant hyperkalemia is best treated by expeditious dialysis. It is, furthermore, somewhat more dangerous to accept a transplant candidate who is quite uremic but has not actually become stable on dialysis for at least 1 to 2 weeks prior to transplant, because of the danger of perioperative fluid overload, hypertension, and hyperkalemia.

EARLY POSTOPERATIVE COMPLICATIONS

Problems With the Transplant Itself

Acute tubular necrosis should be almost nonexistent in uncomplicated transplants if the total period of preservation is less than a few hours. However, after the first few hours, regardless of the excellence of all technical factors, acute tubular necrosis will become a possibility. The incidence will rise with the length of time the kidney has been preserved, whether on pulsatile perfusion or simple cold storage, and, beyond approximately 48 to 60 hours, acute tubular necrosis is frequent or universal. Even after this period of time, some transplants may eventually function quite well. However, at some point beyond 48 to 60 hours, the incidence of primary nonfunction because of severe ischemic damage becomes increasingly important. In the average case, if the transplant either has minimal or no urine output initially and the patient remains in oliguric renal failure postoperatively, an extensive workup should not be undertaken. The transplant is simply followed by routine radionuclide scanning and ultrasonography. A baseline radionuclide scan should be obtained within the first few days posttransplant, and if this study shows reasonable blood flow, then no further invasive studies should be undertaken, even if the patient temporarily has no renal function.[20] When the patient has severe acute tubular necrosis, repeat isotopic scans may be performed at approximately weekly intervals and compared to the initial baseline study. Decreasing flow is taken as evidence for the development of rejection, in the absence of other changes to explain it.[21] There is evidence that accumulation of radionuclide in a technetium 99m sulfur colloid scan is a sensitive indicator of rejection.[22, 23] Ultrasonography is most useful to rule out hydronephrosis and fluid collections, although it has also been suggested that increased size and altered echogenicity may correlate with rejection.[24]

Occasionally, disastrous rupture of the renal allograft may develop early postoperatively, heralded by sudden severe pain in the area of the transplant, plus hypovolemic hypotension. This complication occurs particularly in the setting of hypertension and severe rejection.[25–27] Immediate exploration is indicated, and the allograft may have to be sacrificed. However, a remarkable number of these ruptured grafts have been salvaged and have functioned effectively.[28–30] Patients who have been retransplanted with another kidney after loss due to rupture of the first kidney may have an increased likelihood of a second rupture.[31] A less disastrous complication is spontaneous renal decapsulation with excessive fluid leakage.[32] Some transplant centers routinely incise the capsule along the convex surface to allow pressure to distribute slowly and evenly as a precaution against rupture.

Complications of the Wound

Wound infection is not remarkably more common in renal transplant recipients than in other postoperative patients, although this can be a serious problem.[33] In addition to the usual causes of surgical wound infection, contamination of the kidney from the donor involves a particularly grave prognosis for the graft and the recipient.[34, 35] Contamination of the preservation fluid is much less serious, particularly if careful surveillance cultures allow the institution of antibiotic therapy prior to the development of serious problems in the recipient.[36] Drains in the wound[37] and the presence of urinary tract infection[38] have both been implicated as particular etiologic agents in posttransplant wound infections. Younger patients who have had splenectomy in preparation for transplantation are probably at particular risk for bacterial sepsis.[39] Detection of pelvic abscesses may be aided by ultrasound and gallium scanning,[40] but computed tomography (CT) scan is the most effective diagnostic aid.[41]

Another major issue in the transplant wound is the development of a fluid collection. Ultrasonography is a convenient and accurate method for detection of such fluid collections[24, 42–47] and should be performed as a routine early after transplantation and then subsequently if problems arise. A lucent defect on radionuclide scan is also an accurate indication of a collection.[48, 49] Many small asymptomatic fluid collections thus detected are unimportant.[50, 51] Larger collections may represent a serious problem. Occasionally this fluid collection is due to urinary extravasation that requires repair. However, a large homogeneous collection of fluid in the transplant wound most commonly represents a lymphocele.[52–55] This complication may occur due to lymphatic leakage, both from the donor lymphatics and the recipient lymphatics,[56] but it appears that recipient lymphatics are the most important contributors, since careful ligation of these lymphatics along the iliac vein during the transplant procedure decreases the incidence of lymphocele[57–59]; furthermore, direct isotopic tracer extravasation from iliac lymphatics into the lymphocele has been documented.[60] Lymphoceles that are large enough to cause ureteral or venous obstruction should be treated either by needle aspiration[61, 62] or by direct marsupialization into the peritoneal cavity.[63–66]

Vascular Complications

Possible arterial complications include hemorrhage, infarction, stenosis, and aneurysm formation.[16, 67, 68] In one case, parenchymal compression due to a perinephric hematoma was reported to produce severe transplant dysfunction.[69] If hemorrhage at an anastomosis is to be a problem, it will generally present as the necessity for reexploration within 24 hours. Another common cause for hemorrhage in the early postoperative period is severe infection; if the infection is in the region of the arterial anastomosis it may cause disruption, with sudden, life-threatening hemorrhage.[70, 71] The only other common setting for hemorrhage is after transplant nephrectomy, as described later in this chapter. Aneurysm formation and the anastomotic changes that cause typical renal artery stenosis occur much later. In the rare instance in which an anastomosis has been fashioned so poorly that only minimal flow is present, this defect should be detected at operation and revised prior to closing the patient. If undetected, such a complication might cause infarction of the entire organ some days after the transplant, but this result is remarkably rare. Also rare is the early occlusion of vessels due to the position of the graft, in spite of the fact that, from either the external iliac end-to-side anastomosis or the end-to-end anastomosis with the internal iliac, the artery and vein pursue a somewhat indirect course to the kidney and are not easily arrangeable in a specific fashion prior to placing the kidney in its retroperitoneal pocket and closing the wound. It is important to avoid mistaking the aortic bifurcation for the iliac bifurcation in the retroperitoneum, where landmarks may be misleading.

Perhaps the most common vascular problem in the early postoperative period is the occlusion of one of the multiple arteries in cases where additional minor vessel anastomoses are required. The technique for small-vessel anastomosis is an important skill for all who do renal transplants,[72–74] since occasionally a shared organ will prove to have multiple vessels not described by the referring organ retrieval center. Occlusion of a revascularized small vessel may be purely a technical error at the anastomosis, but there is another potential problem that is obscure and only evident if the surgeon examines the vessels. If there is a moderate degree of atherosclerosis in the renal donor, excessive traction on the kidney during the removal, particularly involving accessory polar vessels that may not be evident early in the dissection, may cause an actual circumferential rent in the intima, leaving the more elastic adventitia intact. An intact thin segment of adventitia is apparent connecting two segments of thicker-appearing artery and may be present anywhere along the course of the vessel. Such areas are likely to cause early postoperative occlusion and should be divided and reanastomosed using microsurgical technique prior to implantation of the kidney. If a failure to revascularize an arterial branch becomes manifest early postoperatively, it usually presents as a urine leak that has resulted from a loss of integrity of a portion of the collecting system.[75–78]

Preservation cannulas inserted into renal arteries cause damage that may result in an intimal tear and early thrombosis[79]; because of this problem and the risk of later stenosis, the renal artery should be trimmed 5 to 10 mm beyond the site of cannula placement. This problem is best avoided by avoiding perfusion, or always perfusing through an aortic cuff rather than with a cannula inserted in the renal artery itself.

Cyclosporine has a renal toxicity that is as yet incompletely understood but is thought to involve progressive interference with renal function. Renal toxicity may occur in the first days or weeks posttransplant or later during administration and is probably dose-related. Although some effect on the microvasculature may be part of this mechanism, this nephrotoxicity has not generally been thought to involve major blood vessels. On the other hand, occasional instances of renal artery thrombosis without warning have been found in patients receiving cyclosporine,[80] and it has been suspected that this might have been due to cyclosporine.

Renal venous thrombosis is an unusual complication in the early postoperative period. Technical problems with the venous anastomosis are quite uncommon as a cause. Some kidneys may appear to have two major venous drainage routes, and it is advisable to anastomose both of these veins if they are of equivalent size and appear to be based in separate regions of the kidney; however, renal venous drainage, unlike the arterial supply to the kidney, is not as anatomically separate, and, generally, anastomosis of one principal renal vein will drain the entire kidney quite adequately, so that this should not be a source of renal venous thrombosis. Deep venous thrombosis can occur[81] and may cause venous outflow obstruction of the transplant as well. Venous thrombosis can be effectively treated by the usual warfarin sodium (Coumadin) anticoagulation.[82] Leg edema, particularly on the side of the transplant, is not uncommon after transplantation and in view of these possible problems should be worked up aggressively. However, in the usual case, in which noninvasive tests or venography exclude thrombophlebitis, the problem is probably due to a combination of altered fluid status, prednisone therapy with salt retention, and lymphatic or relative venous obstruction in the region of the transplant. Leg edema in these cases typically will resolve as the operative inflammation and steroid dosage decrease.

Another vascular problem that may become evident soon after the operation is interference with pelvic arterial flow, producing impotence in men. Several reports document the significant risk of this problem in patients who receive one transplant on each side and in whom both internal iliac arteries are sacrificed to provide end-to-end anastomoses to the transplants.[83–85] The second transplant in the male patient should therefore always employ end-to-side anastomosis of the renal artery to the external iliac artery to preserve pelvic blood flow.

Urologic Complications

The most common urologic problem early during the course of the transplant is a leak, which may occur either from a bladder suture line or from the ureteroneocystostomy site. As noted above, if an accessory vessel occlusion presents early in the patient's course, it usually is manifest as a urine leak at about 1 week, when a necrotic area of pelvis or ureter gives way.[75–78] Urine leak in a transplant recipient has a potentially catastrophic significance, as opposed to the rather less serious consequences of this problem in the patient with an autologous kidney who is not under immunosuppression. Although successful reconstruction of a defect in the urinary tract may be possible with care,[86–88] the development of a leak puts the graft at great risk and is associated with an increased risk of death of the patient.[89–91] This problem is serious in the transplant recipient because of the difficulty with healing and the likelihood of the development of a dangerous urinary tract or wound infection.

A fluid collection found on scan or sonogram should be investigated as a possible leak, particularly if there is increasing renal dysfunction, but it may often represent a benign collection. If the fluid in a collection has had more than 1 to 2 hours to equilibrate, even if it is urine it will have roughly the same blood urea nitrogen and creatinine levels as serum, so that determination of these values on fluid aspirated from a collection does not provide a reliable indicator of whether it is urine or not. In several instances, excretion of urine into a cavity detected on radioisotopic scan has allowed diagnosis of a leak.[77, 92–94] The author has seen one case in which urinary extravasation occurred under the bladder mucosa, traveled via the retroperitoneum to the colonic mesentery, and produced intraabdominal edema, pain, and azotemia without actual extravasation of urine into a cavity.

The treatment of urine leak typically involves exploration and closure of a defect in the bladder, replacement of the ureterocystostomy, or revision or formation of a ureteropyelostomy. Omental flaps have been employed to help provide closure for pelvic and pelvicaliceal leaks.[95] In an effort to avoid urinary tract problems, some groups routinely anastomose the recipient ureter to the donor renal pelvis.[96–98] Occasionally, a direct anastomosis of the bladder to the transplant pelvis, suturing the bladder to the psoas muscle to hold it in place near the transplant, may be employed.[99, 100] Bringing the contralateral ureter across to the transplant may be helpful.[101] Partial or complete diversion with a nephrostomy tube[102–104] and a ureteral stent[105, 106] are important adjuncts to the repair of pelvicaliceal defects.

Early urinary obstruction may occur from ureteral blood clots, which will lyse spontaneously in 24 to 72 hours, or from extrinsic compression,[107] a major cause of which should be avoided by dividing the round ligament or carefully passing the ureter under the spermatic cord to the base of the bladder.

Although some posttransplant urinary tract infections develop in cases of repairs of urinary tract complications involving indwelling stents and pyelostomies, urinary tract infection is also quite common in patients with no apparent anatomical abnormality. Some have observed that asymptomatic urinary tract infections do not represent a serious threat and may not require intensive efforts at eradication,[108] but most centers have advocated vigorous measures to sterilize the urine.[109–111]

Pyelonephritis may be treated successfully if the transplant is viable.[112] The presence of antibody coating on bacteria in the urine has been reported to indicate that the infection is in the kidney, rather than merely in the bladder.[113] Anaerobic infection appears to represent a particular risk to the allograft.[114] Another infection which may represent a special risk is *Streptococcus faecalis* urinary tract infection, which may produce cross-reactive immune stimulation and potentiate allograft rejection.[115]

An Approach to Early Renal Dysfunction

If the transplant procedure was without apparent complications and the patient has begun recuperation with gradually improving function but then develops decreased urine output or worsening renal function, rejection is the most likely source of this problem. Urinary tract and other anatomical problems should be ruled out with an ultrasonic study and a radioisotopic scan. Transplant biopsy may be helpful. Unless hypertension is severe or the flow, as indicated by the scan, is seriously impaired, there is little reason to question the possibility of renal artery stenosis early in the postoperative period. Urinary tract outlet obstruction should be ruled out. Following these maneuvers, if no other source of difficulty is observed, expeditious institution of increased immunosuppression should be undertaken. Vigilance with regard to possible anatomical or infectious problems should not be relaxed during the period of rejection treatment, but reassurance that rejection is the problem will usually be obtained when improved function occurs within a few days after the additional immunosuppression is instituted. More extensive and invasive diagnostic procedures merely subject the patient and the transplant to an increased risk and are unlikely to provide much additional information.

LATE RENAL TRANSPLANT COMPLICATIONS

Late onset of worsening renal failure may represent rejection, but renal artery stenosis or urologic problems may be the culprit and should be thoughtfully sought. Late operative approach to the transplant often is best achieved by the transperitoneal route, since the artery or collecting system may be approached more directly without having to dissect the entire renal parenchyma free from the surrounding scar tissue.

Renal Artery Stenosis

A challenging technical problem is the late development of narrowing in the renal transplant artery. As the stenosis develops, it will cause increasing hypertension, but high blood pressure is very common in renal transplant recipients due to a multiplicity of causes.[116–121] Progressive severe hypertension during the first year after transplantation, particularly if accompanied by a bruit and deterioration of renal failure, should produce a strong suspicion of renal artery stenosis.[122–124] Erythrocytosis may accompany stenosis of native or transplant arteries.[125–127] Arteriography should be performed in suspect cases to determine whether renal artery stenosis has in fact developed.[128–133] The etiology of the stenosis is usually thickening of the arterial wall, either at the anastomosis or nearby in an area of turbulence. Another important, preventable complication is the inclusion of an arterial segment that has had a perfusion cannula placed in it.[134] It has also been suggested that renal artery stenosis may stem from immunologic injury of the arterial intima.[134] A stenosis may form at the site of previous vascular clamps due to traumatic arterial occlusion during the transplant procedure.[136] Even if renal arterial stenosis of a significant degree is noted on angiography, hypertension may be secondary to the autologous kidneys if they have not been removed,[121] and this issue should be considered very carefully before addressing the transplant as the source of hypertension.

If treatment of a transplant arterial stenosis is necessary, the treatment of choice is an interposition bypass graft between the iliac artery and an area of normal renal artery beyond the stenosis[137–139] (Fig 15–2), but revascularization represents some threat to the kidney and therefore is best reserved for cases with unmanageable hypertension, a rather tight stenosis angiographically, or deteriorating renal function due to the stenosis.[140, 141] Furthermore, a remarkable number of cases have documented actual regression of the stenosis; this might occasionally be artifactual due to a misleading arteriogram but seems likely to have actually occurred in several instances.[142–144] The use of transluminal angioplasty is dangerous, because occlusion of the renal artery as a complication of this procedure is more likely to cause renal infarction than in the native state, since there is no collateral flow to the transplant. However, good results have been obtained in many instances with percutaneous transluminal angioplasty.[145]

Ureteral Reflux and Stenosis

The usual ureteroneocystostomy is performed using a tunneled course for the ureter, as in the Leadbetter-Politano technique. There is some suspicion that late ureteral complications occur if this reimplant is not effective in prevention of reflux[146]; however, it is possible to obtain good results with a simple insertion of the ureter into the bladder without an attempt at tunneling,[147] and, furthermore, some centers have documented the fact that reflux does not cause long-term problems.[148, 149] If major reflux either in native ureters or in the transplant ureter seems to be associated with recurrent urinary tract infections, correction may be indicated, but otherwise, if reflux is detected, there is no convincing indication for intervention.

If the arterial supply to the lower ureter is compromised partially, but not suf-

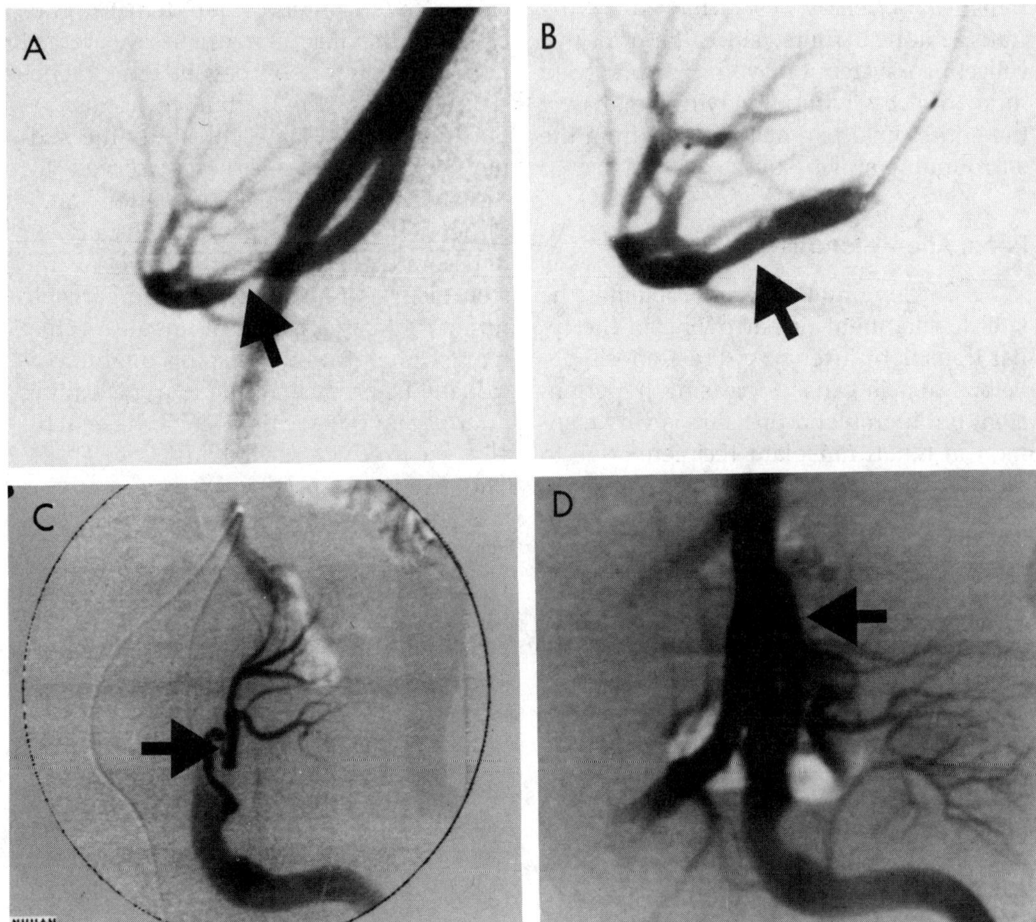

FIG 15–2.
Treatment of renal transplant arterial stenosis. **A,** stenosis in the vicinity of an end-to-end internal iliac-to-renal artery anastomosis (*arrow;* stenotic area); **B,** the lesion shown in **A,** after transluminal angioplasty (*arrow;* site of dilated stenosis); (**A** and **B** from Kadir S: *Angioplasty.* New York, McGraw-Hill Publishers. Used by permission.) **C,** a lesion in a tortuous area of a long renal artery (*arrow:* site of stenosis); **D,** external iliac-to-renal artery saphenous vein bypass graft (end-to-side at both ends) (*arrow* indicates the graft).

ficiently to cause a major renal pelvic or ureteral catastrophe early in the transplant course, then distal ureteric fibrosis may ensue subsequently.[150–153] This diagnosis should always be suspected if late rejection appears to be developing[150] and may be investigated definitively by the use of percutaneous antegrade perfusion, by which it is possible to obtain an excellent pyelogram and measurement of pressure within the collecting system.[154] Risk of late fibrosis due to inadequate blood supply is minimized by making the ureter no longer than necessary. Correction is usually by anastomosis of the recipient ureter to the transplant ureter or pelvis above the strictured area, employing temporary drainage similar to that described above for early urologic complications.

Stones

The development of calculi in the collecting system of the renal transplant is frequently associated with bacteriuria[155, 156] or hypercalcemia due to persistent hyperparathyroidism.[156, 157] Calculi are probably more common in patients with previous lower tract problems and with implantation of the transplant ureter into an ileal conduit.[158] However, calculi may occur in the absence of any apparent underlying cause in the transplant recipient.[159, 160] Extraction of the stones and correction of any other underlying problems is generally reported to produce excellent long-term results.[161, 162]

PERCUTANEOUS BIOPSY OF THE RENAL TRANSPLANT

The renal transplant is almost always easily accessible for percutaneous biopsy at the bedside. Initial palpation should be performed to define the position of the kidney, and the biopsy should be directed toward the upper pole, as depicted in Figure 15–3. After initial preparation and draping, local anesthesia is infiltrated down through the fascial layers. With care, complete anesthesia can be achieved in most patients so that the procedure is quite painless. The peritoneum is best avoided if the biopsy is performed laterally. The biopsy is aided by a previous medial orientation of the original incision at the time of transplantation, so that the fold of peritoneum does not extend over much of the anterior transplant surface. Particular care is necessary in patients whose peritoneal space has been expanded by chronic peritoneal dialysis. A tiny skin incision is made with a No. 11 scalpel blade, and then the biopsy needle (e.g., Tru-Cut, Travenol Laboratories, Inc.) is advanced through the subcutaneous tissue and through the fascia. Particularly after several weeks posttransplant, the tip of the needle meets firm resistance in traversing the lower fascial plane. The needle must be pushed firmly through the fascia, but as soon as it "pops"

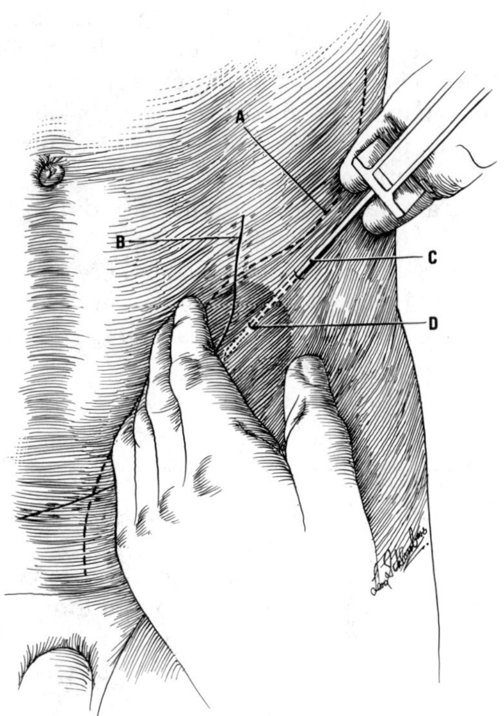

FIG 15–3.
Percutaneous transplant biopsy technique: *A,* fold of peritoneum with needle inserted lateral to this; *B,* healed transplant incision; *C,* biopsy needle; and *D,* insertion site in upper pole of the kidney, well away from the hilum and preferably lateral to the transplant incision and peritoneal fold.

through and again meets little resistance, advancement of the entire assembly is halted. The internal portion is then advanced into the renal parenchyma, followed by advancement of the sleeve and then withdrawal of the entire needle, which contains the biopsy. One or two passes of this sort should suffice, and multiple unsuccessful attempts may endanger the transplant. Transient skin bleeding or hematuria are occasionally produced.

In a large series of such biopsies, including over 30 on a routine protocol,[4] the most serious complication was several hours of anuria due to a ureteral clot, which then passed spontaneously. Damage serious enough to require exploration or even endanger the transplant from urine leak or bleeding is a conceivable complication, and, although it has not been reported, intrarenal aneurysm due to trauma could theoretically occur later. In fact, this is an extremely safe procedure when performed as described. In patients who are quite obese or otherwise difficult to biopsy, sonographic guidance may be useful, but it is not usually necessary. Open biopsy may be performed under local anesthesia if the percutaneous route proves too difficult.

COMPLICATIONS OF LIVE-DONOR TRANSPLANT NEPHRECTOMY

Careful exploration of the live donor and removal of the kidney is performed via a technique similar to that for a radical nephrectomy, but with entry into Gerota's fascia and the perirenal space. Care should be taken not to dissect extensively near the hilum of the kidney, but rather carry the dissection toward the great vessels, liberally including hilar fat so that the aorta on the left or the vena cava on the right is well delineated prior to the division of the vessels. Excessive traction and pressure on the kidney should be avoided to minimize vasospasm in the renal parenchyma. Excellent diuresis should be produced by administration of mannitol or furosemide during the dissection. The ureter should be dissected with the periureteral tissues incorporated liberally, past the level of the iliac artery. After a good length of ureter has been obtained, it can be ligated as distally as possible and divided. The dissection should attempt to provide an adequate length of the donor renal artery and vein without endangering the recipient. Accessory or multiple vessels are generally detected on the preoperative arteriogram, but the nephrectomy should be performed with the expectation of encountering such vessels, since they are not always clearly demonstrated on arteriogram. Accessory vessels should be divided with as much length as possible, and the transplanting surgeon will then have to determine whether anastomosis to the main renal artery or separately to the external iliac artery will be appropriate for revascularization. As with cadaver donor kidneys, accessory vessels to the lower pole are critically important in maintaining good perfusion of the collecting system in the renal transplant, which has no collateral arterial circulation to the ureter. It should next be ensured that the surgeons receiving the transplant are prepared to place it in iced saline and perfuse it appropriately. Careful division of the vessels, using clamps and an unhurried systematic approach, is mandatory for avoiding damage to the kidney or a bleeding catastrophe in the recipient. The minimal warm ischemia that this may entail is of no consequence. Suture ligation plus a tie, or, in some cases on the vein, a running suture closure, are necessary for safe hemostasis.

Common complications after live-donor nephrectomy include myocardial infarction, brachial plexus injury, ileus, pneumonia, and urinary tract infection.[163] Caution with regard to these possibilities will help to minimize the chance of any unfortunate event occurring as a complication of this very special operative procedure.

COMPLICATIONS OF TRANSPLANT NEPHRECTOMY

If the transplant is to be removed within a few days of transplantation, merely reopening the incision and dividing the vessels and ureter between ties is appropriate. If the transplant incision has had more time than this to heal, the technique described by Sutherland et al. is the method of choice.[164] Intracapsular dissection, allowing eventual delivery of the kidney gently through the incision and placement of a large, full-size Kelly clamp on the hilum, followed by resection of most of the renal parenchyma, transforms this otherwise totally unpleasant operation into a rapid, well-controlled procedure involving minimal blood loss. After the parenchyma has been excised, a suture is placed at one end underneath the clamp and tied firmly; it is then run back and forth underneath the clamp to the far end, after which the clamp is released with care. The suture is then run over and back along the line of hilar structures and tied at the original end. Transplant nephrectomy is often performed in a patient at the end of a long course of major immunosuppression, perhaps with infectious or metabolic complications, and this expeditious technique is of great value in minimizing the risk in these ill patients. The small residuum of retained hilar structures has caused no postoperative complication and engendered no difficulty during retransplantation in the author's experience.

The most serious complication after transplant nephrectomy occurs when an external iliac arterial anastomosis was performed at transplantation. Infection extending to this anastomosis in an infected wound after transplant nephrectomy has produced many cases of life-threatening or fatal hemorrhage.[165, 166] Ligation of this artery may often be possible without limb-threatening ischemia, to be followed by later revascularization, in situations where a bleed from the suture line has occurred or is threatened. It should be noted that routine graft nephrectomy is not always necessary after the transplant has undergone terminal rejection, since immunosuppressive therapy can gradually be tapered and withdrawn completely without problems in many patients.

It is hoped that, with improvements in immunosuppression, extensive experience with transplant nephrectomy is becoming an anachronism.

EDITORIAL COMMENT

Perioperative and postoperative complications are outlined in detail in this chapter. The late complications of ureteral stenosis may be mediated by compromise of the microvasculature of the distal ureter, but I have often thought that chronic rejection may be responsible for some of these microvasculature changes in the long-term distal ureteral stenosis of the transplant ureter. Any distal ureteral complication is usually best managed by a pelvis (transplant)-to-ureter (recipient) anastomosis.

In general, it is still probably better to try to obtain an antireflux component to the ureteroneocystostomy rather than just a direct reimplant at the time of the original transplant. Over a period of time, massive reflux can provide stasis in the urinary tract and increase the propensity for infection and subsequent problems. We have also seen stones in patients with renal transplants, including a calculus on small nylon suture in a patient who underwent ureteroureterostomy. Also, we have had patients who have had ileal conduits and renal transplants with calculi. When mucus refluxes from the conduit into the kidney, it can provide a nidus for struvite calculus formation. Finally, we have had one patient with recurrent probable xanthine stones.

Patients with a variety of congenital anomalies of the lower urinary tract have still been transplanted.[*] A patient with previously unrecognized posterior urethral valves has undergone a successful transplant.[†] In addition, a patient with exstrophy has had a transplant with a ureteral anastomo-

[*]Marshall FF, Smolev JK, Spees EH, et al: Urological evaluation and management of patients with congenital lower urinary tract anomalies prior to renal transplantation. *J Urol* 1982; 127:1078.

[†]Marshall FF, Mueller SC: Spectrum of unrecognized posterior urethral valves in the adult. *Urology* 1983; 22:139.

sis to the bladder. Other forms of urinary diversion with ileal conduits have also been employed with renal transplantation.

EDITORIAL COMMENT II

As our population ages, an increasing number of patients will develop chronic renal failure. Even in diabetics survival appears to be improved with the use of renal transplantation rather than chronic dialysis. Cyclosporine has made significant impact in the reduction of rejection.

REFERENCES

1. Morris PJ: *Kidney Transplantation Principles and Practice.* New York, Grune & Stratton, 1984.
2. Najarian JS, Bach FH, Sutherland DER: Proceedings of the Tenth International Congress of The Transplantation Society. *Transplant Proc* 1985; 17(1).
3. Simmons RL, Finch ME, Ascher NL, et al: *Manual of Vascular Access, Organ Donation, and Transplantation.* New York, Springer-Verlag New York, 1984.
4. Burdick JF, Beschorner WE, Smith WJ, et al: Characteristics of early routine renal allograft biopsies. *Transplantation* 1984; 38:679.
5. Banowsky LH: Current results and future expectations in renal transplantation. *Urol Clin North Am* 1983; 10:337.
6. Kahan B (ed): Proceedings of the Second International Congress on Cyclosporine. *Transplant Proc* 1988; 20(suppl 2).
7. Fine RN: Renal transplantation update. *Ann Intern Med* 1984; 100:246.
8. Calman KC, Bell PR, Briggs JD, et al: Bilateral nephrectomy prior to renal transplantation. *Br J Surg* 1976; 63:512.
9. Bennett WM: Cost-benefit ratio of pretransplant bilateral nephrectomy. *JAMA* 1976; 235:1703.
10. Pechan W, Novick AC, Braun WE, et al: Management of end stage polycystic kidney disease with renal transplantation. *J Urol* 1981; 125:622.
11. Maley WR, Williams GM, Colombani P, et al: Simple instrument occlusion of the anterior visceral branches of the aorta during en bloc renal allograft procurement. *Surg Gynecol Obstet* 1988; 167:442.
12. Vaziri ND, Barton CH, Ravikumar GR, et al: Femoral neuropathy: A complication of renal transplantation. *Nephron* 1981; 28:30.
13. Sisto D, Chiu WS, Geelhoed GW, et al: Femoral neuropathy after renal transplantation. *South Med J* 1980; 73:1464.
14. Vaziri ND, Barnes J, Khosrow M, et al: Compression neuropathy subsequent to renal transplantation. *Urology* 1976; 7:145.
15. Solez K, Williams GM: Hyperacute rejection and perfusion injury, in Williams GM, Burdick JFG, Solez K (eds): *Kidney Transplant Rejection: Diagnosis and Treatment,* in press, 1986.
16. Russo VR, Marks C: Renal transplantation: An analysis of operative complications. *Am Surg* 1976; 42:153.
17. Margolis DM, Etheredge EE, Garza-Garza R, et al: Ischemic bowel disease following bilateral nephrectomy or renal transplant. *Surgery* 1977; 82:667.
18. Carson SD, Krom RA, Uchida K, et al: Colon perforation after kidney transplantation. *Ann Surg* 1978; 188:109.
19. Romolo JL, Williams GM: Effect of Kayexalate and sorbitol on colon of normal and uremic rats. *Surg Forum* 1979; 30:369.
20. Kjelstrand CM, Casali RE, Simmons RL, et al: Etiology and prognosis in acute post-transplant renal failure. *Am J Med* 1976; 61:190.
21. Lopatkin NA, Gleizer YY, Jarmolinski JS, et al: Radioisotope studies in the diagnosis of acute complications in the post-transplantation stage. *Int Urol Nephrol* 1980; 12:169.
22. Kim YC, Massari PU, Brown ML, et al: Clinical significance of 99m technetium sulfur colloid accumulation in renal transplant patients. *Radiology* 1977; 124:745.
23. Leonard JC, Baumann WE, Pederson JA, et al: 99m technetium sulfur colloid scanning in diagnosis of transplant rejection. *J Urol* 1980; 123:815.

24. Petrek J, Tilney NL, Smith EH, et al: Ultrasound in renal transplantation. *Ann Surg* 1977; 185:441.
25. van der Vliet JA, Kootstra G, Tegzess AM, et al: Management of rupture in allografted kidneys. *Neth J Surg* 1980; 32:45.
26. Van Cangh PJ, Ehrlich RM, Smith RB: Renal rupture after transplantation. *Urology* 1977; 9:8.
27. Prompt CA, Johnson WH, Ehrlich RM, et al: Nontraumatic rupture of renal allografts. *Urology* 1979; 13:145.
28. Nghiem DD, Corry RJ: Long-term result of conservative surgical management of the ruptured renal transplant. *Am Surg* 1983; 49:392.
29. Susan LP, Braun WE, Banowsky LH, et al: Ruptured human renal allograft. Pathogenesis and management. *Urology* 1978; 11:53.
30. Thukral R, Mir AR, Jacobson MP: Renal allograft rupture: A report of three cases and review of the literature. *Am J Nephrol* 1982; 2:15.
31. Brekke I, Flatmark A, Laane B, et al: Renal allograft rupture. *Scand J Urol Nephrol* 1978; 12:265.
32. Koene RA, Skotnicki SH, Debruyne FM: Spontaneous renal decapsulation with excessive fluid leakage after transplantation. *N Engl J Med* 1979; 300:1030.
33. McHenry MC, Braun WE, Popowniak KL, et al: Septicemia in renal transplant recipients. *Urol Clin North Am* 1976; 3:647.
34. Doig RL, Boyd PJ, Eykyn S: *Staphylococcus aureus* transmitted in transplanted kidneys. *Lancet* 1975; 2:243.
35. Bore PJ, Basu PK, Rudge CJ, et al: Contaminated renal allografts. *Arch Surg* 1980; 115:755.
36. McCoy GC, Loening S, Braun WE, et al: The fate of cadaver renal allografts contaminating before transplantation. *Transplantation* 1975; 20:467.
37. Walter S, Pedersen FB, Vejlsgaard R: Urinary tract infection and wound infection in kidney transplant patients. *Br J Urol* 1975; 47:513.
38. Lobo PI, Rudolf LE, Krieger JN: Wound infections in renal transplant recipients—a complication of urinary tract infections during allograft malfunction. *Surgery* 1982; 92:491.
39. Schroter GP, West JC, Weil R III: Acute bacteremia in asplenic renal transplant patients. *JAMA* 1977; 237:2207.
40. Chiffoleau S, Chatal JF, Talmant C, et al: The respective roles of gallium 67 citrate scanning and diagnostic ultrasound in detecting suppurations in renal allograft recipients. *Pathol Biol* 1980; 28:155.
41. Bia MJ, Baggish D, Katz L, et al: Computed tomography in the diagnosis of pelvic abscesses in renal transplant patients. *JAMA* 1981; 246:1435.
42. Morley P, Barnett E, Bell PR, et al: Ultrasound in the diagnosis of fluid collections following renal transplantation. *Clin Radiol* 1975; 26:199.
43. Lipshultz LI, Barker CF, Wein AJ, et al: Post-transplantation lymphocyst: Use of ultrasound as adjunct in diagnosis. *Urology* 1976; 8:624.
44. Phillips JF, Neiman HL, Brown TL: Ultrasound diagnosis of posttransplant and renal lymphocele. *Am J Roentgenol* 1976; 126:1194.
45. Bartrum RJ Jr, Smith EH, D'Orsi DJ, et al: Evaluation of renal transplants with ultrasound. *Radiology* 1976; 118:405.
46. Burt RW, Reddy RK: Evaluation of nuclear imaging for detecting posttransplant fluid collection. *Am J Res* 1979; 133:91.
47. Spigos DG, Tan W, Pavel DG, et al: Diagnosis of urine extravasation after renal transplantation. *Am J Res* 1977; 129:409.
48. Corcoran RJ, Thrall JH, Kaminski RJ, et al: Body-background defects with 99mTc-DTPA after renal transplantation: Case reports. *J Nucl Med* 1976; 17:696.
49. Bingham JB, Hilson AJ, Maisey MN: The appearances of renal transplant lymphoceles during dynamic renal scintigraphy. *Br J Radiol* 1978; 51:342.
50. Donaldson RA, Jacobson JE, Pontin A: Fluid collections associated with renal allografts. *S Afr Med J* 1978; 53:51.
51. Yap R, Madrazo B, Oh HK, et al: Perirenal fluid collection after renal transplant. *Am Surg* 1981; 47:287.
52. McLoughlin MG, Williams GM: Late perirenal lymphocele causing ureteral and

arterial obstruction in renal transplant patients. *J Urol* 1975; 114:527.
53. Koehler PR, Kanemoto HH, Maxwell JG: Ultrasonic "B" scanning in the diagnosis of complications in renal transplant patients. *Radiology* 1976; 119:661.
54. Brockis JG, Hulbert JC, Patel AS, et al: The diagnosis and treatment of lymphoceles associated with renal transplantation. A report of 6 cases and a review of the literature. *Br J Urol* 1978; 50:307.
55. Kristiansen JH, Rohr N: Lymphocele as a complication of renal transplantation. *Int Urol Nephrol* 1980; 12:225.
56. Pontes JE, McDonald FD, Midgal SD, et al: Lymphatic complications in renal allografts—a new look. *Urology* 1981; 17:26.
57. Howard RJ, Simmons RL, Najarian JS: Prevention of lymphoceles following renal transplantation. *Ann Surg* 1976; 18:166.
58. Lindstedt E, Lindholm T, Gustavson J: Lymphocele: An important posttransplantation complication. *Scand J Urol Nephrol* 1976; 10:94.
59. Griffiths AB, Fletcher EW, Morris PJ: Lymphocele after renal transplantation. *Aust NZ J Surg* 1979; 49:626.
60. Ward K, Klingensmith WC III, Sterioff S, et al: The origin of lymphoceles following renal transplantation. *Transplantation* 1978; 25:346.
61. Spigos D, Capek V: Ultrasonically guided percutaneous aspiration of lymphoceles following renal transplantation: A diagnostic and therapeutic method. *J Clin Ultrasound* 1976; 4:45.
62. McDonald DG, Libertino JA: Ultrasound in diagnosis and evaluation of lymphoceles after renal transplantation. *Urology* 1976; 7:216.
63. Sodal G, Flatmark A: Surgical treatment of lymphoceles. *Scand J Urol Nephrol* 1975; 6:75.
64. Bear RA, McCallum RW, Cant J, et al: Perirenal lymphocyst formation in renal transplant recipients: Diagnosis and pathogenesis. *Urology* 1976; 7:581.
65. Meyers A, Salant D, Rabkin R, et al: Lymphoceles in renal homograft recipients. *Proc Eur Dial Transplant Assoc* 1976; 12:452.
66. Schweizer RT, Bartus SA, Foster JH: Treatment of pelvic lymphoceles after renal transplantation by intraperitoneal marsupialization. *Am Surg* 1976; 42:316.
67. Goldman HM, Tilney NL, Vineyard GC, et al: A twenty-year survey of arterial complications of renal transplantation. *Surg Gynecol Obstet* 1975; 141:758.
68. Palleschi J, Novick AC, Braun WE, et al: Vascular complications of renal transplantation. *Urology* 1980; 16:61.
69. Cromie WJ, Jordan MH, Leapman SB: Pseudorejection: The Page kidney phenomenon in renal allografts. *J Urol* 1976; 116:658.
70. Vidne BA, Leapman SB, Butt KM, et al: Vascular complications in human renal transplantation. *Surgery* 1976; 79:77.
71. Nissen HM, Sorensen BL, Wolf H, et al: Sudden massive hemorrhage after renal transplantation. *Scand J Urol Nephrol* 1975; 9:273.
72. Oesterwitz H, Althaus P, Scholz D, et al: Experimental and clinical application of microsurgery in kidney transplants. *Acta Urol* 1983; 51:385.
73. Fox M, Yalin R: Renal transplantation with multiple arteries. *Br J Urol* 1979; 51:333.
74. Merkel FK, Straus AK, Anderson O, et al: Microvascular techniques for polar artery reconstruction in kidney transplants. *Surgery* 1976; 79:253.
75. Goldman MH, Burleson RL, Tilney NL, et al: Calyceal-cutaneous fistulae in renal transplant patients. *Ann Surg* 1976; 184:679.
76. Palmer JM, Chatterjee SN: Urologic complications in renal transplantation. *Surg Clin North Am* 1978; 58:305.
77. Salvatierra O, Olcott C, Amend WJ, et al: Urological complications of renal transplantation can be prevented or controlled. *J Urol* 1977; 117:421.
78. Schiff M, McGuire EJ, Webster J: Successful management of caliceal fistulas following renal transplantation. *Arch Surg* 1975; 110:1129.
79. Braf ZF, Horowitz A: Intimal tear, cause of transplant failure. *Br J Urol* 1978; 50:52.
80. Green L, Verani R, Schoenberg L, et al: Comparative pathological review of 72

renal transplant nephrectomies of patients treated with cyclosporine or azathioprine (abstract). Presented at the American Society of Nephrology, Dec 9–12, 1984.
81. Joffe SN: Deep vein thrombosis after renal transplantation. *Vasc Surg* 1976; 10:134.
82. Golden J, Stone RA, Goldberger L: Immune-related renal vein thrombosis in a renal allograft. *Ann Intern Med* 1976; 85:612.
83. Burns JR, Houttuin E, Gregory JG, et al: Vascular-induced erectile impotence in renal transplant recipients. *J Urol* 1979; 121:721.
84. Gittes RF, Waters WB: Sexual impotence: The overlooked complication of a second renal transplant. *J Urol* 1979; 121:719.
85. Billet A, Davis A, Linhardt GE Jr, et al: Effects of bilateral renal transplantation on pelvic hemodynamics and sexual function. *Surgery* 1984; 95:415.
86. McLoughlin MG: The ureter in pediatric renal allotransplantation. *J Urol* 1977; 118:1041.
87. Mehta SM, Kennedy JA, Loughridge WG: Urological complications in 119 consecutive renal transplants. *Br J Urol* 1979; 51:184.
88. Dabhoiwala NF, Ten Cate HW, Linschoten H: Conservative surgical management of urological complications after cadaveric renal transplantation. *J Urol* 1978; 120:290.
89. Waltzer WC, Woods JE, Zincke H, et al: Urinary tract reconstruction in renal transplantation. Mayo clinic experience and review of literature. *Urology* 1980; 16:233.
90. Holden S, O'Brien DP III, Lewis EL, et al: Urologic complications in renal transplantation. *Urology* 1975; 5:182.
91. Pfeffermann R, Vidne B, Leapman S, et al: Urologic complications in renal primary and retransplantation. Experience with 202 consecutive transplants. *Am J Surg* 1976; 131:242.
92. Haden HT, Stacy WK, Wolf JS, et al: Scintiphotography in diagnosis of urinary fistula after renal transplantation. *J Nucl Med* 1975; 16:612.
93. Texter JH Jr, Haden H: Scintiphotography in the early diagnosis of urine leakage following renal transplantation. *J Urol* 1976; 116:547.
94. DeLange EE, Pauwels EK, Lobatto S: Scintigraphic detection of urinary leakage after kidney transplantation. *Eur J Nucl Med* 1982; 7:55.
95. Linke CA, Cockett AT, Lai MK, et al: The use of pedicled grafts of omentum in the repair of transplant-related urinary tract problems. *J Urol* 1978; 120:532.
96. Donohue JP, Hostetter M, Glover J, et al: Ureteroneocystostomy versus ureteropyelostomy: A comparison in the same renal allograft series. *J Urol* 1975; 114:202.
97. Greenberg SH, Wain AJ, Perloff LJ, et al: Ureteropyelostomy and ureteroneocystostomy in renal transplantation: Postoperative urological complications. *J Urol* 1977; 118:17.
98. Whelchel DJ, Cosimi AB, Young HH II, et al: Pyeloureterostomy reconstruction in human renal transplantation. *Ann Surg* 1975; 181:61.
99. Cook GT, Cant JD, Crassweller PO, et al: Urinary fistulas after renal transplantation. *J Urol* 1977; 118:20.
100. Lindstedt E, Bergentz SE, Lindholm T: Long-term clinical follow-up after pyelocystostomy. *J Urol* 1981; 126:253.
101. Martelli A, Reggiani A, Buli P: Post-transplantation ureteral stricture: Contralateral pyelocalicostomy. *Eur Urol* 1979; 5:330.
102. Kim CH, Fjeldborg OC: A modified nephrostomy in the management of urinary fistula after renal transplantation. *Scand J Urol Nephrol* 1975; 9:269.
103. Brockis JG, Golinger D, Haywood EF, et al: The management of urinary fistulae following cadaveric renal transplantation. *Br J Urol* 1975; 47:371.
104. Goldstein I, Cho SI, Olsson CA: Nephrostomy drainage for renal transplant complications. *J Urol* 1981; 126:159.
105. Tremann JA, Marchioro TL: Gibbons ureteral stent in renal transplant recipients. *Urology* 1977; 9:390.
106. Berger RE, Ansell JS, Tremann JA, et al: The use of self-retained ureteral stents in the management of urologic complications in renal transplant recipients. *J Urol* 1980; 124:781.

107. Donaldson RA, Jacobson JE, Pontin AR: Ureteric obstruction in renal allograft recipients. *S Afr Med J* 1977; 52:1077.
108. Griffin PJ, Salaman JR: Urinary tract infections after renal transplantation: Do they matter? *Br Med J* 1979; 1:710.
109. Krieger JN, Tapia L, Stubenbord WT, et al: Urinary infection in kidney transplantation. *Urology* 1977; 9:130.
110. Krieger JN, Brem AS, Kaplan MR: Urinary tract infection in pediatric renal transplantation. *Urology* 1980; 15:362.
111. Ramos E, Karmi S, Alongi SV, et al: Infectious complications in renal transplant recipients. *South Med J* 1980; 73:751.
112. Pearson JC, Amend WJ Jr, Vincenti FG, et al: Posttransplantation pyelonephritis: Factors producing low patient and transplant morbidity. *J Urol* 1980; 123:153.
113. Keren DF, Nightingale SD, Hamilton CL, et al: Antibody-coated bacteria as an indicator of the site of urinary tract infection in renal transplant recipients receiving immunosuppressive agents. *Am J Med* 1977; 63:855.
114. Krieger JN, Senterfit L, Muecke EC, et al: Anaerobic bacteriuria in renal transplantation. *Urology* 1978; 12:635.
115. Byrd LH, Tapia L, Cheigh JS, et al: Association between *Streptococcus faecalis* urinary infections and graft rejection in kidney transplantation. *Lancet* 1978; 2:1167.
116. Bachy C, van Ypersele de Strihou C, Alexandre GP, et al: Hypertension after renal transplantation. *Proc Eur Dial Transplant Assoc* 1976; 12:461.
117. Jacquot C, Idatte JM, Bedrossian J, et al: Long-term blood pressure changes in renal homotransplantation. *Arch Intern Med* 1978; 138:233.
118. Sufrin G, Kirdani R, Sandberg AA, et al: Studies of renin-aldosterone axis in stable normotensive and hypertensive renal allograft recipients. *Urology* 1978; 11:46.
119. Ingelfinger JR, Grupe WE, Levey RH: Post-transplant hypertension in the absence of rejection or recurrent disease. *Clin Nephrol* 1981; 15:236.
120. Kim KE, Bates O, Lyons P, et al: Haemodynamics of stable renal transplant recipients. *Clin Sci* [Suppl] 1980; 6:377s.
121. McHugh MI, Tanboga H, Marcen R, et al: Hypertension following renal transplantation: The role of the host's kidney. *Q J Med* 1980; 49:395.
122. Pedersen EB, Kornerup HJ: The renin-aldosterone system and renal hemodynamics in patients with posttransplant hypertension. *Acta Med Scand* 1976; 200:501.
123. Whelton PK, Russell RP, Harrington DP, et al: Hypertension following renal transplantation. Causative factors and therapeutic implications. *JAMA* 1979; 241:1128.
124. Stribrna J, Zabka J, Belan A, et al: Renal artery stenosis of the transplanted kidney. Diagnosis and therapy of the hypertension. *Czech Med* 1981; 4:55.
125. Bacon BR, Rothman SA, Ricanati ES, et al: Renal artery stenosis with erythrocytosis after renal transplantation. *Arch Intern Med* 1980; 140:1206.
126. Dagher FJ, Ramos E, Erslev A, et al: Erythrocytosis after renal allotransplantation: treatment by removal of the native kidneys. *South Med J* 1980; 73:940.
127. Dagher FJ, Ramos E, Erslev A, et al: Are the native kidneys responsible for erythrocytosis in renal allorecipients? *Transplantation* 1979; 28:496.
128. Boltuch RL, Alfidi RJ: Selective renal angiography: Its value in renal transplantation. *Urol Clin North Am* 1976; 3:611.
129. Levin E, Meyers AM, Salant DJ, et al: Angiography after renal homotransplantation. *S Afr Med J* 1976; 50:1295.
130. Schacht RA, Martin DG, Karalakulasingam R, et al: Renal artery stenosis after renal transplantation. *Am J Surg* 1976; 131:653.
131. Beachley MC, Pierce JC, Boykin JV, et al: The angiographic evaluation of human renal allotransplants. Functional graft deterioration and hypertension. *Arch Surg* 1976; 111:134.
132. Klarskov P, Brendstrup L, Krarup T, et al: Renovascular hypertension after kidney transplantation. *Scand J Urol Nephrol* 1979; 13:291.
133. Jones BJ, Palmer FJ, Charlesworth JA, et al: Angiography in the diagnosis of renal allograft dysfunction. *J Urol* 1978; 119:461.
134. Oakes DD, Spees EK Jr, Light JA, et al: Renal perfusion preservation without

cannulation. Prevention of posttransplantation renal artery stenosis. *Arch Surg* 1978; 113:654.
135. Kaufman JJ, Ehrlich RM, Dornfeld L: Immunologic considerations in renovascular hypertension. *Trans Am Assoc Genitourin Surg* 1975; 67:40.
136. Frodin L, Thorarinsson H, Willen R: Preanastomotic arterial stenosis in renal transport recipients. A report of four cases. *Scand J Urol Nephrol* 1975; 9:66.
137. Lindfors O, Laasonen L, Fyhrquist F, et al: Renal artery stenosis in hypertensive renal transplant recipients. *J Urol* 1977; 118:240.
138. Ricotta JJ, Schaff HV, Williams GM, et al: Renal artery stenosis following transplantation: Etiology, diagnosis, and prevention. *Surgery* 1978; 84:595.
139. Hsu AC, Balfe JW, Olley PM, et al: Allograft renal-artery stenosis: Increased peripheral plasma renin activity as an early indicator of uncontrollable hypertension. *Clin Nephrol* 1978; 10:232.
140. Smith RB, Cosimi AB, Lordon R, et al: Diagnosis and management of arterial stenosis causing hypertension after successful renal transplantation. *J Urol* 1976; 115:639.
141. Jachuck SJ, Wilkinson R, Uldall PR, et al: The medical management of renal artery stenosis in transplant recipients. *Br J Surg* 1979; 66:19.
142. Cautrebande J, Pirson Y, van Ypersele de Strihou C, et al: Reversible renal artery stenosis in renal transplantation. *Urology* 1979; 13:529.
143. Vegter AJ, Bosch E, Westra D, et al: Spontaneous reversible renal artery stenosis after renal allotransplantation. *Br Med J* 1978; 1:1028.
144. Stensma-Vegter AJ, Krediet RT, Westra D, et al: Reversible stenosis of the renal artery in cadaver kidney grafts: A report of three cases. *Clin Nephrol* 1981; 15:102.
145. Gerlock AJ Jr, MacDonell RC Jr, Smith CW, et al: Renal transplant arterial stenosis: Percutaneous transluminal angioplasty. *Am J Res* 1983; 140:325.
146. Mathew TH, Kincaid-Smith P, Vikraman P: Risks of vesicoureteric reflux in the transplanted kidney. *N Engl J Med* 1977; 297:414.
147. McDonald JC, Rohr MS, Frentz GD: External ureteroneocystostomy and ureteroureterostomy in renal transplantation. *Ann Surg* 1979; 190:663.
148. Debruyne FM, Wijdeveld PG, Koene RA, et al: Ureteroneocystostomy in renal transplantation: Is an antireflux mechanism mandatory? *Br J Urol* 1978; 50:378.
149. McMorrow RG, Curtis JJ, Lucas BA, et al: Does vesicoureteric reflux result in renal allograft failure? *Clin Nephrol* 1980; 14:89.
150. Zincke H, Woods JE, Hattery RR, et al: Late ureteral obstruction mimicking rejection after renal transplantation. *Urology* 1977; 9:504.
151. Schweizer RT, Bartus SA, Kahn CS: Fibrosis of a renal transplant ureter. *J Urol* 1977; 117:125.
152. Smolev JK, McLoughlin MG, Rolley R, et al: The surgical approach to urological complications in renal allotransplant recipients. *J Urol* 1977; 117:10.
153. LaMasters D, Katzberg RW, Confer DJ, et al: Ureteropelvic fibrosis in renal transplants: Radiographic manifestations. *Am J Res* 1980; 135:79.
154. Schiff M Jr, Rosenfield AT, McGuire EJ: The use of percutaneous antegrade renal perfusion in kidney transplant recipients. *J Urol* 1979; 122:246.
155. Brien G, Scholz D, Oesterwitz H, et al: Urolithiasis after kidney transplantation—clinical and mineralogical aspects. *Urol Res* 1980; 8:211.
156. Lucas BS, Castro JE: Calculi in renal transplants. *Br J Urol* 1978; 50:302.
157. Christensen MS, Nielsen HE, Torring S: Hypercalcemia and parathyroid function after renal transplantation. *Acta Med Scand* 1977; 201:35.
158. Rattiazzi LC, Simmons RL, Markland C, et al: Calculi complicating renal transplantation into ileal conduits. *Urology* 1975; 5:29.
159. Braren V, McNamara TC, Johnson HK, et al: Urinary tract calculous disease after renal transplantation. *Urology* 1978; 12:402.
160. Shackford S, Collins GM, Kaplan G, et al: Idiopathic ureterolithiasis in a renal transplant patient. *J Urol* 1976; 116:660.
161. Leapman SB, Vidne BA, Butt KM, et al:

Nephrolithiasis and nephrocalcinosis after renal transplantation: A case report and review of the literature. *J Urol* 1976; 115:129.

162. Schweizer RT, Bartus SA, Graydon RJ, et al: Pyelolithotomy of a renal transplant. *J Urol* 1977; 117:665.
163. Jacobs SC, McLaughlin AP III, Halasz NH, et al: Live donor nephrectomy. *Urology* 1975; 5:175.
164. Sutherland DER, Simmons RL, Howard RJ, et al: Intracapsular technique of transplant nephrectomy. *Surg Gynecol Obstet* 1978; 146:950.
165. Mosley JG, Castro JE: Arterial anastomoses in renal transplantation. *Br J Surg* 1978; 65:60.
166. Walsh TJ, Zachary JB, Hutchins GM, et al: Mycotic aneurysm with recurrent sepsis complicating post-transplant nephrectomy. *Johns Hopkins Med J* 1977; 141:85.

CHAPTER 16

Ureteral Injuries

Fray F. Marshall, M.D.

Ureteral injuries have been a feared complication. If the ureteral and associated injuries are diagnosed accurately, they can be managed promptly and appropriately without significant morbidity. There are two general types of ureteral injuries: blunt or penetrating trauma, usually associated with injuries to other organs, and iatrogenic surgical injury to the ureter. If basic principles of surgical management are applied to the operative reconstruction, a successful outcome will be the usual result.

ANATOMY

The surgical anatomy of the ureter is most important and explains periodic injury to the ureter; this fibromuscular tube has a close relationship to a number of important organs (Fig 16–1). The average ureter is 25 to 30 cm in length and starts at the junction of the renal pelvis at the renal hilum. The ureter then descends inferiorly over the psoas muscle and is surrounded by retroperitoneal fat. As it descends, it usually becomes closely adherent to the peritoneum, and it crosses the genitofemoral nerve, which lies on the body of the psoas muscle. The ureter then courses under the gonadal vessels at the level of L_3. The duodenum is adjacent to the superior portion of the right ureter, and the remaining upper portion of the right ureter is covered by the right colon or right colonic mesentary with its associated vessels. The ileum crosses over the ureter as it inserts into the cecum. The left colon and left colonic mesentary lie above the left ureter, and the sigmoid colon crosses over a lower portion of the ureter as it descends.

As the ureter courses into the pelvis, it crosses the iliac artery at the junction of the internal and external iliac arteries. This landmark is important, and the ureter will usually lie in close proximity to the hypogastric artery. This relationship can aid the surgeon in the identification of either the ureter or the hypogastric artery at that level. The ureter then drops into the pelvis and courses posteriorly and inferiorly as it follows the curvature of the pelvis down to the levator ani musculature. Then it obliquely enters the posterior aspect of the bladder. The ductus deferens in the male crosses over the ureter and then descends inferiorly behind it. In the female, the pelvic ureter courses behind the ovary and lies in the uterosacral ligaments. It then continues inferiorly in a portion of the broad ligament. The ureter lies anterior to the iliac vessels and is initially medial to the uterine artery higher in the pelvis but is lateral in the lower pelvis where the uterine artery crosses the ureter. The uterine artery can provide significant vascular supply to the pelvic ureter.

The vascular supply to the ureter is usually divided into three portions. The

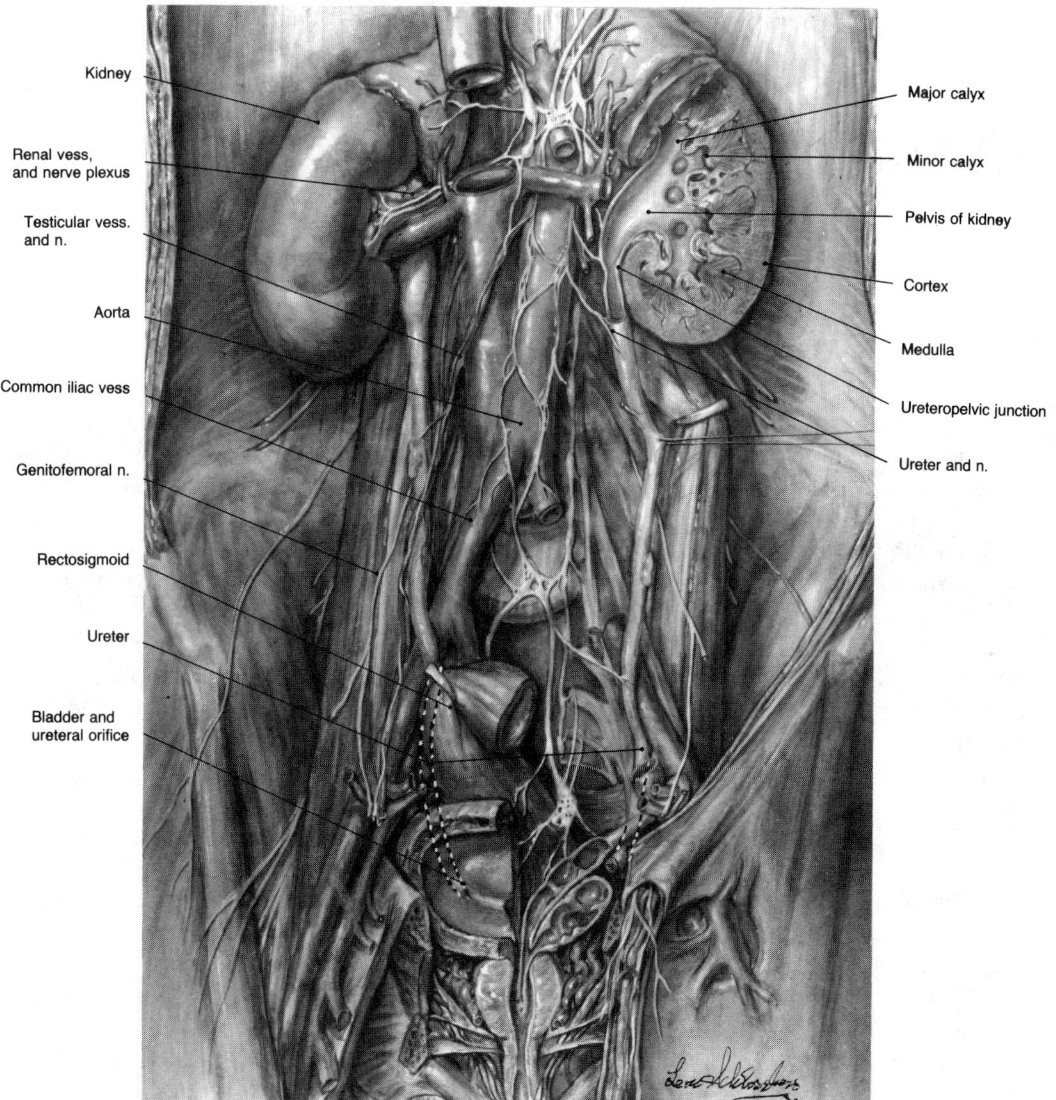

FIG 16–1.
The course of the ureter is identified in the retroperitoneum.

superior portion of the ureter derives blood supply from the renal artery and renal pelvic branches. Some of these small important vessels run in the peripelvic fat surrounding the renal pelvis. The middle portion of the ureter receives supply from the aorta, gonadal, and iliac branches, but the midportion of the ureter appears to have a poorer blood supply than the most superior or inferior ureteral segments. The most inferior portion of the ureter can receive arterial supply from the vesical branches of the hypogastric artery.

The ureter may reside in unusual anatomical locations in association with a variety of renal anomalies such as horseshoe kidney or a pelvic kidney. In addition, ureteral duplication is a common anomaly and can present a confusing clinical picture if not appreciated.

CAUSES OF URETERAL INJURY

Trauma

The ureter enjoys a protected anatomical position within the retroperitoneum and is surrounded by heavy muscle posteriorly, the abdominal contents, and abdominal wall anteriorly. For these reasons it is not injured frequently in blunt abdominal trauma. Occasionally, a shearing force at the ureteral pelvic junction or just below it can disrupt the ureter at that level.[1] A large extrarenal pelvis full of urine may provide for a greater shearing force in some patients. Blunt injuries to the ureter involve severe blunt trauma such as an automobile accident. In general, there is a high association of injuries to other organ systems.

The majority of traumatic ureteral injuries are caused by penetrating injuries. The incidence of ureteral injuries has been reported from 0% to 4% of injuries involving the genitourinary system.[2] Usually a gunshot wound or knife is responsible for the injury. Some estimate of the velocity and size of the missile is important, because wounds resulting from the higher-velocity missiles, as seen in wartime or from high-powered rifles, will require much more extensive debridement. In addition, there is a very high rate of associated injury. The course of the missile is sometimes difficult to determine, and a systematic investigation is required, both preoperatively with an intravenous pyelogram and intraoperatively with careful investigation of all abdominal viscera. All associated injuries, such as frequent bowel perforations, are repaired. When the ureteral injury is identified, resection usually has to be carried out before an anastomosis can be performed. Mobilization of the kidney can compensate for loss of ureteral length and provides for an anastomosis of the ureter without tension. Although not always advocated, a proximal urinary diversion as well as the necessary wound drainage can provide greater protection for the operative repair.

Case Report of Penetrating Injury.—A 26-year-old man presented with a gunshot wound to the right lower quadrant following an altercation. The patient was in good health without any significant medical problems. On physical examination the entrance wound could be visualized in the right lower quadrant, and there was diffuse abdominal tenderness but the vital signs were stable. No exit wound was appreciated. There was no gross hematuria, but microscopic analysis of the urine revealed hematuria. His blood urea nitrogen (BUN) and serum creatinine were normal. An intravenous pyelogram (IVP) was obtained, and extravasation was noted within the retroperitoneum.

At exploration, multiple holes were closed in the small bowel. The right colon was reflected, and the ureteral injury was clearly identified. This portion of the ureter was resected, and a spatulated end-to-end anastomosis was performed with interrupted, absorbable 5-0 sutures. A retroperitoneal drain was placed and brought out through a separate stab wound in the flank. In this patient an 8 F feeding tube was placed in the ureter to drain the kidney and function as a stent. It was brought out through the bladder. The feeding tube was removed on the ninth postoperative day, and at ten days an IVP was normal (Fig 16–2). Other options might have included no stent, the use of a proximal formal nephrostomy tube, or double-J catheter as an internal stent.

Surgical

Obstetrics and Gynecological Ureteral Injury

Ureteral injuries are uncommon. Unfortunately, they are not always recognized at the time of surgery, and the pa-

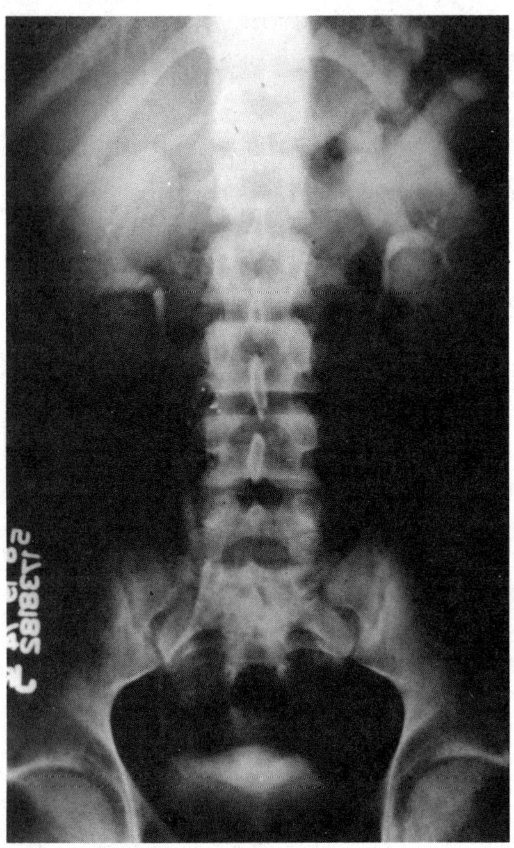

FIG 16–2.
Postoperative IVP reveals good function of the right kidney with no obstruction or extravasation. Bullet fragments seen at bottom of third lumbar vertebra.

tient presents in the postoperative period with usually either urinary leakage from the drain or with symptoms of ureteral obstruction.[3] Since most of these operations occur within the pelvis, it is the pelvic ureter that is at greatest risk for ureteral injury. More extensive surgery, especially with complicating features, such as infection, previous radiation, adhesions, or intraoperative bleeding, increases the likelihood of ureteral injury. Additional problems such as endometriosis may also obscure normal anatomical landmarks within the pelvis and make surgery more difficult and ureteral injury more likely.

There have been reports of a 0%[4] to 3%[5] incidence of ureteral injury during radical hysterectomy. With the wider dissection in a radical hysterectomy, the incidence of ureteral injury is higher than in a simple abdominal hysterectomy. Ovarian surgery can result in ureteral injury, since the ovarian vessels cross over the ureter. If there is troublesome bleeding in this area, again the ureter is in close anatomical proximity to the ovary and ovarian vessels. In a vaginal hysterectomy, the most inferior portion of the ureter can be occluded with a clamp or suture, and obstruction or a fistula may result. In addition, patients undergoing cesarean section or even difficult forceps delivery have been reported to have ureteral injury. In one recent series of iatrogenic ureteral injuries, hysterectomy and gynecologic surgery accounted for 26 of 52 patients, so it appears that patients undergoing gynecologic surgery represent the largest group of patients with iatrogenic surgical injury to the ureter.[3]

Since these patients usually present with either a leak of urine or urinary obstruction with pain, an IVP can be diagnostic and will demonstrate obstruction or extravasation. Cystoscopy and retrograde pyelography can demonstrate extravasation from a ureteral fistula. The use of intravenous methylene blue or indigo carmine with a tampon in the vagina will sometimes demonstrate the site of the fistula. More recently, computered tomography (CT) scans can also demonstrate areas of inflammation and possible extravasation.

Once the diagnosis of ureteral injury has been made, any associated urinary tract infection or metabolic or medical problems should be corrected. In several instances, there have been reports of bilateral ureteral obstruction, and patients have required dialysis before operative repair. Obviously, in such patients it was important not to ascribe their anuria to acute tubular necrosis. Establishment of subsequent ureteral drainage corrected the renal failure. If the patient is in reasonable condition and the anatomical defect is clearly demonstrated, an operative repair is usually performed. In recent years percutaneous nephrostomy has been employed successfully to provide for urinary drainage for an obstructed ureter when there was no extravasation and absorbable suture material had been utilized.[6, 7] On the other hand, if a urinary fistula is present with constant drainage, potential problems remain with infection and septicemia if this situation cannot be brought under control with passage of a ureteral catheter or placement of a nephrostomy.

If operative intervention is indicated, the psoas hitch reimplant is often very successful in these gynecologic, pelvic, ureteral injuries.[8] The use of a Boari flap[3] or a transureteroureterostomy[9] has also been advocated. Rarely, a simple ureteroneocystostomy can be performed without a submucosal tunnel,[10] but an antireflux feature should be incorporated into the repair. The percutaneous nephrostomy can be utilized as a form of proximal urinary diversion. The complications of ureteral repair include recurrent fistula, ureteral obstruction, infection, and reflux.

General Surgery

Ureteral injuries can occur in a wide variety of general surgical procedures, including resections of the colon, especially the left colon and sigmoid.[11] Operations on the colon for diverticulitis or even operations for rectal prolapse can be associated with ureteral injury. Abdominal perineal resection for rectal carcinoma also has an incidence of ureteral injury. Abdominal explorations in a trauma patient with a fractured pelvis can sometimes result in ureteral injury, because normal anatomical relationships may be disturbed with hematoma. Again, an intravenous pyelogram will demonstrate ureteral obstruction or urinary extravasation. These injuries may occur because the ureter is often immediately adherent to the peritoneum and on the other side of the mesocolon. The ureter can also be injured where it crosses the great vessels or deeper in the pelvis when clamps are placed on the lateral pedicle of the bowel. In addition, the ureter may be injured during an appendectomy, especially if there is a retrocecal appendix. Lastly, excision of large retroperitoneal tumors often requires careful, extensive dissection of the ureters. Devascularization of the ureter may also cause postoperative fistula formation or subsequent ureteral obstruction.

Placement of ureteral catheters has been advocated to help in localizing the ureters during surgery, but bilateral ureteral catheterization can sometimes have significant morbidity. We have had experience with at least one patient who developed transient anuria following bilateral ureteral catheterization, so ureteral catheterization is not strongly advocated.

Vascular Surgery

With an increasing number of vascular procedures for occlusive and aneurysmal disease, there is obvious potential for ureteral injury. The ureter can be associated intimately with the aorta or the iliac artery as it crosses over the common iliac artery. During vascular bypass procedures or aneurysm surgery,[12] a fibrotic, desmoplastic response around the aneurysm can be encountered, probably related to small leaks of blood. Retroperitoneal fibrosis can occur with medial displacement of the ureter even in the presence of a dilated aortic aneurysm. These ureters become entrapped in this desmoplastic tissue. Aneurysmal disease of the iliac artery has also been associated with ureteral entrapment. Although not performed often, bilateral lumbar sympathectomy or vena caval ligation can be associated with ureteral injury.

Again, these patients who have undergone vascular surgery usually have evidence of fistula formation or ureteral obstruction on intravenous pyelography. Any patient with a fistula and a vascular prosthetic graft is most worrisome because of potential infection of the graft. For that reason, immediate treatment with a percutaneous nephrostomy urinary diversion and institution of antibiotics might be needed for a severely ill patient. If the patient is otherwise stable, surgical exploration should achieve a water-tight closure of the urinary tract. An attempt should be made to interpose tissue between the graft and the repaired ureter. Proximal urinary diversion in the form of a nephrostomy is usually performed in this higher-risk group. If the patient is severely ill and has a reasonable contralateral kidney, a nephrectomy might be considered.[3] Occasionally, if there is no evidence of urinary extravasation and a suture is found, simple deligation will suffice.

Genitourinary Surgery

The upper ureter can be injured during calculus surgery, especially pyelolithotomy. This complication usually occurs in a patient with an intrarenal pelvis and following a difficult dissection. Devascularization and trauma of the ureteral pelvic junction may result in a later significant stenosis. A ureterolithotomy can also result in obstruction at any point in the ureter. The mid ureter may be slightly more prone to injury because of the more precarious vascular supply in this area. In addition, difficult dissections can occur following irradiation, infection, or previous surgery. Large retroperitoneal lymphadenopathy from testicular tumors or large sarcomas can create precarious dissection of the ureter. Ureteral dissection in retroperitoneal fibrosis also risks ureteral injury. Any surgery on the bladder, such as a partial cystectomy or, in particular, a vesical diverticulectomy, may be associated with a lower ureteral injury. Vesical diverticula often occur around the ureteral orifice and may be adherent to a portion of the ureter, making the dissection more difficult.

Ureteral obstruction can occur with a Marshall-Marchetti procedure.[7] Deep bites of suture may actually go through the bladder and entrap the distal portion of the ureter. Usually, absorbable suture has been utilized, and percutaneous nephrostomy has allowed for the conservative management of some of these patients.[7]

Ureteral obstruction and perforation from ureterorenoscopy will increase with more endoscopy. A ureter has to be dilated to 14 or 16 French to allow passage of a rigid instrument up the ureter. Perforation can occur and subsequent ureteral obstruction can ensue.

Even simple bilateral retrograde pyelography has resulted in transient anuria. Clearly, manipulation of a ureteral calculus with a stone basket carries the risk of ureteral avulsion or ureteral injury with subsequent fibrosis. Certain principles should be followed in stone basket manipulation. In general, the calculus should be below the iliac vessels. It should not be more than 8 to 10 mm in diameter. Radiographic verification of the manipulation with the use of a fluoroscopic C-arm is helpful. Fluoroscopy provides much greater control than periodic plain x-ray studies. In addition, the use of ureteral dilation with balloons or ureteral dilators may also facilitate removal.

Transurethral resection of the prostate or a bladder tumor may result in ureteral injury. The resection of a large median lobe of the prostate can be carried up on the trigone inadvertently, and the ureteral orifice can be resected. More commonly, problems arise in the transurethral resection of transitional cell carcinoma of the bladder around the ureteral orifice. It is said that cutting current causes less fibrosis and ureteral obstruction than the fulgurating current. In general, we have found ureteral reflux more likely than ureteral obstruction after such a procedure.

PRINCIPLES OF SURGICAL REPAIR

Accurate diagnosis and management of ureteral and associated injuries are paramount. In the patient with ureteral trauma, there is a very high association of injury to other organs. These other injuries also require careful management. Location of the ureteral injury and the possibility of injury to either ureter is usually well identified by intravenous pyelography. Cystoscopy and retrograde pyelography can also provide accurate assessment of the ureter. Computed tomographic scans are increasingly utilized to provide additional information about associated injuries.

Once the ureteral injury is accurately delineated, operative repair can be performed, but in some instances percutaneous drainage and manipulation may provide for more conservative management. At surgical exploration, a systematic investigation is performed for any associated injuries. The damaged ureteral segment and adjacent area are debrided. An anatomical water-tight reconstruction or anastomosis is performed without tension. If there has been a significant loss of ureter, mobilization of the kidney can be performed and large defects in the ureter can be repaired without tension.[13] In one instance of major loss of the ureter, we have mobilized the kidney down and utilized a psoas hitch to bring the bladder up, and the superior aspect of the bladder was at the same level as the lower pole of the kidney. An antireflux ureteroneocystostomy was accomplished with only a few centimeters of ureter below the ureteral pelvic junction.

Once the anatomical water-tight reconstruction has been performed, then the area of the anastomosis is drained, usually with a Penrose drain through a separate flank stab wound. In difficult cases, proximal urinary diversion can be maintained through a nephrostomy tube. In other instances, a stent has been left draining the kidney through the ureter, and it is brought out through the bladder. Internal stents such as double-J catheters can also be used although sometimes they can become occluded or migrate. In the more difficult patients, it is better to provide greater protection with both a proximal urinary diversion (nephrostomy tube) and a stent as well.

OPERATIVE RECONSTRUCTION

In situ deligation

If there is no evidence of ureteral extravasation and the ureter appears to be only obstructed, ureteral deligation can be performed.[14] We have performed this procedure in several patients in whom a suture could be easily identified and the ureter appeared to be absolutely intact.

Percutaneous Manipulation (Fig 16–3)

There have been several reports indicating use of percutaneous techniques, especially with a percutaneous nephrostomy to allow for dissolution of absorptive suture material.[6,7] There has also been a case report of a ureteral dilation with intraureteral balloons to create ureteral patency.[15] We have increasingly resorted to the initial use of percutaneous manipulations in all sorts of ureteral injuries associated with obstruction and extravasation following a variety of surgical procedures (urologic, gynecologic, general surgical). If these patients are severely debilitated with ureteral obstruction or slight urinary extravasation, they can be managed conservatively with a percutaneous proximal nephrostomy tube

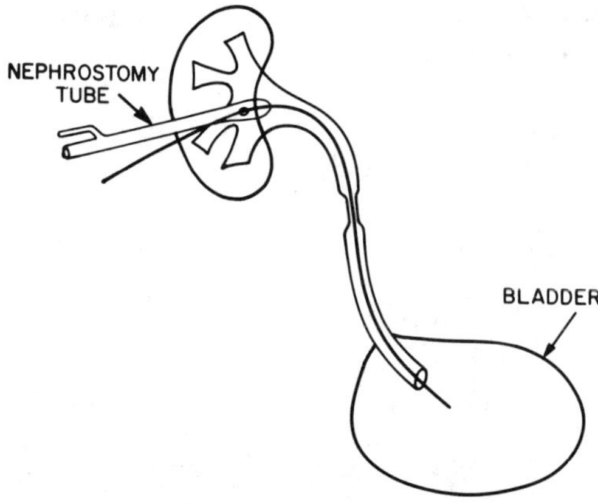

FIG 16–3.
Percutaneous management frequently includes placement of both a nephrostomy tube and stent.

diversion and the placement of a ureteral stent to reduce the likelihood of a subsequent ureteral fibrosis and stricture formation at the site of urinary extravasation. Although not all patients are managed this way, many can be managed with initial percutaneous manipulation until control of the patient is obtained. If necessary, surgical treatment can be performed when medical conditions have improved.

In our experience, the patients who profit most with the percutaneous technique have had fairly recent iatrogenic injuries. These patients have a more favorable prognosis. On the other hand, delayed ureteral obstruction from ureteral ischemia, infection, or long-term problems are usually less amenable to percutaneous manipulation.

Ureterocalycostomy (Figs 16–4 and 16–5)

In patients who have complete obstruction of an intrarenal ureteropelvic junction from calculus surgery, a ureterocalycostomy provides a reasonable alternative in the management of these patients. Ureterocalycostomy can sometimes be a difficult procedure but can produce excellent results. In these procedures it is necessary to resect the parenchyma around the most inferior calyx because if this resection is not done, stenosis occurs at this site.[16] In order to accomplish this resection accurately, it is often necessary to control the renal vasculature and temporarily occlude it. Then the mucosa of the calyx can be dissected from the parenchyma to provide an accurate calyceal to ureteral anastomosis with interrupted absorbable suture. A nephropexy is performed. Generally, a nephrostomy tube as well as a stent are utilized. The stent may be left in place for two to four weeks. Upon its removal, a nephrostogram will verify the patency of the anastomosis and the lack of any urinary extravasation.

Ureteroureterostomy (Fig 16–6)

If there has been a relatively short ureteral injury, a ureteroureterostomy can be performed.[17] The tissue is debrided back to good, bleeding, viable ureteral tissue on each side. The ends of the ureter are spatulated to provide a generous oblique anastomosis. Usually, interrupted sutures have been utilized, so there is no narrowing of the suture line with a running suture. A running suture can be utilized if stay sutures are placed, so there is no telescoping of the anastomosis. A run-

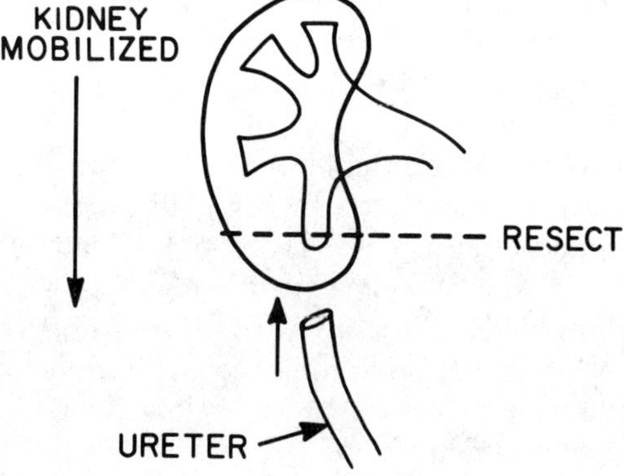

FIG 16–4.
A direct anastomosis of the ureter to the most inferior calix.

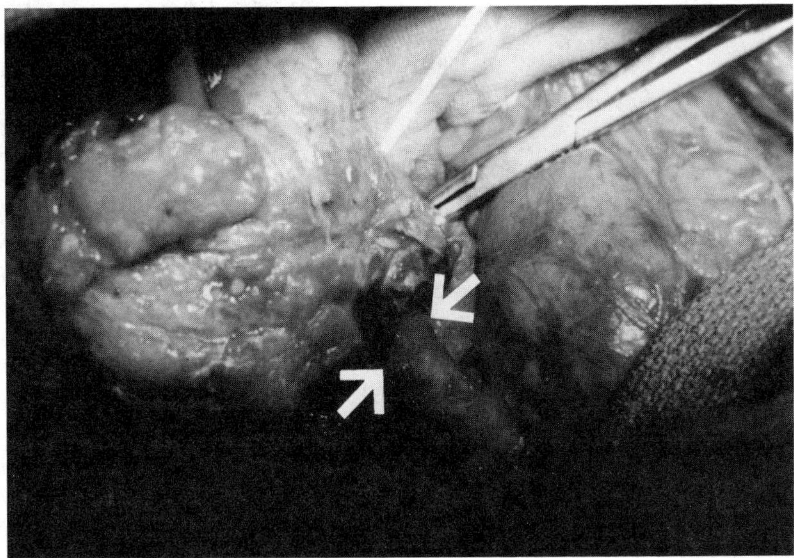

FIG 16–5.
After loss of the ureteropelvic junction following pyelolithotomy, the ureter is anastomosed directly to the inferior calix. (*Arrows* indicate junction of ureter and calix.)

ning locked suture will also be less likely to reduce the diameter of the anastomosis. Although no form of diversion or stenting has been recommended,[18] a proximal urinary diversion with or without a stent can provide greater protection for the patient and surgeon.

Transureteroureterostomy (Fig 16–7)

If there is extensive injury of the lower ureter, a transureteroureterostomy can provide excellent drainage of both kidneys.[9, 19] The affected ureter can be brought under or above the inferior mesenteric artery, depending on the length of ureter available. The ureter then passes anterior to the vena cava and aorta and is brought to the contralateral side and sutured in place, end to side. A vertical incision of about 15 mm is employed in the side of the ureter, and a running 5-0 absorbable suture has been advocated for the anastomosis.[9] It is important to be sure that the ureter is not kinked under the inferior mesenteric artery and has a smooth course to the level of the anastomosis, which is performed without any tension. Some physicians have employed stents.[19] Others have not utilized any stents or urinary drainage.[9] In general, the results have been excellent. There is at least the theoretical risk of injury to an already intact, normal collecting system, and for that reason we have sometimes avoided the use of transureteroureter-

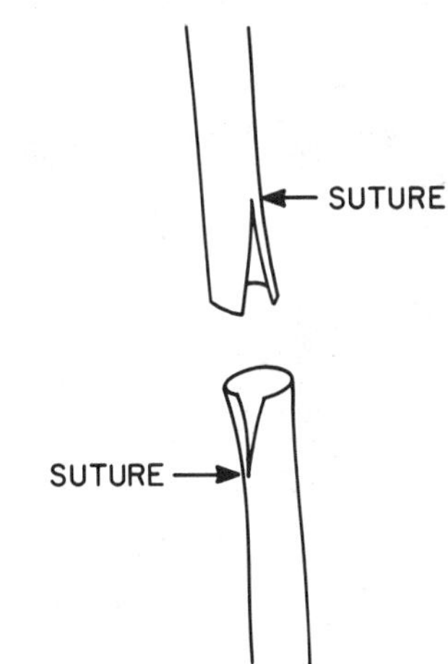

FIG 16–6.
The spatulated end-to-end uretero-ureterostomy.

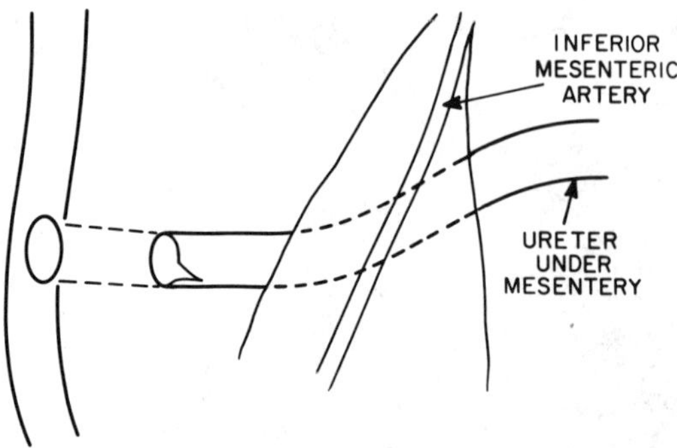

FIG 16–7.
The contralateral ureter is brought under the vascular supply to the bowel and anastomosed end to side.

ostomy, but it certainly remains a good operation in selected patients. Stone disease remains a contraindication and intraperitoneal malignancy a relative contraindication.

Boari Flap, Psoas Hitch (Figs 16–8 and 16–9)

The Boari or bladder flap has been utilized in many patients with ureteral injury.[3] Lower ureteral injuries are the primary injuries necessitating the use of this repair. Sometimes it can be difficult to obtain a good submucosal tunnel in a Boari flap after the bladder is closed, but certainly the Boari flap can remain an option for the surgeon.

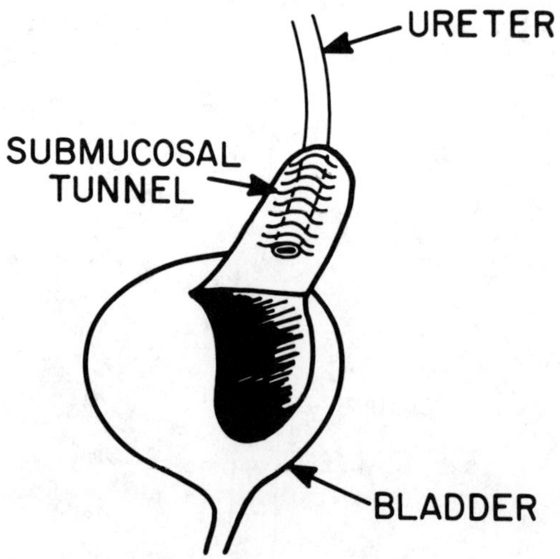

FIG 16–8.
The vesical flap is demonstrated.

The psoas hitch will usually provide almost as much length as a Boari flap. With good fixation of the bladder to the psoas muscle above the iliac vessels, the entire pelvic ureter can be bypassed. Frequently, this is the operation of choice when there has been extensive previous pelvic surgery. The use of this technique allows reimplantation of the ureter with a submucosal tunnel well away from sites of ureteral injury and obviates the need for dissection in previously operated or irradiated areas. Results from the use of the psoas hitch for ureteral replacement have been excellent.[8, 20] It can sometimes be utilized in conjunction with a transureteroureterostomy.

The important technical features include ligation and division of the obliterated umbilical vessels, and sometimes the contralateral superior vesical vasculature, to provide adequate mobilization of the bladder. The bladder then can be pulled up to the level of the psoas muscle and carefully secured with heavier absorbable sutures. We have reimplanted the ureter with a submucosal tunnel to provide an antireflux anastomosis of the ureter. In general, we have also left a feeding tube as a stent in the ureter and brought it out through the contralateral wall of the bladder. This stent also provides for urinary drainage and is usually removed on about the tenth postoperative day. A nephrostogram or intravenous pyelogram is obtained at that time.

Bowel Replacement (Fig 16–10)

When there has been extensive loss of the ureter, many of the previously described procedures may not be sufficient. In that circumstance, the ileum has been the most commonly utilized segment of bowel for ureteral substitution.[21] At times

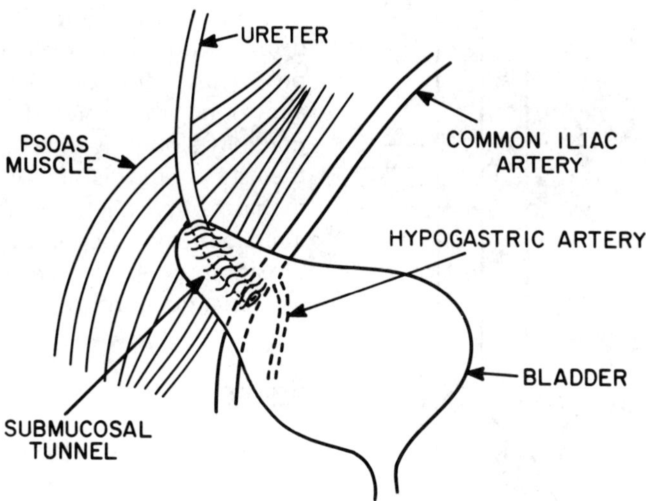

FIG 16–9.
The bladder is dissected free and sutured to the psoas muscle.

it has also been utilized with the cecum, which has been applied to the bladder as a patch.[22] If the entire ureter is replaced, an ileal segment of 25 cm is required. A bowel prep preoperatively is in order. The ileum is isolated on its mesenteric pedicle. An ileal-renal pelvic anastomosis is performed. The distal ileum can be reimplanted directly into the bladder.[21] Others have advocated tapering the distal ileum and creating a submucosal tunnel to provide for an antireflux anastomosis.[19] This tunnel can be technically difficult because of the bulk of the ileum and the necessity for preservation of its blood supply. Intussusception of the ileocecal valve[23] can provide an antireflux component to the system. If the ileum is employed for reconstruction or replacement of the left ureter, it must be brought through the mesocolon.

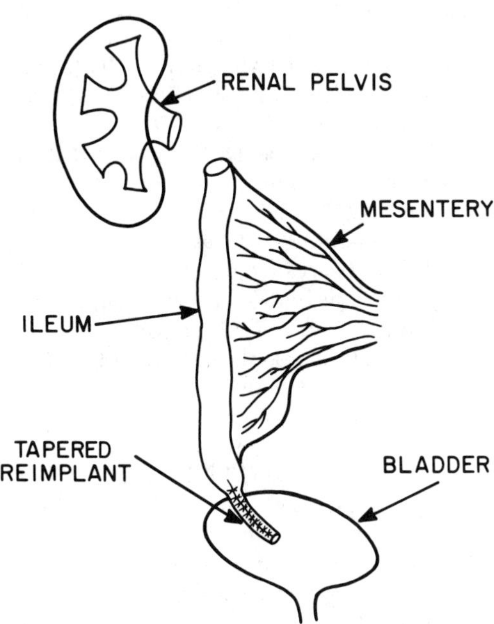

FIG 16–10.
The ileum can be utilized for extensive ureteral replacement.

Renal Autotransplantation (Fig 16–11)

In the extensively destroyed ureter, renal autotransplantation has also been utilized to restore continuity of the urinary tract.[24–26] This procedure is more extensive than some of the previously described techniques and should be used only when these techniques do not work and there is a long ureteral deficit. Care must be taken especially in patients who have azotemia or urinary tract infections.

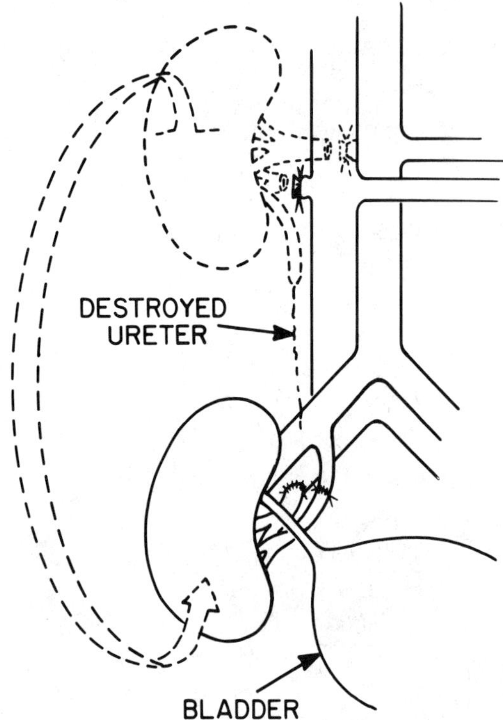

FIG 16–11.
An autotransplanted kidney is placed in the pelvis.

A kidney that is infected does not tolerate an ischemic insult well. Short and long-term vascular complications appear to be rare. In general, patients with extensive ureteral injury with a reasonably healthy kidney in the absence of infection are possible candidates for this operation.

Nephrectomy

When all else has failed or if the patient is very ill, a nephrectomy may provide a more certain recovery with a paucity of complications. A nephrectomy is indicated in selected circumstances with the recognition of an excellent kidney on the contralateral side. Although a fundamental urologic tenet is preservation of renal tissue, there are circumstances in which the general poor condition of the patient or associated injuries might dictate the use of this option.

In general, it is not a good idea to ligate a ureter and hope it will become hydronephrotic and create later renal atrophy. This option can be very dangerous, and, often, the ureter at the point of ligation may slough with resultant urinary extravasation and fistula formation. The potential complications of fistula formation, infection, and septicemia can be life-threatening, so ureteral ligation is not usually a good option.

REFERENCES

1. Stone HH, Jones HQ: Penetrating and nonpenetrating injuries to the ureter. *Surg Gynecol Obstet* 1962; 114:52.
2. Persky L, Hoch WH: Iatrogenic ureteral and vesical injuries, in Karafin L, Kendall AR (eds): *Urology*. New York, Harper & Row, 1974.
3. Flynn JT, Tiptaft RC, Woodhouse CRJ, et al: The early and aggressive repair of iatrogenic ureteric injuries. *Br J Urol* 1979; 51:454.
4. Park RC, Patow WE, Rogers RE, et al: Treatment of stage I carcinoma of the cervix. *Obstet Gynecol* 1973; 41:117.
5. Rusche C, Morrow JW: Injury to the ureter, in Campbell MF, Harrison JH (eds): *Urology*. Philadelphia, WB Saunders Co, 1970, p 811.
6. Persky L, Hampel N, Kedia K: Percutaneous nephrostomy and ureteral injury. *J Urol* 1981; 125:298.
7. Harshman MW, Pollack HM, Banner MP, et al: Conservative management of ureteral obstruction secondary to suture entrapment. *J Urol* 1982; 127:121.
8. Prout GR Jr, Koontz WW Jr: Partial vesical immobilization: An important adjunct to ureteroneocystostomy. *J Urol* 1970; 103:147.
9. Hodges CV, Moore RJ, Lehman TH, et al: Clinical experiences with transuretero-ureterostomy. *J Urol* 1963; 90:552.
10. Beland G: Early treatment of ureteral injuries found after gynecological surgery. *J Urol* 1977; 118:25.
11. Hughes ESR, McDermott FT, Polglase AL, et al: Ureteral damage in surgery for cancer of the large bowel. *Dis Colon Rectum* 1984; 27:293.

12. Schapiro HE, Li R, Gribetz M, et al: Ureteral injuries during vascular surgery. *J Urol* 1981; 125:293.
13. Harada N, Tanimura M, Fukuyama K, et al: Surgical management of a long ureteral defect: Advancement of the ureter by descent of the kidney. *J Urol* 1964; 92:192.
14. Herman A, Guerries K, Persky L: Delayed ureteral deligation. *J Urol* 1972; 107:723.
15. Reimer DE, Oswalt Jr, GC: Iatrogenic ureteral obstruction treated with balloon dilation. *J Urol* 1981; 126:689.
16. Levitt SB, Nabizadeh I, Javaid M, et al: Primary calycoureterostomy for pelvioureteral junction obstruction: Indications and results. *J Urol* 1981; 126:382.
17. Fry DE, Milholen L, Harbrecht PJ: Iatrogenic ureteral injury—options in management. *Arch Surg* 1983; 118:454.
18. Carlton CE Jr, Scott R Jr, Guthrie AG: The initial management of ureteral injuries: A report of 78 cases. *J Urol* 1971; 105:335.
19. Hendren WH, Hensle TW: Transureteroureterostomy: Experience with 75 cases. *J Urol* 1980; 123:826.
20. Warwick RT, Worth PHL: The psoas bladder hitch procedure for the replacement of the lower third of the ureter. *Br J Urol* 1969; 41:701.
21. Goodwin WE, Winter CC, Turner RD: Replacement of the ureter by small intestine: Clinical application and results of ileal ureter. *J Urol* 1959; 81:406.
22. Gil-Vernet JM: The ileocolic segment in urologic surgery. *J Urol* 1965; 94:418.
23. Gittes RF: Bladder augmentation procedures, in Libertino JA, Zinman L (eds): *Urologic Surgery, Pediatric and Adult.* Baltimore, Williams & Wilkins Co, 1977, p 222.
24. Marshall VF, Whitsell J, McGovern JH, et al: The practicality of renal autotransplantation in humans. *JAMA* 1966; 196:1154.
25. Hodges CV, Lawson RK, Pearse HD, et al: Autotransplantation of the kidney. *J Urol* 1973; 110:20.
26. Stewart BH, Hewitt CB, Banowsky LHW: Management of extensively destroyed ureter: Special reference to renal autotransplantation. *J Urol* 1976; 115:257.

CHAPTER 17

Complications of Cystectomy

David P. Wood, Jr., M.D.
William R. Fair, M.D.

Partial or radical cystectomy is the treatment of choice for the majority of deeply invasive bladder cancers. These operations are some of the longer and more difficult procedures a urologist performs. Additionally, some patients have had prior definitive external beam radiation or chemotherapy, which compounds the difficulty of the operation and leads to a myriad of complications, some common to any major abdominal operation and others unique to cystectomy.

The axiom "an ounce of prevention is worth a pound of cure" clearly applies to surgical complications. The preoperative optimization of a patient's cardiovascular, pulmonary, and nutritional status and the postoperative medical and surgical care common to major surgery are discussed in other chapters. Intraoperatively, the utilization of a systematic approach to surgery by completing one phase of the operation before starting another will minimize the chance of complications. This is particularly relevant to cystectomy because of the many steps involved and the rapid blood loss that can occur during certain phases of the procedure.

In this chapter we will discuss the specific operative complications associated with partial and radical cystectomy. Special attention will be given to the problems associated with cystectomy following chemotherapy or definitive radiotherapy.

IMPACT OF COMPLICATIONS

Morbidity rates of 25% to 40% have been reported following cystectomy but the mortality rate is only 1% to 3%.[1–4] The low mortality rate attests to modern medicine's ability to control previously life-threatening complications such as infection and malnutrition. However, the high morbidity rate is disturbing and highlights the difficulty of this operation. Although the majority of complications are minor (superficial wound separation, ileus, urinary tract infection) any complication can significantly prolong the patient's hospital stay.[1] This is often because one complication leads to another more serious complication. To prevent this cascade of complications, rigorous attention to the smallest problem both intraoperatively and postoperatively is necessary.

Intraoperative complications can cause short-term morbidity and have long lasting consequences. Fistulae or hernias, for example, may require reoperation several months after the cystectomy. These additional procedures may result in more complications and ultimately in a disabled or dissatisfied patient. Considering the elderly age group that undergo cystectomy, lingering problems can diminish the patient's quality of life during their remaining years and strengthens the notion that prevention is the key.

PARTIAL CYSTECTOMY

Partial cystectomy is indicated to treat solitary invasive bladder cancers provided a 2-cm rim of surrounding normal bladder mucosa and bladder wall can be resected. The bladder capacity should be 300 mL or more and without carcinoma in situ in the bladder or prostatic urethra. Prior to Cisplatin-based combination chemotherapy, a minority of patients met these criteria for partial cystectomy. We have found 68% of bladder tumors treated with neoadjuvant MVAC (Methotrexate, Vincristine, Adriamycin, and Cisplatin) and transurethral resection will have a partial or complete response.[5] For some of these patients, formerly requiring a radical cystectomy to adequately resect the cancer, a partial cystectomy may be possible if the bladder tumor regresses enough following chemotherapy.

A urinary fistula is the major technical complication of a partial cystectomy. This occurs from incomplete closure of the cystotomy incision, leakage from the site of a ureteral implantation or unrecognized injury to the ureter or bladder. Several factors can increase the risk of urinary fistulae. Previous radiation therapy to the pelvic area can lead to ischemia and poor wound healing. Prior surgery to the bladder increases the possibility of bladder or ureteral injury during the dissection. Finally, when removing tumors near the bladder base, a watertight closure of the cystotomy incision can be difficult.

Urinary fistulae are recognized by an increased output from the perivesical drain and/or a decreased urine output. Increased drainage can be either urine or lymphatic fluid. Determination of the electrolyte, blood urea nitrogen (BUN), and creatinine concentrations can differentiate between the two; a low sodium concentration, combined with high BUN and creatinine levels, is indicative of urine. If a perivesical drain is not present, the patient will often develop ileus, abdominal distension, and fever. The patient's serum BUN and creatinine levels will rise; the BUN will be 20- to 40-fold higher than the creatinine level as a result of the greater systemic reabsorption of the low molecular weight urea.

The time of fistula formation implicates the cause of the fistula. Urine leaks from inadequate cystotomy closure result in immediate and persistent drain output. Fistulae secondary to inadequate healing of ischemic tissue usually manifest 4 to 6 days after the procedure. Finding the exact cause or site of the fistula may not be necessary to treat the problem. A cystogram may introduce bacteria, or if done under high pressure, can make a small fistula into a large one. If the fistula is persistent or worsens, radiologic investigation with a gravity cystogram, including a drainage film, is helpful to rule out any surgically correctable cause for the fistula.

Prevention of a urine leak is dependent on obtaining a watertight cystotomy closure and ensuring that the bladder is well drained. We perform a two-layer closure of the bladder with an absorbable suture; the first layer is a continuous closure of the full thickness of the bladder and the second layer is an interrupted suture which imbricates the bladder wall over the first layer. A #22 F Foley catheter and a #24 F suprapubic tube will allow maximal drainage of the bladder and provide two avenues of drainage in case one tube becomes clotted or inadvertently removed. We do not irrigate the Foley catheter or suprapubic tube unless blood clots form in the bladder. In this case, passive irrigation into the urethral Foley catheter (which has the smaller lumen) and gentle suction on the suprapubic tube is indicated. Finally, a closed suction drain provides excellent perivesical drainage and should be used routinely. If there is no urine leak, we clamp the suprapubic tube on the 7th to 10th postoperative day and remove the Foley catheter. If the patient voids well with no leakage from the perivesical drain, the suprapubic tube is first removed and then the drain, 24 hours later.

The management of urinary fistulae is basically adequate drainage. Reinsertion of the catheter is sufficient in most cases to provide bladder drainage. Occasionally, the fistula will persist if the cystotomy is near the bladder base. With a standard Foley the balloon occupies the base of the bladder and this area is not well drained. Insertion of a straight catheter without a balloon will provide maximal bladder drainage for the floor of the bladder. If the perivesical drain has been removed a CT scan or ultrasound is necessary to determine if a fluid collection is present. If there is no collection and the patient is stable, reinsertion of the perivesical drain is not necessary. If a large fluid collection is present drainage is required. This can often be accomplished percutaneously. With adequate drainage the fistula should close but it may take weeks. In these cases, a cystogram should be performed prior to removing the Foley catheter.

RADICAL CYSTECTOMY

Radical cystectomy is the treatment of choice for the majority of invasive bladder cancers. It is one of the more difficult operations performed by urologists. To prevent complications, divide the operation into a series of steps and complete each step before advancing to the next one. This not only establishes a routine that allows assistants to anticipate your next move, but decreases the likelihood of missing a step in a long operation.

The operative procedure to perform a radical cystectomy has been described in detail.[6] A few relevant points that can make the operation easier will be highlighted. First, we routinely use epidural anesthesia as a supplement to general endotracheal anesthesia. This appears to decrease the blood loss and supplies a means of providing postoperative pain relief without large doses of systemic narcotics. Second, patients are placed in the modified lithotomy position with the legs slightly abducted on spreader bars. This allows room for the second assistant to stand. With female patients it also provides access to the perineum to remove the urethra and anterior vaginal wall. With the female, it is essential to have the pelvis extend slightly beyond the edge of the table to provide room for the weighted speculum. Third, blood loss can be diminished by tying the internal iliac arteries. It is important to ligate the artery beyond the superior gluteal branch because there is a risk of gluteal claudication if this branch is occluded bilaterally. Finally, we leave a #24 F Foley catheter in the urethra on slight traction for 12 to 16 hours to help identify a large postoperative hemorrhage and provide hemostasis of the urogenital diaphragm.

COMPLICATIONS

There are three complications following a radical cystectomy that are intraoperative in nature: hemorrhage, rectal injury, and pelvic abscess. Although these problems cannot always be prevented, the morbidity to the patient can be minimized by early recognition and prompt intervention.

Massive blood loss is one complication that can result in an intraoperative death. To prevent this occurrence, knowledge of the blood supply to the bladder and prostate is important. The major arterial blood supply is via the visceral branch of the internal iliac artery which includes the inferior vesical and the middle rectal arteries. This branch arises beyond the takeoff of the parietal arterial branch and, in particular, the superior gluteal artery. By ligating the visceral branch of the internal iliac artery much of the blood supply to the bladder is diminished. Additionally, a large plexus of arteries and veins feed the bladder that have no discrete origin. Therefore, we separate the blood supply into the lateral and posterior pedicles. By ligating these pedicles between sequential Kelly clamps under direct vision blood loss can be controlled. There is little necessity for "blind clamping" of the pedicles, which can result in damage to surrounding structures. Finally, the dorsal vein complex courses through the urogenital diaphragm and anterior to the urethra and prostate. If this venous complex is entered a large amount of blood loss can occur in a short period of time. We utilize the technique popularized by Walsh[7] to control the dorsal vein complex. In this procedure, the puboprostatic ligaments are sharply divided and the dorsal vein complex is dissected from the anterior urethra with a right angle clamp and ligated with a #1 silk suture. This is particularly important to do in patients undergoing an orthotopic bowel reservoir to the urethra.

If a hemorrhage occurs the first move is to compress the bleeding site manually and the second is to notify the anesthetist. Visualization and control of the bleeding site should not be attempted until enough blood products are in the operating room and the patient is well hydrated. Trying to control the bleeding without these maneuvers can lead to disastrous consequences. If the bleeding is from the pedicles, the bladder should be mobilized as quickly as possible in order to identify the bleeding site. If the dorsal vein complex is bleeding, it is best to try to find the exact site of bleeding and control it. If this is not possible, suturing the edges of the urogenital diaphragm may control the bleeding. To improve visualization of this area the second assistant can push up on the perineum with a sponge stick. If all else fails, the bleeding can usually be controlled by placing a #24 F 30-mL catheter in the urethra and filling the balloon to 50 mL and placing it on traction.

PELVIC ABSCESS

Pelvic abscesses occur in 1% to 3% of radical cystectomy cases.[1, 3] The signs and symptoms are nonspecific and include ileus, fatigue, lower abdominal pain, spiking fever, and leukocytosis. In some cases the abscess can be palpated on rectal examination or via the vagina. However, the best method to diagnose an abscess is with a CT scan or ultrasound examination (Fig 17–1) An abscess is predominantly fluid-filled and has a thick rim of inflammatory tissue surrounding it. On ultrasound, the abscess usually has echogenic foci within the mass. These findings are in contrast to those found in lymphoceles or urinomas which are typically homogeneous, anechoic fluid filled cavities with minimal inflammatory reaction. Not all abscesses fit this picture and clinical judgment should prevail.

Most pelvic abscesses are caused by aerobic and/or anaerobic enteric bacteria. If a pelvic abscess is suspected, broad spectrum antibiotics should be started after blood and urine cultures are obtained. Very few abscesses will resolve with antibiotics alone and adequate drainage is essential. In the majority of cases percutaneous drainage should be attempted first. In females, a catheter can be inserted through the vaginal cuff and in men a urethral

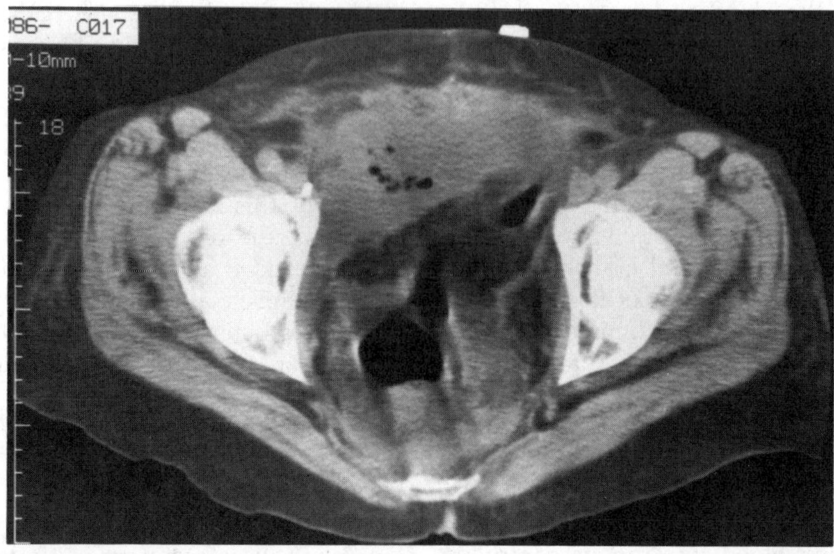

FIG 17–1.
CT scan of a large pelvic abscess following cystectomy. The cavity is predominately fluid-filled with evidence of gas formation by anaerobic bacteria.

Foley catheter can be inserted to drain the abscess. If these procedures are unsuccessful, a percutaneous catheter can be placed under radiographic guidance (Fig 17–2). These measures, in combination with specific antibiotic therapy, will resolve most abscesses within 5 to 10 days. Some do not respond to percutaneous drainage and an exploratory laparotomy is necessary. In these situations, the pelvis should be irrigated with normal saline and large closed suction drains placed.

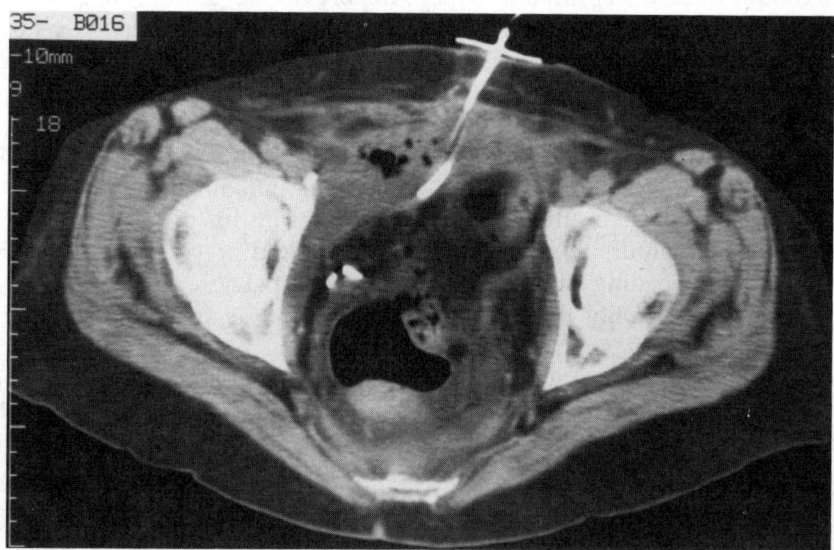

FIG 17–2.
A percutaneous drain has been placed into an abscess cavity. After the drainage stopped the drain was removed without sequelae.

RECTAL INJURY

Rectal lacerations have been reported in 0% to 2% of cystectomy series with a higher incidence following salvage cystectomy.[1, 3, 4, 8] As mentioned earlier, one complication often leads to another and rectal injuries certainly exemplify this concept. Of 21 reported rectal injuries, there was a 19% mortality rate and a 57% incidence of another complication occurring.[8–13] Clearly, rectal injuries can lead to serious postoperative problems particularly if there is a delay in recognition of the injury.

Rectal injuries usually occur either during the ligation of the distal aspect of the posterior bladder pedicle or in the dissection of the prostate off the rectum. Occasionally the rectum can be tented up with the posterior pedicle and an enterotomy made if the pedicles are not ligated under direct vision. The most common time for rectal injuries to occur is during the dissection of the prostate off the rectum. In the majority of cases the posterior portion of the bladder, seminal vesicles and prostate can be dissected away from the rectum bluntly by entering the plane behind Denonvillier's fascia anterior to the rectum. Rectal injuries often occur by blunt digital probing in an attempt to identify the proper plane. If there is any difficulty in entering this plane from above we recommend a retrograde dissection of the prostate and seminal vesicles as if performing a radical prostatectomy.

The most important aspect of limiting the consequences of a rectal injury is early identification. The surgeon must be honest with himself; if you think there is a rectal injury, there probably is one. Assuming the patient has undergone an adequate preoperative bowel prep, the intraoperative management of a rectal injury is dependent on the size and location of the enterotomy and whether a tension-free closure can be obtained. All rectal injuries should be closed in two layers and encircled with omentum. Small enterotomies can be closed primarily without a diverting colostomy. In patients with a large rectal injury, inadequate bowel prep, or with perirectal fibrosis from radiation or chemotherapy, a diverting colostomy may be necessary. Large closed-suction drains should be used to help prevent a pelvic abscess. By following these recommendations the subsequent morbidity from a rectal injury can be minimized.

CYSTECTOMY FOLLOWING CHEMOTHERAPY

Sixty-eight percent of bladder tumors will exhibit some response to MVAC chemotherapy plus transurethral resection, but only 20% will achieve a complete response.[5] To complicate matters, there is a 28% clinical staging error with the vast majority of tumors being understaged. This understaging can be significant; 40% of patients clinically staged TO with negative transurethral resection biopsies before surgery had residual tumor in the surgical specimen.[14] Therefore, all patients treated with neoadjuvant chemotherapy require a full thickness resection of the area where the bladder lesion was located. Because there is no factor that predicts which patient will completely respond to MVAC, coupled with the difficulty in accurately staging these patients, we believe neoadjuvant MVAC is currently experimental therapy to be used in investigative protocols and should not be routinely utilized.

Radical cystectomy after chemotherapy can be difficult because of the fibrosis that occurs in the perivesical tissue. This is particularly evident in patients with nodal disease or perivesical tumor extension. The chemotherapy can shrink involved lymph nodes which then form a dense reactive tissue adherent to the iliac vessels similar to the reaction following chemotherapy for testis cancer. Unless an obvious enlarged lymph node or mass is present it may not be possible to perform a pelvic lymph node dissection in these cases.

The fibrotic reaction following chemotherapy in patients with extravesical tumor can obliterate the normal planes of dissection. In these cases the fibrotic tissue needs to be cut sharply in order to remove the bladder. Biopsies of the remaining tissue should be taken to rule out residual cancer. Although we have not noticed an increase in the complication rate following postchemotherapy cystectomy the potential is clearly there.

SALVAGE CYSTECTOMY

Cystectomy following definitive radiotherapy is associated with a higher complication rate compared to cystectomy alone. Many authors have reported morbidity rates of approximately 45% and mortality rates of 5% to 8%.[8, 10, 11, 15] This increased complication rate is secondary to the fibrosis, ischemia, and tissue destruction caused by radiation. To decrease the chance of a complication, a few points should be kept in mind. First, the bladder will often be adherent to the pelvic sidewall and blunt dissection may result in a vesicostomy; sharp dissection with the electrocautery knife or surgical blade is then necessary. Second, the prostate can become adherent to the rectum following radiation therapy which may result in a rectal injury during the dissection. To prevent this, the prostate should be dissected off the rectum in a retrograde manner similar to a radical prostatectomy. Finally, the small bowel is at risk for ischemic injury when it is packed out of the field. Care should be taken to minimize the tension on the mesentery and to check the small bowel for ischemia periodically during the case.

The main complications that are more prevalent during salvage cystectomy compared to cystectomy alone are wound infections and rectal injuries. Radiation causes decreased wound healing and increases the incidence of wound infections with half of these, resulting in a wound dehiscence.[8] To prevent this complication we use an interrupted mattress closure of the full thickness of the abdominal wall excluding the subcutaneous fat and skin. We do not routinely use retention sutures.

Rectal injuries have been reported in 3% to 10% of salvage cystectomy series.[9, 10, 11, 16] This increased incidence is because the fibrotic reaction from the radiation obliterates the plane between the prostate and the rectum. If a rectal laceration occurs the same criteria for management should be employed as discussed earlier but the surgeon should not hesitate to perform a diverting colostomy.

CONCLUSION

Cystectomy is associated with a significant morbidity rate but some complications can be prevented by dividing the operation into a series of steps and completing one step before starting the next. Cystectomy following chemotherapy or external beam radiation are more difficult because of the fibrotic reaction that can occur in the perivesical tissue. If a complication does occur prompt recognition and treatment are imperative to stop further problems from developing.

EDITORIAL COMMENT

The complications of cystectomy, particularly radical cystectomy, are generally bleeding, rectal injury, or infection as indicated. A self-retaining retractor that provides extensive peripheral as well as deep retraction can be helpful in the anatomical dissection. I have not ligated the hypogastric artery but usually a dissection can be performed along the hypogastric artery with division of individual vesical branches. The apical prostatic dissection usually controls the dorsal vein of the penis. Dissection of the bladder from above can be carried down to the seminal vesicles in some patients and again the neurovascular bundle can be spared if the dissection is kept adjacent to the seminal vesicle.

Impotence remains another complication but now the majority of patients can have potency maintained following radical cystoprostatectomy with preservation of the neurovascular bundle. Urethrectomy tends to produce a higher incidence of impotence. This impotence may be reduced by careful dissection of the urethra with urethrectomy at the time of radical cystoprostatectomy. Some of these findings have been substantiated by Doctors Walsh and Brendler in our department.

I do not think there is enough good evidence to consider utilizing neoadjuvant chemotherapy in many patients. The overall staging accuracy and response rates are not high enough. Certainly this population represents a population that is also more likely to have complications.

REFERENCES

1. Wood DP, Jr, Montie JE, Maatman TJ, et al: Radical cystectomy for carcinoma of the bladder in the elderly patient. *J Urol* 1987; 138:46.
2. Whitmore WF, Jr, Marshall VF: Radical total cystectomy for cancer of the bladder: 230 consecutive cases five years later. *J Urol* 1962; 87:853.
3. Skinner DG, Crawford ED, Kaufman JJ: Complications of radical cystectomy for carcinoma of the bladder. *J Urol* 1980; 123:640.
4. Montie JE, Wood DP, Jr: The risk of radical cystectomy. *Br J Urol* 1989; 63:483.
5. Scher HI, Yagoda A, Herr HW, et al: Neoadjuvant M-VAC (Methotrexate, Vinblastine, Doxorubicin and Cisplatin) effect on the primary bladder lesion. *J Urol* 1988; 139:470.
6. Whitmore WF, Jr: Total cystectomy, in Cooper EH, Williams RE (eds): *The Biology and Clinical Management of Bladder Cancer.* Oxford, Blackwell Scientific, 1975, pp 193–227.
7. Walsh PC, Lepor H, Eggleston JC: Radical prostatectomy with preservation of sexual function: Anatomical and pathological considerations. *Prostate* 1983; 4:473.
8. Smith JA, Jr, Whitmore WF, Jr: Salvage cystectomy for bladder cancer after failure of definitive irradiation. *J Urol* 1981; 125:643.
9. Winter CC, Gluesenkamp EW: Management of intraoperative proctotomy incidental to total cystectomy for bladder carcinoma. *J Urol* 1973; 109:62.
10. Freiha FS, Faysal MH: Salvage cystectomy. *Urology* 1983; 22:496.
11. Konnack JW, Grossman HB: Salvage cystectomy following failed definitive radiation therapy for transitional cell carcinoma of bladder. *Urology* 1985; 26:550.
12. Bracken RB, McDonald M, Johnson DE: Complications of single-stage radical cystectomy and ileal conduit. *Urology* 1981; 17:141.
13. Flechner SM, Spaulding JT: Management of rectal injury during cystectomy. *Urology* 1982; 19:843.
14. Fair WR, Scher HI, Herr HW, et al: Clinical pathological downstaging of bladder preservation in patients receiving neoadjuvant M-VAC. Read at the Annual meeting of the American Urological Association, Dallas, Texas, Abstract. *J Urol* 1989; 141:245A.
15. Crawford ED, Skinner DG: Salvage cystectomy after irradiation failure. *J Urol* 1980; 123:32.
16. Swanson DA, von Eschenbach AC, Bracken RB, et al: Salvage cystectomy for bladder carcinoma. *Cancer* 1981; 47:2275.

CHAPTER 18

Complications of Urinary Diversion

Jerome P. Richie, M.D.

For more than a century, surgeons have grappled with the need to achieve an effective bladder substitute for patients with malignancy or malfunction of the lower urinary tract due to a variety of diseases or injuries. Urinary diversion has advanced through four basic eras of evolution in the maturation of diversionary procedures in conjunction with bowel.

The ureterosigmoidostomy era led to the development of antirefluxing techniques such as the direct buried anastomosis of Coffey, the elliptic mucosal anastomosis of Nesbit, and finally, the combined technique of Leadbetter and Clarke. In the early 1950s, Eugene Bricker popularized the development of ileal conduit urinary diversion, avoiding some of the complications that had been seen with ureterosigmoidostomy. This innovation seemed a far superior technique and rapidly gained acceptance for diversion for both malignant and benign lesions. Problems with deterioration of the upper tracts, in conjunction with free reflux, led Mogg and others to use the techniques of antireflux learned from ureterosigmoidostomy and apply these to isolated sigmoid colonic conduits or ileocecal conduits with antireflux valves. This change ushered in the third era of the nonrefluxing conduit. More recently, with the acceptance of intermittent self-catheterization, continent diversions, as described by Kock and Camey, have become popular. Thus, continent urinary diversions represent the fourth era of urinary diversion.

Each of these types of urinary diversion is associated with its own particular complications, and some complications are related to urinary diversion in general. The delicate nature and potential hazards of a major procedure such as urinary diversion require meticulous attention to every minute detail in order to prevent early or late complications. Each of the types of urinary diversion will be considered in detail in terms of early and late complications.

BASIC PREPARATION

Patient Preparation

In any elective procedure in which bowel will be utilized, bowel preparation, both mechanical and antibiotic, should be instituted preoperatively in order to minimize potential complications of infection. A standard bowel preparation that has worked well is that described by Nichols and associates.[1] A clear liquid diet is initiated 24 hours preoperatively and 60 mL castor oil is given 24 hours prior to the operation for mechanical cleansing. Oral neomycin (1 g/hr for four doses followed by 1 g/4 hr) and erythromycin base (1 g/6 hr) are given, beginning at 10 A.M. the morning prior to operation. Erythromycin base is added to neomycin to inhibit effectively the growth of colonic anaerobic organisms, particularly *Bacteroides fragilis*. If a colonic segment is to be incorporated, neomycin retention enemas are used the night prior to operation.

An equally effective outpatient bowel preparation consists of a castor oil preparation given 3 days preoperatively, along with clear liquids for the ensuing 3 days. In addition, 1 g neomycin and 1 g erythromycin base are each given by mouth four times daily for 2½ days prior to operation. This regimen seems to be better tolerated and can be done entirely on an outpatient basis rather than having the patient admitted early the day prior to operation in order to receive medications.

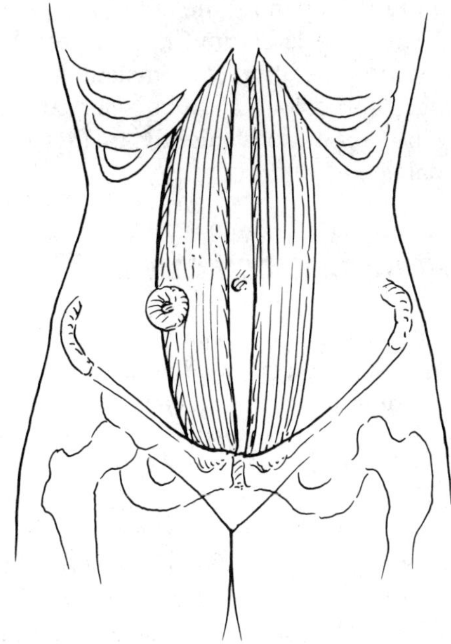

FIG 18–1.
Ideal stomal placement site. The stoma should be located just inside of the border of the rectus muscle and midway between the umbilicus and the anterior superior iliac spine. (From Richie JP, Skinner DG: Complications of urinary conduit diversion, in Smith RB, Skinner DG (eds): *Complications of Urologic Surgery*. Philadelphia, WB Saunders Co, 1976. Used by permission.)

Stomal Placement

From the patient's point of view, the stoma will be the single most important part of the surgical procedure. The success of the patient's adaptation to a new life will be governed by his ability to wear an external appliance and his relief from the problems of urinary leakage. It is incumbent upon the surgeon to exercise sound judgment in the construction and placement of a stoma that will function in the most appropriate manner. The stomal site should not impinge on any adjacent bony structure nor should it be near any abdominal deformity such as the umbilicus or a previous surgical scar (Fig 18–1). The abdominal incision should be chosen relative to the anticipated stomal site, with care being taken to keep the incision, retention sutures, and drains well away from the stoma. The site should be relatively flat, at least an inch and a half in diameter, and free of any surrounding scars or wrinkles in the abdominal wall. It is advisable to have an enterostomal therapist evaluate the patient preoperatively, both for patient education as well as selection of an appropriate stomal site. The ideal site is usually just below the center of a line connecting the umbilicus with the anterior superior iliac spine. In a relatively obese patient, the stoma should be placed somewhat more craniad than usual to allow visualization, which is an important aspect in the proper positioning of the appliance. The patient should be examined in the supine, sitting, and standing positions in order to be certain that no deformities or changes will cause stomal problems. The selected site should be marked with indelible ink or scratched preoperatively to prevent accidental erasure during preoperative shaving and preparation for operation. I prefer to make the stomal opening near the conclusion of the operative procedure rather than prior to opening the anterior abdominal wall. The later time is preferred because intraoperative circumstances may change, and a loop may be selected that may not reach conveniently to the ideal stomal site.

URETEROSIGMOIDOSTOMY

Ureterosigmoidostomy is historically the first type of urinary diversion that has been attempted, dating back to John Simon in 1851. Ureterosigmoidostomy was a logical first attempt to answer the problems of urinary diversion, relying upon the inherent advantage of an intact anal sphincter mechanism to control both urinary and fecal streams. Ureterosigmoidostomy was the procedure of choice from the 1880s until 1950, when Bricker described the isolated ileal conduit diversion. Many of the complications of ureterosigmoidostomy are related to the problem of admixture of urine with the fecal stream and the presence of fecal bacteria which may ascend to the upper tracts. Even though good techniques have been described for antirefluxing procedures, the complications of ureterosigmoidostomy continue to be a major concern to urologists. In addition, data concerning subsequent development of colonic tumors following ureterosigmoidostomy call attention to potentially significant or life-threatening long-term complications.

Early Complications

The most feared early complication of ureterosigmoidostomy is anuria, usually secondary to edema or obstruction of rectal drainage by fecal matter or mucus plugs. The use of two rectal tubes with multiple perforations will generally eliminate the problem. Anuria secondary to obstruction of the stents can be alleviated by removing the stents. If anuria persists, however, radiographic studies should be performed to search for a urinary leak.

The most distressing complication is leakage of urine from the ureterocolonic anastomosis or from the colotomy suture line. Abdominal distention, an increasing blood urea nitrogen ratio compared to serum creatinine, and poor urinary output signify such a complication. A small leak will usually seal without surgical intervention; however, a major leak necessitates immediate reoperation, drainage, reanastomosis, and possibly cutaneous diversion or nephrectomy.

Pelvic abscess may be heralded by spiking fevers. Ultrasonography, or, more recently, computed tomography, are valuable in diagnosing and localizing a pelvic abscess. Drainage should be performed through the lower abdominal incision or through a perineal stab wound.

Late Complications

Even with the use of the combined technique as described by Leadbetter and Clarke in 1954[2] or the transcolonic technique as described by Goodwin et al. in 1953,[3] pyelonephritis continues to be a significant problem. Wear and Barquin[4] reported an 81% incidence of acute pyelonephritis in patients with ureterosigmoidostomy using the older refluxing techniques of Coffey or Nesbit as compared to a 57% incidence using the combined technique of Leadbetter. Therefore, all patients should receive antibacterial medication for the first 3 months after surgery. Many patients should be advised to remain on antibiotics permanently.

Ureteral obstruction at the ureterocolonic anastomotic site may occur in 30% to 60% of patients. This condition can be minimized by use of a careful mucosa-to-mucosa anastomosis.

Renal calculi may occur as a late complication, usually associated with stasis and recurrent pyelonephritis. The incidence increases with the length of follow-up and is of the same magnitude as that observed after ileal loop cutaneous diversion.

Electrolyte disturbance after ureterosigmoidostomy was well described by Ferris and Odel in 1950.[5] This electrolyte disturbance is characterized by hypokalemia, hyperchloremia, acidosis, and absorption of ammonia from the rectal bladder. This electrolyte abnormality is seen in approximately 50% of patients undergoing ureterosigmoidostomy, more so in those with poor renal function. Supplementation with sodium potassium citrate will usually correct the abnormality.

Colonic neoplasia at the site of ureterosigmoidostomy has become an increasing problem in recent years. Hammer first reported the association of ureterosigmoidostomy with tumor in 1929.[6] In the ensuing 50 years, 45 documented cases have been reported.[7] The majority of these have been adenocarcinoma of the colon. There is a mean lag of 8.7 years in patients older than 40 years of age and 21 years in patients under 40. The patient with ureterosigmoidostomy has about a 5% risk of developing cancer of the colon at the implant site within 6 to 50 years.[8] Therefore, follow-up should include periodic tests for occult blood in the stool and yearly colonoscopy in order to detect changes at an early time.

DIVERSION INVOLVING ISOLATED BOWEL SEGMENTS

Acute Intestinal Obstruction.—The most common cause of early postoperative bowel obstruction is related to adhesions. Intestinal hernia may occur through a mesenteric defect after bowel anastomosis. Anastomotic obstruction may occur as a result of excessive narrowing of the stoma, especially with small bowel anastomoses. Angulation of distended loops may create a partial volvulus that may lead to obstruction as well. Postoperative bowel obstruction must be differentiated from adynamic ileus. Pain from acute abdominal obstruction is more likely to be intermittent and colicky, whereas adynamic ileus generally produces continuous abdominal discomfort of less intensity. Radiographic films of the abdomen reveal air-fluid levels and a stepladder appearance of the bowel, as well as an absence of gas in colon and rectum, when small intestinal obstruction exists.

Intestinal Leak.—Leakage from the enteric anastomosis should be extremely rare, regardless of the type of anastomosis utilized. The most likely site of a leak would be at the antimesenteric border of the enteroenterostomy. Overzealous and extended removal of the mesentery prior to diversion of the bowel predisposes to ischemia at the anastomotic site.

Intestinal fistulas usually respond to drainage, decompression with a long Miller-Abbott tube, and intravenous hyperalimentation. Occasionally, reexploration is necessary.

Vascular Thrombosis of Intestinal Conduit.—Excessive tension on the mesentery to the chosen bowel segment, hematoma in the mesentery, or inadvertent ligation of the major blood supply to the loop may result in ischemia, or, rarely, necrosis of the stoma or the entire bowel segment. The stoma, which may normally appear dusky at the termination of a procedure, fails to regain its healthy appearance over the ensuing hours or days. Endoscopy of the segment can be used to ascertain the extent of involvement. Although rarely resulting in urinary leakage in the first week, this complication should be recognized and corrected on a semiemergent basis, preferably at the time of the initial operation. Reexploration and reconstruction of an entire new segment are the treatments of choice, depending on the extent of thrombosis.

Wound Infection.—Wound infection may be related to spillage of contaminated bowel contents and is more common in a patient who has not received preoperative bowel preparation as well as intraoperative antibiotics. Patients who undergo urinary diversion in conjunction with radical cystectomy have a higher incidence of wound infection and potential dehiscence. Preoperative radiation therapy may well increase the rate of this complication. Wound infection can be minimized by appropriate preoperative and intraoperative antibiotics, careful irrigation of the subcutaneous tissues, and closure of the anterior abdominal wall with anterior fascial retention sutures.

URETEROILEAL CUTANEOUS DIVERSION

The isolated ileal conduit, popularized by Bricker in 1950,[9] has been by far the most common type of supravesical urinary diversion, and there have only been a few surgical modifications of Bricker's original description. These modifications relate predominantly to ureteral implantation into the isolated ileal segment. Barzilay and Wallace have described methods of joining the two ureters and implanting them together either into the side or the end of the ileal segment. However, it is my preference to close the butt end of the ileal conduit and anchor the conduit to the sacral promontory or right psoas muscle and then implant the ureters end-to-side just above the closed end of the segment.

Technique

Several aspects of ileal conduit urinary diversion need emphasis in order to minimize complications. Mobilization of the ureters should be adequate to achieve implantation without tension yet preserve adequate blood supply to the ureters. The ureters are usually identified where they cross the common iliac arteries and are traced into the pelvis and then ligated. Mobilization should be carried further craniad for the left ureter, since increased length is necessary in order to pass the ureter underneath the sigmoid mesocolon. Proximal mobilization of the ureter is facilitated by placement of a stay suture of 4-0 chromic catgut. A tunnel is then created beneath the sigmoid mesentery, preferably by blunt dissection, usually just below the level of the inferior mesenteric artery. The tunnel should be of adequate dimension for the left ureter to pass freely in a gentle arc to join the right ureter.

In preparation of the bowel segment, care should be taken to select a segment which will adequately reach to the surface without tension. Heavily irradiated intestine, identified by edematous muscularis with ischemic appearance of the serosa, should not be selected. Sufficient length of the segment must be utilized so the skin can be reached and an everting bud formed without tension. Attention should be paid to the arcades giving blood supply for the segment, and a base of mesentery should be selected wide enough for adequate venous return. Mesenteric incisions need be only 2 to 4 cm deep for the proximal segment, which will be anchored near the root of the mesentery. The distal segment, however, will require a longer mesenteric incision. Once the bowel segment has been selected, standard enteroenterostomy is performed and the butt end of the isolated bowel segment closed. Early closure of the proximal end of the bowel segment ensures an isoperistaltic segment.

The ureteroileal anastomosis is the crucial part of the operation, and meticulous attention must be paid to detail. The ureter should be spatulated along its medial surface and anastomosed end-to-side by means of closely spaced mucosa-to-mucosa interrupted sutures. My preference is to use 4-0 Vicryl absorbable sutures. Placement of the sutures in the ileum should incorporate the edge of the mucosa with a generous cuff of serosa. This cuff of serosa prevents tension on the mucosal anastomosis. Trauma to the ureter by forceps should be avoided. With the use of a stay suture and open forceps, no grasping of the ureteral mucosa should be necessary.

Creation of the stoma at the previously selected site is another major aspect of the procedure, insofar as the problems stemming from stomal placement place a major onus on the patient and the enterostomal therapist. I prefer to mark the stomal site with an "X" but not to excise an ellipse of skin until the conduit has been prepared and anchored and the ureteroileal anastomoses are performed. Therefore, if a change in site of the stoma becomes necessary, an alternate site can then be selected with no other incisions in the abdominal wall.

Prior to excising a button of skin and subcutaneous tissue, all layers of the abdominal wall are grasped with heavy clamps to avoid shuttering of the muscle layers. An elliptic incision, oriented craniad-caudad and approximately the size of a quarter, is excised at the predetermined location. The skin edges should not be undermined. Subcutaneous fat is excised in a wedged or cone-shaped fashion. A cruciate incision is made longitudinally in the anterior rectus fascia, the rectus muscle is split, and a longitudinal incision is made in the posterior fascia and peritoneum. The segment is then brought through the opening and should protrude at least 2 to 3 cm above the skin. If this cannot be accomplished without undue tension on the conduit mesentery, a loop stoma should be created according to the method of Turnbull and Fazio.[10]

Prior to bringing the ileal conduit through the ostomy opening, four stay sutures of 3-0 chromic catgut are passed through the anterior and posterior rectus fascia and temporarily clamped. This method excludes the rectus muscle from the area of the anastomosis and allows approximation of anterior and posterior fascia directly to the serosa of the bowel, thereby allowing firm anchoring and preventing herniation. The segment is brought through the opening with care that the mesentery is not rotated or compromised. The four tag sutures are then placed through the seromuscular layer to fix the bowel in place.

Eversion of the stoma is created by a modified Brooke technique. Quadrant sutures are placed through the subcuticular tissue at the cutaneous margin, through the seromuscular level of the ileum approximately 1 cm above the fascia fixation and through the full thickness of the ileum at the top of the loop. Tying these quadrant sutures will produce an everting cuff or sleeve, allowing the stoma to turn upon itself and creating a bud or everting stoma.

In patients who are obese or with a short, thick mesentery, the ileal segment often cannot be brought to the skin level without undue tension. In such patients, the end-loop ileostomy of Turnbull is performed. The distal end of the conduit is closed in standard fashion and a Penrose drain placed through the most mobile part of the ileal loop mesentery, approximately 3 to 4 cm from the closed distal end of the conduit. This section can be easily brought to the skin because it does not depend upon resection of the distal ileal segment (Fig 18–2). The terminal end of the loop is then delivered through the abdominal wall, with at least several centimeters protruding above the skin level. The functional limb of the loop is oriented caudad and the nonfunctioning limb cephalad. The loop is opened transversely four-fifths of the way around the circumference near the junction of the de-

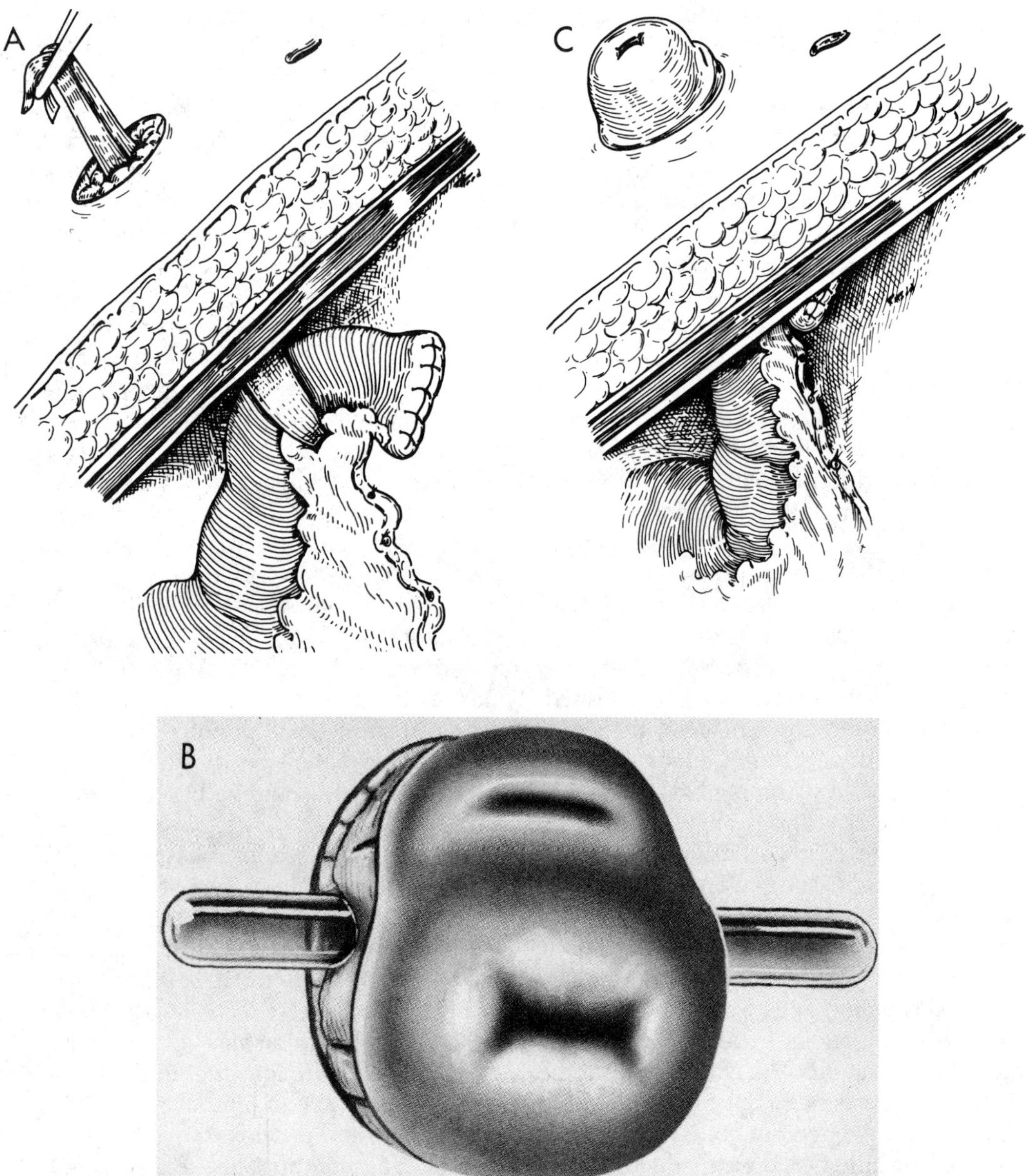

FIG 18–2.

Turnbull end-loop ileostomy. **A,** the end of the loop has been prepared and a tape passed through the mesentery in preparation for delivery of the loop. Note orientation of functional end of the limb in caudad position. **B,** loop has been opened four-fifths of the way across the nonfunctional segment, creating a protuberant functional and a recessive nonfunctional limb. Glass rod is optional. **C,** completed Turnbull stoma with the functioning loop pointed caudad and a short nonfunctioning loop pointed craniad. (From Weakley FL, Turnbull RB: Special intestinal procedures, in Stewart BH (ed): *Operative Urology.* Baltimore, Williams & Wilkins Co, 1975. Used by permission.)

functionalized limb and the skin, and the mucosa is everted, creating a large functionalized limb and a small defunctionalized limb ostomy.

Early Complications

Urinary or fecal leakage is the most dreaded and lethal of the early complications of urinary diversion. Leakage may occur in the early postoperative period, because of technical error, or it may be delayed, because of necrosis at the anastomosis. Various methods of treatment may be instituted for urinary leakage and/or fistula, depending upon the severity of the leak and the general condition of the patient. In a patient following cystectomy, in whom drainage has been provided, urinary leakage may be detected early by an increased output from the drain or hemovac sites. If the patient is stable and nonseptic, conservative therapy can be instituted with catheter drainage and low, intermittent sump suction.

If conservative management fails, percutaneous nephrostomy with antegrade passage of stents may be attempted. If this maneuver fails, however, exploration and revision are necessary. These procedures are necessarily difficult secondary to reaction from urinary extravasation. Occasionally, nephrectomy may be a more prudent choice. Other options include closure of the leakage site, resection of the leakage site, and reanastomosis to the bowel in a different area, or transureteroureterostomy.

(Other early complications are covered in the section on general bowel complications.)

Late Complications

Stomal Complications.—Stomal problems continue to be the most common complication of urinary diversion. Several reviews have disclosed that stomal stenosis develops in up to 25% of children that have undergone urinary diversion. The overall incidence of stomal complications ranges from 15% to 45%. Some of these complications relate to errors in construction of the stoma and correction may require reconstruction or repositioning of the stoma to the other lower abdominal quadrant. Some problems can be related to poor hygiene and can be corrected by proper instruction. Conservative measures should be given a trial in the management of problems such as dermatitis, encrustation, and even stenosis before surgical intervention is considered.

Education of the patient and his family must be initiated prior to the operation. Thorough understanding of and familiarity with all the requirements of stomal management will virtually eliminate complications stemming from neglect, poor hygiene, or misunderstanding. This education must be continued through the postoperative and convalescent periods, preferably with the aid of an enterostomal therapist, until the patient is thoroughly versed in the management of his appliance. Ideally, the collecting device should not require changes more frequently than every 5 to 7 days.

Stomal bleeding, encrustation, and plaque are problems that are almost always secondary to alkaline urine and poor hygiene. Acidification should be instituted and sometimes a bedside collecting device must be utilized to prevent bathing of the stoma in alkaline urine.

Peristomal Herniation.—This complication results from inadequate fascial fixation. There is obvious evidence of a hernia, and the patient has difficulty maintaining an appliance. Treatment generally requires open reduction and proper fixation at the fascial level. Careful suturing of the bowel serosa to both fascia layers in all quadrants will effectively prevent this complication. In a patient with poor muscle tone, synthetic fascial replacement material, such as Marlex or Proline mesh, occasionally may need to be incorporated into the fascial closure.

Ureterointestinal Obstruction.—Predominantly because of its silent nature, ureteral obstruction can be a significant and ominous complication which, if undiscerned, leads to progressive renal deterioration. Therefore, careful follow-up—either by excretory urograms or, recently, ultrasound—is the best way to recognize this problem early.

Obstruction occurs most commonly at the level of the ureteroileal anastomosis or where the left ureter crosses underneath the sigmoid mesocolon. Stenosis of the ureteroileal anastomosis may be caused by technical failure at the original anastomosis, ischemia with subsequent fibrosis, recurrent tumor, or abscess formation with scarring. Rarely, a calculus may lodge at the ureteroileal junction. Evaluation should include excretory urography, retrograde loopogram, and possible antegrade pyelogram.

Options for surgical repair include local incision with reanastomosis to the ileum, transureteroureterostomy, or a Heineke-Mikulicz type of pyloroplasty at the ureteroileal junction. Repair must be individualized, depending upon the circumstances causing the obstruction, the time after surgery, and a variety of other factors.

Pyelonephritis.—In a collected series of ileal diversions, pyelonephritis occurred in 5.8% of patients. This complication occurs more frequently in patients with previously damaged upper tracts. Treatment consists of administration of fluids and appropriate antibiotics. Evaluation should be carried out to exclude obstruction or other contributing anatomical factors. Recurrent bouts of pyelonephritis indicate long-term antibiotic therapy or consideration of conversion of the conduit to a nonrefluxing system.

Calculi.—Renal calculi occur in 5% of patients undergoing urinary diversion for benign disease. Calculi are seen more commonly in children after prolonged periods after urinary diversion, usually greater than 5 years. Dretler[11] in 1973 postulated that the pathogenesis of renal calculi formation relates to obstruction, hyperchloremic acidosis, buffering by calcium absorption from bone, and precipitation of calcium in the acid urine.

The mainstay of therapy for calculi is directed toward prophylaxis—adequate fluid intake, vigorous treatment of infection, and close surveillance. Large calculi may require removal or dissolution by a variety of techniques.

SIGMOID/ILEOCECAL CONDUIT

As increasing numbers of ureteroileal cutaneous diversions were performed, and patients were followed for longer periods of time, disappointment with the long-term effects of ileal conduit became more and more obvious. Reflux of infected urine produces chronic pyelonephritis in patients with an intact urinary system. Attention was thus turned to the development of more effective conduit systems, and Mogg[12] in 1967 reverted to the use of sigmoid colon as a conduit rather than reservoir. The colon offers major theoretical advantages: it has less absorption and the capability of creating antirefluxing tunnels because of the thicker musculature. Experimental animal models have shown an increased incidence of histologic pyelonephritis in freely refluxing ileal conduits when compared with nonrefluxing colonic conduits.[13]

Technique.—The redundant sigmoid colon is mobilized, and the redundant portion is incorporated into the conduit, with the blood supply derived from the last sigmoid artery or the superior hemorrhoidal artery. A standard colocolostomy is performed, and creation of submucosal tunnels is performed by the method described by Leadbetter and Clarke in 1954 for ureterosigmoidostomy. The stoma may be brought out in the left lower quadrant, shielded from the remainder of the bowel contents by the sigmoid mesocolon.

Early Complications.—The early complications are similar to those of ileal conduit or the ones covered in the general bowel section, with urinary leakage being somewhat less common than with ileal conduit diversion. However, early obstruction may occur and stenting may be preferable for these patients.

Late Complications.—Stomal complications are uncommon because of the larger size and better capability of the sigmoid colon to form an enterostomy. Likewise, stomal bleeding, encrustation, and plaque are less common problems. However, obstruction is more likely to be a problem because of the tunneled anastomosis. Another potential complication with sigmoid conduit is reflux from failure of the antireflux mechanism. In a review of 31 adults with nonrefluxing colon conduits, Hagen-Cook and Althausen[14] found that 28 of 31 patients had stable or improved upper tracts when followed for up to 3½ years postdiversion. Seven of 10 patients with preexisting reflux and pyelonephritis had no recurrences. In a review of Mogg's original series by Elder and associates, with an average follow-up of 13 years, renal deterioration was noted in 73% of the units with reflux compared with 21% of nonrefluxing units.[15] The isolated sigmoid conduit with antirefluxing ureterocolonic anastomosis may be a preferable form of permanent cutaneous diversion in children, but is performed rarely, because of success with intermittent catheterization, ureteral reimplantation, and artificial sphincters for the management of neurogenic bladder in children.

The transverse colon conduit, similar in construction to the sigmoid colon conduit, is useful in patients with extensive prior pelvic irradiation. The greatest benefit of the transverse colon is that a more proximal ureterocolonic anastomosis generally is used. Beckley and associates[16] reported the data on 30 patients who underwent transverse colon conduit after heavy irradiation, with no operative mortality and no complications in 86% of patients. The most frequent complication was peristomal hernia or stenosis.

JEJUNAL CONDUIT

In patients with prior heavy pelvic irradiation, the high jejunal conduit has been advocated as an alternative to the use of the transverse colon conduit. Morales and Whitehead[17] have had the most experience with this satisfactory alternative in patients with high-dose irradiation to the true pelvis. Surgical technique is similar to that for ileal conduit diversion, with a segment of the jejunum isolated approximately 5 to 10 cm distal to the ligament of Treitz. A standard enteroenterostomy is performed and end-to-side ureterojejunal anastomoses are performed high up in the retroperitoneum, well above the field of radiation therapy. The method of stomal creation and maturation is identical to that of ileal conduit.

The major complication from jejunal conduit diversion has to do with a unique electrolyte abnormality, the jejunal loop syndrome.[18] The syndrome is characterized by hypochloremia, hyponatremia, hyperkalemia, and acidosis. The jejunal conduit excretes sodium and chloride into the lumen and absorbs potassium, resulting in hyperkalemia. The syndrome is more prevalent in patients with diminished creatinine clearance. Patients who have undergone jejunal conduit diversion should add more salt to their diets in order to prevent hyponatremia and hyperkalemia. Jejunal conduits are generally contraindicated in patients with creatinine clearance less than 50 mL/min.

CONTINENT URINARY DIVERSIONS (KOCK POUCH, CAMEY PROCEDURE)

The innovative descriptions for continent forms of ileal diversion represent an exciting step forward in the evolution of urinary diversion. The procedures are not new, as attested to by the continent ureterocecocutaneous ileostomy of Gilchrist et al. over 30 years ago.[19] Continent methods of diversion logically should have sodium and chloride absorption and bicarbonate loss similar to ureterosigmoidostomy. Reflux must be prevented either by the ileocecal valve, an intussuscepted ileal nipple, or a tunneled ureterocolonic anastomosis. The advent of intermittent catheterization, along with suppressive antibiotics, has made many of these techniques now acceptable. Patient acceptance of the continent forms of urinary diversion seems to ensure that these types of procedures will continue to be performed and improved with time.

A variety of techniques are available to provide continent forms of urinary diversion, with the stoma brought out to the skin for intermittent catheterization or anastomosed directly to the urethra for normal voiding function. The early forms of continent diversion were the Kock pouch and the Camey procedure. Newer modified techniques have included use of the ileocecal segment with detubularization and a fluted ileal segment (Indiana pouch), detubularization of the ileocecal segment with interposition of an ileum (Mainz) pouch, or anastomosis of some of these detubularized segments directly to the urethra. Each of these methods of continent urinary diversion may have complication in general, as well as specific complications related to the type of diversion.

The Kock pouch form of continent ileal reservoir involves the use of a U-shaped segment of ileum approximately 80 cm in length to create a pouch with two intussuscepted nipples, one to provide the continence mechanism and the second to prevent reflux. In order to prevent extrasusception of the nipples, staples have been utilized in four quadrants in addition to incorporation of a Marlex mesh to serve as a collar and anchor the nipples to the serosa and to the anterior abdominal wall. Although long-term follow-up data are available only on the original patients operated on by Kock, certain potential complications unique to the Kock pouch do exist.

In addition to standard types of complications, including electrolyte absorption, five potentially distinct complications exist for the Kock pouch. The first is potential malabsorption related to the long segment of ileum removed. However, no problems with respect to absorption of bile salts or vitamin B_{12} have been reported with the use of this considerable length of small bowel. The second potential complication is reflux, which should be prevented by effective nipple valve construction. In a series of 12 patients studied by Kock and co-workers, reflux because of sliding of the reflux-protecting nipple valve was noted in three patients and subsequently corrected surgically.[20] In a report of Skinner et al., of 51 patients with Kock pouch continent ileal reservoir, early complications were seen in 10 patients.[21] There were no instances of reflux, however. One of the 51 patients was noted to have hyperchloremic acidosis. Five patients required reoperation and revision of the continence valve mechanism, and three required hospitalization for pyelonephritis. Thus, with attention to detail and the staples and collar, reflux should be prevented effectively in almost all patients. The third complication is loss of continence, which was seen in five of the patients in the series of Skinner et al. The nipple valve construction must include at least a 5-cm nipple, with staples interspersed to prevent extrasusception. A fourth complication is obstruction or failure to catheterize the pouch. Careful construction necessitates fixation of the collar to the anterior abdominal wall fascia so that a straight catheterization is effected. The fifth complication, unique to the Kock pouch, is potential stone formation on the staples that are used to prevent extrasusception of the nipple. Skinner et al. reported stone formation in two patients on exposed staples at the end of the nipples. Staples near the base of the nipple become buried in the mucosa, and stones have not been observed at that location. Skinner's current practice is to remove several distal staples from the end of the stapling device nearest to the end of the nipple. However, long-term follow-up of these patients will be necessary to see the effects of stone formation.

In the Camey procedure, a long segment of ileum is anastomosed directly to the urethra, with flap valve mechanisms to prevent reflux. Therefore, one segment is isoperistaltic and one segment antiperistaltic. Sagalowsky and associates in 1985 reported their preliminary experience.[22] Eight male patients underwent the Camey procedure, which involved the use of a U-shaped ileal segment, ureteroileal reimplantation in antirefluxing fashion, and urethroileal anastomoses. Ureteral reflux was seen in three patients. The most significant complication is daytime frequency and nocturnal enuresis. One enteric ileal bladder fistula was also reported in their series.

The Indiana urinary reservoir, consisting of tunneled ureteral implantations along the tenia for antireflux and a plication or tapering of the terminal ileal segment, has the advantage of a detubularized segment with continence created by the ileocecal valve. The technique, described by Rowland and associates, has the advantage that the use of the cecoileal continent reservoir is technically easier to perform than the Kock pouch urinary diversion.[23] Potential complications include difficulty with catheterization if the ileal segment has not been appropriately plicated, and incontinence. This technique depends upon the native ileocecal valve, either with reinforcement or intussusception of the ileum through the ileocecal valve, with the attendant disadvantage of staples.

Rowland and associates[23] reported their early experience with 29 patients. Initial procedures with no attempt at disrupting the tubular configuration of the cecum led to significant incontinence, which has been ameliorated by detubularization. The Mainz pouch, described by Thuroff and associates, involves splitting a rather long segment of ileum and the right colon with subsequent reanastomosis.[24] Antireflux mechanisms are created by tunneled implants into the colon. Continence is created by the ileoileal intussusception valve. This technique is applicable to diversion to the skin or reanastomosis to the urethra. Preliminary results are encouraging. Leakage may occur if the intussuscepted valve is not completely continent. Staples are used for the ileoileal intussusception technique, and these have the potential disadvantage of stones as well. A fascial strip around the base of the intussusception to secure the base to the abdominal wall has the potential for erosion.

All of these forms of continent diversion have potential metabolic complications. McDouglas reported significant hyperchloremic metabolic acidosis when bowel was used as a reservoir.[25] This acidosis can be reduced by the use of chlorpromazine or nicotinamide. Ammonia intoxication, osteomalacia, total body potassium depletion, and growth retardation are also possible consequences of continent forms of urinary diversion. Furthermore, the potential for defective vitamin B_{12} absorption has been reported.[26] In the pediatric age range, the use of this much bowel in a growing child may be a source of concern as well. Functional metabolic deficiencies can occur in children that may not become apparent for years. Because these problems are subtle, long-term observation will be necessary to establish the safety of continent urinary diversions in the pediatric age range.

The concept of a continent form of urinary diversion is certainly attractive. It must be emphasized, however, that all forms of urinary diversion seem to look good on short-term results. However, the lessons learned from the past indicate that long-term results are necessary in order to assess efficacy. Long-term follow-up data are not really available on the continent forms of urinary diversion, and the operations certainly are more time-consuming than other forms of urinary diversion. New and better forms of urinary diversion will certainly be described in the future, attesting to the innovative skills of the urologist in searching for an ideal substitute when the bladder needs to be removed or bypassed.

EDITORIAL COMMENT

Dr. Richie has outlined the evolution of urinary diversion, from ureterosigmoidostomy to ileal conduits, antirefluxing colon conduits, and, most recently, intestinal reservoir procedures such as the Camey procedure and the Kock pouch. A few personal impressions will be outlined. Although we rarely perform ureterosigmoidostomies we occasionally see such patients. We recently reconstructed a ureterosigmoidostomy in a 65-year-old exstrophy patient because of chronic pyelonephritis from massive coloureteral reflux. The patient was thought incorrectly to have urinary obstruction. He has done well.

Several points will be mentioned on ileal conduits. The Wallace ureteroileal anastomosis has never been as appealing because of its long suture line. For stomas, we usually do not excise any subcutaneous tissue in the formation of the ileal conduit stoma, because it is important to prevent any dimpling or inversion of the skin at the ileocutaneous junction. Peristomal hernias usually occur close to the mesentery at the superior aspect of the incision.[1] If local reconstruction of the stoma fails, it can be sometimes moved to the opposite side of the abdomen and brought through the contralateral rectus muscle. Jejunal conduits may be theoretically easy, but the mesentery of the small bowel is often shorter when higher small bowel segments are utilized. In obese patients it can sometimes be impossible to place the stoma easily with a high small bowel segment. Last, although Dr. Dretler's well-conceived explanations* for stone formation in ileal conduits certainly outline some factors that contribute to stone formation, the persistence of bacteria in a freely refluxing system with the nidus of mucus provides an excellent environment for struvite stone formation. It is surprising that struvite stone formation is not more common.

*Marshall FF, Leadbetter WF, Dretler SP: Ileal conduit parastomal hernias. *J Urol* 1975; 114:40.

EDITORIAL COMMENT II

There has been tremendous interest in continent urinary diversion in the past few years, with many new operations. The Kock pouch was one of the first operations to change urinary diversion from the concept of a conduit to that of a reservoir, although reservoirs have been constructed intermittently for some time. It is not clear that continent urinary diversion, particularly with a cutaneous anastomosis, is appropriate for all patients. Older debilitated patients may have difficulty catheterizing a stoma every 4 to 6 hours and a longer operation may increase the complication rate. If possible, we have emphasized a urethral anastomosis employing a detubularized ileocolic segment with a cecal urethral anastomosis.[†] In 20 patients we have been very pleased with our results. In general, these patients have continence at night. In addition, with preservation of the neurovascular bundle, potency can be maintained in the majority of patients. It is then possible to have patients void with excellent continence and have almost normal sexual function postcystectomy.

[†]Marshall FF: Creation of an ileocolic urinary bladder postcystectomy. *J Urol* 1988; 139:1264.

REFERENCES

1. Nichols RL, Broido P, Condon RE, et al: Effect of preoperative neomycin-erythromycin intestinal preparation on the incidence of infectious complications following colon surgery. *Ann Surg* 1973; 178:453.
2. Leadbetter WF, Clarke BG: Five years' experience with uretero-enterostomy by the 'combined' technique. *J Urol* 1954; 73:67.
3. Goodwin WE, Harris AP, Kaufman JJ, et al: Open, transcolonic ureterointestinal anastomosis; new approach. *Surg Gynecol Obstet* 1953; 97:295.
4. Wear JB, Jr, Barquin OP: Ureterosigmoidostomy: Long-term results. *Urology* 1973; 1:192.
5. Ferris DO, Odel HM: Electrolyte pattern of the blood after bilateral ureterosigmoidostomy. *JAMA* 1950; 142:634.
6. Hammer E: Cancer du colon sigmöide dix ans après implantation des ureteres d'une vessie exstrophiée. *J Urol Nephrol* 1929; 28:260.
7. Leadbetter GW, Jr, Zickerman P, Pierce E: Ureterosigmoidostomy and carcinoma of the colon. *J Urol* 1979; 121:732.
8. Preissig RS, Barry WF Jr, Lester RG: The increased incidence of carcinoma of the colon following ureterosigmoidostomy. *Am J Roentgenol* 1974; 121:806.
9. Bricker EM: Bladder substitution after pelvic evisceration. *Surg Gynecol Obstet* 1950; 30:1511.
10. Turnbull RB Jr, Fazio V: Advances in the surgical technique and ulcerative colitis surgery, in Nyhus L (ed): *Surgery Annual.* New York, Appleton-Century-Crofts, 1975, p 315.
11. Dretler SP: The pathogenesis of urinary tract calculi occurring after ileal conduit diversion: I. Clinical study. II. Conduit study. III. Prevention. *J Urol* 1973; 109:204.
12. Mogg RA: The treatment of urinary incontinence using the colonic conduit. *J Urol* 1967; 97:684.
13. Richie JP: Intestinal loop urinary diversion in children. *J Urol* 1974; 111:687.
14. Hagen-Cook K, Althausen M: Early observations on 31 adults with nonrefluxing colonic conduits. *J Urol* 1979; 121:13.
15. Elder DD, Moisey CU, Rees, RWM: A long-term followup of the colonic conduit operation in children. *Br J Urol* 1979; 51:462.
16. Beckley S, Wajsman W, Pontes JE, Murphy G: Transverse colon conduit: A method of urinary diversion after pelvic irradiation. *J Urol* 1982; 128:464.
17. Morales PA, Whitehead ED: High jejunal conduit for supravesical urinary diversion. Report of 25 cases. *Urology* 1973; 1:426.
18. Golimbu M, Morales P: Electrolyte disturbances in jejunal urinary diversion. *Urology* 1973; 1:432.
19. Gilchrist RK, Merricks JW, Hamlin HH, et al: Construction of a substitute bladder and urethra. *Surg Gynecol Obstet* 1950; 90:752.
20. Kock NG, Nilson AE, Nilsson LO, et al: Urinary diversion via a continent ileal reservoir: Clinical results in 12 patients. *J Urol* 1982; 128:469.
21. Skinner DG, Boyd SD, Lieskovsky G: Clinical experience with the Kock continent ileal reservoir for urinary diversion. *J Urol* 1984; 132:1101.
22. Sagalowsky I, Allen TD, Chinn HK, et al: Preliminary experience with the continent

ileal bladder (Camey procedure) (abstract 219). Presented at American Urological Association 80th Annual Meeting, Atlanta, May 13–18, 1985.

23. Rowland RG, Mitchell ME, Bihrle R, et al: Indiana continent urinary reservoir. *J Urol* 1987; 137:1136.
24. Thuroff JW, Alken P, Riedmiller H, et al: Mainz pouch (mixed augmentation ileum and cecum) for bladder augmentation and continent diversion. *J Urol* 1986; 136:17.
25. McDougal WS: Bladder reconstruction following cystectomy by ureteroileocolourethrostomy. *J Urol* 1986; 156:698.
26. Kinn AC, Lantz B: Vitamin B_{12} deficiency after radiation for bladder carcinoma. *J Urol* 1984; 131:888.

CHAPTER 19

Complications of Simple and Radical Prostatectomy

Alex F. Althausen, M.D.

When it has been determined that the patient's symptoms of urinary outlet obstruction secondary to prostatic hyperplasia warrant operative treatment, several different surgical techniques can be used: suprapubic, retropubic, perineal, and transurethral.[1-8]

No single method has established itself as the best operation for the relief of prostatism. The choice of any of these procedures should be determined by the surgical anatomy of the prostate, bladder, and urethra as well as the patient's general physical condition.

Suprapubic prostatectomy is the procedure of choice when the patient requires simultaneous excision of bladder diverticula or removal of vesical calculi too large or dense to be taken care of by endoscopic methods. A prostatic gland that is mainly intravesical also lends itself easily to this technique.

The retropubic approach has the advantage of direct access to the prostatic bed, allowing "cleaner" enucleation of a large intraurethral gland with subsequent better hemostatic control than the suprapubic technique. The operative time is usually longer but may afford fewer complications in the end.

H. H. Young[9] refined and popularized the perineal approach to prostatectomy. This technique is still preferred by many senior urologists in treating hyperplasia as well as prostatic cancer. However, impotence is usual and urinary incontinence and rectal injury may occur with the inexperienced perineal surgeon.[9]

Better optics and instrumentation have greatly increased the safety of transurethral surgery. Urethral stricture, ankylosis of the hip, certain penile prostheses, and other less common conditions may preclude transurethral surgery and require open prostatectomy. (Indications and complications of transurethral surgery are discussed in Chap. 20.)

HEMORRHAGE

Knowledge of the prostatic blood supply is mandatory for the control of bleeding at the time of surgery. R. H. Flocks described the distribution of the arteries within the prostate in his classic 1937 monograph.[10]

The inferior vesical artery divides into a branch supplying the vas deferens and seminal vesicle and branches supplying the prostate and bladder base. The prostatic arteries enter the capsule and the prostate at the level of the bladder neck, in front of the seminal vesicle. There are usually four vessels on either side which break up into the external capsular group and the internal urethral group. The capsular group passes along the outer surface of the gland posterolaterally. The internal urethral vessels penetrate the gland at the vesicoprostatic junction between the median and lateral lobes. They supply the majority of the hyperplastic prostate. These vessels are fairly large and usually recognizable after enucleation (Fig 19–1).

It is, therefore, sound surgical judgment to suture-ligate these vessels even if they are not actively bleeding. Most often the internal urethral vessels are seen coming out from the bladder neck at 5- and 7-o'clock.

The deep dorsal vein of the penis may also be a troublesome source of bleeding, especially in retropubic prostatectomy. This vein appears in the retropubic space on the anterior aspect of the prostatic capsule between the puboprostatic ligaments and then branches at the bladder neck. It is wise to suture-ligate and divide the vein before it branches and electrocoagulate the tributaries if they interfere with retropubic capsulotomy.[11]

A tear in the prostatic capsule may occur when the surgeon loses the necessary landmarks or has the misfortune of trying to enucleate a small fibrous gland. This complication may also occur when carcinomatous enlargement of the prostate is missed prior to surgery.

Tearing of the capsule not only causes excessive bleeding but may lead to rectal damage as well as urinary incontinence. Part of the seminal vesicles usually comes with the specimen.

The first priority in this situation is to suture the prostatic vessels as they emerge from the area of the vesical neck and, if possible, suture the external prostatic arteries as they branch posterolaterally from the seminal vesicles. If bleeding still persists, then ligation of the inferior vesical artery on either side of the bladder neck becomes necessary.

When the bleeding is under control, the remaining prostatic tissue can be removed by making an incision at 12 o'clock through the bladder neck into the anterior prostatic capsule. This allows greater exposure of the prostatic bed (if the original attempt was at suprapubic enucleation).

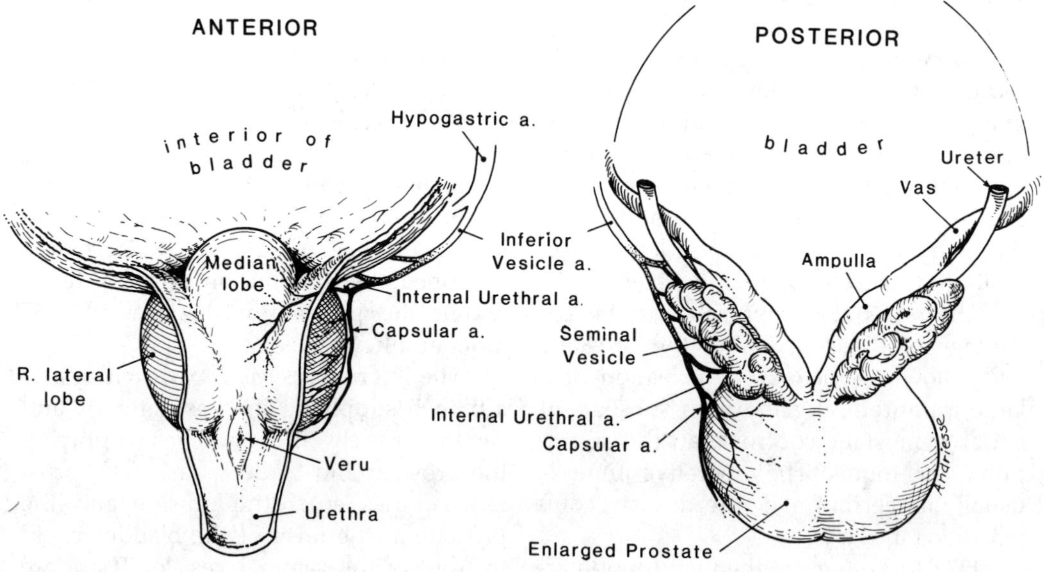

FIG 19–1.
Anatomy of prostate: anterior and posterior views.

Sharp dissection of the obstructing prostatic tissue is necessary. The inadvertent capsular tears may then be better closed. A suprapubic tube as well as a Foley catheter is used to achieve adequate urinary drainage and minimize extravasation and clot retention.

Occasionally, a large prostate is enucleated and the capacious bed fails to contract. A constant venous ooze ensues. In this instance, imbrication of the posterior prostatic capsule with heavy chromic sutures stops further bleeding.

Finally, intraoperative as well as postoperative hemorrhage may occur if the patient has a bleeding disorder that was not recognized when his history was taken at admission or if the patient has been receiving medicine that may promote poor clotting (see Chap. 10). Routine bleeding studies should be obtained for all patients prior to surgery.

FISTULAS

Urinary extravasation occurring early in the postoperative period in patients who have undergone open prostatectomy usually decreases with time. However, if it persists beyond the first postoperative week, a cystogram is performed to locate the site of leakage.

Most often the extravasation is due to poor operative technique in closing the bladder or the prostatic capsule. The tissues may have become devitalized from dissection and not debrided properly before closure. Inadvertent capsular tears or bladder calculi may have been missed.

The position and patency of the Foley catheter must also be checked. If the position and drainage are adequate, then the urethral catheter may be left in place for 2 or 3 more weeks. Most fistulae will close.

When a repeated cystogram continues to show a fistula, cystoscopic evaluation is necessary. If the fistulous tract is large, immediate reoperation with adequate debridement and closure, rather than waiting months for spontaneous closure, will greatly shorten the patient's distress. Small urinary fistulas will eventually close spontaneously. Curetting the superficial tract will remove excessive granulation tissue, allowing faster closure. Silver nitrate stick application may also help.

With radical prostatectomy, urinary extravasation for the first week or 10 days is not unusual. Tissue drains are left until the drainage stops. Occasionally, putting the catheter to chest suction at 15 cm decreases the drainage more quickly.

Fecal fistulas occur most often when the perineal surgeon is inexperienced and loses sight of the standard anatomical landmarks. Intraoperative recognition of rectal trauma is most helpful. The musculomucosal tear can then be closed primarily in standard surgical fashion and the rectal sphincter dilated gradually to four fingers. Antibiotics to help with bowel sterilization and prolonged urethral catheter drainage are necessary.

If the fecal drainage is discovered postoperatively, prolonged catheter drainage usually will not allow spontaneous closure. A diverting colostomy is performed, and further evaluation and closure of the fistula are attempted at least 3 months after initial injury. This treatment allows the development of better tissue planes for future repair and the very occasional spontaneous closure of the fistula. Standard surgical texts and numerous articles in the urologic literature will aid the reader in developing the best techniques in handling this disastrous complication.

URETERAL OBSTRUCTION/REFLUX

Postoperative flank pain or colic associated with fever should alert the urologist to the possibility of ureteral obstruction. This complication may be due to inadvertent suture ligation of the ureteral orifice at the time of placement of bladder neck sutures for hemostasis after enucleation of the prostate. To avoid this complication, intravenous injection of methylene blue or indigo carmine will allow visualization of the orifices as "blue urine" effluxes from them. Placement of catheters into the ureters is another method for continuous identification of the intravesical ureters.

Ureteral reflux as well as obstruction may result from acute inflammation of the trigone. This can occur from urinary tract infection as well as urethral catheter–induced cystitis. Postsurgical trigonitis from manipulation of the bladder neck is another cause. Severe inflammation causes the ureteral tunnels to stiffen, resulting in reflux. However, vesicorenal reflux in the immediate postoperative period occurs more commonly than is believed and is usually asymptomatic. It is the obstructed ureter that produces renal colic and/or pyelonephritis.

An intravenous pyelogram is necessary to confirm the clinical suspicion of ureteral obstruction. Cystoscopy, with placement of a ureteral stent or catheter for a week to 10 days, usually takes care of the problem. When the orifices cannot be identified or catheterized, a percutaneous nephrostomy is done with a follow-up nephrostogram and pressure studies 1 week later. Persistent ureteral obstruction with high antegrade flow pressures will require surgical correction when the tissues have adequately healed from the initial prostatectomy.

STRICTURE

Urethral stricture and bladder neck contracture occur more commonly as complications of transurethral surgery than as the result of open prostatectomy because of longer intraurethral instrumentation and the electrical current of injury.

Terrence Millin[7] reported a 6% to 7% incidence of bladder neck contracture in patients after retropubic prostatectomy prior to his routine use of resecting a segment of posterior bladder neck. Since then, contractures have diminished to less than 2%. Removing a segment of the bladder neck can be done in suprapubic prostatectomy as well. Suturing the posterior bladder neck to the posterior prostatic capsule will also help to avoid this complication.[7]

Bladder neck contractures are not uncommon in radical prostatectomy if the reconstructed bladder neck is less than a 26F diameter. In patients with a prolonged urine leak at the site of the vesicourethral anastomosis, a contracted bladder neck may also develop.

The incidence of bladder neck contracture is higher in patients whose prostatic tissue is inflamed, as in cases of acute abscess or calculous prostatitis. Healing may then result in excessive fibrous scar formation.

The treatment of bladder neck contractures should be transurethral incision or transurethral resection of the scarred tissue. If this procedure fails, open bladder neck revision with a Y-V plasty becomes necessary.

Urethral strictures result most often from urethritis caused by the Foley catheter. The three most common sites are the bulbomembranous, distal bulbar, and meatal urethral segments. Urethral dilatation is the initial treatment. If the strictures recur, then an internal urethrotomy under direct endoscopic vision should be done. Further failures may require urethroplasty.

When a postprostatectomy patient presents with voiding dysfunction or develops the same symptoms that he had prior to surgery, anatomical outlet obstruction needs to be excluded. This evaluation is accomplished by a voiding cystourethrogram, followed by a retrograde urethrogram at the time of cystoscopic evaluation. Once the diagnosis is made, treatment is usually obvious.

INCONTINENCE

Transient loss of urinary control is common in the early postprostatectomy patient. When the urethral catheter is out, urinary urgency with urge incontinence occurs. The prostatic bed is still not urothelialized. This raw surface causes severe urgency with incontinence secondary to detrusor hyperreflexia. Edema of the external sphincter and partial incompetence of the internal sphincter (bladder neck) aid in producing urinary stress incontinence. Stress and urgency incontinence of this nature usually disappear within the first postoperative month.[12]

Total urinary incontinence following subtotal prostatectomy is disastrous, though extremely rare; its incidence is less than 1%. This complication occurs when the external sphincter has been damaged permanently in association with surgical trauma to the bladder neck and prostatic capsule.

A voiding cystourethrogram, retrograde urethrogram, and cystoscopy must all be done prior to urodynamic evaluation. Urodynamic studies will evaluate bladder sensation, capacity, compliance, and contractions. The urethral pressure profile helps determine the extent of sphincteric efficiency.[13]

Preservation of urinary continence is in the hands of the urologist. Basic tenets of prostatic surgery must be followed: the urethra is severed just at the apex of the prostate prior to removing the adenomatous tissue; no adenoma is left behind; no sutures are placed or dissection done at the urogenital diaphragm; and care is taken in placing instruments and catheters into the bladder transurethrally.

Conservative measures in treating postprostatectomy incontinence are tried first. Perineal exercises in combination with pharmacologic agents are used. Knowledge of the neurophysiology of voiding is mandatory for the intelligent application of the many drugs that inhibit or stimulate bladder, bladder neck, and urethral contractions.

If a patient's incontinence 1 year after prostatectomy is still disabling, surgical correction, using the multiple prosthetic devices available, is then tried. Penile clamps, condom drainage, and supravesical urinary diversion are all methods that can be used if everything else fails. Artificial sphincters will usually solve incontinence.

RETENTION

Urinary retention following subtotal prostatectomy is most often due to retained adenomatous tissue or a hypotonic bladder from chronic vesical overdistention.

When a patient fails his first voiding trial, the urethral catheter is reinserted for 2 or 3 more days. The second failure requires cystoscopy, preceded by a urethrogram to look for retained adenoma or a flap of tissue that could create a ball valve effect obstructing the bladder outlet in an antegrade fashion. If no obvious anatomical causes for retention are found, urodynamic studies are indicated. For the hypotonic bladder, pharmacologic treatment is used, combining medications that stimulate bladder contractions with those that inhibit the function of the bladder neck and urethra. If this line of treatment fails, a reduction cystoplasty can be successful in selected patients.

IMPOTENCE

Erectile impotence following prostatectomy should be considered a complication only if the urologist has failed to discuss this possibility with the patient prior to surgery.

The organic causes of nonperineal, subtotal prostatectomy impotence are poorly understood, unless the posterior and lateral parts of the capsule have been violated. The pelvic plexus that provides autonomic innervation to the corpora cavernosa passes between the rectum and urethra through the urogenital diaphragm. This plexus may be injured at the time of radical prostatectomy when the lateral pedicles of the prostate are divided or at the time of apical prostatic dissection and urethral transection.[14, 16] Loss of ejaculation in the subtotal prostatectomy patient is usually a constant finding. The bladder neck is made partially incompetent, the ejaculatory ducts are removed or injured, and the majority of the fluid-producing tissues are no longer there. Again, this is not a complication if the patient is made aware of this preoperatively. Drugs to "tighten" the bladder neck have not been successful in creating adequate antegrade ejaculation in the postprostatectomy patient.

TABLE 19–1.
Complications of Radical Retropubic Prostatectomy (%)

	Lieskovsky and Skinner (1983)[17]	Middleton (1987)[18]	Peters (1988)[19]
Pulmonary embolism	4.6	5.3	3.6
Rectal injury	3.0	3.1	3.6
Lymphocele	3.0	0.8	0.0
Bladder neck contracture	N/A	4.5	4.0
Chronic incontinence	3.2	3.1	1.2
Mortality	1.5	0.0	N/A

N/A = not available.

RADICAL RETROPUBIC PROSTATECTOMY

Walsh and Donker and associates have created a renaissance in the surgical treatment of localized cancer of the prostate with their potency-sparing technique described in 1982.[16] A modified pelvic lymph node dissection is done prior to the prostatectomy in order to stage the disease. Once the surgical anatomy is understood and the prescribed surgical techniques are followed, the complications become more acceptable (Table 19–1).

Impotence

The pelvic plexus is most commonly injured at the time of urethral transection or when the lateral pelvic fascia and pedicles are divided. When strict attention is paid to detail, potency returns in over 80% of patients within 1 year of surgery. The older a patient is and the more advanced the local pathologic stage of the cancer, the less chance there is of preserving sexual potency. Patients 70 years of age or older with B2 disease have about a 50% postoperative potency rate. If one neurovascular bundle is sacrificed the potency rate does not drop proportionately but does fall 10% to 20% more than the expected figure.

Another surgical cause of impotence can occur at the time the posterior row of sutures are placed in the urethra for the vesicourethral anastomosis. Care must be taken to avoid entrapment of the cavernous nerves and the neurovascular bundles by the stitches.

It is important to emphasize that the priority of radical retropubic prostatectomy is not the preservation of potency but the extirpation of local disease. This tenet should not be compromised if nerve-sparing leaves tumor behind.

Incontinence

Total urinary incontinence following radical surgery is, fortunately, less than 4%. Again, good surgical technique will allow for a visual placement of the urethral sutures. Occasionally partial pubectomy becomes necessary to perform the anastomosis. Tumor at the urethral resection margin may be a cause of persistent incontinence as it grows to involve the fibers of the external sphincter. Artificial sphincters should be considered when the degree of incontinence is socially crippling.

Urinary stress incontinence is seen in the majority of early postoperative patients. Perineal exercises and the occasional use of pharmacologic agents help resolve this problem within 3 to 6 months.

Bladder Neck Contracture

Contracture of the bladder neck is caused by a non–mucosa-to-mucosa anastomosis of the bladder to the urethra. Walsh has advocated eversion of the mucosa at the newly formed bladder neck prior to the vesicourethral approximation. This has minimized leakage and subsequent fibrosis. The bladder neck should be no larger than a 20F to 26F opening. Fibrosis also may potentiate urinary incontinence by the resultant stiffness of the posterior urethra. Cystoscopic evaluation of the postoperative patient with symptoms of bladder outlet obstruction and/or urinary incontinence allows for a rational approach to a potentially difficult problem.

PELVIC LYMPHADENECTOMY

The major long-term complication of a pelvic lymphadectomy is genital or lower extremity edema. This usually occurs less than 2% of the time but may be problematic. Since the removal of pelvic lymph nodes for the prostatic cancer patient is only a staging procedure rather than a "curative" one, it becomes necessary to avoid major complications. We have left most of the external iliac chain behind unless the adenopathy is palpable. This allows for adequate drainage and helps avoid edema if adjuvant pelvic irradiation is deemed necessary.

A lymph leak or lymphocele is avoided by carefully ligating or cauterizing all lymphatic channels that have been severed.

Thrombophlebitis and pulmonary embolism can be largely avoided by fitting the patient with pneumatic antiembolism boots prior to the induction of anesthesia. The boots are left in place for the first 4 to 5 postoperative days. This simple procedure diminishes a potentially fatal outcome to less than 1% and obviates the worry of prophylactic anticoagulation. Intraoperative injury to the ureters can be prevented by the temporary insertion of ureteral catheters until the bladder neck is refashioned. Rectal tears are closed in the standard fashion and should be accompanied by a diverting colostomy.

EDITORIAL COMMENT

Fortunately, the complications of open prostatectomy, especially bleeding, can be managed satisfactorily. Other complications, such as urinary fistulas and ureteral obstruction, are rather rare. Incontinence can be a tragic complication but the use of the artificial sphincters has greatly aided the urologist with this catastrophic complication when all other conservative treatments have failed. Urinary retention may reflect detrusor dysfunction if all obstructive tissue has been removed. Occasionally, a patient will present with a very hypotonic bladder, and intermittent self-catheterization following prostatectomy will be required.

EDITORIAL COMMENT II

Radical prostatectomy is performed more frequently because the refinement of the technique as described by Walsh and others has greatly reduced the incidence of complications. Control of the dorsal vein of the penis is one of the most important steps in the operation because, if not controlled, injury to the neurovascular bundle, rectal injury, or a poor anastomosis are more likely to ensue. I have never had to perform a pubectomy for a radical prostatectomy but I have taken the orthopedic chisel and removed an osteophyte on the posterior aspect of the symphysis. This maneuver greatly improved visualization of the apex of the prostate. If a bowel preparation is given routinely, a small rectal tear can sometimes be repaired primarily with interposition of omentum between the urethral anastomosis and the rectum. If there is any question, a colostomy should be performed.

REFERENCES

1. Belfield WT: Operations on the enlarged prostate, with a tabulated summary of cases. *Am J Med Sci,* 1890; 100:439.
2. Belt E, Ebert CE, Surber AC Jr: A new anatomic approach in perineal prostatectomy. *J Urol* 1939; 41:482.
3. Flocks RH (ed): The prostate. *Urol Clin North Am* 1975; 2:1.
4. Freyer PJ: A new method of performing prostatectomy. *Lancet* 1900; 1:774.
5. Hudson PB, Stout AP: *An Atlas of Prostatic Surgery.* Philadelphia, WB Saunders Co, 1962.
6. Lowsley O.S.: Total perineal prostatectomy. *J Urol* 1940; 43:275.
7. Millin T: *Retropubic Urinary Surgery.* Edinburgh, E & S Livingstone Ltd, 1947.
8. O'Conor VJ Jr, Bulkley GJ, Sokol JK: Low suprapubic prostatectomy: Comparison of results with the standard operation in two comparable groups of 142 patients. *J Urol* 1960; 84:493.
9. Young HH, Davis DM: *Young's Practice of Urology.* Philadelphia, WB Saunders Co, 1926, pp 497–500.
10. Flocks RH: The arterial distribution within the prostate gland: Its role in transurethral prostatic resection. *J Urol* 1937; 37:524.
11. Malament M: Maximal hemostasis in suprapubic prostatectomy. *Surg Gynecol Obstet* 1965; 120:1307.
12. Kaufman JJ, Raz S (ed): Male incontinence. *Urol Clin North Am* 1978; 5:2.
13. Turner-Warwick R, Whiteside CG (ed): Clinical urodynamics. *Urol Clin North Am* 1979; 6:1.
14. Finkle AL, Taylor SP: Sexual potency after radical prostatectomy. *J Urol* 1981; 125:350.
15. Furlow WL (ed): Male sexual dysfunction. *Urol Clin North Am,* 1981; 8:1.
16. Walsh PC, Donker PJ: Impotence following radical prostatectomy: Insight into etiology and prevention. *J Urol* 1982; 150:492.
17. Lieskovsky G, Skinner DG: Technique of radical retropubic prostatectomy with limited pelvic node dissection. *Urol Clin North Am* 1983; 10:187.
18. Middleton AW Jr: Radical prostatectomy for carcinoma in men more than 69 years old. *J Urol* 1987; 138:1185.
19. Peters PC: Complications of radical prostatectomy and lymphadenectomy. *Urol Clin North Am* 1988; 15:219.

CHAPTER 20

Complications of Transurethral Resection of the Prostate

Arnon Krongrad, M.D.
Michael J. Droller, M.D.

Transurethral prostatectomy (TURP) is the most common urologic operation done in the United States.[1] Interestingly, the rates at which TURP is performed show great regional and even international variability.[2, 3] This probably reflects, at least in part, the perceived utility of this treatment. While most patients undergoing TURP experience long-term improvement in symptoms and quality of life, short-term complications (such as clot retention) and occasional long-term complications (such as incontinence and impotence) may occur.[4, 5] Thus variability in perception of risk may also contribute to variability in TURP rates.

Risk on an individual basis is not necessarily predicted by large-scale epidemiologic data. However, several general observations are of interest. In the United States, for example, mortality is inversely correlated to surgical volume.[6] Mortality is also nearly twice higher in smaller hospitals and more than three times higher in non–university hospitals.[7] For a given age group, a man having a TURP is almost three times more likely to die the same year as a man not having a TURP.[3] Nearly two thirds of post-TURP deaths in the first 3 months occur following discharge.[7, 8] Compounding the initial risk is a 20% eight-year probability of reoperation.[7] With advancing age, operative mortality may increase by almost six times.[8] Age also determines postoperative ability to void, complications, and length of stay.[9]

Notwithstanding the above, overall mortality and morbidity associated with TURP have decreased over the last three decades.[9] Better recognition of individual risk factors, perioperative prophylaxis, and management of these, and advances in instrumentation have been responsible. This chapter reviews the fundamentals of perioperative and intraoperative safety for TURP in the context of the potential complications that may occur.

PREOPERATIVE CONSIDERATIONS

Seventy-five percent of men undergoing TURP have a history of other medical problems.[9] Since TURP is an elective procedure, concurrent medical problems which might complicate anesthesia or promote bleeding should be addressed and minimized preoperatively.

Particular attention must be paid to cardiac and respiratory function, as dramatic fluid shifts and circulatory alterations may accompany TURP. In one study, eight of 12 unselected men experienced a mean decrease in cardiac index of 37%.[10] This was in the absence of hyponatremia. As documented by intracardiac catheterization, vital signs were maintained by elevation of peripheral resistance. Patients at risk for endocarditis must receive appropriate prophylaxis (Table 20–1).

Azotemia has also been shown to herald increased risk, perhaps as a sign of a compromised, chronically ill patient.[9, 11] Bladder drainage should precede TURP by a period sufficient to allow serum creatinine to stabilize if urinary retention with outlet obstruction transmitted to the upper tracts is responsible for this. Interestingly, however, no study has shown that correction of preoperative azotemia for a given patient will diminish that risk.

TABLE 20–1.

Endocarditis Prophylaxis in Transurethral Prostatectomy

Adults: Aqueous crystalline penicillin G (2 × 10^6 IM or IV)

OR

Ampicillin (1.0 g IM or IV)

PLUS

Gentamicin (1.5 mg/kg [not to exceed 80 mg] IM or IV)

OR

Streptomycin (1.0 g IM)

Give initial doses 30 min to 1 hr prior to procedure. If gentamicin is used, give a similar dose of gentamicin and penicillin (or ampicillin) every 8 hr for two additional doses.* If streptomycin is used, give a similar dose of streptomycin and penicillin (or ampicillin) every 12 hrs for two additional doses*

*For those patients who are allergic to penicillin**

Adults: Vancomycin (1.0 g IV given over 30 min to 1 hr)

Plus

Streptomycin (1.0 g IV)

A single dose of these antibiotics begun 30 min to 1 hr prior to the procedure is probably sufficient, but the same dose may be repeated in 12 hr*

*During prolonged procedures, or in the case of delayed healing, it may be necessary to provide additional doses of antibiotics. For brief outpatient procedures, such as uncomplicated catheterization of the bladder, one dose may be sufficient.

In patients with significantly compromised renal function, it may be necessary to modify the dose of antibiotics used. Some of these doses may exceed manufacturer's recommendations for a 24-hr period. However, since they are only recommended for a 24-hr period, in most cases it is unlikely that toxicity will occur.

Preoperative evaluation of clotting mechanisms is mandatory. Patients with known bleeding disorders, such as hemophilia, may successfully undergo TURP with appropriate precautions and prophylactic therapy.[12, 13] Although use of nonsteroidal anti-inflammatory drugs does not appear to increase blood loss,[14] the use of aspirin is to be avoided. Intraoperative transfusions are given 2.5% of the time,[9] but recommendations regarding routine preoperative cross-matching are contradictory.[15, 16]

Concurrent urologic problems, such as bladder stones, may be managed at the time of TURP. However, this approach may also occasionally be associated with premature termination of the prostatectomy, necessitating a repeat procedure.[17]

Neurologic disease associated with bladder dysfunction must be addressed when the decision to operate is made. Sixty percent of patients with postprostatectomy incontinence have been found to have some form of dysfunction.[18]

PERIOPERATIVE ANTIBIOTICS

The indications for perioperative antibiotics remain controversial, and extensive reviews on the subject have been published.[19] Although perioperative sepsis is rare, it is the leading cause of death from TURP.[9, 20] Other infectious complications, such as bacteriuria and epididymitis, have also been the focus of a large number of studies, with divergent results.

In evaluating the clinical relevance of published studies, one must distinguish between laboratory and clinical abnormalities. For instance, in one study, four out of 14 patients undergoing TURP became bacteremic.[21] However, bacteremia was uncovered only because of study design, and not because of clinical sepsis. Similarly, a study of prophylactic cefotaxime showed a diminution of bacteremia in the treatment arm, with no change in length of hospital stay, febrile episodes, or incidence of bacteriuria at discharge.[22] Bacteriuria moreover has usually been observed to clear spontaneously.[23]

One might intuitively suspect that patients with infected urine should be treated preoperatively. A recent study of infected patients randomized either to receive preoperative treatment or not demonstrated a significant benefit of treatment in decreasing postoperative bacteriuria, sepsis, and length of hospital stay.[24] Such differences were also achieved with as little as a single preoperative dose of aztreonam or gentamicin.[25, 26] On the other hand, prophylactic piperacillin significantly lowered the 3-day incidence of bacteriuria, but had no effect on the 3-week incidence.[27]

Particular difficulty arises in determining whether preoperative antibiotics should be given to patients with sterile urine, since the absence of infection preoperatively does not preclude perioperative bacteremia.[21, 28] The source of infection in these patients may well be a prostatic reservoir. A recent bacteriologic study of TURP chips showed that in 82% of patients with infected prostates the preoperative urine was sterile.[29] At least 21% of the patients undergoing TURP had positive, single-organism prostate chip cultures. The most common organisms were *Escherichia coli* (44%), *Streptococcus faecalis* (23%), and *Staphylococcus epidermidis* (18%).

In the study of Gorelick et al.,[29] the only statistically significant indicator of prostate infection was the presence preoperatively of an indwelling urethral catheter. The study made no attempt to define postoperative complications, and definite recommendations regarding prophylactic antibiotics were not made. Since the organisms cultured generally vary in their sensitivities to antibiotics, prophylactic antibiotics, if given, would need to be very broad-spectrum to address this variation effectively. Catheterized patients have been shown to have a higher incidence of preoperative bacteriuria.[26, 28, 30] They are also thought to be at a higher risk for epididymitis.[31] Interestingly, previous TURP appears to diminish the risk of epididymitis.[32]

Short-term use of antibiotic prophylaxis in patients with sterile urine has generally not demonstrated an influence on ultimate clinical course.[25, 33, 34] Two recent studies have shown a more highly significant impact of the integrity of the postoperative drainage system on postoperative bacteriuria than the use of prophylactic antibiotics.[23, 35] In addition, long-term evaluation demonstrates a high incidence of bacteriuria following TURP, regardless of perioperative prophylaxis.[20] Of note, patients in the nontreatment group were given more antibiotics during a 3-year follow-up and had a much higher incidence of urethral stricture.

Clinical experience with the relatively new quinolone antibiotics is limited, although three recent studies in patients with sterile urine indicate a significant diminution of postoperative bacteriuria.[24, 36, 37] In one of these studies,[37] a single preoperative 500-mg dose of ciprofloxacin was associated with a greatly diminished likelihood of septicemia.

CHOICE OF ANESTHESIA

In the United States, TURP is done with spinal (77%), general (20%), and other unspecified (3%) anesthetics.[9] Spinal anesthesia is generally considered safer because of its lower propensity to suppress respiration. In addition, mental status changes and complaints of abdominal discomfort in an awake patient may serve as early signs of the TURP syndrome.

Spinal anesthesia offers other advantages over general anesthesia for patients undergoing TURP. Two studies have confirmed a significant reduction of blood loss.[38, 39] This is presumably associated with an increase in lower-limb blood flow with spinal anesthesia, suggesting a reduced lower-limb blood pressure.[40] With general anesthesia, patients undergoing TURP experience a 72% early postoperative fall in lower-limb blood flow, suggesting vasoconstriction and hypoperfusion.

General, but not spinal, anesthesia has been shown to increase early postoperative plasma epinephrine and oxygen uptake.[41] While the two techniques provide similar intraoperative heat loss, heat production is diminished with general anesthesia.

Complete analgesia is achieved at the third lumbar segment with spinal anesthesia.[42] Long-acting drugs significantly diminish the need for postoperative analgesia,[43] although this may be of limited practical relevance, as 80% of patients deny perineal or abdominal pain following TURP, while 20% have minimal discomfort.[14]

In patients considered at risk for spinal or general anesthesia, local anesthesia via perineal and transurethral routes, or intravenous sedation alone, may be viable options.[44–46] In the series by Sinha et al.[45] there were no instances of hyponatremia, no mortality, and 98% of the patients said they would undergo the procedure again. There were instances of leg twitching with high settings of the cutting current, as well as discomfort with bladder distention.

INTRAOPERATIVE COMPLICATIONS

The unique nature of transurethral surgery may predispose a patient to certain complications during the course of the procedure that are not seen with other forms of surgery. These comprise both the technical aspects of the procedure as well as its potential side effects, both of which may result in medical conditions that can be prevented or that can be more readily reversed if recognized early in their development.

Introducing the Resectoscope

The prevention of intraoperative difficulties and postoperative complications requires that the resectoscope be introduced into the bladder with a minimum of trauma to the urethra. While this is readily achieved in most instances in which patients have not had previous urologic difficulties or instrumentation, there are certain conditions that present potential problems in this area.

Phimosis may not only cause difficulty in introducing the instrument, but it may also prevent adequate aseptic preparation of the glans. This problem may result in severe urethritis, stricture formation, and possibly sepsis during the postoperative period due to trapping of secretions and poor urethral drainage around the indwelling catheter. In such instances, circumcision may be the prudent course to follow before initiating transurethral resection.

Meatal stenosis may be of inflammatory, traumatic, congenital, or iatrogenic origin. It may not only prevent the introduction of the resectoscope, but it also may cause severe trauma to the mucosal lining of the urethra and ultimately result in severe meatal stricture formation. Preoperative calibration of the urethra will permit definition of the extent of the stenotic segment. A ventral meatotomy is generally sufficient to relieve the stenosis. Internal urethrotomy or perineal urethrostomy will only occasionally be required in this setting.

Urethral strictures or false passages more proximally are not uncommon, especially if the patient has had prior catheterization because of obstructive problems. When encountered, mild strictures can be dilated gently with curved sounds prior to introduction of the resectoscope. More extensive strictures may require internal urethrotomy under direct vision. This should be done prior to attempts to introduce the resectoscope, since attempts at blind dilatation of such strictures may result in the creation of false passages, excessive hemorrhage, and progressive stricture formation postoperatively. Occasionally, filiforms and followers can be used. The followers will dilate the stricture to a diameter that is adequate to permit introduction of the resectoscope sheath. In these situations, however, it is prudent to introduce the sheath under direct vision so that the false passages can be identified and avoided.

If the urethra cannot be negotiated, a perineal urethrostomy may be necessary to accomplish resection. In these circumstances, however, it may be wiser to postpone the procedure rather than risk further injury. Certainly, the more distal strictures should be addressed prior to transurethral resection, since resection will not accomplish the purpose of relieving obstruction if a more distal stricture remains untreated. Moreover, the delay will permit a false passage to heal, and the stricture can then be more readily visualized and will be amenable to direct introduction of the resectoscope at a later time with less trauma.

Erections during transurethral resection can occur regardless of the type of anesthesia used. Techniques that have been used to produce detumescence have included wrapping the base of the penis with gauze soaked in ice water, or using hypotensive anesthesia, curarelike substances, muscle relaxants, sympatholytic and parasympatholytic agents, ketamine, or amyl nitrite. None has been predictably effective. An extreme case has been described in which a patient required three trips to the operating room and seven separate anesthetics before having TURP via perineal urethrostomy.[47] Recently, intracorporal injections of ephedrine have been shown to cause prompt intraoperative detumescence with no apparent postoperative complications.[48]

Attempts to introduce a resectoscope or perform resection while the patient has an erection is bound to lead to trauma to the urethra and excessive hemorrhage by such trauma, and the operation will be inadequate as a result. Continued stimulation will only result in further tumescence and further trauma.

Intraoperative Hemorrhage

Intraoperative hemorrhage has been found to constitute the single most important determinant in potentially compromising visualization and the adequacy of resection. Assuming that a complete preoperative coagulation profile has been found to be normal or that coagulopathies have been corrected prior to surgery, intraoperative bleeding comes from either open venous sinuses or unrecognized arterial bleeding sites.

Generally, the bladder neck represents the predominant site of arterial bleeding, the major source being prostatic branches of the inferior vesical arteries. These vessels must be carefully fulgurated immediately upon uncovering them when the adenoma overlying the bladder neck is resected. In addition, they must be reinspected at the termination of the procedure to decrease the likelihood that delayed hemorrhage will occur in the postoperative period. The pulsatile blood flow that is characteristic of arterial bleeding is easily recognized, and careful attention to the source of such bleeding will ultimately assist in general visualization during resection.

Venous bleeding need not be troublesome during resection. Generally, cauterization will control such bleeding while contraction of the prostatic capsule during the course of resection will assist in decreasing the volume of bleeding as the resection proceeds.

Occasionally, a venous sinus will be unroofed. Cauterization in these instances may only extend the defect in the vessel wall and compound this bleeding. However, such bleeding will occur only if the tissue bite has been taken too deeply before other planes of tissue have been removed. Therefore, deep resection without paying attention to the maintenance of the smooth planes of resection should be avoided.

If a venous sinus is opened during resection, the major risk to the patient is the increased amount of irrigating fluid likely to be absorbed through the patent sinus (see later) rather than the amount of hemorrhage that is occurring. Decreased visibility from increased bleeding is likely to encourage the use of an increased fluid flow to assist in resection. This temptation should be avoided, and the resectoscope should be placed so as to produce direct pressure on the vessel wall and compensate for and control the bleeding that is taking place. When a venous sinus has been opened toward the end of resection, capsular contraction will generally compress the opened vessel and limit blood loss. Placing the urethral catheter balloon so that it lies gently against the bladder neck postoperatively will then also assist in hemostasis for bleeding from this source. Although this is generally a safe practice, strong traction on the catheter balloon has been associated with reflex hypotension and bradycardia.[49]

Other attempts to diminish intraoperative hemorrhage have included the use of cold irrigant. However, this has also been shown to augment heat loss and shivering, and in one study the surgeons had difficulty handling the cooled instruments.[50] A recent study has shown no increase in blood loss when irrigant was warmed to 33° C. Heat loss was decreased and patient and surgeon comfort were improved.[51]

Estimation of blood loss by visual inspection of irrigant is grossly inaccurate.[52] As such, several methods of intraoperative calculation of blood loss have been described.[53, 54] Whether this is necessary, however, is unclear, as a large series has shown that only 2.5% of patients undergoing TURP receive intraoperative transfusions.[9] Bleeding has been reported to range from 1.9 to 36.7 cc/g of tissue resected.[53, 55] As a general rule, total blood loss correlates to weight resected and may increase significantly with the preoperative presence of an indwelling urethral catheter.[16, 53]

Trauma

Advances in optics and fiberoptic lighting systems have permitted far better visualization of urethral, prostatic, and vesical structures than has been possible in years past. Better visualization has helped to prevent the damage caused by inadvertent manipulation of the resectoscope and resection of normal or critical structures. In addition, various teaching attachments have also helped by permitting the demonstration of urethral anatomy and potential resection pitfalls, so that students may better learn the technique of TURP. The recent addition of video large-screen visualization of prostatic resection should further enhance the teaching of TURP technique and further decrease the risk of technical complications.

Trauma to Landmarks

Trauma to the ureteral orifices may occur in cases of trigonal hypertrophy with apparent displacement of the orifices toward the prostate. In these instances, the adenoma may obscure the orifices, and severe trabeculation with the formation of cellules and diverticula may further hide the orifices from view. Ureteral resection, and more commonly fulguration, can then result in ureteral stricture and obstruction with consequent hydronephrosis. The use of indigo carmine to assist in visualization of the orifices may be necessary to avoid such trauma. The verumontanum is the critical landmark lying proximal to the external sphincter. Maintenance of its integrity, with awareness of its location relative to the sphincter, will prevent trauma to the sphincter during transurethral resection. The critical points in any resection in this regard are at the apex of the prostate adjacent to the verumontanum, where residual flaps of tissue can occasionally cause persistent voiding problems postoperatively, and at the anterior portion of the adenoma at the level of the verumontanum, where resection can often be extended too far distally in repositioning the resectoscope. The presence of striated muscle in the resection specimen, however, does not necessarily indicate clinically significant sphincter injury.[56]

Urethral Perforation

Perforation of the urethra or the prostate may occur during the passage of the resectoscope before as well as during resection from inadvertent movements of the instrument.[57] Perforation may be especially likely if the patient has had previous stricture disease or the urethra has false passages. These events can be avoided by passing the resectoscope under direct vision. Perforation of the bladder neck occurs most commonly during deep resection of adenomatous tissue at the bladder neck, which is not protected by a large amount of hypertrophied adenoma. When deep resection is performed at this site, it is easy to undermine the bladder neck and trigone. This complication can be prevented by resecting this area when the bladder is partially filled, taking care to resect only the adenoma.

Lateral or anterior perforations of the bladder neck are more likely than posterior perforations to be associated with substantial extravasation of irrigating fluid. Visualization of such perforations at these sites is more difficult, but a clue is provided by the absence of fluid return and occasionally by the apparent fixation and decreased maneuverability of the resectoscope. Additional signs of bladder neck perforation and fluid extravasation include elevation and compression of the lateral borders of the bladder and poor visualization of the bladder neck. The posterior wall of the bladder and the trigone may appear more distant.

Still later signs include apparent decreased bladder capacity, increased intravesical pressure, and generally decreased visualization. As absorption of the extravasated fluid takes place, the so-called TUR (transurethral resection) syndrome (see later) will occur with restlessness, nausea, vomiting, abdominal pain, pallor, diaphoresis, tachycardia, dyspnea, and hypotension as the predominant manifestations. Abdominal tenderness and a rigid abdominal mass may then be palpable.

Once the TUR syndrome is recognized, the procedure should be terminated, after adequate hemostasis has been obtained and prostatic chips have been evacuated. A urethral catheter needs to be inserted. In addition, suprapubic drainage of the retroperitoneum should be instituted to minimize further fluid absorption. Suprapubic bladder drainage rarely is necessary.

Perforation of the prostatic capsule as a result of failure to recognize the circular capsular fibers that identify this landmark may produce the same signs and symptoms as perforation of the bladder neck. In addition, however, excessive bleeding from an exposed venous sinus may occur. In this case, resection should be completed as expeditiously as possible, and the patient should be managed in the same manner as described above.

Inadvertent perforation of the bladder during prostatic resection may result in intraperitoneal extravasation. An abnormal irrigating pattern will be apparent as more fluid enters the bladder than can be recovered. The signs and symptoms are similar to those described for extraperitoneal extravasation but are more pronounced. Evaluation and management are also the same as those described for extraperitoneal extravasation (see fluid and electrolyte management later). Although some have advocated open exploration with closure of the perforation in cases of large intraperitoneal extravasations, laparotomy and drainage of the peritoneal cavity are not needed in all cases.[9] These operations should probably be reserved for those patients with respiratory embarrassment and for those in whom trauma to the bowel is suspected. Smaller perforations and lesser extravasation can generally be managed with catheter drainage and diuretics.

Excessive Fluid Absorption

Overabsorption of irrigation fluid during TURP can lead to the so-called post-TUR syndrome. This clinical entity is manifested by hypertension, bradycardia, restlessness, muscle twitching, apprehension, disorientation, visual alterations, seizures, and vascular collapse. Factors responsible for overabsorption include intraoperative bladder pressure, perforation or entry into venous sinuses, and duration of operation.[9, 58] Unfortunately, reducing the head of pressure of the irrigating fluid and limiting the time used for resection have been only partly successful in eliminating this syndrome. In one highly monitored case, absorption was more rapid at a later stage in the operation, when intravesical pressures were actually lower.[59]

Although much effort has been directed at minimizing intravesical pressures through the use of continuous flow resectoscopes,[60, 61] these have not been shown to diminish fluid absorption.[62,63] Certain authors advocate the use of suprapubic punch catheters as adjuncts to resection.[64, 65] The advantages would include continuous low bladder pressures and uninterrupted resection. However, blood loss may be higher and fluid absorption might not necessarily be less.

Other prophylactic measures have included frequent bladder emptying during resection and postoperative measurements of intravenous input and urinary output.

Recently, intravascular sodium-sensitive electrodes have been used to detect large variations in plasma sodium concentration during transurethral resection, and these have provided a continuous monitoring to give early warning of hemodilution. In a related manner, some have used a double-isotope technique to determine the amount of irrigating fluid absorbed during resection. Colorimetric and gravimetric methods have demonstrated that the major portion of irrigation fluid is absorbed extravascularly into the perivesical and retroperitoneal spaces (71%), while only 29% of the total amount of fluid is absorbed intravascularly.[66]

Most monitoring methods are cumbersome. A recent simple, inexpensive introduction is the incorporation of ethanol into irrigation solution.[67] Expired ethanol, monitored easily by the anesthesiologist, has been found to correspond to serum glycine and serum sodium concentrations.

A significantly lower absorption of irrigating fluid has been found to occur when the height of the fluid is no greater than 60 cm above the operating table. Central venous pressure and cardiac index might be used as a measure of fluid absorption, especially in patients who have compromised cardiac or renal function. Most patients with normal cardiac function or compensated cardiac function tolerate the added fluid load well; they generally excrete this fluid while maintaining nearly normal serum electrolyte concentrations and normal serum osmolarity.

The anesthesiologist can be particularly helpful in the identification of the development of TUR syndrome. A patient's restlessness and confusion, together with an increase in central venous pressure and findings associated with hypoxemia (muscle twitching, seizure activity, and cardiac arrhythmia), may indicate the possibility that fluid overload and electrolyte imbalance have occurred. Such findings are generally more noticeable under spinal anesthesia. Under these circumstances, increased systolic and diastolic pressures in the presence of increased central venous pressure and bradycardia are indicative of the fluid overload that is taking place. Corresponding changes on the electrocardiogram include widening of the QRS complex, possible elevation of ST segments, and bradycardia. If these symptoms are recognized, the resection should be terminated.

Thermal Burns and Intravesical Explosions

Each of these problems has become relatively rare. The former results from inadequate grounding of the patient, and care should be taken to ensure that there is no contact between the patient and any metallic parts of the operating table. Proper grounding and maintenance of cables and connectors in good condition will successfully avoid this problem.

Electrolysis and thermolytic decomposition of tissue may liberate hydrogen gas which, when combined with air in the bladder, may explode upon ignition by the electric current used for resection. Frequent emptying of the bladder to remove all air and gases will prevent such explosions from taking place.

Postresection Catheter Insertion

Although catheter insertion after resection is usually easily accomplished, occasional difficulties are encountered if the bladder neck has been resected too deeply, leaving a posterior ridge, or if false passages have been created in prior catheterization attempts. Under such circumstances, a catheter guide may extend a traumatic passage. Use of a catheter coudé may avoid the posterior obstruction. Often useful is the insertion of a ureteral catheter into the bladder under direct vision with insertion of a Council urethral catheter over it.

A 22-F or 24-F urethral catheter with a 30-cc balloon inflated to 40 to 50 cc is generally sufficient for irrigation of clots if these occur postoperatively. The catheter should be positioned with the balloon resting against the bladder neck (but not under traction) so that clots that develop in the prostatic fossa are expelled rather than allowed to accumulate in the bladder. Under these conditions, continuous bladder irrigation is generally unnecessary, and two-way catheters can be used for drainage.

POSTOPERATIVE COMPLICATIONS: IMMEDIATE

TUR Syndrome

The manifestations of TUR syndrome and the means of its prevention have been described in the previous section. Although it is advantageous to recognize the signs and symptoms of this condition as early as possible in order to prevent its fullest expression, the effects of overabsorption of the irrigating fluids often do not become manifest until the immediate postoperative period. In these situations, assessment must be made of the lower abdomen and the possible need for retroperitoneal drainage to prevent further fluid absorption. Early recognition will permit early treatment, and may completely prevent this sydrome from occurring. Such treatment is readily accomplished by a small suprapubic incision and the insertion of a Penrose drain into the perivesical space. Extravesical extravasation has been shown to have a 17% mortality.[32] Since all deaths occurred in the subgroup explored more than 2 hours following perforation, early drainage is strongly indicated.

Attention should also be given to initiating the mobilization of fluid that has been absorbed to prevent further sequelae of the syndrome and reverse its effect. The production of a net loss of water from the intravascular and extravascular spaces can be accomplished by administering hypertonic saline (250–500 mL of a 3%–5% solution) and intravenously administering 40 to 100 mg of furosemide (Lasix). The clinical response to these measures can then be used as a guide for further administration of these substances. The major disadvantage of the use of hypertonic saline has been ascribed to its side effect of adding more volume to an already heavily compromised circulatory system. This side effect can be controlled, however, by careful monitoring of central venous pressure and urinary output. Throughout treatment, serum osmolarity and serum electrolytes should also be monitored, especially during the first few hours after the onset of the syndrome. In end-stage renal disease, symptomatic hyponatremia may occur in the absence of hypo-osmolality.[68] Dialysis may be effective, at least in part, in elevating serum sodium and lowering the osmolar gap caused by uncleared sorbitol.

The development of encephalopathy has been ascribed not only to fluid absorption and central nervous system hypervolemia but also to the development of hyperammonemia, which may result from hyperabsorption of glycine irrigating solution.[69, 70] Encephalopathy has generally been found to occur largely in a subset of patients who have shunted absorbed glycine into a metabolic pathway by which ammonia is cleaved from the glycine residue. One should consider avoiding glycine irrigating solutions in patients with liver disease, who may be especially susceptible to this complication. Similarly, visual disturbances following TURP may be related to the direct inhibitory effects of glycine on retinal neurotransmitters.[71–73] Hyperoxaluria may result from metabolism of glycine, and may interfere with renal function.[74]

Excessive fluid absorption during TURP may lead to massive diuresis. This has been thought to be the result of the relief of chronic urinary obstruction with the concomitant manifestation of a sodium-wasting nephropathy. In addition, the retained sodium, urea, and water from the obstructive uropathy may contribute to an osmotic diuresis. In these instances, damage to the renal tubule may be manifest in a decreased concentrating ability, decreased responsiveness to antidiuretic hormone, and a resultant decrease in sodium reabsorption. This sequence can lead to dehydration and/or hyponatremia. Appropriate replacement is dependent upon recognition of this potential problem.

The most likely patients at risk for this complication are those with severe obstructive changes of the upper urinary tracts as demonstrated on preoperative intravenous pyelography. The diuresis that develops in such patients appears to be entirely dependent upon the severity of renal damage as well as the amount of fluid that has been used to replace the diuresis.

Replacement with 5% dextrose/0.5N saline has been suggested for the management of this syndrome. If the hourly urine output is less than 250 mL/hr, the entire amount should be replaced. If the output is 250 to 500 mL/hr, fluid replacement should be two thirds of this volume. When urine output is greater than 500 mL/hr, one-half the hourly volume should be replaced. With careful monitoring, total fluid replacement should not be 1,500 to 2,000 mL less than the total urine output. Frequent measurement of urinary and serum electrolyte levels is important. Serum levels of magnesium, calcium, and phosphorous should also be obtained, and these substances should be replaced as necessary.

Preoperative stabilization of renal function is critical if this syndrome is to be avoided in patients with apparent obstruction of the upper urinary tract. On the other hand, postresection diuresis in the absence of prior obstruction may be the result of fluid absorption. In either instance, care must be taken not to overload a patient's circulatory system further.

Diabetics may be at special risk for developing nonketotic hyperosmolar syndromes with hyponatremia. The high serum osmolarity in these patients causes water to shift from intracellular to extracellular spaces, producing a relative decrease in serum osmolarity as well as a decrease in serum sodium concentration. Treatment should be addressed to the lowering of serum concentration of osmotically active substances. For each 100 g/dL of glucose above 200, serum sodium concentration should be decreased in such instances by 1.6 m/dL.

The syndrome involving apparently inappropriate secretion of antidiuretic hormone, which can cause water retention and expansion of extracellular spaces (with resultant relative hyponatremia and low serum osmolarity), is most commonly seen postoperatively in patients who have suffered acute volume depletion. The development of this syndrome may be diagnosed by the presence of a relative hyponatremia and low serum osmolarity upon extracellular fluid expansion. In these instances, urine osmolarity will be increased.

Although this syndrome may resemble post-TUR syndrome clinically in that patients may experience headaches, irritability, nausea, vomiting, and confusion, this form of water retention usually responds promptly to fluid restriction rather than to stimulation of water loss. Although the administration of sodium may increase plasma sodium concentration, the sodium is then rapidly excreted in the urine. Intravenous diuretics will then generally produce a loss of water and an eventual increase in plasma sodium concentration, thereby reversing the syndrome. One must be aware of the possible development of this syndrome in contrast to that represented by overabsorption of fluid to prevent the perpetuation of morbidity by the institution of inappropriate therapies.

In the context of the TUR syndrome, it is important to discuss the various irrigation solutions that are commonly used in resection and which ones may predispose a patient to a particular risk depending upon the presence of underlying medical conditions (Table 20–2). All commercially available irrigating solutions are *hypo*-osmolar (normal serum osmolality is 280/310 mOsm/L) and acidic (normal serum pH is 7.35–7.45).

The use of distilled water may improve visibility through the lysis of red cells, but hemolysis and hemoglobinemia may lead to renal failure. One should keep in mind that serum sodium is minimally effected by water irrigation.[75] In fact, one fatal case of water absorption has been described in which serum sodium was 134 mEq/L,[76] potassium was 9.8 mEq/L, and serum hemoglobin was 1,350 mg/dL. TUR syndrome variants are also seen with nonhemolytic solutions. In such instances, similarities of the predisposing factors include massive absorption of hypo-osmolar irrigating solutions, resulting in acute volume expansion, sudden alterations in serum electrolytes and proteins, and disturbances in acid-base balance.

Patients with preexisting liver function impairment may be at increased risk if glycine (1.5% aminoacetic acid) is used for irrigation. This substance is rapidly excreted by the kidneys and metabolized by the liver to ammonia. Hyperammonemic

TABLE 20–2.
Irrigating Solutions in Transurethral Resection (TUR) of Prostate

Solution	Osmolality (mOsm/L)	Advantages	Disadvantages
Distilled water	0	Improved visibility	Hemoglobinemia; hyponatremia; hemolysis; TUR syndrome
Sorbitol (3.3%)	165–180	Less likelihood of TUR syndrome unless massive fluid overload	Hyperglycemia (metabolized to glucose); possible lactic acidosis; risk to diabetics
Glycine (1.5%) (aminoacetic acid)	200	Same as sorbitol	Hyperammonemia (ammonia is metabolic by-product) in patients with hepatic dysfunction
Mannitol (5%)	275	Isomolar solution	May cause massive diuresis; possible acute intravascular volume expansion if absorbed intravenously

encephalopathy may occur as the result of acute volume expansion, not only on the basis of the volume changes described for the TUR syndrome, but also possibly on the basis of a prolonged toxic effect of glycine and ammonia.

Diabetics may be particularly susceptible to side effects when sorbitol solution is used for irrigation (this solution has a concentration of 3.0%–3.3%, is acidic with an average pH of 5.5, and has an osmolality of 165–180). It is rapidly excreted by the kidneys but is also metabolized to glucose, which may lead to hyperglycemia. Sorbitol may also be metabolized from pyruvate to lactate and may therefore be a cause of lactic acidosis. The possibility of intraoperative or postoperative sepsis, especially in diabetics who may be more susceptible to infection, may also lead to lactic acidosis and therefore be compounded by the overabsorption of sorbitol solution.

When mannitol is used in the irrigation solution, creating an iso-osmolar solution, marked intravascular volume expansion may be compounded by the osmotic effect of mannitol when the irrigation fluid is absorbed. Furthermore, since the mannitol is not distributed evenly throughout the total body fluid space, hypervolemic changes may be compounded and further contribute to manifestations of the TUR syndrome. The mannitol may subsequently induce a profound diuresis, causing difficulties in the replacement of fluids.

Taken together, each irrigating fluid has its advantages and disadvantages. The use of a particular irrigating solution must be based on the specific clinical situation. Attention to minimizing the degree of fluid absorption by adjusting the mechanics of resection is probably the most effective way of decreasing the likelihood that TUR syndrome may occur.

Fever

The development of fever immediately following TURP suggests bacteremia. Any suggestion of preoperative urinary infection, prior indwelling catheter, or prior instrumentation suggests the need for antibiotics prior to surgery to prevent potential bacteremia from occurring. If this has been done, a change in antibiotics in response to postoperative fever is not necessarily indicated.

When antibiotics have not been used preoperatively, subsequent bacteriuria can be prevented by preserving a closed drainage system, avoiding frequent catheterization, and eliminating continuous bladder irrigation as a routine in postoperative care. In the event that continuous bladder irrigation is needed to decrease clot formation postoperatively, acetic acid

(0.125%–0.25%, with pH less than 5.0) may be added to the irrigation solution to prevent introduction and colonization of bacteria.

Acute prostatitis and pyelonephritis are unusual in the immediate postoperative period. Acute epididymitis, on the other hand, may occur within several days of resection and is especially likely if a catheter has been indwelling for a lengthy period both pre- and postoperatively. Some have suggested that ligation of the vas deferens should be performed intraoperatively prior to initiating resection to prevent acute epididymitis by preventing reflux of urine and bacterial organisms into the vas deferens during the resection. Evidence to support this contention, however, is lacking.

Another cause of fever postoperatively but usually not occurring until 4 to 5 days after resection is the development of staphylococcal urethritis. This infection is presumably the result of the presence of an indwelling catheter. Its prevention by the application of antibiotic ointments at the urethral meatus has not been demonstrated to be effective. Treatment, however, is readily accomplished by simply removing the indwelling catheter and instituting appropriate antibiotics (penicillin or cephalexin). Most patients express their relief almost as soon as the catheter has been removed and normal voiding has started. (See also Chap. 4, Infectious Diseases.)

Shock

When fever occurs in association with bacteremia, one should also anticipate the potential development of hypovolemic shock. While shock is a rare occurrence in elective urologic surgery, the elderly patient may be at special risk because the initial appearance of sepsis is occasionally not clinically obvious. The usual cause of septic shock seen after resection is prior infection with either *Escherichia coli, Klebsiella, Bacteroides,* or *Pseudomonas,* organisms that easily gain access to the bloodstream during resection or postoperatively.

Such patients generally present with fever, rigors, altered mental status, hypotension, oliguria, decreased central venous pressure, decreased cardiac output, tachycardia, elevated peripheral resistance, respiratory alkalosis, metabolic acidosis, and, occasionally, disseminated intravascular coagulation (occurring in 10% of these patients).

Added complications of septic shock include respiratory distress syndrome ("shock lung"), acute renal failure, and heart failure. Since mortality rates may vary between 50% and 70%, the prevention of bacteremia is preferable to treatment after septic shock has taken place.

Elderly patients in septic shock may be more likely to demonstrate subtle clinical changes without fever until electrolyte and fluid disturbances are severe enough to produce cardiogenic shock. The presence of prior coronary artery disease may contribute to this risk, and such patients may frequently manifest a variety of cardiac arrhythmias during both early and late postoperative periods. Continuous cardiac monitoring in such patients is therefore mandatory. Treatment is based on rapid administration of intravenous fluids, broad-spectrum antibiotic coverage, correction of electrolyte abnormalities, and, though still controversial, high-dose steroids (predicated on the putative stabilization of lysosomal and cellular membranes).

Intravascular Coagulation and Fibrinolysis

Intravascular coagulation and fibrinolysis are among the most serious complications that can occur immediately following TURP. In disseminated intravascular coagulation, a state of hypercoagulability causes an abnormal increase in fibrin thrombi. This condition leads to decreases in platelet number and fibrinogen levels through their consumption in the process of thrombus formation. Prolonged bleeding times occur with decreased prothrombin and partial thromboplastin times. Secondary fibrinolysis may then occur.

This situation is more commonly seen when transurethral resection of prostate cancer is performed. It is thought to reflect the release of thromboplastin, which is found in high concentrations in prostate cancer cells. Trauma, sepsis, and transfusion reactions may also contribute to this syndrome.

Patients who present with unexplained increased postoperative bleeding accompanied by the development of petechiae, purpura, hematomas, and acral cyanosis may be manifesting this syndrome. Laboratory data include decreased platelet count, hypofibrinogenemia, prolonged partial thromboplastin and prothrombin times, and an increase in fibrin split products.

Aggressive treatment is mandatory as soon as the syndrome is recognized and is directed at both treating the primary disease and providing total support (blood replacement, platelet transfusions, crystalloids, pressor agents, and oxygenation). Oral or intravenous administration of ϵ-aminocaproic acid (EACA, Amicar) and inhibitors of plasminogen activator can also be used, as these have been shown to significantly diminish blood loss.[77, 78]

Although these agents theoretically may prevent local fibrinolysis, their systemic use may be complicated.[79, 80] These agents should not be used routinely, even though an increased incidence of deep venous thrombosis has not been proved.[81] Moreover, intravesical irrigation with EACA has not been found to produce significant differences.[82, 83] More recently, a fibrin adhesive which may be directly instilled into the prostatic fossa has been described.[84] This material has been shown to reduce postoperative blood loss with no apparent complications. Indications in the case of fibrinolysis, however, are unclear. (See also Chap. 5, Hematologic Complications.)

Bacterial Cystitis

Postoperative cystitis secondary to bacterial contamination is readily treated by appropriate antibiotics. Cystitis secondary to colonization by yeast may be seen in diabetics who have had indwelling urethral catheters and have been treated with broad-spectrum antibiotics. Such patients can be treated with amphotericin B or 5-fluocytosine, either orally or by intravesical irrigation, to eliminate the infecting organism. Prevention of this development involves early removal of an indwelling catheter in patients who may be at risk.

Treatment with each of these agents, however, may have side effects. The 5-fluocytosine (at a dose of 100–150 mg/kg/day) may induce leukopenia and hepatic dysfunction, and approximately 50% of yeast organisms may be resistant to this agent. Amphotericin B is usually the treatment of choice for infections confined to the bladder and is administered as a solution of 50 mg in 500 to 1000 mL of sterile water by continuous intravesical irrigation over a 24-hour period. Systemic absorption is minimal by this route, but the drug is potentially nephrotoxic if absorbed.

DELAYED POSTOPERATIVE COMPLICATIONS

After transurethral resection, patients may complain of frequency, urgency, dysuria, occasional urgency incontinence, and a weak stream. These symptoms often last 6 to 8 weeks and do not require further investigation or treatment other than reassurance.

Several problems that may, however,

arise do require immediate attention. These include symptoms associated with inadequate resection, urinary tract infections, epididymitis, and urinary incontinence.

Inadequate Resection

Symptoms of either continuous or intermittent obstruction suggest that the resection of obstructive tissue was incomplete. Treatment must consist of repeat resection with removal of residual tissue. To prevent this complication, the extent of resection at the time of surgery must be assessed, with careful attention to apical tissue, anterior tissue, and the bladder neck.

Abnormal Sediment

An abnormal urinary sediment may persist for several months following prostatic resection. Sloughing of cauterized and necrotic residual prostatic tissue accounts for the frequent presence of white blood cells and red blood cells in the examination of urinary sediment. On the other hand, persistence of white blood cells beyond 3 months after resection may indicate the presence of an infection.

Irritative Symptoms

Irritative symptoms with or without hematuria 6 months following resection is a worrisome finding. In these instances, neoplasm of the bladder or of the upper tracts must be excluded, and intravenous pyelography, cystourethroscopy, and urinary cytology should be obtained. Rarely, tuberculosis or fungal cystitis are causes of these symptoms. Persistent hematuria despite normal evaluation requires reevaluation for these possibilities every 6 months until the source of these findings is either identified or resolved.

A subgroup of patients who undergo TURP for irritative symptoms continue to complain of their symptoms postoperatively, even though urine cultures are negative and cystoscopy discloses only inflammatory changes of the prostatic urethra and trigone. Such patients may benefit from conservative measures (sitz baths, antispasmotics). However, such patients should also be evaluated neurologically and with urinary cytology to rule out carcinoma.

Incontinence

Urinary incontinence may be a late sequela of prostate surgery. The several etiologies of such incontinence are inflammatory, neoplastic, mechanical (residual tissue or stricture), and neurogenic (weakness of the external sphincter, detrusor instability). When urinary incontinence is seen, its evaluation requires urinalysis, urine culture, cystourethroscopy, neurologic evaluation, urodynamics, sphincter electromyography, and urethral pressure profilometry.

The most common type of delayed incontinence after resection is urgency incontinence. It is seen in association with inflammatory or infectious mucosal lesions, neoplasms, or calculi. Although strictures can contribute to the urgency that is seen, the primary source of this urgency is a raw, healing prostatic fossa. While persistence of urgency and incontinence beyond 2 months indicates the need to evaluate these possibilities, the diminution of such symptoms with time implies healing of the resected fossa.

Stress incontinence may occur if the external sphincter and tissue surrounding the verumontanum have been weakened either iatrogenically or neurologically. Damage to the external sphincter intraoperatively may lead to scarring of the membranous urethra, with stricture formation. Severe scarring will prevent complete urethral sphincter closure. In this instance, incontinence will result.

Urethral dilatation with curved sounds

may satisfactorily disrupt any scar tissue that has developed, thereby permitting improved pliability of the tissues and total sphincter closure. On the other hand, the blind nature of this procedure may undermine the bladder neck, create false passages, and extend the degree of trauma. Direct-vision, internal urethrotomy is a more satisfactory way of resolving this problem. When minor urinary stress incontinence is seen, exercises in voluntary closure of the external sphincter may be initiated. Generally, these exercises will lead to resolution of symptoms. Pharmacologic agents such as α-adrenergic sympathomimetics (chlorpheniramine maleate–phenylpropanolamine hydrochloride, ephedrine) may also increase urethral resistance proximally and thereby relieve mild degrees of stress incontinence.

For those in whom these measures are not successful, external collection devices (condom catheter urosheath, Cunningham clamp) may be required. In elderly patients, an indwelling urethral catheter may be preferable if external devices cannot be well tolerated. Suprapubic drainage may be even more beneficial than a urethral catheter.

Several anti-incontinence surgical procedures have also been developed. Urethral compression with a variety of prostheses has proved successful in 30% to 50% of patients. More successful have been a variety of artificial sphincters, but mechanical malfunctions have been common. Injection of Teflon particles has recently been found to achieve some success. However, potential thromboembolic phenomena with Teflon have tempered initial enthusiasm for this technique. A new alternative is the periurethral injection of collagen, which may create a partial obstruction at the level of the external sphincter and relieve the incontinence.[85]

Because of the risk of total urinary incontinence, special care is required when transurethral resection for prostate cancer is undertaken. Normal voiding patterns may never be restored in these instances, since malignant involvement of the external sphincter may be responsible for the symptoms.

Similarly, there are some patients with neurogenic bladders in whom putative obstructive symptoms are only assumed to be caused by an enlarged prostate. In the presence of the prostatism, detrusor decompensation may occur and transurethral resection will not relieve the voiding symptoms. An areflexic or hyperreflexic bladder, with or without incontinence, may be seen in these instances to have no readily apparent cause, and the diagnosis of neurogenic bladder should therefore be considered.

Taken together, preoperative assessment for causes of apparent outlet obstruction other than an enlarged prostate should always be considered before resection of the prostate is undertaken. This precaution will prevent needless surgery and permit other therapeutic options to be considered.

Bladder Neck Contracture

Primary bladder neck contracture is usually the manifestation of adenomatous hyperplasia of the posterior lobe of the prostate and is only rarely due to a true fibrous median bar. Both of these are an indication for resection and do not represent a complication of resection.

In contrast, secondary bladder neck contracture is iatrogenic as a result of circumferential resection of the bladder neck at the time of prostatectomy. Surgical relief by transurethral incision is usually sufficient to correct the contracture. Occasional injection of steroids may assist in preventing recurrence.[86] Open Y-V plasty may be a suitable alternative, but generally it is not required in the context of improved transurethral visualization and urethrotomy procedures.

Neurogenic dysfunction of the bladder neck may contribute to bladder neck obstruction following resection. Because it is a purely functional obstruction, differentiation of this entity from true anatomical obstruction is required for accurate patient selection preoperatively. Pharmacologic agents (β-blockers) may obviate the need for bladder neck resection in these cases. Detrusor hypertrophy as a concomitant of spastic neurogenic bladder is often seen in such instances.

Urethral Stricture

Up to 9% of patients who undergo TURP later develop urethral strictures.[87] The most common sites are the membranous urethra, the bulbar urethra at the level of the penoscrotal junction, and the fossa navicularis. Symptoms reflect progressive obstruction. Treatment requires urethral dilatation or internal urethrotomy under direct vision. Open urethroplasty is rarely indicated.

In cases done through perineal urethrostomy, the incidence of urethral stricture is 0.6%.[88] Similarly, preliminary internal urethrotomy to 32 F to 36 F produces a 1% stricture rate.[89] Patients with preoperative instrumentation have a higher risk of stricture.[90] In addition, size of gland correlates with stricture rate. Duration of resection, patient's age, and pathologic diagnosis do not.[91]

Prevention requires attempts to minimize trauma to the urethra during prostatic resection. Strictures at the meatus or in the fossa navicularis can often be minimized by meatotomy prior to instrumentation. Visual assessment of the entire urethra by panendoscopy before attempting to insert a resectoscope blindly will permit a more accurate navigation of the urethral channel. Attempts to decrease the incidence of urethritis and meatitis both pre- and postoperatively may also be important in the prevention of stricture formation.

Identification of a stricture prior to resection is an indication for internal urethrotomy before the attempted resection is begun. If the urethral channel is too small to accommodate an appropriate resectoscope, a perineal urethrostomy may permit a less traumatic resection. Finally, the type of catheter used postoperatively may be important in preventing the likelihood of later stricture formation. A Silastic catheter is less traumatic to the urethral mucosa. The caliber of catheter is important and should be consistent with the size of the urethra and the adequate drainage of any postoperative bleeding. The catheter should be taped to the thigh without tension on the bladder neck to avoid bladder neck contracture and to prevent pressure from being created within the urethra at the penoscrotal angle. In addition, the catheter should not be permitted to remain indwelling for an excessive time.

Sexual Function

Virtually the only effect of prostatic resection on sexual activity is the development of retrograde ejaculation. Patients who desire additional children should be warned that recovery of semen after prostatectomy by catheterization may be less than satisfactory and that insemination of multiple semen collections may be necessary for conception. Some have suggested that if the bladder neck need not be resected and tissue along the verumontanum is not cauterized, antegrade ejaculation may be maintained. However, because of the contribution of the bladder neck itself to outlet obstruction, most will consider retrograde ejaculation a necessary concomitant of effective transurethral resection.

α-Adrenergic agents have been suggested as a means of preventing retrograde ejaculation, but it is probably impossible to accomplish this effect pharmacologically once the bladder neck has been resected.

Transurethral resection will ordinarily

not affect potency on a physiologic basis and will not diminish a patient's ability to achieve erection and orgasm, even in the absence of antegrade ejaculation. There is little argument, however, that some patients may become impotent after TURP. Indeed, a recent study of impotence before and after TURP showed a significantly higher incidence than with other forms of surgery.[92] Cauterization of nerves in their course at the distal prostate, or at the bladder neck, has been suggested to account for this rare albeit documented occurrence.

Perineal Pain

The development of perineal pain following TURP is an uncommon occurrence, especially when it has not been present preoperatively. Although such pain may mimic that of prostatitis, a bacterial etiology is usually not found. Scarring and stenosis of the ejaculatory ducts have been suggested as contributing to this problem. In such cases, orgasm may be painful and seminal vesicle emission may be absent. Care should thus be taken during the procedure not to cauterize or resect at the ejaculatory ducts. Generally, resection in these areas is not necessary to accomplish satisfactory tissue excision, may introduce the risk of "overresection" with violation of the sphincter (leading to the development of incontinence), and may induce prostatic congestion and perineal pain.

Treatment of this pain consists of sitz baths and analgesics. Although antibiotics may be used even if bacteria are not isolated from the prostatic secretions, such antibiotics may actually have only a placebo effect. Injection of 5% argyrol has been suggested to palliate such discomfort because of the mild cauterization of the surface of the resected prostatic urethral fossa. However, reports of the efficacy of this approach have been mixed. It would appear that the most important aspect of treatment of this potential complication is reassurance that such pain generally resolves with time.

CATHETER CARE

Urethral catheters are standard following TURP, although their care is variable. In one large series, 82% of catheters were removed by postoperative day 3 and 2.4% of patients were discharged with an indwelling catheter.[9] Complications, such as clot retention or failure to void, which presumably required recatheterization, totaled 10%. In another study, catheters were routinely removed the morning after surgery, even in the presence of hematuria, with the patients discharged the following day.[93] Fifteen percent of these patients required recatheterization. Whether or not early catheter removal predisposes to recatheterization or other long-term complications is unclear.

Techniques of maintaining catheter patency postoperatively are generally poorly described. Some centers do not use continuous irrigation, preferring instead to induce diuresis.[16, 35] Indications for either continuous irrigation or simple diuresis-induced drainage technique are unclear. In our experience, adequate intraoperative hemostasis frequently obviates the need for either.

RECENT TECHNICAL INNOVATIONS

Recent advances in video technology have led to the development of cameras which will attach directly to the resectoscope.[94, 95] These cameras allow more comfortable viewing for the surgeon, as well as simultaneous viewing by many. In one study of 50 patients treated with video monitoring, results were similar to those in patients treated by conventional method.[94] The author notes that rotation of the camera may be disorienting, and that depth perception may be altered.

Dynamic imaging of TURP by transrectal sonography has also been described.[96] This technique offers the ability to assess tissue thickness in all dimensions. Its practical clinical application and safety with existing equipment have not been studied. Along these lines, computer-monitored tissue conductivity measurements have been implemented to diminish capsule perforation.[97] The practical benefit of this in relation to clinical application remains to be determined.

SUMMARY

In view of all of the possible pitfalls that can be encountered during TURP, it is remarkable how low the morbidity and mortality actually are. In those instances where potential morbidity can be recognized, avoidance by precautionary measures will in most instances be readily accomplished. Occasionally more problematic are those instances in which the procedure itself has led to intraoperative, immediate postoperative, or delayed postoperative complications. In many of these cases, simple attention to detail and avoidance of trauma to the urethra during resection will generally provide a satisfactory result both immediately and in the long term.

The performance of TURP is one of those operations unique to urology and is a procedure for which nearly all patients will be grateful. The opportunity to administer such treatment safely through minimizing potential morbidity is an option readily available to all urologic surgeons.

EDITORIAL COMMENT I

The complications of transurethral resection of the prostate have been covered in depth in this chapter. A few comments are outlined.

A coagulation profile is not necessary in routine cases, but obtaining a history of aspirin consumption is increasingly important, since we have seen some bleeding from patients on aspirin. Small amounts of extravasation, especially retroperitoneal, are commonplace after TURP. It is only the gross extravasations that require more than catheter drainage. Although a standard Foley catheter is used by many urologists, a three-way Foley catheter for irrigation has worked well in my hands, and I think, because of it, there are fewer calls for catheter irrigations in the first postoperative night. If multiple attempts at endoscopic resection or incision of bladder neck contractures fail, a Y-V plasty will usually be successful.

EDITORIAL COMMENT II

In spite of all of the outlined complications of TURP, it remains a well-tolerated procedure with a relative paucity of complications in the appropriately managed patient. We have routinely utilized the 26 F resectoscope sheath and occasionally the 24 F sheath rather than the 28 F sheath. The use of a smaller instrument may reduce the likelihood of postoperative urethral stricture.

REFERENCES

1. Rutkow IM: Urological operations in the United States: 1979 to 1984. *J Urol* 1986; 135:1206–1208.
2. McPherson K, Wennberg JE, Hovind OB, et al: Small-area variations in the use of common surgical procedures: an international comparison of New England, England, and Norway. *N Eng J Med* 1982; 307:1310–1314.
3. Wennberg J, Gittelsohn A: Variations in

medical care among small areas. *Sci Am* 1982; 246:120–134.
4. Bruskewitz RC, Larsen EH, Madsen PO, et al: 3-year followup of urinary symptoms after transurethral resection of the prostate. *J Urol* 1986; 136:613–615.
5. Fowler F, Wennberg JE, Timothy RP, et al: Symptom status and quality of life following prostatectomy: *JAMA* 1988; 259:3018–3022.
6. Riley G, Lubitz J: Outcomes of surgery among the medicare aged: surgical volume and mortality. *Health Care Finan Rev* 1985; 7:37–47.
7. Wennberg JE, Roos N, Sola L, et al: Use of claims data systems to evaluate health care outcomes: mortality and reoperation following prostatectomy. *JAMA* 1987; 257:933–936.
8. Lubitz J, Riley G, Newton M: Outcomes of surgery among the Medicare aged: mortality after surgery. *Health Care Finan Rev* 1985; 6:103–105.
9. Mebust WK, Holtgrewe HL, Cockett ATK, et al: Transurethral prostatectomy: immediate and postoperative complications. A cooperative study of 13 participating institutions evaluating 3,885 patients. *J Urol* 1989; 141:243–247.
10. Garcias VA, Mallouh C, Park T, et al: Depressed myocardial function after transurethral resection of prostate. *Urology* 1981; 17:420–427.
11. Melchior J, Valk WL, Foret JD, et al: Transurethral prostatectomy in the azotemic patient. *J Urol* 1974; 112:643–646.
12. Kernoff PBA: Prostatectomy in haemophilia and Christmas disease. *Br J Urol* 1972; 44:51.
13. Kirby K, Mesrobian HG, Fried F: Prostatectomy in patients with bleeding disorders. *J Urol* 1988; 140:87–90.
14. Bricker SRW, Savage ME, Manning CD: Peri-operative blood loss and nonsteroidal anti-inflammatory drugs: an investigation using diclofenac in patients undergoing transurethral resection of the prostate. *Eur J Anaesthesiol* 1987; 4:429–434.
15. Jenkins AD, Mintz PD: Optimal blood use in genitourinary surgery. *J Urol* 1981; 126:497–499.
16. Faber JE, Hansen M, Genter HG: Use of blood in transurethral prostatectomy—routine or selective cross-matching? *Scand J Urol Nephrol Suppl* 1987; 104:73–75.
17. Nseyo UO, Rivard DJ, Garlick WB, et al: Management of bladder stones: Should transurethral prostatic resection be performed with cystolitholapaxy? *Urology* 1987; 24:265–267.
18. Leach GE, Yip CM, Donovan BJ: Postprostatectomy incontinence: The influence of bladder dysfunction. *J Urol* 1987; 138:574–578.
19. Grabe M: Antimicrobial agents in transurethral prostatic resection *J Urol* 1987; 138:245–252.
20. Grabe M, Hellsten S: Long-term followup after transurethral prostatic resection with or without a short perioperative antibiotic course. *Br J Urol* 1985; 57:444–449.
21. Arpi M, Werner C, Timmermann B: Bacteremia following transurethral instrumentation. *Scan J Urol Nephrol* 1986; 20:169–176.
22. Nielsen PB, Lawssen H, Hansen RI, et al: Effective perioperative prophylaxis with a single dose of cefotaxime in transurethral prostatectomy. *Clin Ther* 1987; 9:167–173.
23. Stricker PD, Grant ABF: Relative value of antibiotics and catheter care in the prevention of urinary tract infection after transurethral prostatic resection. *Br J Urol* 1988; 61:494–497.
24. Murdoch DA, Badenoch DC, Gatchalian ER: Oral ciprofloxacin as prophylaxis in transurethral resection of the prostate. *Br J Urol* 1987; 60:153–156.
25. Millar MR, Inglis T, Ewing R: Double-blind study comparing aztreonam with placebo for prophylaxis of infection following prostatic surgery. *Br J Urol* 1987; 60:345–348.
26. McEntee GP, McPhail S, Mulvin D, et al: Single dose antibiotic prophylaxis in high risk patients undergoing transurethral prostatectomy. *Br J Surg* 1987; 74:192–194.
27. Hoogkamp-Korstanje JAA, de Leur EJA, Franssens D: The influence of prophylactic piperacillin on the postoperative course of transurethral prostatectomy. *J Antimicrobiol Chemother* 1985; 16:773–779.
28. Hansen M, Genster HG, Thordsen C: Urinary infections in connection with trans-

urethral resection of the prostate. *Scan J Urol Nephrol Suppl* 1987; 104:65–68.

29. Gorelick JI, Senterfit LB, Vaughan ED: Quantitative bacterial tissue cultures from 209 prostatectomy specimens: Findings and implications *J Urol* 1988; 139:57–60.
30. Grabe M, Forsgren A: The effectiveness of a short perioperative course with pivampicillin/pivmecillinam in transurethral prostatic resection: Clinical results. *Scand J Infect Dis* 1986; 18:567–573.
31. Melchior J, Valk WL, Foret JD, et al: Transurethral prostatectomy and epididymitis. *J Urol* 1974; 112:647–650.
32. Holtgrewe HL, Valk WL: Factors influencing the mortality and morbidity of transurethral prostatectomy: A study of 2,015 cases. *J Urol* 1962; 87:450–459.
33. Fair WR: Perioperative use of carbenicillin in transurethral resection of prostate. *Urology Suppl* 1986; 27:15–18.
34. Conn IG, Moffat LEF: Short term cephradine prophylaxis in elective transurethral prostatectomy. *J Hosp Infect* 1988; 11:373–375.
35. Fahal AH, Ibrahim A: Post prostatectomy auto-irrigation with furosemide in the tropics. *Pharmatherapeutica* 1986; 4:590–594.
36. Desai KM, Abrams PH, White LO: A double-blind comparative trail of short term orally administered enoxacin in the prevention of urinary infection after elective transurethral prostatectomy: A clinical and pharmokokinetic study. *J Urol* 1988; 139:1232–1234.
37. Shearman CP, Silverman SH, Johnson M, et al: Single dose, oral antibiotic cover for transurethral prostatectomy. *Br J Urol* 1988; 62:434–438.
38. Madsen RE, Madsen PO: Influence of anesthesia forms on blood loss in transurethral prostatectomy. *Anesth Analg* 1967; 46:330–332.
39. Abrams PH: Blood loss during transurethral resection of the prostate. *Anaesthesia* 1982; 37:71–73.
40. Foate JA, Horton H, Davis FM: Lower limb blood flow during transurethral resection of the prostate under spinal or general anesthesia. *Anaesth Intensive Care* 1985; 13:383–386.
41. Stjernstrom H, Henneberg S, Eklund A, et al: Thermal balance during transurethral resection of the prostate. *Acta Anaesthesiol Scand* 1985; 29:743–749.
42. Evans TI: Regional anesthesia for transurethral resection of the prostate—which method and which segments? *Anaesth Intensive Care* 1974; 2:240–242.
43. Millar JM, Jago RH, Fawcett DP: Spinal analgesia for transurethral prostatectomy: Comparison of plain bupivacaine and hyperbaric lignocaine.*Br J Anaesth* et al: 1986; 58:862–867.
44. Lichtwardt JR, Girgis S: Transurethral resection of prostate with intravenous sedation. *Urology* 1985; 26:112–113.
45. Sinha B, Haikel G, Lange PH, et al: Transurethral resection of the prostate with local anaesthesia in 100 patients. *J Urol* 1986; 135:719–721.
46. Loughlin KR, Yalla SV, Belldegrun A, et al: Transurethral incisions and resection under local anaesthesia. *Br J Urol* 1985; 60:185–188.
47. Van Arsdalen KN, Chen JW, Smith MJV: Penile erection complicating transurethral surgery. *J Urol* 1983; 129:374–376.
48. Sundein E, Kolmert T: Ephedrine: A possible alternative for treatment of penile erection in connection with transurethral resection of prostatic or bladder tumors. *J Urol* 1987; 138:411.
49. Ignatoff JM, Haupt M, Ampel LL: Hemodynamic instability associated with balloon catheter traction after transurethral surgery. *Heart Lung* 1985; 14:357–358.
50. Kulatilake AE, Roberts PN, Evans DF, et al: The use of cooled irrigating fluid for transurethral prostatic resection *Br J Urol* 1981; 53:261–262.
51. Heathcote PS, Dyer PM: The effect of warm irrigation on blood loss during transurethral prostatectomy under spinal anaesthesia. *Br J Urol* 1986; 58:669–671.
52. Desmond JW, Gordon RA: Bleeding during transurethral prostatic surgery. *Can Anaesth* 1969; 16:217–224.
53. Freedman M, Van der Molen SW, Makings E: Blood loss measurement during transurethral resection of the prostate gland. *Br J Urol* 1985; 57:311–316.
54. Hahn RG: A haemoglobin dilution method (HDM) for estimation of blood volume variations during transurethral

prostatic surgery. *Acta Anaesthesiol Scand* 1987; 31:572–578.
55. Mackenzie AR, Levine N, Scheinman HF: Operative blood loss in transurethral prostatectomy. *J Urol* 1979; 122:47–48.
56. Graversen PH, England DM, Madsen PO, et al: Significance of striated muscle in curretings of the prostate. *J Urol* 1988; 139:751–753.
57. Morse RM, Spirnak JP, Resnick MI: Iatrogenic colon and rectal injuries associated with urological intervention: Report of 14 cases. *J Urol* 1988; 140:101–103.
58. Madsen PO, Naber KG: The importance of the pressure in the prostatic fossa and absorption of irrigating fluid during transurethral resection of the prostate. *J Urol* 1973; 109:446–452.
59. Hahn R, Berlin T, Lewenhaupt A: Rapid massive irrigating fluid absorption during transurethral resection of the prostate. *Acta Chir Scand [Suppl]* 1986; 530:63–65.
60. Rao PN: Fluid absorption during urological endoscopy. *Br J Urol* 1987; 60:93–99.
61. Bretan PN, Carroll PR, McClure RD: Improved continuous flow transurethral prostatectomy. *J Urol* 1985; 134:77–80.
62. Stephenson TP, Latto P, Bradley D, et al: Comparison between continuous flow and intermittent flow transurethral resection in 40 patients presenting with acute retention. *Br J Urol* 1980; 52:523–525.
63. Flechner SM, Williams RD: Continuous flow and conventional resectoscope methods in transurethral prostatectomy: Comparative study. *J Urol* 1982; 127:257–259.
64. Madsen PO, Frimodt-Moller PC: Transurethral prostatic resection with suprapubic trocar technique. *J Urol* 1984; 132:277–279.
65. Stamey TA: Percutaneous suprapubic continuous-flow transurethral prostatectomy. *Monogr Urol* 1987; 8:4–13.
66. Oester A, Madsen PO: Determination of absorption of irrigating fluid during transurethral resection of the prostate by means of radioisotopes. *J Urol* 1969; 102:714–719
67. Hahn RG: Ethanol monitoring of irrigating fluid absorption in transurethral prostatic surgery. *Anaesthesiology* 1988; 68:867–873.
68. Campbell HT, Fincher ME, Sklar AH: Severe hyponatremia without severe hypoosmolality following transurethral resection of the prostate (TURP) in end-stage renal disease. *Am J Kidney Dis* 1988; 12:152–155.
69. Hoekstra PT, Kahnaski R, McCamish MA, et al: Transurethral prostatic resection syndrome—a new perspective: Encephalopathy with associated hyperammonemia. *J Urol* 1983; 130:704–707.
70. Shepard RL, Kraus SE, Babayan RK, et al: The role of ammonia toxicity in the post transurethral prostatecotomy syndrome. *Br J Urol* 1987; 60:349–351.
71. Gillett W, Grossman HB, Lee R: Visual disturbances in TUR resection. *Urology* 1985; 25:573–575.
72. Alexander JP, Polland A, Gillespie IA: Glycine and transurethral resection. *Anaesthesia* 1986; 41:1189–1195.
73. Casey WF, Hannon V, Cunningham A: Visual evoked potentials and changes in serum glycine concentration during transurethral resection of the prostate. *Br J Anaesth* 1988; 60:525–529.
74. Fitzpatrick JM, Kasidas GP, Alan Rose G: Hyperoxaluria following glycine irrigation for transurethral prostatectomy. *Br J Urol* 1981; 53:250–252.
75. Norlen H, Allgen LG, Vinnars E, et al: Plasma haemoglobin concentrations and other influx variables in blood in connection with transurethral resection of the prostate using distilled water as an irrigating fluid. *Scand J Urol Nephrol* 1987; 21:161–168.
76. Madsen PO, Madsen RE: Clinical and experimental evaluation of different irrigating fluids for transurethral surgery. *Invest Urol* 1965; 3:122–129.
77. Fetter TR, Tocantins LM, Cottone RN, et al: Effect of epsilon aminocaproic acid on bleeding after prostatectomy. *J Urol* 1961; 85:970–972.
78. Ladehoff AA, Otte E: Inhibitory effect of epsilon amminocaproic acid on fibrinolytic activity and bleeding in transvesical prostatectomy. *Scand J Clin Lab Inves* 1963; 15:239–247.
79. Ratnoff OD: Epsilon aminocaproic acid—a dangerous weapon. *N Engl J Med* 1969; 280:1124–1125.
80. Kursh ED, Ratnoff OD, Persky L: Current

clotting concepts in urology. *J Urol* 1976; 116:214–217.

81. Sinclair J, Forbes CD, Prentia CRM, et al: The incidence of deep vein thrombosis in prostatectomised patients following the administration of the fibrinolytic inhibitor, aminoaproic acid (EACA). *Urol Res* 1976; 4:129–131.
82. Flanigan RC, Butler KM, O'Neal W, et al: Comparison of epsilon amniocaproic acid and normal saline for postoperative bladder irrigation following transurethral resection of prostate. *Urology* 1985; 26:227–228.
83. Sharifi R, Lee M, Ray P, et al: Safety and efficacy of intravesical aminocaproic acid for bleeding after transurethral resection of prostate. *Urology* 1986; 27:214–219.
84. Luke M, Kvist E, Anderson F, et al: Reduction of post-operative bleeding after transurethral resection of the prostate by local instillation of fibrin adhesive (Beriplast). *Br J Urol* 1986; 58:672–675.
85. Walker RD: The injection of Teflon paste to correct urinary incontinence and vesicourethral reflux. *AUA Update Series*, lesson 20, vol 8, 1989.
86. Sikafi Z, Butler MR, Lane U, et al: Bladder neck contracture following prostatectomy. *Br J Urol* 1985; 57:308–310.
87. Jorgensen PE, Weis N, Bruun E: Etiology of urethral stricture following transurethral prostatectomy. *Scand J Urol Nephrol* 1986; 20:253–255.
88. Melchoir J, Valk WL, Foret JD, et al: Transurethral resection of the prostate via perineal urethrostomy: Complete analysis of 7 years of experience. *J Urol* 1974; 111: 640–643.
89. Emmett JL, Roos SN, Greene LF, et al: Preliminary internal urethrotomy in 1036 cases to prevent urethral stricture following transurethral resection: Caliber of normal adult urethra. *J Urol* 1963; 89:820–835.
90. Lundhus E, Dorflinger T, Moller-Madsen B, et al: Significance of the extent of transurethral prostatic resection for postoperative complications. *Scand J Urol Nephrol* 1987; 21:9–12.
91. Holtgrewe HL, Valk WL: Late results of transurethral prostatectomy. *J Urol* 1964; 82:51–55.
92. Bolt JW, Evans C, Marshall VR: Sexual dysfunction after prostatectomy. *Br J Urol* 1987; 59:319-322.
93. Feldstein MS, Benson NA: Early removal and reduced length of hospital stay following transurethral prostatectomy: A retrospective analysis of 100 consecutive cases. *J Urol* 1988; 140:532–534.
94. Widran J: Video transurethral resection using controlled continous flow resectoscope. *Urology* 1988; 31:382–386.
95. Allhoff E, Bading R, Hoene E, et al: The chip camera: perfect imaging in endourology. *World J Urol* 1988; 6:6–7.
96. Krongrad A, Stone NN: Sonographic imaging of prostatectomy (abstract V-48). Presented at American Urological Association Annual Meeting, Dallas, Tex, 1989.
97. Chang LS, Young ST: Transurethral prostatectomy with computer-monitored resectoscope. *Br J Urol* 1988; 62:54–58.

CHAPTER 21

Complications of Surgery for Male Urinary Incontinence, Including the Artificial Urinary Sphincter

J. Keith Light, M.D.

Surgery for the correction of male urinary incontinence has advanced significantly over the past decade. The improvement in the artificial urinary sphincter and the introduction of Teflon injections are two important additions to the surgeon's armamentarium. Each patient needs to be assessed individually and the least invasive procedure that will succeed chosen.

Surgical procedures to correct male urinary incontinence can be divided into two broad groups: (1) *reconstruction of a new sphincteric mechanism,* in which the patient's own tissues are used to reconstruct a new sphincteric mechanism; and (2) *substitution for the damaged sphincteric mechanism,* in which the tissues are compressed with either a device or injected materials.

RECONSTRUCTION OF A NEW SPHINCTERIC MECHANISM

Inherent to the success of sphincteric reconstruction is the normality of the bladder's vascular and nerve tissue. Reconstruction of the bladder neck to form a new functioning sphincter utilizes the anterior or posterior (i.e., trigone) bladder wall.

The trigonal tubularization described by Young[1] and by Leadbetter[2] is seldom applicable to the adult man, since the most common cause of incontinence in this group is prostatectomy. The posterior or trigonal bladder wall is inevitably damaged by the procedure to some extent. The majority of prostatectomies are now performed transurethrally, and this results especially in scarring of the trigone, rendering the tissues unsuitable for reconstruction. More recently, Tanagho et al. have described reconstructing a new sphincter using the anterior bladder wall.[3] This method avoids scar tissue resulting from the prostatectomy. In essence, a tube is formed from the anterior bladder wall which is anastomosed to the prostatic capsule.

The success rate following reconstruction of the bladder neck is variable. The failure rate with the Tanagho anterior bladder tube ranges from 30% to 50%.[4, 5] Leadbetter in 1985 reported a 43% failure rate in adults after a 10- to 20-year follow-up using his technique.[6] Other complications include stenosis of the reconstructed tube, resulting in obstruction. It is therefore not uncommon to see patients who have a combination of urinary incontinence and urinary retention.

The initial reconstruction stands the best chance of success. Multiple operations in attempting to reconstruct the bladder neck are to be condemned.

SUBSTITUTION OF THE SPHINCTERIC MECHANISM

Substitution for a damaged or nonfunctioning sphincteric mechanism implies the use of compression, either with a device or injected substances. Inherent to the success of this approach is the normal vascularity of the tissue and the use of compressive forces less than the systolic blood pressure. The ability to compensate for sudden increases in intraabdominal pressure to avoid stress incontinence is only possible with the artificial urinary sphincter.

Injections

Sachse in 1963 reported on the use of sclerosing injections to cure urinary incontinence.[7] The occurrence of pulmonary emboli, however, led to its abandonment. Politano[8] refined this technique by injecting polytef (Teflon) paste around the urethra to increase outflow resistance. Success rates of 73% in men have been reported.[8] Frequently, however, more than one injection is required. The simplicity of the procedure is indeed attractive. The occurrence of emboli to distant organs has been reported, but the clinical significance of these emboli at present is unsettled. Other complications have been few in number and limited to infection, low-grade fever, and prolonged urinary retention.

Contrary to popular belief, insertion of the artificial urinary sphincter following a failed Teflon injection is almost always doomed to failure. Two reasons account for this failure. The first is the presence of a subclinical infection at the injection site so that the artificial urinary sphincter is contaminated at insertion. The second is the difficulty of defining tissue planes for accurate placement of the cuff due to the fibrosis or the amount of Teflon present.

Devices

Berry in 1961 described using an acrylic block placed under the bulbocavernosus muscle to compress the bulbar urethra.[9] Kaufman, from 1968 to 1974, described several models of a silicone gel prosthesis that were designed to obtain continence by passive compression of the bulbous urethra.[10] At best, the long-term results were only moderate, with a 61% success rate. The reasons for failure were infection; urethral erosion, since the pressure was not satisfactorily controlled; and recurrent incontinence, which was probably secondary to pressure atrophy of the tissue beneath the device. Both the Berry and Kaufman devices are no longer in widespread use. Rosen introduced his prosthesis in 1976.[11] The device was inflated by means of a pump reservoir, located in the scrotum, connected to an inflatable "cuff" which was placed around the bulbar urethra and held in place with two prongs. Although initial results were encouraging, late complications were common. These included infection and, particularly, urethral erosion. The erosion occurred because the pressure in the cuff was controlled by the patient and not the device. The patient continued to fill the cuff under pressure until continence was achieved. Unfortunately, this was at the expense of urethral viability. This device, like those described above, now belongs in the archives.

THE AMS 800 ARTIFICIAL URINARY SPHINCTER

The first AMS artificial urinary sphincter was implanted by Scott in 1973.[12] Numerous refinements have culminated in the current device, the AMS 800 series (Fig 21–1). The main advantages of this device over previous devices are

1. Pressure regulation by the balloon and not the patient
2. Prevention of stress incontinence with placement of the balloon in the submuscular, extraperitoneal position
3. Applicability to sphincteric incontinence of diverse etiology
4. May be implanted at the bladder neck in both sexes or the bulbar urethra in males
5. Ability to deactivate the device without surgery
6. Unobstructed urination

This device has proved thus far to be the most reliable method for restoring urinary continence in men. Two factors have, however, emerged, pelvic irradiation and previous urethral damage, that place the patient in a high-risk category. Previous irradiation to the pelvic area invariably diminished the blood supply to the urethra and bladder neck. The incidence of cuff erosion in this group of patients is therefore significantly increased, being approximately 60%. Previous urethral damage, e.g., stricture or reconstruction, similarly impairs the blood supply and therefore increases the risk of erosion. Although the bladder neck is the preferred site for the cuff placement, this is seldom possible in the adult man, since previous operative procedures or trauma usually involve this site. The bulbous urethra therefore is used to place the cuff if the bladder neck is unsuitable. With the new artificial urinary sphincter, the incidence of cuff erosion is definitely related to the balloon pressure and tissue vascularity. With normal vascularity, a 61- to 70-cm balloon is used for a bulbar sphincter and a 71- to 80-cm balloon for a bladder neck sphincter. If the tissues, however, appear suspect at surgery, lower-pressure balloons are recommended. It should be remembered that the artificial urinary sphincter is used to treat urinary incontinence secondary to sphincteric weakness and not abnormalities of bladder function. Appropriate urodynamic evaluation is therefore essential prior to surgery to characterize bladder function. The success with the artificial urinary sphincter is directly related to the type of bladder function present.[13] Standardization of the surgical technique and improved reliability of the device have significantly decreased the complications.[14] Problems may still occur, however, and can prove frustrating to both physician and patient. The results of the artificial urinary sphincter in patients with post-prostatectomy incontinence indicate a 91% chance of success.[15]

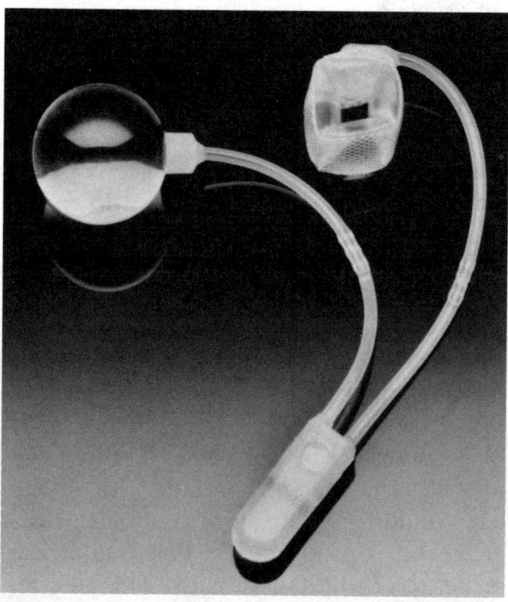

FIG 21–1.
AMS 800 artificial urinary sphincter. (Courtesy of American Medical Systems, Inc.)

An understanding of the device mechanism is important when considering causes of malfunction. The control pump assembly contains the fluid resistors and one-way and poppet valves. The balloon pushes fluid across the resistors to first fill the pump and then the cuff. The rate of fluid transfer in a controlled situation is 0.5 mL/min at a constant driving pressure of 100 cm of water. This, however, does not occur in a clinical situation, since the balloon volume decreases with cuff filling, thereby decreasing the driving pressure. In addition, balloon pressures of 100 cm of water are no longer in use. It takes approximately 10 to 15 minutes for the cuff to become fully pressurized in vivo for any given balloon pressure. On squeezing the pump, fluid passes easily and immediately to the balloon. On releasing the pump, fluid is sucked from the cuff to immediately refill the pump. When the cuff is empty, the pump no longer reexpands and therefore stays "flat." Gradual refilling of the pump and then the cuff occurs as the cycle is repeated. The following clinical and surgical protocol is used by the author to diagnose complications resulting from the artificial sphincter.

Clinical Protocol

A urine culture is performed to ensure that the urine is sterile. If not, the appropriate antibiotic treatment is given. Examination and manipulation of the pump is the single most important aspect of the clinical examination (Fig 21–2). Induration and/or hyperemia surrounding the pump suggest underlying infection with the possibility of cuff erosion. This complication will be discussed later. The most common problem occurring postop-

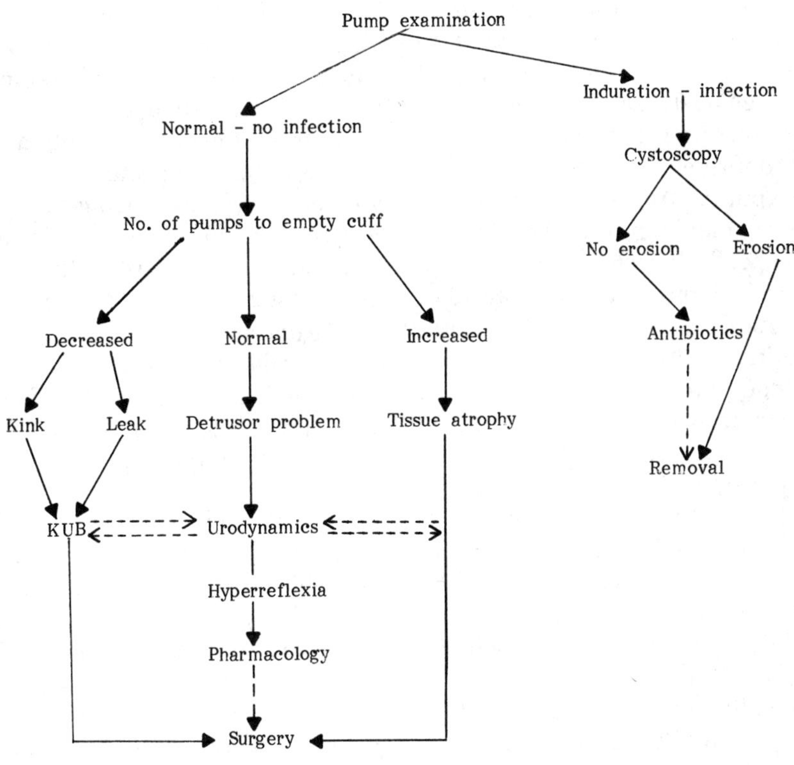

FIG 21–2.
Clinical protocol. *KUB* = kidney-ureter-bladder.

eratively, however, is urinary incontinence. There are two basic causes for persistent or recurrent urinary incontinence following insertion of the artificial sphincter. The first involves the device itself and the second is related to abnormal tissues, usually the bladder.

Causes of Device Failure

The most frequent complication involving the device is a decrease in the closing pressure of the cuff. The two most common causes for this are a leak in the device and pressure atrophy of the tissue beneath the cuff. Other problems include tube kinks, debris in the system, and a restrictive sheath around the reservoir.

Leak in the Device.—The fluid loss may be gradual or sudden depending on the size of the leak and may occur at any stage following implantation of the device. Characteristically, the patient states that the number of pumps required to empty the cuff has decreased from that observed previously or that the pump does not refill, i.e., stays flat. This can easily be confirmed on clinical examination of the pump. An x-ray of the pelvis may show an alteration or decrease in the balloon shape, but it should be remembered that a balloon volume of only 10 cc may look radiologically normal. A normal-appearing balloon radiographically therefore does not exclude a slow leak. The cuff has been the most common site for a leak, followed by the balloon. In previously reported series where repeat surgery was required for a mechanical problem, a cuff leak was responsible in 56% of instances and a balloon leak in 13%.[16] The introduction of the new silicone-coated cuff is expected to sharply diminish the incidence of cuff leaks by preventing friction between the inner soft and outer firm backing of the cuff. The site of the leak is determined at surgery.

Pressure Atrophy.—A variable degree of pressure atrophy inevitably occurs beneath the cuff, the severity of which is related to the balloon pressure. This problem is becoming recognized more frequently and results in the cuff volume increasing at the expense of the balloon volume. The pressure-volume relationship on the deflate curve of the balloon is sigmoid (Fig 21–3). The pressure will drop sharply for a relatively small decrease in volume below a critical balloon volume of approximately 14 cc. Significant pressure atrophy will decrease the cuff closing pressure by "siphoning" fluid from the balloon. Other factors that play a part when considering an incompetent cuff include cuff size, tissue compliance, and the shape the cuff assumes on inflation. The AMS 800 control pump assembly expresses approximately 0.75 cc with each pump. This is in contrast to the AMS 791/2, which has a pump volume of 0.5 cc. Assuming no leak, counting the number of pumps required to empty the cuff allows a reasonably accurate estimate of cuff volume to be made. The residual balloon volume can now be estimated by subtracting this cuff volume from the original balloon volume. Generally, a snug-fitting cuff will contain 0.75 to 2.0 cc depending on the position, i.e., bulbous urethra or bladder neck, respectively. A cuff volume of 6 cc or greater at the bladder neck or 3 cc at the bulbar urethra usually indicates that the cuff is too large. This can be determined clinically by counting the number of pumps required to empty the cuff.

In a recently reported series, a leak in the device and pressure atrophy were responsible for 88% of the malfunctions that required repeat surgery following insertion of the artificial sphincter.[16] It is therefore possible to diagnose 88% of the possible mechanical malfunctions that require further surgery simply by clinical examination of the pump. If doubt is still

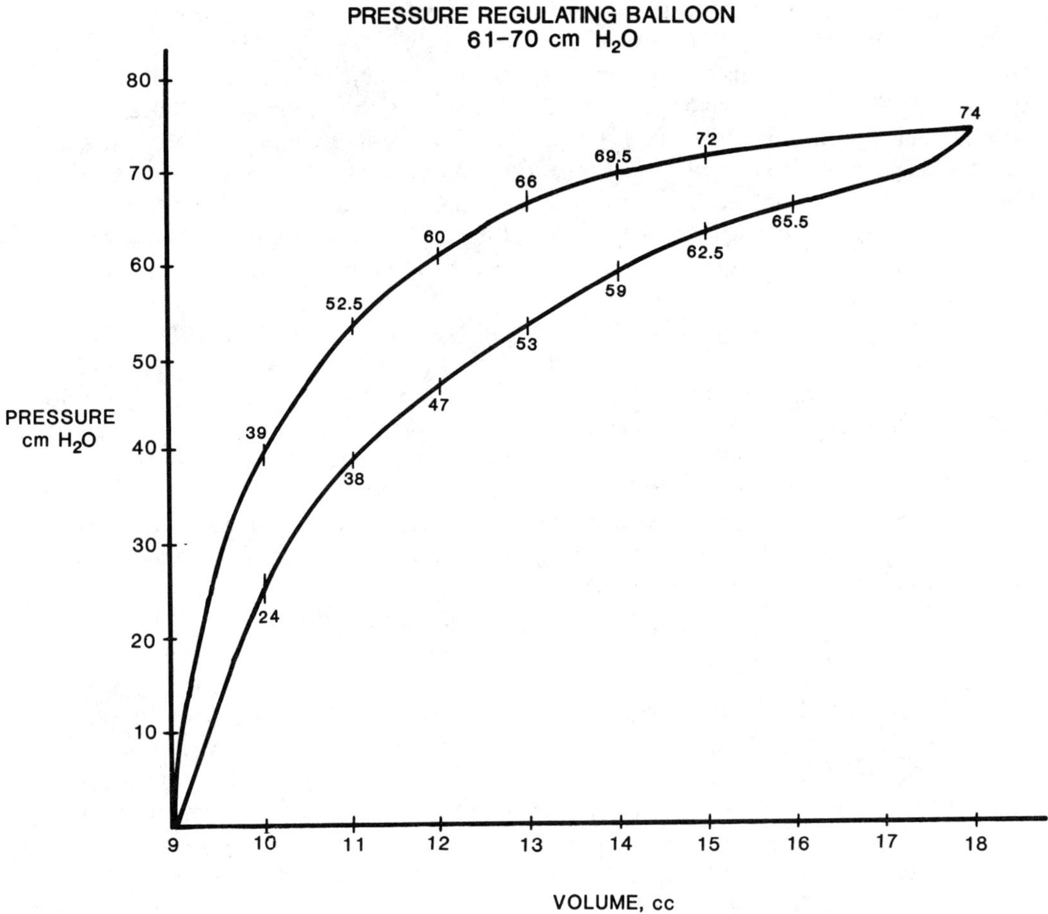

FIG 21–3.
Pressure-volume relationship for 61- to 70-cm water balloon showing inflate curve *(top)* and deflate curve *(bottom)*.

present, urodynamic evaluation can be performed to confirm that the cuff is inefficient.

Debris.—Occasionally, debris within the system can simulate a leak. The patient usually says that the number of pumps required to empty the cuff varies, as does the continence status, which is due to the intermittent obstruction of the resistors by the debris. This obstruction prevents full cuff pressurization. Primary malfunction of the control assembly is extremely rare, and it follows that the introduction of debris occurs at the time of surgery or following a leak.

Kink.—A kink in the tubing may also simulate a leak, due to incomplete refilling of the cuff. A straight x-ray of the pelvis will often identify the site of the kink in addition to showing dye within the system. The specific abnormality found on pump manipulation will depend on the site of the kink. If a kink occurs between the cuff and pump, extremely slow refilling of the pump occurs following the first manipulation. If, however, the kink lies between the pump and balloon, difficulty will be experienced pumping the device with the very first manipulation.

Restrictive Reservoir Sheath.—Occasionally, a restrictive sheath forms around the reservoir postoperatively. This results in the inability of the reservoir to distend to accept all the fluid from the cuff. Characteristically, the first couple of pumps are easy, but are followed by a progressive increase in the resistance as the elasticity of the sheath is exceeded. The significance of a restrictive reservoir sheath is that it may prevent complete cuff deflation and therefore interfere with adequate urination. Urinary incontinence associated with this type of problem is usually an overflow type of incontinence secondary to incomplete bladder emptying. This can be avoided by ensuring that the patient completely empties the cuff on a frequent basis in the postoperative period.

Abnormal Tissues

If there is no change in the pumping characteristics of the device, the reason for the incontinence usually lies within the tissues. Detrusor hyperreflexia or poor bladder compliance are two common causes. Both conditions result in an increase in intravesical pressure at variable volumes. If this intravesical pressure exceeds the cuff pressure, fluid will move out of the cuff, resulting in a decrease in the closing pressure and therefore urinary leakage. Urodynamic evaluation has been essential. Cystometry is routinely performed postoperatively in this situation to categorize bladder type. Frequently, preoperative hyperreflexia is aggravated or detrusor instability is precipitated by the surgery. This problem is treated initially with anticholinergics. A flow rate and postvoid residual are also performed to exclude the presence of an outflow obstruction and/or inefficient bladder emptying. An overflow-type incontinence can thus be excluded. Static urethral pressure profilometry with the cuff open and closed adds a further dimension to the evaluation. Because of cuff efficiency, the intraurethral pressure beneath the cuff generally closely approximates or exceeds that of the balloon pressure. If the problem lies with the bladder, the maximum urethral pressure obtained with the cuff closed will be close to or will exceed the balloon pressure. If the maximum urethral pressure is significantly lower than the balloon pressure, the cuff is inefficient. Profilometry with the cuff open is a general measure of outflow resistance and may indicate an inadequate sphincterotomy or poor cuff opening. Pressure-flow studies with simultaneous video cystourethrography performed transurethrally is an excellent means of confirming abnormal detrusor function or outlet obstruction as a cause for the urinary leakage.

Surgical Protocol

The first step is to perform retrograde gas sphincterometry to determine the opening pressure of the cuff (Fig 21–4). This measures essentially the same parameters as the urethral pressure profilometry does but is more accurate than the latter in assessing cuff efficiency. The opening pressure of the cuff should normally be equal to or greater than the stated balloon pressure. This measurement also serves as a baseline for comparison following "corrective" surgery (Fig 21–5). Cystoscopy is performed to assess the cuff site and exclude an erosion.

The electrical test is performed following exposure of the connectors to determine the presence or absence of a leak.[17] If a leak is found, the damaged component is exchanged, and the system is refilled. In the absence of a leak, the balloon volume is measured. With significant pressure atrophy around the bladder neck, this volume will be 14 cc or less. Finally, the cuff volume is measured. The total volume of the cuff and balloon should add up to the original volume inserted if the inefficient cuff is secondary to pressure atrophy. A smaller cuff will correct the problem, and repeat gas

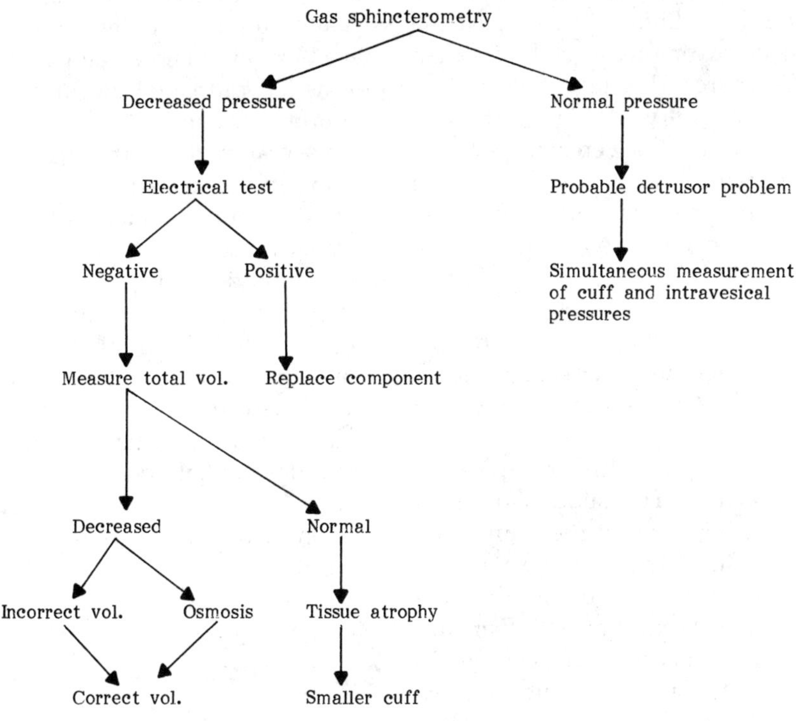

FIG 21–4.
Surgical protocol.

sphincterometry will show the expected increase in the opening pressure (Fig 21–6). Rarely, the total volume will have decreased in the absence of a leak. Original insertion of the incorrect volume is one possibility; so is fluid loss secondary to osmosis from a hypo-osmolar mixture. Replacement of the fluid will solve the problem. In the event that the opening pressure is normal, the problem will usually be the tissues. A problem with the tissues, however, should have been suspected on preoperative evaluation. In this instance, it may be necessary to measure simultaneous pressures of the cuff and

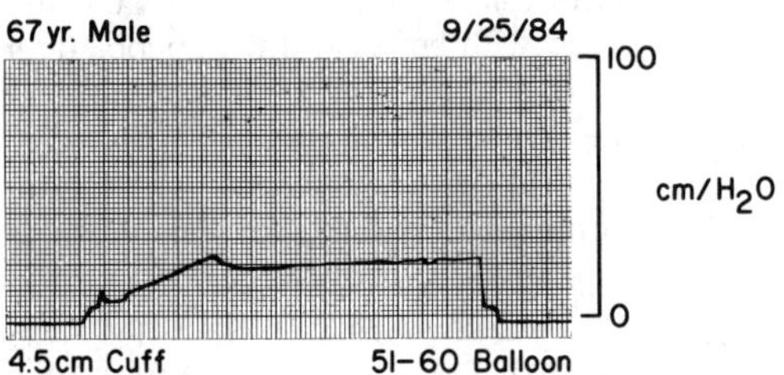

FIG 21–5.
Low opening pressure of the cuff, preoperative.

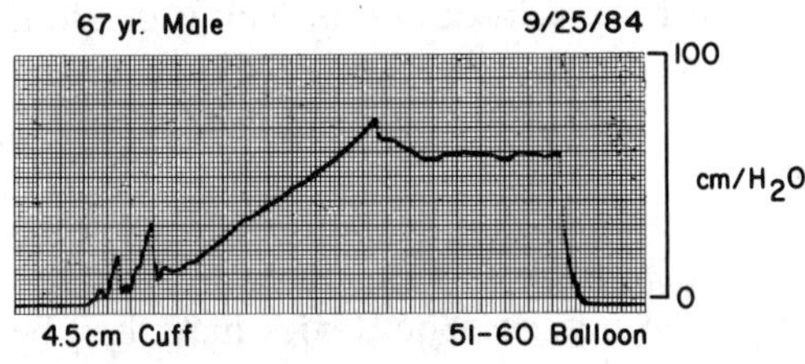

FIG 21–6.
Increase in cuff opening pressure following repair surgery.

bladder to confirm poor tissue compliance as the cause for the incontinence. If the problem lies with poor tissue compliance beneath the cuff, fluid will leak past the cuff, with detrusor pressures lower than the cuff pressure. This test, however, is only rarely necessary. A higher-pressure balloon is inserted to overcome poor tissue compliance of the cuff area, while an augmentation cystoplasty may be necessary with poor bladder compliance.

Infection

Infection involving the artificial sphincter is a serious complication, since removal of the device is inevitable. Any induration around the pump, local skin hyperemia, or pain with manipulation suggests infection. The sudden onset of pain and swelling around the pump suggests cuff erosion. In addition, a persistent, burning type of pain in the perineum in the presence of a bulbar cuff points to an impending cuff erosion. In the presence of a suspected infection, exclusion of a cuff erosion is imperative. This is best done with a cystoscopy in the operating room, with arrangements being made to proceed with removal if necessary. A urethrogram is contraindicated, since this may contaminate a sterile erosion or fail to show extravasation if the erosion is small. The cuff only may be removed with a sterile erosion of the bladder neck or relocated if possible with a bulbar sphincter. Removal of the entire device is necessary, though, with an erosion in the presence of infected urine. Cystoscopy may reveal mucosal edema at the cuff site without an apparent erosion. In this situation, the device should be deactivated and a full course of intravenous and then oral antibiotics given. Repeat cystoscopy should be performed 6 weeks later to ensure that a small erosion has not been missed. The device may then be reactivated if the mucosa overlying the cuff site appears healthy.

Patients with an infected device rarely present with the usual systemic signs of an infection, such as leukocytosis or fever. The key symptoms and signs are usually confined to the pump area and have been enumerated above. If the infection is left untreated, eventual erosion of the pump or cuff will occur.

Several methods that have been tried to salvage an infected device include long-term antibiotic treatment, irrigation of the prevesical space with the appropriate antibiotic solution, and exchange of the infected device. This author, however, has not succeeded in salvaging an infected device using all three of the above methods and therefore has abandoned this approach for the artificial sphincter. An infected device that does not respond to antibiotic treatment or is associated with erosion of the cuff or pump must always be removed.

CONCLUSION

The adult man with urinary incontinence has a far greater chance of achieving continence now than ever before. The surgical procedure to be performed must be meticulously chosen after due consideration of all the complications and the procedure's success rate. Correction of incontinence will probably earn the patient's eternal gratitude.

EDITORIAL COMMENT

Artificial sphincters have been utilized with bowel and with neobladder reconstruction or continent urinary reservoirs in some patients. Although an artificial sphincter may provide for continence in this situation, erosions and problems have occurred in a significant percentage of these patients. There is often more tissue around the urethra that allows for better perfusion than having a sphincter placed around the bowel. The use of a sphincter with the bowel should be utilized with caution.

REFERENCES

1. Young HH: An operation for the cure of incontinence of urine. *Surg Gynecol Obstet* 1919; 28:84.
2. Leadbetter GW Jr: Surgical correction of total urinary incontinence. *J Urol* 1964; 91:281.
3. Tanagho EA, Smith DR, Meyers FH et al: Mechanism of urinary continence: II. Technique for surgical correction of incontinence. *J Urol* 1958; 101:305.
4. Tanagho EA: Bladder neck reconstruction for total urinary incontinence: Ten years of experience. *J Urol* 1981; 125:321–326.
5. Light JK: Personal observation, 1985.
6. Leadbetter GW Jr: Surgical reconstruction for complete urinary incontinence. 10- to 22-year follow-up. *J Urol* 1985; 133:205.
7. Sachse H: Sclerosing therapy in urinary incontinence: Indications, results, complications. *Urol Int* 1963; 15:225–244.
8. Politano VA: Periurethral Teflon injection for urinary incontinence. *Urol Clin North Am* 1978; 5:415–422.
9. Berry JL: A new procedure for correction of urinary incontinence: Preliminary report. *J Urol* 1961; 85:771.
10. Kaufman JJ: Treatment of postprostatectomy incontinence using a silicone-gel prosthesis. *Br J Urol* 1973; 45:646.
11. Rosen M: A simple artificial implantable sphincter. *Br J Urol* 1976; 48:675.
12. Scott FB: Treatment of urinary incontinence by implantable prosthetic sphincter. *Urology* 1973; 1:252.
13. Light JK, Scott FB: Use of the artificial urinary sphincter in spinal cord injury patients. *J Urol* 1983; 130:1127.
14. Scott FB, Light JK, Fishman IJ, et al: Implantation of an artificial sphincter for urinary incontinence. *Contemp Surg* 1981; 18:11–34.
15. Scott FB, Light JK, Fishman IJ: Postprostatectomy incontinence: The artificial sphincter, in Hinman F Jr (ed): *Benign Prostatic Hypertrophy*. New York, Springer-Verlag, 1983, pp 1008–1022.
16. Light JK, Scott FB: The artificial urinary sphincter in children. *Br J Urol* 1984; 56:54–57.
17. Webster GD, Sikelnich SA: Troubleshooting the malfunctioning Scott artificial urinary sphincter. *J Urol* 1984; 131:269.

CHAPTER 22

Complications of Incontinence Surgery in Women

Jacek L. Mostwin, M.D., D.Phil.

Many of the expected and avoidable complications of incontinence surgery have been previously discussed in the context of the operations in which they are likely to occur[1–3] and in the previous edition of this book.[4] Specific complications of vaginal surgery have recently been discussed in an issue of *Seminars in Urology* devoted to the subject.[5] Most operations designed to correct incontinence take place with very few complications. The most feared and most common complication is probably the failure to obtain the desired result, either because incontinence due to hypermobility or sphincteric dysfunction persists or returns or because incontinence due to bladder instability is unrecognized preoperatively or appears de novo. Recent classifications of incontinence in women have emphasized the importance of distinguishing incontinence associated with prolapse or hypermobility of the bladder (types I and II) from incontinence due to intrinsic dysfunction of the sphincteric mechanism (type III).[6] A similar approach is presented in this chapter along with a discussion of preoperative evaluation. The importance of female pelvic and vaginal anatomy is emphasized along with the contributions made by gynecology to the understanding and management of this condition. Most of the more common surgical approaches and their indications are discussed, along with general and specific complications.

DIFFERENCES IN APPROACH BY UROLOGISTS AND GYNECOLOGISTS

One rarely hears the name of Howard Kelly today when discussing innovation in female urology, but it must be remembered that he was a major leader in gynecologic practice and teaching throughout most of this century. Kelly was greatly interested in urology.[7] He was a *general* surgeon for women, in the truest sense of the word.

As a result of their tradition and historical background, many gynecologists in America have assumed responsibility for the urologic care of their patients except where major surgery for cancer, transplantation, or reconstruction has been required. Many still perform cystoscopic examination of their patients.

The accumulated experience and insight of the gynecologic profession regarding the management of stress incontinence in women is enormous, especially among older, more experienced surgeons who have specialized in this area for some years. Gynecologists have the advantage of general familiarity with the vaginal approach and have a greater familiarity with the spectrum of vaginal disorders, including major or minor degrees of prolapse. For many, the complaint of stress incontinence will be seen in the context of some degree of vaginal prolapse, and repair of stress incontinence will be incidental to repair of vaginal prolapse. Any urologist wishing to undertake the urologic care of women must be willing to recognize the great contribution of gynecologists to pelvic surgery and anatomical understanding in general and to their role as primary care providers for women.

Since World War II, urologists have pioneered the urodynamic approach to the problem of incontinence in men, women, and children. The urodynamically and anatomically oriented urologist is an excellent physician to evaluate and treat the incontinent woman, provided that he can familiarize himself with the spectrum of vaginal pathology affecting the parous or aging female, and that he can learn the necessary abdominal and vaginal techniques. The modern urologist is an experienced endoscopist and a general surgeon of the pelvis. He should be able to master the details required to evaluate and treat female incontinence. He is an ideal specialist to provide leadership in this developing area of urology.

GENERAL CLASSIFICATION OF INCONTINENCE IN ADULT WOMEN

In women without congenital defects such as ureteral ectopia or epispadias, urinary incontinence will be due either to hypermobility of the bladder neck with or without an associated degree of vaginal prolapse, intrinsic dysfunction of the urethra, or neuromuscular dysfunction of the bladder.

A *normal bladder* is one which has normal sensation, stability, compliance, and capacity and empties primarily by intrinsic muscular contraction without associated abdominal straining. Any other bladder requires further consideration. Urodynamic evaluation is often required.

A *normal urethra* is one in which the intrinsic sphincteric mechanism is intact. At present the sphincteric mechanism is thought to be composed of a number of factors, each of which contributes to overall urethral integrity. If one or more of these factors fails, urethral incompetence results. The urethra should be at least 2.5 cm long, the mucosal walls well vascularized and coapted, and the bladder neck closed at rest as judged either by standing cystogram or cystoscopy. The symptom of *total urinary incontinence,* the constant leakage of urine at rest or during straining, whether supine or standing, implies intrinsic sphincteric dysfunction. This abnormality will not respond to the conventional suspensory operations. This is the most difficult form of incontinence to correct surgically. The management of this problem is discussed below.

Hypermobility refers to detachment of the lateral bladder neck from the arcus tendineus fasciae pelvis from either or both internal lateral pelvic walls. This is the typical pathologic finding in 85% to 90% of women complaining of stress incontinence. This type of hypermobility represents herniation of an otherwise normally functioning bladder and intrinsic sphincteric unit into the vaginal vault. This type of patient is an ideal candidate for a purely suspensory operation. It is important to realize that this herniation can frequently be associated with other types of vaginal prolapse, including cystocele, rectocele, and attenuation of the perineal body. It is less common to find stress incontinence in superior vaginal wall prolapse (prolapse of the uterus with or without enterocele and a high rectocele). It is important to understand that such advanced prolapse can mask stress incontinence due to minor bladder neck hypermobility because the prolapsed bladder is hinged at the bladder neck and absorbs the downward thrust of intraabdominal straining. Consideration should be given to suspending the bladder neck when such patients undergo vaginal reconstruction.

It is important to distinguish among these three contributing factors. The majority of suspensory operations available for the treatment of stress incontinence today rely on prevention of hypermobility during increased intraabdominal pressure. They will only work if hypermobility alone is responsible for the problem. For a patient with intrinsic sphincteric damage, a sling or similar variant will be required.

EVALUATION OF THE INCONTINENT WOMAN

A majority of patients who complain primarily of leakage on stress really do have stress incontinence, probably due to simple hypermobility, and it probably will be corrected by any one of a number of operations with 85% to 90% chance of complete success if it is the first operation. Evaluation should be aimed at identifying and separating these patients from others with more complicated etiologies or histories.

History

The patient with hypermobility will complain of leakage during vigorous activity, and when coughing, sneezing, or laughing. In more advanced stress incontinence, patients will leak with minimal movements, such as getting out of bed or changing position in bed. The number of pads worn or changed per day gives a good indication of the severity of the incontinence. Although some patients with hypermobility have bladder instability, most do not. Symptoms suggestive of instability include urgency or urge incontinence provoked by the sound of running water or testing the bath water with the foot, urgency upon awakening in the morning when the feet first touch the floor, or nocturia. Patients with urethritis, urethral syndrome, or early interstitial cystitis are rarely incontinent and may often have pain as a major feature of their complex. Pain is almost never associated with simple stress incontinence. A voiding diary and schedule of medications can be helpful in evaluating the complaints of the elderly.[8] It is important to know if the patient has had previous surgery for incontinence. Such patients are more likely to have dysfunctional sphincters or distorted vaginal, urethral, or bladder neck anatomy. If the patient is postmenopausal, preoperative estrogens may be required. In some cases of urethral incompetence, estrogens alone may solve the problem or make it tolerable enough that the patient will forego surgery. (Breast or endometrial cancer is a contraindication to estrogen administration.)

Physical Examination

A gynecologic examination table, adequate lighting, and a female assistant are necessary. The patient should be examined in both the supine and standing position. (This examination can often be repeated immediately following cystoscopy with the bladder full.) The urologist's vaginal examination is different from the gynecologist's. From Dr. Shlomo Raz I learned the technique of using only the posterior blade of a pediatric vaginal speculum to displace the posterior vaginal wall, directly observing the mobility of the anterior vaginal wall. I find this most helpful. This blade will fit into all but the most stenotic introitus. One should inspect the urethra to ensure that it is fully formed and the meatus is correctly positioned. The lateral attachments of the bladder neck to the arcus tendineus fasciae pelvis can be seen and felt and their integrity determined during coughing or straining. When incontinence is seen in association with hypermobility, an attempt should be made to prevent it by laterally supporting the vaginal wall without occluding the urethra (Bonney or Marshall test). As Dr. Victor Marshall has written: "In addition to this so-called stress test the vaginal placement of a sponge tampon (usually made up of four to eight 4- × 4-in. gauze sponges) should support the vesical base to provide dramatic relief while the tampon is in place during the next 10 to 12 hours."[9] Correction of the incontinence suggests the likelihood of successful surgical repair, but the examination will not always precisely distinguish between incontinence due to hypermobility and that due to intrinsic sphincteric incompetence. Uterine or superior vaginal vault prolapse, cystocele, enterocele, rectocele, and perineal attenuation should be identified. Ideally, all these defects can and should be corrected at the time of stress incontinence repair. The degree of bladder neck hypermobility should be interpreted within the context of overall vaginal prolapse. Many urologists are not very comfortable recognizing and identifying these abnormalities, but some additional reading and consultation with more experienced colleagues can be very helpful. Even if the urologist is not prepared to perform all necessary reconstructive vaginal procedures, at least he can make a complete anatomical diagnosis and recognize the need for additional intervention.

The presence of a full bladder, either naturally or following cystoscopy, will aid in the direct identification of urinary leakage during straining and confirm the diagnosis of *stress* incontinence. Examination in the knee-chest position can help to exclude vesicovaginal fistula if suspected. Inspection of the anterior abdominal wall will reveal previous surgical incisions and give an indication of the strength of abdominal fascia.

Radiologic Imaging

Most of the techniques described are meant to substantiate the clinician's impression. All can be a valuable source of additional information and will help to reinforce and constantly educate the clinician interested in this problem. The bead-chain cystogram relies on the image of the urethra relative to the symphysis pubis at rest and during straining to identify hypermobility. It is rarely used today. A similar examination can be performed with a simple catheter in the urethra. It is important that the examination be performed at rest and during straining. It is important to get a view of the bladder neck in the erect position at rest to determine its competence. An actively interested radiologist is most helpful. We have recently explored the use of dynamic fast-scan magnetic resonance imaging (MRI) to image the entire pelvis at rest and during straining.[10] This allows us to see all the pelvic compartments in motion and determine the full extent of prolapse and associated pathology prior to planning reconstructive surgery.

If previous stress incontinence surgery has been performed, an intravenous pyelogram (IVP) or other upper tract imaging study should be performed to ensure that the ureters are normal prior to undertaking a second operation.

Urodynamics

A bad bladder will ruin the outcome of the best incontinence repair, rendering miserable both patient and surgeon. It is important that the surgeon be satisfied with his understanding of the patient's bladder function. A simple approach for the examining room suggested by Blaivas[11] is to fill the bladder slowly by gravity through the open chamber of a 60-cc piston-tipped syringe attached to a catheter, observing for signs of steady filling at a steady rate with no evidence of spontaneous or unstable contractions. This also provides an estimate of sensation and capacity. This method of "eyeball cystometry" provides very adequate screening in the hands of a clinician who understands bladder function.[11] If there is doubt, more complete urodynamic testing can be performed. Whatever the urodynamic technique or instruments used, the result should be a complete understanding of the patient's bladder cycle including sensation, stability, capacity, compliance, presence of intrinsic detrusor contraction and relative absence of straining, adequate flow, and absence of significant residual.

In patients with total incontinence due to intrinsic sphincter damage or urethral dysfunction in whom a sling operation is likely to be selected, it is important to have an idea of how the bladder will perform *after* the urethra is obstructed by the sling. McGuire has described pulling the balloon of the urodynamic catheter against the bladder neck to allow greater filling unlimited by incontinence to assess capacity and compliance.[12] As in children prior to undiversion, however, urodynamic evidence of small capacity and poor compliance should not necessarily be taken as indicators of poor postoperative performance. This is an area requiring future investigation.

McGuire has previously discussed the relationship of instability to stress incontinence, suggesting both that instability may accompany stress incontinence and disappear following surgical repair in 80% of cases.[13, 14] Instability may also follow the correction of the stress incontinence, but it is possible that the incidence does not exceed the incidence in the general population. The exact relationship is yet to be understood. At present it is fair to say that most women who have instability associated with stress incontinence should be permitted to undergo corrective surgery with the expectation that their urgency will also be corrected, but they must be counseled about the possibility of persistent postoperative urgency and possible urge incontinence.

The value of preoperative urethral pressure profiles has not been generally accepted. Studies comparing pre- and postoperative profiles have failed to demonstrate a clear relationship between good results and anticipated changes in pressure profiles. A very low preoperative pressure may suggest the need for supportive sling surgery, but in general the technique is not widely used in the evaluation of stress incontinence.

Cystoscopy

Urethral length, vascularity, and coaptation are examined. Bladder neck position and mobility during stress are examined. Bladder neck closure at rest and muscular tone of the bladder neck are examined. These are all indirect ways to ascertain that the intrinsic sphincteric mechanism is intact. Combined cystoscopic examination and digital manipulation of the bladder neck and the trigone through the anterior vaginal wall will precisely pinpoint the location of the ureteral orifices and the extent of cystocele and urethrocele.

SELECTING THE OPERATION

Anatomical Considerations

A complete discussion of the anatomy of bladder and bladder neck support is beyond the scope of this chapter. There is still much active investigation in this area.[2, 15–20] There are four major supporting structures preventing bladder hypermobility: (1) the extrapelvic urogenital diaphragm, consisting primarily of the deep transverse perineal muscle and its superficial fascia; (2) intrapelvic condensations of the endopelvic fascia near the bladder neck, manifested medially as the pubourethral ligaments and more laterally as the arcus tendineus fasciae pelvis, which attaches the lateral bladder to the obturator internus and pubococcygeus muscles; (3) the pubocervical fascia separating the anterior vaginal wall from the bladder between the cervix and bladder neck; and (4) the high indirect bladder supports near the cervix consisting of the cardinal and uterosacral ligaments. The relationship of anatomical support to the evolution and selection of operations has been recently reviewed.[21]

Kelly Plication

This operation,[22, 23] and its more modern modification by Nichols and Randall,[2] uses the superficial fascia of the deep transverse perineal muscle of the urogenital diaphragm to tighten the attenuated lateral attachments of the bladder neck by a pants-over-vest method in the midline. A ridge is formed across the posterior bladder neck preventing further descent during stress. Unless the plication is performed too tightly, obstruction is unlikely.

Transabdominal Suspensions

The procedure best known to the urologist is the retropubic urethropexy or Marshall-Marchetti-Krantz (MMK) procedure.[24, 25] This operation fixes the proximal urethra and bladder neck in a retropubic position by placing sutures into the pubocervical fascia on both sides of the urethra and bladder neck, securing them to the periosteum of the posterior symphysis pubis. In the original description, chromic catgut sutures were used and the attenuated endopelvic fascia attaching the bladder neck to the inferior edge of the symphysis was divided. If the periurethral sutures are placed too far medially or too high against the symphysis, obstruction will result which will later be seen in lateral cystograms as kinking or excessive angulation of the urethra.

Although the urethra is not directly mobilized, the most popular abdominal gynecologic procedure of this sort is the Burch colposuspension.[26] In Burch's original description, he describes placing his suspensory sutures into Cooper's ligament because symphyseal periosteal sutures often came out. His paraurethral sutures are also placed into the pubocervical fascia lateral to the bladder neck. The most recent and not generally well-known procedure in this group is the repair developed by Cullen Richardson.[27] Based on extensive anatomical dissection illustrating the importance of arcus tendineus fasciae pelvis separation in the genesis of vaginal herniation, he has designed a retropubic operation in which this defect is repaired by replacing the lateral border of the bladder and bladder neck using sutures connecting the pubocervical fascia to the original insertion of the arcus tendineus along the pelvic side wall.

In all of these operations, the goal is to prevent hypermobility during stress, *not* to increase the resistance of the urethra. After one of these operations, the thin female bladder is very tightly adherent to the symphysis and the undersurface of the rectus abdominis fascia, making subsequent transabdominal operations to get at the bladder neck much more difficult and bladder perforation common.

Needle Suspensions

These operations attempt to perform by a vaginal route exactly what is performed by the transabdominal route: prevent hypermobility. All of the operations to be discussed rely on vaginal identification and/or exposure of paravesical structures into which sutures are placed and then passed by means of a needle introduced through a small superficial suprapubic incision into a position just anterior to the rectus abdominis fascia where they are tied.

The first of these was the Pereyra procedure.[28] The vaginal wall is incised on either side of the bladder neck and urethra and a helix of suspensory sutures is placed into the pubocervical fascia and deep transverse perineal muscle and its superficial fascia. The endopelvic fascia is entered vaginally near the lateral reflections of the arcus tendineus fasciae pelvis and the Pereyra needle passed into this incision through a superficial skin incision near the symphysis. The sutures are passed into these incisions anterior to the intact rectus abdominis fascia where they are tied. The rectus abdominis provides the support to hold the sutures. This operation was modified and brought to the attention of the urologic community by Stamey.[29, 30] Stamey introduced the use of the cystoscope to aid in determining the amount of bladder neck elevation required to restore the correct vesicourethral angle. He simplified the dissection at the bladder neck, using a Dacron pledget placed against the intact pubocervical fascia, held in place by the two ends of a suspensory suture passed by needle through the pubocervical fascia 1 cm apart into suprapubic incisions where they were tied while the assistant determined position by cystoscopic inspection. This operation was further simplified by Gittes,[31] placing suspensory sutures into the pubocervical fascia adjacent to the bladder neck through the intact vaginal wall, allowing the vaginal wall to epithelialize over the sutures.

The most comprehensive of the needle suspensions has been developed by Raz.[32] Beginning with the dissection of Pereyra, the endopelvic fascia is entered just medial and adjacent to the insertion of the arcus tendineus. The suspension is created with sutures incorporating the medially displaced endopelvic fascia, which can be seen with suitable retraction and lighting against the lateral wall of the bladder when the bladder is retracted away from the lateral pelvic side wall to the pubocervical fascia lying just underneath the bladder neck itself. These sutures are then passed by means of a newly developed double-pronged needle creating two evenly spaced punctures 1 cm apart in the rectus abdominis fascia through which the suspensory sutures are delivered and tied.

All of the operations discussed thus far, whether transabdominal or vaginal, are meant only to *support the bladder neck and prevent hypermobility*. This is accomplished not by occluding the urethra but by supporting the paraurethral and bladder neck tissues sufficiently lateral to provide support without kinking, excessively elevating, or occluding the urethra. The surgeon should not feel he has to provide "the right amount of tension," because *support*, not tension, is the desired result of the operation.

Operations for Intrinsic Urethral Damage

In patients in whom urethral dysfunction is identified, correction of hypermobility alone, if it is also present, will not solve the problem. These patients often complain not only of stress incontinence but of *total incontinence*. They include those who have an atrophic or fibrotic urethra, previous radiation, or multiple vaginal operations or neurologic disease. The vaginal wall may be fixed or distorted following previous surgery and hypermobility need not be evident on examination. The cystoscopic appearance may show a "drainpipe" urethra with a clear view into the bladder from the meatus. A standing cystogram will show contrast in the urethra or obvious leakage. Operations designed to correct this problem all create urethral compression.

Fascia Lata Sling

This is the operation of "next resort" for many gynecologists dealing with stress incontinence. It is selected in cases of failure or recurrence following previous repair. Very few urologists are familiar with this procedure. It is often used by gynecologists for severe or recurrent hypermobility, when a Burch or Kelly will not suffice or has failed, or when there is general doubt about the integrity of fascial structures that will have to hold the suspensory sutures.

The operation as introduced by Goebell[33] and later modified by Frangenheim[34] and by Stoeckel,[35] presently uses a strip of fascia lata obtained with a special instrument, the Masson stripper, through a small suprapatellar incision on the lateral thigh. The urethrovesical junction is exposed through a vaginal incision. Suprapubic exposure is made either by transabdominal or transvaginal dissection. The sling is passed up along either side of the bladder, seated at the urethrovesical junction, and sewn to the anterior abdominal wall fascia or Cooper's ligament, depending on the surgeon's preference and the strength of the patient's abdominal wall fascia.[36] Most authorities caution against excessive elevation of the urethra by the sling. When the patient assumes an upright position, the urethra will rest against the sling, providing the necessary coaptation and compression. During stress, the urethra will be pressed down against the sling with more force, preventing stress incontinence.

Variations on the Sling

Several variations on the Goebell-Stoeckel sling have been described. Each attempts to produce compression and coaptation of the dysfunctional urethra. These include (1) rectus abdominis fascia, separated from its attachment or left as a flap in situ,[37, 38] (2) a small patch of rectus abdominis fascia supported by sutures,[3] or (3) a sling or suture-supported patch of Marlex mesh.[2, 39]

Most recently, Raz et al. have introduced an anterior vaginal wall sling[40] in which an island of full-thickness vaginal wall is separated from the rest of the vaginal wall and suspended by means of suspensory sutures passed anterior to the rectus abdominis muscles as in Raz's other needle suspensory procedures. This procedure releases the posterior wall of the urethra and allows it to be compressed against the anterior wall with support provided by the sling. The full thickness of the vaginal wall sling is buried beneath the remaining anterior vagina wall, which is closed over it.

The sling, in any of its configurations, is not an operation to be undertaken casually. Technical difficulties of the operation include mobilization of the adherent or frozen urethra and bladder neck, the seating of the sling and the judgment required to tighten the sling correctly. Also, the patient for whom this operation is usually selected may often have a dysfunctional bladder or multiple previous operations, making postoperative rehabilitation difficult and time-consuming for both patient and physician.

Periurethral Injection

Based on the assumption that the dysfunctional urethra can be compressed by submucosal injection of artificial material, first Teflon,[41] and more recently, glutaraldehyde cross-linked collagen[42, 43] have been injected cystoscopically at the bladder neck and urethra for the correction of incontinence due to urethral incompetence. Teflon has fallen into disfavor because it has been shown to migrate throughout the body following injection and there is fear of pulmonary embolization. It is not inert within the body and granuloma formation has been reported, leading to unpredictable results.[44] Nonetheless, the principle of increasing urethral resistance by submucosal injection has been incorporated into reconstructive technique.[45, 46] Bovine collagen has been used for some time by dermatologists for cosmetic correction of skin defects. The glutaraldehyde cross-linked product has not yet been approved by the Food and Drug Administration. Long-term evaluation is awaited, but initial trials are encouraging.[42]

Artificial Sphincter

This device, in its latest configuration, the AMS 800, has become popular in the treatment of postprostatectomy incontinence in men. Its use has been reported in complicated stress incontinence in women with variable results. Both Appel[47] and Light and Scott[48] have reported 90% success in women, but there has been a high reoperation rate, and other smaller series reporting experience with stress incontinence have reported unacceptably high rates of erosion, infection, and removal, whether inserted by the vaginal or suprapubic route.[49] It has not gained widespread acceptance among urologists or gynecologists managing women with total urinary incontinence, but in the hands of someone familiar with the device, it can be considered an alternative in incontinence due to sphincteric incompetence.

Urinary Diversion

Although not generally considered part of the management of incontinence, the use of indwelling catheter and surgical diversion in the form of vesicotomy or urostomy should not be forgotten. These procedures may significantly improve the life of a patient totally disabled by incontinence and may be required if severe incontinence is associated with general debility or a bladder that is not likely to function after reconstruction, or if the patient is a poor candidate for surgery and the bladder retraining that will likely follow.

COMPLICATIONS

Preoperative Considerations

With careful preoperative evaluation and intraoperative monitoring, operative mortality for older patients has not been shown to be greater than for younger patients. In a review of 84 of 130 elderly women undergoing elective gynecologic surgery, primarily for prolapse, there were no deaths, but there was an increase in associated medical illnesses and such complications as falling out of bed, acute glaucoma, and pneumonia.[50] Special attention should be paid to history of varicose veins, deep venous thrombosis, or pulmonary embolus. Prophylaxis in the form of subcutaneous heparin or intraoperative pneumatic antiembolism stockings should be considered. Preoperative antibiotics should be considered to prevent against subsequent pelvic abscess. Broad-spectrum coverage is advised to cover vaginal anaerobic bacteria. Postoperative antibiotics help in healing of suture lines. When rectocele or enterocele repair is contemplated, or if there is a risk of enteric perforation, preoperative bowel preparation by mechanical lavage, hyperosmotic oral solutions, and oral antibiotics should be considered. If bleeding is anticipated, such as for repeat operations or more extensive repairs, the patient should be offered the chance to donate autologous blood for transfusion to minimize the risk of bloodborne contamination.[51, 52] One unit a week may be donated to the blood bank for 3 weeks beginning 1 month prior to surgery. Supplemental iron is taken during this time.

Intraoperative Considerations

The use of a suprapubic tube placed in the operating room to avoid the problems of immediate postoperative urinary retention has both advantages and disadvantages. This catheter can be placed at the beginning of a vaginal case or the end of a transabdominal case. The advantages of suprapubic drainage are more rapid and easy mobilization and hospital discharge after more complicated repairs such as vaginal slings, or more extensive cystocele repairs when prolonged retention is anticipated. For simple urethropexy and needle suspension, if done with attention to suspension and not obstruction, many women will void following removal of the catheter, and suprapubic drainage is unnecessary.

There are many types of suprapubic tubes: prepackaged small silicon trocar-inserted catheters (Bonano, Stamey), open inserted Malecot catheters, or Foley catheters inserted in a retrograde manner through the abdominal wall using a Lowsley curved prostatic retractor or a Turner-Warwick curved trocar. The Foley has the advantage that the balloon can be placed on traction and temporary bleeding arrested by compressing the bladder wall between the balloon and the skin. For postoperative leakage around the catheter, traction often will solve the problem.

Problems specific to the suprapubic tube are increased postoperative urgency, leakage of urine around the catheter, and delayed bleeding from the suprapubic tract.

Surgical Instruments and the Preparation of the Surgical Field

For transabdominal surgery, separating the patient's legs on padded supports allows perioperative vaginal access. The vagina is prepared and draped into the sterile field. The urethra is catheterized *after* draping so that bladder and vaginal access are sterile. A padded retractor or lubricated sponge stick is an excellent vaginal retractor which allows identification of the vesicouterine fold intraabdominally or tension to be placed on the lateral wall for the placement of urethropexy or colposuspension sutures.

For vaginal surgery a weighted vaginal speculum is needed. Specialists such as Nichols have modified this to include lateral drill holes to allow suturing to drapes, with suction attached.[2] Some have attached fiberoptic light sources. Headlights are excellent sources of directional lights for deep cavitary surgery, but experience is required to use them well. The angle required for direct vision in vaginal surgery and the need to use a cystoscope may make a headlight awkward and a separate overhead or handheld fiberoptic light source preferable.

The vaginal route offers cystoscopic access during surgery to examine urethral position, suture laceration of the bladder, or urethral patency. (If the legs are separated and the vagina prepared for transabdominal surgery, this is also possible.) Usually, only a limited cystoscopic assortment is needed. Indigo carmine in 5-mL ampules can be injected intravenously by the anesthesiologist before the conclusion of the case to ensure that both ureters are patent. Dye can be seen effluxing from the ureters 3 to 5 minutes after injection.

Monofilament sutures should be selected for repairs because of their resistance to infection. Nylon or polypropylene are the choices of most urologists. Many gynecologists are now using monofilament absorbable polydioxanone suture, which is similar to polyglycolic acid but retains its tensile strength in the body for several months.

Inadvertent Intraoperative Injuries

Bladder.—Small lacerations of the bladder in otherwise healthy tissue will heal, given several days of catheter drainage with antibiotic coverage and freedom from suture line tension. Closure of the laceration may be accomplished with fine absorbable sutures placed into the bladder, or, if the bladder is very thin or attenuated, into the surrounding tissues. Interposition of layers between the bladder injury and the vaginal wall will help in the prevention of fistula. The thin female bladder does not hold sutures well, especially the extraperitoneal portion. Excessive suture material encourages inflammation and tissue necrosis, retarding healing and favoring fistula formation.

Ureter.—A ureteral injury in the form of transection, crushing, or ligation may be difficult to identify at the time of surgery. Blue dye seen effluxing from both ureteral orifices 3 to 5 minutes after intravenous administration of indigo carmine dye will reassure the surgeon that the ureter is probably patent. Hypertension in the recovery room may suggest unilateral ureteral ligation. Investigation of postoperative fistula should include IVP to exclude the possibility of ureteral involvement. If the ureter is injured at the time of the operation and the injury recognized, reimplantation or de-ligation with long-term stenting should be performed at once. If the injury is recognized in the immediate postoperative period, immediate repair should be undertaken. If urinoma has accumulated after a period of unrecognized ureteral or vesical extravasation, open or percutaneous drainage of the collection may be required with temporizing urinary diversion by retrograde or percutaneous antegrade catheter. After a particularly difficult dissection, the surgeon may wish to obtain renal sonography or IVP 3 to 5 days postoperatively to satisfy himself that there is no obstruction. It is the *unrecognized* ureteral injury which will lead to renal loss.

Urethra.—A catheter placed in the urethra during surgery will aid in its identification. If a small laceration occurs, stenting over the catheter for 10 to 14 days may allow cleaner reepithelialization than suturing. Attempt at suturing may produce a stricture, and absorbable sutures will produce greater inflammation and tissue necrosis, making the risk of fistula greater. When suturing is required, clean well-visualized edges reapposed without tension offer the best chances for success. If at all possible, preserve the urethral meatus.

Peritoneum.—If entered transabdominally, closure without tension using absorbable suture is sufficient. If entered vaginally, the surgeon has probably pursued a cystocele or rectocele high enough into the vaginal vault to encounter the peritoneal reflection. If there has been previous hysterectomy, there may be a small enterocele. Closure of the edges with pursestring sutures of absorbable material is sufficient. More important is the reapproximation of supporting tissues of sufficient strength, the cardinal and uterosacral ligaments, to prevent subsequent herniation.

Bowel.—Bowel injury may occur during enterocele or rectocele repair, and should be anticipated when undertaking repeat repairs. Injury can theoretically occur during percutaneous puncture of the bladder with a trocar or during passage of needles for the delivery of suspensory sutures above the symphysis. The risk is greater after previous surgery, but bowel injury has rarely been reported as a complication of surgery for incontinence. Preoperative bowel preparation by lavage and antibiotics should be considered when there is risk of perforation. Sharp division of intestinal adhesions is preferable to blunt separation, which increases the risk of tearing the bowel. A rectal injury is most likely to take place below the peritoneal reflection, and in this setting can be closed in two layers and the anal sphincter manually dilated at the conclusion of the procedure. Diverting colostomy should not be required if the injury is below the peritoneal reflection, even in the unprepared bowel. If the defect is large and cannot be closed without tension, closure with omental interposition will be required. If unprepared bowel is injured above the peritoneal reflection, diverting sigmoid colostomy may be required.[1]

Postoperative Complications

Septic Complications.—Infectious complications in the form of urinary infection and urosepsis may be expected if prohylactic antibiotics are not used. Less common complications which may develop include septic pelvic thrombophlebitis or pelvic abscess. For a complete discussion of these and other unusual surgical complications of gynecologic pelvic surgery, the excellent reference by Nichols[1] should be consulted.

Osteitis Pubis.—This is an unusual but recognized complication of pelvic trauma, surgery, or childbirth. It may represent noninfectious periosteal inflammation. The cardinal findings are suprapubic pain, tenderness, adductor spasm, fever, leukocytosis, and elevated erythrocyte sedimentation rate. A bone scan will show increased activity. Characteristic roentgenographic findings include irregularity and "step lesions" of the symphysis, increased bone density, or occasionally, mothball areas of rarefaction. There is no agreement as to etiology. Bone biopsy may be necessary to exclude the diagnosis of septic osteomyelitis or abscess. When cultures are negative, improvement with heparin has been reported, leading to the suggestion that the condition is a result of pelvic thrombophlebitis. Bed rest and anti-inflammatory drugs will be required. Resolution in the past has been spontaneous after an indolent course of many weeks.[53–56]

Ogilvie's Syndrome.—The unusual condition of acute intestinal pseudoobstruction (Ogilvie's syndrome) should be suspected in a patient with progressive postoperative ileus. Plain abdominal roentgenograms will show the dilatation of the cecum and ascending colon which is thought to be due to autonomic imbalance in the usual regulation of bowel motility. Bowel rest and nasogastric suction may be sufficient to allow spontaneous resolution if the degree of cecal dilatation on x-ray is less than 11 to 13 cm. Serial films should be obtained to ensure resolution. If dilatation exceeds 13 cm, colonoscopic or, rarely, surgical decompression will be required.[57, 58]

Pelvic Hematoma.—The space of Retzius may permit sudden or gradual accumulation of several units of blood following surgery unless there has been careful attention to hemostasis or if there is a bleeding diathesis. Evacuation and reexploration may be required if blood loss is rapid and hemodynamic instability develops. If the bleeding develops slowly in the few days following surgery, only a falling hematocrit may indicate a problem. Transfusion may be required. It is better to allow the bleeding to tamponade spontaneously as resolution will eventually occur. The bleeding may cause mechanical disruption of the repair.

Sutures and Pledgets.—If these erode or become infected they need to be removed. Often the surrounding fibrosis will maintain the support and resuspension may not be required.

Long-term Postoperative Complications

Urinary Retention.—Depending upon the type of operation undertaken, suprapubic drainage may be selected. Patients can be taught to clamp and unclamp these catheters after every void until a regular pattern of voiding that eliminates 75% of the bladder contents can be established. The tube should not be removed before 10 to 14 days to allow the tract to mature and prevent extravesical intraabdominal extravasation. The presence of this tube in the bladder increases urgency and the patient may spend a frustrating week or two handling the catheter. It may be particularly difficult for the elderly. An alternative is to have the patient perform self-catheterization. The technique can be taught preoperatively.

If only a urethral catheter is used and retention occurs following removal, phenoxybenzamine 10 mg orally as a single dose has been used following gynecologic surgery with good results.

Prolonged retention in the absence of neurogenic bladder dysfunction when the restoration of normal voiding is desired implies surgical obstruction, especially after vaginal sling surgery. Time limits of 2 to 6 months have been suggested for normal voiding to reappear. Urodynamic confirmation of low flow with high voiding pressure may be helpful in making the diagnosis. Bladder instability may develop due to obstruction, or there may be urinary retention without evidence of voluntary contraction on cystometry. Urethrolysis may be required and will depend on the type of surgery causing the obstruction and the original pathology. After simple urethropexy, transvaginal release of adhesions of the urethra to the symphysis can be accomplished and simultaneous resuspension of more laterally located nonobstructing supports may be required. After needle suspension, one suspensory suture may be released and the results assessed before releasing the other. After sling surgery, the sling may be released on either side of the urethra at the point where it passes from under the urethra to just behind the inferior ramus of the pubis. More extensive dissection of the sling in the midline with division at the urethrovesical junction has been advocated, but this may increase the chances of urethral perforation, devascularization, and fistula. The fibrosis that has taken place following these original operations will usually prevent further hypermobility and may suffice to keep the urethra competent even when a sling is released.

Bladder Instability.—The emergence of this symptom following otherwise successful stress incontinence surgery is very distressing for both patient and physician. It cannot always be prevented. Its presence should be sought preoperatively and the patient counseled regarding anticipated results. New onset instability following repair may be due to various factors. A relative degree of obstruction may be present following repair. The bladder may be adjusting to a new volume after years of reduced capacity produced by incontinence. This may be especially true of the totally incontinent patient with small reduced capacity and compliance. It may take several months for the compliance characteristics of the bladder to adjust to new volumes. Surgical injury may be responsible for the symptoms: damage to perivesical or periurethral nerves during dissection or irritation or destruction by suture placement. The usual parasympatholytic medications should be offered: oxybutynin, flavoxate, imipramine. Adrenolytic agents such as prazosin can be offered as it has been shown that there may be an α-agonist contribution to the unstable and noncompliant bladder.

Progression of Associated Vaginal Prolapse.—If associated vaginal pathology is not repaired at the time of stress incontinence surgery, it may become worse afterward. The unrepaired prolapsing bladder neck absorbs and dissipates some of the intraabdominal pressure exerted during straining, preventing other structures from bearing the full force. If the bladder neck is immobilized by successful surgery, a greater amount of stress will be directed at the remaining structures. If there is already a mild enterocele, rectocele, or cystocele, these may become worse when intraabdominal pressure is more concentrated after bladder neck surgery. For this reason, associated vaginal prolapse should be corrected at the time of initial bladder neck resuspension.

Failure to Achieve the Desired Result.— Incontinence may persist or a new problem such as bladder instability, bladder dysfunction, or deterioration of previously mild vaginal prolapse may result. A certain amount of urgency is to be expected for 1 or 2 months following repair, but prolonged urgency or urge incontinence should raise the suspicion of obstruction or emergence of new bladder instability. Urodynamic examination with possible cystoscopy and radiographic imaging may be required. The patient may require antimuscarinic or antispasmodic medication. If obstruction can be identified, partial release of the repair or urethrolysis may be required. Persistent incontinence may be due to failure to recognize a deficient intrinsic sphincter mechanism preoperatively or distortion caused by the new repair. Persistent incontinence may also be due to an incorrectly performed repair, sutures which have pulled out of attenuated fascia, or infection which has destroyed the fascia where anchoring sutures have been placed.

SUMMARY

Most of these operations take place with few complications. Failure to achieve a satisfactory result is probably the most feared complication. Familiarity with the underlying pathology—hypermobility, bladder dysfunction, and urethral dysfunction—and the ability to select candidates for a suitable operation, based on the identified abnormality, is a most helpful preoperative consideration. It is also important to recognize the difference between suspension and urethral occlusion by sling during the operation. With greater experience will come improved insight and more predictable results.

EDITORIAL COMMENT

Dr. Mostwin has covered extensively the operations frequently utilized for incontinence in the female. Most of these operations are for hypermobility of the bladder. As pointed out, the objective is to obtain fixation of the bladder neck but not occlusion of the urethra. The urologist needs to be careful when performing these operations in patients in whom urgency and detrusor instability seem to be the primary problems. Correction of a cystocele, enterocele, or other anatomical abnormalities should be performed at the same time.

REFERENCES

1. Nichols DH (ed): *Clinical Problems, Injuries and Complications of Gynecologic Surgery,* ed 2. Baltimore, Williams & Wilkins Co, 1988.
2. Nichols DH, Randall CL: *Vaginal Surgery,* ed 3. Baltimore, Williams & Wilkins Co, 1989.
3. Raz S: *Female Urology,* Philadelphia, WB Saunders Co, 1985.
4. Goldstein, MS, Droller MJ: Complications of female urinary incontinence surgery, in Marshall FF (ed): *Urologic Complications.* Chicago, Year Book Medical Publishers, 1986, pp 257–266.

5. Schmidbauer CP, Hadley H, Staskin D, et al: Complications of vaginal surgery. *Semin Urol* 1986; 4:51.
6. Blaivas JG, Olsson CA: Stress incontinence: classification and surgical approach. *J Urol* 1988; 139:727.
7. Kelly HA, Burnham CF: *Disease of the Kidneys, Ureters and Bladder.* New York, D. Appleton & Co, 1922.
8. Resnick NM, Yalla SV, Laurino E: The pathophysiology of incontinence among institutionalized elderly persons. *N Engl J Med* 1989; 320:1.
9. Marshall VF: Editorial comment re:Hancock R, Brandstetter LH, Hodgins TE: Transpubic suspension of the bladder neck for urinary incontinence. *J Urol* 1980; 123:667.
10. Yang A, Mostwin JL, Radebaugh LC, et al: Dynamic evaluation of pelvic prolapse using fastscan magnetic resonance imaging (MRI) and cinematic display, comparison with cystometrogram. *J Urol* 1989; 141:200A.
11. Blaivas JG: Techniques of evaluation, in Yalla SV, McGuire EJ, Elbadawi A, et al (eds): *Neurology and Urodynamics: Principles and Practice.* New York, Macmillan, 1988, pp 155–198.
12. McGuire EJ: *Clinical Evaluation and Treatment of Neurogenic Vesical Dysfunction.* Baltimore, Williams & Wilkins Co, 1984.
13. McGuire EJ: Bladder instability and stress incontinence. *Neurourol Urodyn* 1989; 7:563.
14. McGuire EJ, Savastano JA: Stress incontinence and detrusor instability/urge incontinence. *Neurourol Urodyn* 1985; 4:313.
15. DeLancey JO: Structural aspects of urethrovesical function in the female. *Neurourol Urodyn* 1989; 7:509.
16. DeLancey JOL: Correlative study of paraurethral anatomy. *Obstet Gynecol* 1986; 68:91–97.
17. DeLancey JOL: Structural aspects of the extrinsic continence mechanism. *Obstet Gynecol* 1988; 72:296–301.
18. Klutke C, Golomb J, Mostwin JL, et al: The anatomy of stress incontinence. *J Urol* 1989; 141:200A.
19. Richardson AC, Lyon JB, Williams NL: A new look at pelvic relaxation. *Am J Obstet Gynecol* 1976; 126:565.
20. Zacharin RF: *Pelvic Floor Anatomy and the Surgery of Pulsion Enterocele.* New York, Springer-Verlag, 1985.
21. Siegel AL, Raz S: Surgical treatment of anatomical stress incontinence. *Neurourol Urodyn* 1988; 7:569.
22. Kelly HA: *Operative Gynecology,* vol 1. New York, Appleton, 1907.
23. Kelly HA, Dumm WM: Urinary incontinence, without manifest injury to the bladder. *Surg Gynecol Obstet* 1914; 18:444.
24. Marshall VF, Marchetti AA, Krantz KE: The correction of stress incontinence in the female by simple vesicourethral suspension. *Surg Gynecol Obstet* 1949; 88:509.
25. McGuire EJ: Abdominal procedures for stress incontinence. *Urol Clin North Am* 1985; 12:285.
26. Burch JC: Urethrovaginal fixation to Cooper's ligament for correction of stress incontinence, cystocele and prolapse. *Am J Obstet Gynecol* 1949; 81:281.
27. Richardson AC, Edmonds PB, Williams NL: Treatment of urinary incontinence due to paravaginal fascial defect. *Obstet Gynecol* 1981; 57:357.
28. Pereyra AJ: Simplified surgical procedure for the correction of stress incontinence in women. *West J Surg* 1959; 67:223.
29. Stamey TA: Endoscopic suspension of the vesical neck for urinary incontinence. *Surg Gynecol Obstet* 1973; 136:547.
30. Stamey TA: Endoscopic suspension of the vesical neck for urinary incontinence in females, report on 203 consecutive patients. *Ann Surg* 1980; 81:281.
31. Gittes RF, Loughlin KR: No-incision pubovaginal suspension for stress incontinence. *J Urol* 1987; 120:418.
32. Raz S: Modified bladder neck suspension for female stress incontinence. *Urology* 1984; 23:484.
33. Goebell R: Zur operativen Beseitigung der angeborenen Incontinentia vesicae. *Zentralbl Gynakol* 1910; 2:187.
34. Frangenheim C: *Zur operativen Behandlung der Inkontinenz männlichem Harnröhre.* 43rd Congress. *Verh Dtsch Ges Chir* 1949; 149.
35. Stoeckel W: Über die Verwendung der Musculi pyramidalis bei der operativen Behandlung der Incontinentia urinae. *Zentralbl Gynakol* 1917; 14:11.
36. Ridley JH: Appraisal of the Goebell-

Frangenheim-Stoeckel sling procedure. *Am J Obstet Gynecol* 1966; 95:714.
37. Aldridge A: Transplantation of fascia for relief of urinary stress incontinence. *Am J Obstet Gynecol* 1942; 44:398.
38. McGuire EJ, Bennett CJ, Konnak JA, et al: Experience with pubovaginal slings for urinary incontinence at the University of Michigan. *J Urol* 1987; 138:525–526.
39. Morgan JE: A sling procedure using Marlex polypropylene mesh for treatment of recurrent stress incontinence. *Am J Obstet Gynecol* 1970; 106:369.
40. Raz S, Siegel AL, Short JL, et al: Vaginal wall sling. *J Urol* 1989; 141:43.
41. Kaufman M, Lockhart JL, Silverstein MJ, et al: Transurethral polytetrafluoroethylene injection for post-prostatectomy urinary incontinence. *J Urol* 1984; 132:463.
42. Appel RA, Goodman JR, McGuire EJ, et al: Multicenter study of peri- and transurethral GAX-collagen injection for urinary incontinence. *J Urol* 1989; 141:359A.
43. Shortliffe LM, Freiha S, Kessler R, et al: Treatment of urinary incontinence by the periurethral implantation of glutaraldehyde cross-linked collagen. *J Urol* 1989; 141:538–541.
44. Boykin W, Rodriguez FR, Brizzolara JP, et al: Complete urinary obstruction following periurethral polytetrafluoroethylene injection for urinary incontinence. *J Urol* 1989; 141:1199–2000.
45. Horbach NS, Blanco JS, Ostergard DR, et al: A suburethral sling procedure with polytetrafluoroethylene for the treatment of genuine stress incontinence in patients with low urethral closure pressure. *Obstet Gynecol* 1988; 71:648–652.
46. Lockhart JL, Walker RD, Vorstman B, et al: Periurethral polytetrafluoroethylene injection following urethral reconstruction in female patients with urinary incontinence. *J Urol* 1988; 140:51–52.
47. Appel RA: Techniques and results with implantation of the artificial urinary sphincter in women with type III stress urinary incontinence by a vaginal approach. *Neurourol Urodyn* 1989; 7:613.
48. Light JK, Scott FB: Management of urinary incontinence in women with the artificial urinary sphincter. *J Urol* 1985; 134:476.
49. Fuchs EF, Forsyth MJ, Hatch TR: Artificial urinary sphincters: The Oregon Health Sciences University experience. *J Urol* 1989; 141:359A.
50. Tancer ML, Matseoane SL: Gynecological surgery in patients over 65. *Geriatrics* 1966; 21:189.
51. Lee D: Autologous blood transfusion. *Br J Haematol* 1988; 70:135.
52. Council on Scientific Affairs: Autologous blood transfusions. *JAMA* 1986; 256:2378.
53. Nissenkorn I, Servadio C, Lubin E: The treatment of osteitis pubis with heparin. *J Urol* 1981; 125:528.
54. Burns JR, Gregory JG: Osteomyelitis of the pubic symphysis after urologic surgery. *J Urol* 1977; 118:803.
55. Gilbert DN, Azorr M, Gore R, et al: The bacterial causation of postoperative osteitis pubis. *Surg Gynecol Obstet* 1975; 141:195.
56. Mynors JM: Osteitis pubis. *J Urol* 1973; 112:664.
57. Wegener M, Borsch G: Acute colonic pseudo-obstruction (Ogilvie's syndrome). Presentation of 14 of our own cases and analysis of 1,027 cases reported in the literature. *Surg Endosc* 1987; 1:169.
58. McVary KT, Dalton DP, Blum MD: Acute intestinal pseudo-obstruction (Ogilvie's syndrome) complicating radical retropubic prostatectomy. *J Urol* 1989; 141:1210.

CHAPTER 23

Complications in the Management of Erectile Dysfunction

Drogo K. Montague, M.D.

Today a variety of treatment options are available for the man suffering from erectile dysfunction. Sex therapy remains the treatment of choice for sexual problems of psychogenic origin; and some men can be helped by changing life style, altering medications, or treating endocrine disorders. For most men with erectile dysfunction owing to organic disorders, however, treatment options will include one of the following: penile prosthesis implantation, intracavernous pharmacotherapy, penile arterial revascularization, or penile venous ligation. The complications associated with these latter forms of management will be considered.

PENILE PROSTHESIS IMPLANTATION

General Considerations

Penile prosthesis implantation is indicated in the treatment of organic erectile dysfunction not reversible by other means. Alternatively, prosthesis implantation may be chosen by a man who has rejected another form of treatment such as intracavernous pharmacotherapy, penile arterial revascularization, or penile venous ligation. Psychogenic erectile dysfunction is best treated by sex therapy, marital therapy, or psychotherapy; however, penile prosthesis implantation may be considered in cases refractory to these usual treatment modalities provided that psychologic clearance is obtained.

Penile prosthesis implantation is usually performed under general, spinal, or epidural anesthesia; however, in selected cases it may be performed under local anesthesia.[1] The duration of the operation is generally 1 or 2 hours depending on the type of prosthesis selected. Surgical approaches commonly used for penile prosthesis implantation are shown in Table 23–1. Tissue removal is usually not necessary, and blood loss is minimal. Penile prosthesis implantation has been performed in selected cases on a outpatient basis; however, most implant recipients are admitted to the hospital and discharged on the first or second postoperative day.

There are more than a dozen different penile prostheses in common use today (Table 23–2). Nonhydraulic prostheses are all totally implantable within the corpora cavernosa. With the exception of the OmniPhase prosthesis, all of these devices impart a permanent degree of rigidity to the penis. Hydraulic prostheses after implantation are less detectable to pal-

TABLE 23–1.
Surgical Approaches for Penile Prosthesis Implantation

Dorsal subcoronal	Transverse scrotal
Dorsal penile shaft	Infrapubic
Ventral penile shaft	Suprapubic
Penoscrotal	Perineal

pation than a nonhydraulic device, and they allow varying degrees of control of erection and flaccidity. In general, mechanical failures with hydraulic devices are higher than with nonhydraulic devices, primarily because of fluid leaks. One-piece hydraulic prostheses are totally implantable within the corpora; two-piece hydraulic devices consist of paired cylinders connected to a scrotal pump-reservoir; and three-piece hydraulic implants consist of paired cylinders, a scrotal pump, and a retropubic reservoir.

Nonmechanical Complications

Sizing for penile prosthesis is done intraoperatively by careful intracorporal measurements. An error in sizing resulting in a prosthesis that is either too long or too short can cause postoperative difficulties. Nonhydraulic prostheses that are too long may, because of their constant rigidity, cause either persistent pain or prosthesis erosion. Hydraulic prostheses that are too long can also cause problems. The AMS Hydroflex prosthesis has a lateral channel which transfers fluid from a rear tip reservoir into a central chamber to provide rigidity. If the Hydroflex device is too long for the corpora, crimping of this channel occurs, and inflation and deflation of the prosthesis may be impaired. Two- and three-piece inflatable prosthesis cylinders that are too long create cylinder folds which may produce abnormal wear leading to early cylinder leakage.

Prostheses that are too short provide inadequate support for the glans penis. This deformity is named *SST* after the *s*upersonic *t*ransport aircraft's nose cone configuration for landing. Correction of an SST deformity is not difficult. The body reacts to silicone by forming a fibrous pseudocapsule around it.[2] A prosthesis may be easily removed by opening the original incision and then using the electrosurgical scalpel to reopen the corporotomies and the pseudocapsule down to the prosthesis; the electrosurgical scalpel will not harm the silicone. After the prosthesis is removed, long Metzenbaum

TABLE 23–2.
Penile Prostheses in Common Use Today*

Type	Name	Manufacturer
Nonhydraulic		
Semirigid	Small-Carrion	Mentor
Hinged	Flexi-Rod II	Surgitek
Malleable	AMS Malleable 600	AMS
	Jonas	Bard
	Mentor Malleable	Mentor
Positionable	DuraPhase	Dacomed
Mechanically activated	OmniPhase	Dacomed
Hydraulic		
One-piece	AMS Hydroflex	AMS
	Flexi-Flate	Surgitek
Two-piece	GFS	Mentor
	Uni-Flate 1000	Surgitek
Three-piece	AMS 700CX	AMS
	Mentor Inflatable	Mentor

*American Medical Systems.

scissors are inserted distally (toward the glans), and they are then used to perforate the distal end of the pseudocapsule. The scissors dissect through the distal corporal tissue which was not previously dilated. Through the glans penis the surgeon can palpate the tips of the scissors in the end of the corpus cavernosum; and following removal of the scissors, the distal corporal tissue is progressively dilated with Hegar dilators. New corporal measurements are made and an appropriately sized implant, usually 1 to 2 cm longer than the original implant, is inserted.

While the corpora cavernosa are being dilated during an implant procedure, perforation may occur and the dilating instrument may inadvertently enter the urethra. If this is recognized, the implant should be abandoned, and a urethral catheter should be left in for 7 days while the urethra is healing; repair of the urethra under these circumstances is not necessary. If perforation of the tunica albuginea occurs either distally or proximally, it is usually not necessary to abandon the implant if the remaining portion of the corpus cavernosum can be adequately dilated and the prosthesis can be inserted past the point of perforation. Healing of the perforation over the prosthetic implant then usually occurs.

Migration of a prosthesis into the perineum occurs when unrecognized perforation of the crus takes place during prosthesis implantation. This false passage into the perineum may be repaired at a later date by making a perineal incision, exposing and opening the crus, and then removing the prosthesis. The false passage is repaired from inside the crus, and the prosthesis is then replaced. Alternatively, a sock for the proximal end of the prosthesis may be fashioned from polytetrafluorethylene (Teflon)[3] or Dacron.[4] This sock, containing the proximal end of the implant, is then inserted into the corpus cavernosum, and the top of the sock is anchored with nonabsorbable sutures to the edge of the tunica albuginea at the corporotomy. This prevents migration of the prosthesis into the perineum.

Erosion of a prosthesis may occur outside the body or internally into an adjacent organ. There are multiple etiologies for erosion; unrecognized intraoperative perforation, an oversize prosthesis, and infection are the main causes. Erosion of prosthetic components has been reported into the bladder,[5, 6] ileal conduit,[7] rectum,[8] and peritoneal cavity.[9]

Since erosion is often either caused by infection or associated with secondary infection, the usual treatment has been removal of all prosthetic components with reimplantation at a later date. Furlow and Goldwasser have shown that a salvage procedure consisting of removal of the eroded component, replacement and repositioning of a new component, and closed drainage with antibiotic irrigation may be successful.[10]

Penile prosthesis implantation usually results in no permanent alteration in penile sensation. Patients experience discomfort for an average of 4 to 6 weeks, but this is quite variable. Pain persisting well beyond this time is usually the result of infection, a sensory neuropathy, or it may have a psychogenic basis. Permanent decrease in penile sensation after prosthesis implantation occurs rarely and is usually unexplainable.

Most implant recipients, provided they receive a properly sized prosthesis, will have adequate penile rigidity for coitus. However, different types of prostheses supply varying degrees of rigidity, and men with longer and larger-girth phalluses require more rigidity for adequate function. An experienced implanter can judge whether a prosthesis recipient's complaint of inadequate rigidity is reasonable and whether conversion to another prosthesis type will correct the complaint.

Different types of prostheses vary in the ease with which they are concealed, and this should be one of the factors considered when a patient and his urologist select a prosthesis preoperatively. After an implant many patients will change their underwear style to help conceal the penis; jockey-style underwear or occasionally an athletic supporter may be necessary.

If a penis containing a hydraulic prosthesis is tucked down into the underwear in the immediate postoperative period while the fibrous pseudocapsule is forming, a ventral chordee requiring surgical correction may result.[11, 12] For this reason all prostheses, especially hydraulic ones, should be kept up on the lower abdomen for 4 to 6 weeks during the healing process. Implantation of a prosthesis into a penis which already has chordee, owing to Peyronie's disease, for example, may by itself partially or fully correct the curvature. Prostheses vary in the degree to which they will help correct penile curvature; the malleable prostheses and the positionable DuraPhase prosthesis provide the best correction in this regard. If chordee correction is incomplete with prosthesis implantation alone, a corporoplasty will usually be necessary.[13]

If an implant recipient is uncircumcised, routine circumcision at the time of prosthesis implantation is not necessary unless the dorsal subcoronal approach is used in which case circumcision is desirable to avoid having a buried incision. However, if preoperative assessment reveals early phimosis, a circumcision at the time of prosthesis implantation should be done since the bulk of the implant may make foreskin retraction difficult postoperatively.

The incidence of urinary retention following penile prosthesis implantation is very low unless the implant recipient has been having voiding difficulties preoperatively. For this reason, in the patient with symptomatic prostatism, subtotal prostatectomy should be considered prior to penile prosthesis implantation.

The incidence of periprosthetic infections after penile prosthesis implantation varies from 0.7% to 16.7%, although most implant series have infection rates of 2% to 5%.[14] Most infections begin at the time of prosthesis implantation; however, seeding of the periprosthetic space with microorganisms from a distant source of infection can occur postoperatively.[15] For this reason these distant infections should be promptly treated, and prophylactic antibiotic usage prior to dental and surgical procedures should be considered.

To reduce the possibility of perioperative infection, the patient's urine should be sterile, and prophylactic antibiotics should be given preoperatively. Performing the implant inside a plastic barrier inflated with filtered air, (Surgical Isolation Bubble System, Lonestar Medical Products, Houston, Texas) may help to reduce the incidence of *Staphylococcus epidermidis* infection which is felt to result from airborne particles and is a frequent cause of prosthesis infection.[14–16]

Standard treatment for periprosthetic infection has been removal of all prosthetic material followed by reimplantation at a later date. An alternative form of management, the salvage procedure previously described, may be successful in some cases.[10]

Periprosthetic infection has replaced priapism as the leading cause of cavernosal fibrosis; other causes are listed in Table 23–3. Penile prosthesis implantation into fibrotic corpora can be very difficult,[17, 18] and attempts to dilate these corpora from a standard corporotomy often result in perforation. An alternative approach is to make extended corporotomies, resect the fibrotic cavernosal tissue, and then lay in the prosthesis. Primary

TABLE 23–3.
Causes of Cavernosal Fibrosis

Periprosthetic infection	Priapism
Peyronie's disease	Idiopathic
Intracavernous pharmacotherapy	

closure of the tunica albuginea is then usually possible; if tunical closure cannot be completed, a Dacron or Gore-Tex patch can be used to complete the closure.[19]

Rarely, penile periprosthetic infection may be associated with tissue loss.[20, 21] Other causes of tissue loss are injury to the dorsal penile arteries, compression dressings that are too tight, and Foley catheters. When ischemia is evident following prosthesis implantation, the implant should be removed; if catheter drainage is needed, a suprapubic tube should be inserted, and any associated infection should be treated. After tissue demarcation occurs, necrotic tissue is debrided and subsequent penile reconstruction may be necessary.

Spinal cord injury patients present special problems with respect to penile prosthesis implantation. Infection and extrusion rates may be as high as 16.5%.[22] Lack of genital sensation, associated urinary tract infections, and atrophy of the tunica albuginea all appear to be factors contributing to this high complication rate. Despite these complications and lack of any sensation, spinal cord injury patients and their partners can still benefit from prosthesis implantation; in addition to benefits with respect to sexual function, some of these patients will be able to more easily wear an external catheter because of the support a prosthesis supplies.

Mechanical Complications

Although rare, fractures of the Small-Carrion and Finney prostheses have been reported.[23] Breakage of the silver wire in the core of the Jonas prosthesis has occurred[24]; however, since the wire strands and the entire malleable core of this prosthesis have been coated with Teflon, no further breakage has been evident. Cable breakage in the OmniPhase device[25, 26] and separation of the Hydroflex prosthesis has also occurred.[27]

Spontaneous deflation of the Flexi-Flate prosthesis during coitus may occur.[28] Deflation of this device is normally accomplished by bending the prosthesis; this increases pressure inside the central rigidity chamber, and a pressure relief valve permits fluid to escape from the central chamber causing loss of rigidity. Spontaneous deflation occurs because similar pressure increases are sometimes reached during coitus.

Spontaneous inflation of three-piece hydraulic prostheses is included in this section because many mistakenly consider this to be a mechanical complication. In reality autoinflation of these devices occurs either because of an error in the implant technique or in postoperative care. Fluid pressure in the reservoirs of these devices is intended to be zero. If an adequate space is not created for the reservoir, or if the reservoir is overfilled, pressure in the reservoir will be higher than zero and autoinflation of the cylinders will occur. If the reservoir is correctly placed and filled, but the cylinders are left fully or partially inflated while healing takes place, the fibrous pseudocapsule that forms around the partially empty reservoir will impede subsequent attempts to fully deflate the cylinders. Deflation can still be accomplished by holding in the deflation valve and squeezing the cylinders; however, this forces fluid back into the reservoir under pressure and autoinflation will subsequently occur. This problem can be avoided by proper operative technique and postoperative care. If autoinflation does occur, correction involves lysis of the capsule surrounding the reservoir and refilling of the reservoir to zero pressure while the cylinders are deflated.

Prior to the advent of the AMS 700CX three-piece inflatable prosthesis (American Medical Systems), the previous AMS three-piece inflatable prosthesis had cylinders whose expansion depended on the elastic characteristics of the recipient's corpora. Because of this, cylinder aneurysms were a frequent complication. The triple-layer, controlled expansion (CX) cylinder, which is supplied with the AMS 700CX prosthesis, has eliminated this problem and has also decreased the rate of cylinder leaks.[29, 30] In this cylinder a woven, expandable fabric is sandwiched between two layers of silicone. This fabric controls cylinder expansion so that each cylinder has a diameter of 12 mm when deflated and a diameter of 18 mm when fully inflated.

Tubing kinks can occur in multiple-component inflatable prostheses, and these kinks can impair either inflation, deflation, or both processes. The recent development and use of kink-resistant tubing will, however, eliminate this complication in the future. Repair of a tubing kink is accomplished by using the electrosurgical scalpel to open the capsule around the tubing, thus releasing the kink. Then, to prevent a recurrent kink, excess tubing is removed and a tubing splice is made over an extra connector. In an area where a tubing kink is likely, the use of a right-angle connector rather than a straight one will decrease the probability of a kink developing.

Fluid loss from hydraulic prostheses is possible and because of this the mechanical failure rate in general is higher with these prostheses than it is with nonhydraulic devices. Within the category of hydraulic prostheses the likelihood of fluid loss is theoretically proportional to the number of components, although experience with the newer one- and two-piece hydraulic implants is relatively limited.

In the early period of inflatable penile prosthesis implantation, isotonic contrast was used as the filling medium so that x-ray could be used as part of trouble-shooting in the case of mechanical failure. Radiographic control proved, however, to be unnecessary and today normal saline is used almost universally as the filling agent. Silicone is semipermeable and the fluid used to fill a hydraulic device must be isotonic.

If fluid escapes from a hydraulic prosthesis, it is harmlessly absorbed by the body. In the case of a three-piece prosthesis, fluid loss will result in an empty reservoir with some fluid remaining in the pump and cylinders. When the pump is cycled, fluid in the pump will move into the cylinders; but because the reservoir is empty, the pump will not refill. Refill of the pump from the cylinders can be accomplished by depressing the deflation mechanism.

To revise a three-piece hydraulic prosthesis, the original implant incision should be opened, and the electrosurgical scalpel used to expose the tubing and all three connectors. The cautery will not damage the silicone. If the tubing and all three connectors appear intact, the connection between the reservoir and the pump is removed and a 50-mL syringe filled with normal saline is substituted for the reservoir. The pump is then cycled while the tubing leading to each cylinder is observed for evidence of fluid escaping around it; this would indicate a cylinder leak. If one of the cylinders has failed, both are routinely replaced. During this process, the cylinder compartments should be remeasured; occasionally a cylinder that is 1 cm longer will be needed.

If the cylinders are intact, the pump is removed from its compartment and carefully inspected while it is cycled. Pump leaks are rare but tubing leaks near the pump are not. Either of these occurrences requires pump replacement.

Next, the 50-mL syringe on the reservoir tubing is reversed so that it is leading to the reservoir. The reservoir is inflated under pressure to rupture the contracted capsule around it. All of the fluid injected into the reservoir is aspirated from it. This is repeated several times with fresh fluid to demonstrate that the reservoir is intact, to flush it, and to fully expand the reservoir so that it can hold at least 50 mL of normal saline under zero pressure. If a reservoir leak is found (they are rare), the reservoir is replaced.

There are two connector systems for the AMS 700CX prosthesis. Plastic tie-on connectors are supplied with the prosthesis, and an optional Quick Sutureless Connect System is available as well. The sutureless connectors can be used for a primary implant or for a revision in which all prosthetic material is replaced; however, this system cannot be used for other revisions because a lipid coating on implanted silicone tubing prevents a secure connection from being made.

INTRACAVERNOUS PHARMACOTHERAPY

Papaverine Hydrochloride and Phentolamine Mesylate

Since reports concerning intracavernous injection of papaverine by Virag in 1982[31] and phenoxybenzamine by Brindley in 1983,[32] intracorporal injection of vasoactive agents has become very popular for both the diagnosis and treatment of erectile dysfunction. Papaverine hydrochloride is a potent smooth muscle and vascular relaxant and may produce erection when injected intracavernously. However, anxiety-mediated sympathetic tone can maintain the corporal smooth muscle in a state of contraction, partially or fully blunting the effects of papaverine. The addition of the α-adrenergic blocking agent, phentolamine mesylate, to papaverine hydrochloride results in better erections than does the intracavernous injection of either of these agents alone.[33] Zorgniotti and Lafleur in 1985 reported their experience with the treatment of erectile dysfunction by intracorporal injection of papaverine and phentolamine,[34] and since that time this has been the most frequently used drug combination for intracavernous pharmacotherapy.

The direct injection of vasoactive drugs into the corpora cavernosa bypasses the nervous system control of erection, and thus intracavernous pharmacotherapy is ideal for men with erectile dysfunction owing to neurogenic causes.[35, 36] Many of these men respond to papaverine alone and require relatively small doses. Approximately 60% to 80% of men with erection difficulties of other diverse causes will also respond to papaverine, usually in higher doses and in combination with phentolamine.[37–39] This method of treatment, in conjunction with sex therapy, has also been used in men with psychogenic impotence.[38]

Complications of intracavernous pharmacotherapy are shown in Table 23–4. Since small needles are used (usually 26- to 30-gauge), the needle insertion causes very little pain. The injection of papaverine and phentolamine, however, has been reported to cause moderate to severe pain in 22% of patients in one series,[37] although most other investigators either do not mention pain as a complication or report a very low incidence of this side effect.[33–36, 38–42]

Prolonged erection, or priapism, has been found in 1.6% to 23% of patients.[33–42] This wide variability is due in part to differing doses of the drugs, varying definitions for prolonged erections, and diverse etiologies for the erectile dysfunction. To avoid priapism, the lowest effective dose of medication should be used. When injection is followed by sexual stimulation, a better erection is obtained, and one group has found that the test dose that produced a full erection in a medical setting could be reduced by a mean of 35% when self-injection at home was followed

TABLE 23–4.
Complications of Intracavernous Pharmacotherapy

Pain	Systemic effects
Priapism	Tachyphylaxis
Ecchymosis	Penile ulcers
Infection	Fibrosis

by sexual stimulation.[41] Priapism following intracavernous drug injection has been reversed in nearly every case by corporal aspiration alone or together with injection of an adrenergic agent.[43]

Penile ecchymosis is a common but minor complication and can be avoided by using a small needle, making the needle puncture through areas free of superficial veins, and applying pressure to the injection site for several minutes. Infection is a possible complication of any injection but has not yet been reported in patients undergoing intracavernous drug injection.

Systemic side effects (flushing, dizziness, nausea) occasionally occur[42] and are thought to result from entry of the drugs into the systemic circulation in patients with moderate to severe corporal-venous occlusive dysfunction. A decrease in the quality of erection over time in spite of an increase in the dose of injected drug (tachyphylaxis) has occasionally been reported.[37] Penile ulcers have been reported in two men after inadvertent subcutaneous injection of drug,[44] and we have seen one case of distal penile ulcer in a man who denied subcutaneous injection and who stated he had made all of his injections in the proximal shaft of the penis, well away from the site of subsequent ulcer formation. After temporary cessation of injection therapy, the ulcers healed, and all three men were able to resume injection therapy.

Anecdotal cases of penile fibrosis occurring in men on intracavernous injection therapy with papaverine and/or phentolamine have been reported.[45–48] In one series of 111 men on intracavernous pharmacotherapy with papaverine and phentolamine, fibrosis increased with length of time on therapy: 8% at 1 month, 17% at 3 months, 32% at 6 months, and 57% at 12 months.[49] In one patient in whom extensive fibrosis developed after papaverine-induced priapism where attempted reversal was delayed, the patient was able to successfully inject papaverine and phentolamine for a total of 70 injections over a period of 9 months without tachyphylaxis or further demonstrable fibrosis developing.[50] When papaverine was injected intracavernously in monkeys, fibrosis at the injection sites and smooth muscle hypertrophy elsewhere in the corpus cavernosum developed.[51] The fibrosis was attributed to trauma and inflammation from repeated injection and to the low pH (3.2) of papaverine.

Prostaglandin E_1

Prostaglandin E_1 occurs naturally in many tissues and is found in high concentrations in seminal vesicles and seminal plasma. Prostaglandin E_1 causes relaxation of smooth muscle and arterial vasodilation; thus its injection intracorporally might prove useful in the diagnosis and treatment of erectile dysfunction. Because this agent is rapidly cleared in a single passage through the lungs, systemic side effects should not be seen when it is injected intracorporally, even in men with corporal-venous occlusive dysfunction. Prostaglandin E_1 is probably metabolized in the corpus cavernosum; therefore, priapism following its intracavernous injection is not likely. Finally, this substance, which is found naturally in body tissues, has a neutral pH, and its continued injection intracavernously is not likely to cause fibrosis.

Early experience with the intracorporal injection of prostaglandin E_1 has been reported. Intracavernous injection of this agent is more effective in producing erections than papaverine alone[52] or papaverine plus phentolamine.[53] Prostaglandin E_1 was injected intracavernously for diagnostic purposes in 135 men; 62% obtained a full erection and 24% obtained a partial erection that was nevertheless judged adequate for coitus.[54] In another series of 210 men, 20 μg of prostaglandin E_1 were injected intracorporally for diagnostic purposes. A positive test, defined as a full erection produced without sexual stimulation and lasting 30 minutes, was obtained in 68.1%.[55]

Intracavernous prostaglandin E_1 has been used therapeutically in one series of 112 men.[55] Dosages varied from 5 to 40 μg. Frequency of coitus varied from once a month to four times weekly. The longest follow-up was 8 months with a mean of 4.5 months; the greatest total number of injections was 90 and the mean number of injections was 15. The only side effect was ecchymosis in 9.8% of patients. There were no systemic side effects, pain, prolonged erections, or fibrosis. Lue, however, in approximately 150 patients noted prolonged erections in two (0.02%) patients, mild pain in 25%, and severe pain in 4.7%. He did not observe any systemic reaction or fibrosis.[56] Preliminary experience with intracavernous prostaglandin E_1 suggests that it is at least as effective or more effective than intracavernous papaverine and phentolamine, and that it may be safer. More experience with this substance, however, is needed before we can be certain of these statements.

PENILE ARTERIAL REVASCULARIZATION

Penile arterial revascularization by a direct anastomosis of the inferior epigastric artery to the corpus cavernosum was described by Michal et al. in 1980[57]; however, most procedures done with this technique ultimately failed because of the development of fibrosis within the cavernous tissue just distal to the anastomosis. This procedure, later known as the Michal I operation, was replaced by the Michal II operation, which involved an anastomosis between the inferior epigastric artery and the dorsal penile artery.[57] McDougal and Jeffery reported successful coitus 1 year postoperatively in six of eight patients treated with the Michal II operation.[58] Anastomosis of the inferior epigastric artery to the central artery of the corpus cavernosum has also been described.[59] Virag described arterialization of the deep dorsal vein of the penis by anastomosis with the inferior epigastric artery or by saphenous vein interposition between the femoral artery and the deep dorsal vein.[60, 61] There are three modifications of each of these two operations, and they are known as the Virag 1 through Virag 6 procedures. Arterialization of the deep dorsal vein of the penis may be effective in some cases because it relieves impotence owing to corporal-venous occlusive dysfunction; however, Virag believes that it can also correct penile arterial insufficiency.

The efficacy of these various penile arterial revascularization procedures needs to be demonstrated by large-scale clinical trials with adequate postoperative controls and long-term follow-up. Complications of these procedures include corporal fibrosis, thrombosis of the donor or recipient vessel, priapism, and hypervascularity of the glans penis. When a bypass is performed between the femoral artery and a recipient vessel in the penis, lower extremity thrombotic and embolic complications can be added to this list.

PENILE VENOUS LIGATION

Men with erectile dysfunction owing to failure to store blood in the corpora cavernosa (corporal-venous occlusive dysfunction) may benefit from procedures designed to increase venous outflow resistance from the corpora cavernosa.[62–65] Candidates for these procedures should have corporal-venous occlusive dysfunction as defined by dynamic infusion cavernosometry[66] and confirmed by dynamic cavernosography.[66, 67] Furthermore, normal arterial status should be demonstrated by a procedure such as duplex ultrasonography.[68]

Penile venous ligation procedures vary from simple ligation and division of the deep dorsal vein at the base of the penis to the more extensive procedure developed by Lue.[69] In Lue's procedure, a unilateral inguinoscrotal incision is made and the distal corpora cavernosa and spongiosum are delivered by inversion of the penile skin. The hilum of the penis is exposed by taking down the suspensory ligament of the penis. The deep dorsal vein and its tributaries, the circumflex and emissary veins, are removed from the inferior pubic arch to a distal point about 2 cm from the edge of the glans penis. The fascia beneath the resected deep dorsal vein in the hilum of the penis is opened, and with the aid of optical magnification, the cavernous veins are suture-ligated. If dynamic cavernosography revealed leakage from the crural veins, the anterior surface of the crura can be plicated.

Complications of penile venous ligation surgery include edema, sensory disturbance, priapism, tissue loss, and penile shortening. As in the case of penile arterial revascularization, large clinical studies with adequate postoperative controls and long-term follow-up are needed before an accurate assessment can be made regarding the proper place for this operation in the treatment of erectile dysfunction.

EDITORIAL COMMENT

There are an increasing number of options in the treatment of the patient with erectile dysfunction. Presuming there is no psychologic component and after appropriate evaluation I have recommended that the management of the typical impotent patient start with a trial of a vacuum device. Second, intracorporal injections are often helpful if the vacuum device fails. Lastly, a prosthesis will generally work in almost all cases if other maneuvers fail. Difficulties in the management of the penile prosthesis are described in lucid detail by Dr. Montague in this chapter.

REFERENCES

1. Kaufman JJ: Penile prosthetic surgery under local anesthesia. *J Urol* 1982; 128:1190–1191.
2. Habal MB: The biological basis for the clinical application of the silicones. *Arch Surg* 1984; 119:843–848.
3. Mulcahy JJ: A technique of maintaining penile prosthesis position to prevent proximal migration. *J Urol* 1987; 137:294–296.
4. Fritzler M, Flores-Sandoval FN, Light JK: Dacron "sock" repair for proximal corporeal perforation. *Urology* 1986; 28:524–526.
5. Dupont MC, Hochman HI: Erosion of an inflatable penile prosthesis reservoir into the bladder, presenting as bladder calculi. *J Urol* 1988; 139:367–368.
6. Fitch WP, Roddy T: Erosion of inflatable penile prosthesis reservoir into bladder. *J Urol* 1986; 136:1080.
7. Godiwalla SY, Beres J, Jacobs SC: Erosion of an inflatable penile prosthesis reservoir into an ileal conduit. *J Urol* 1987; 137:297–298.
8. Montague DK: Penile prostheses, in Montague DK (ed): *Disorders of Male Sexual Function,* Chicago, Year Book Medical Publishers, 1988, pp 154–191.
9. Nelson RP: Small bowel obstruction secondary to migration of an inflatable penile prosthesis reservoir: recognition and prevention. *J Urol* 1988; 139:1053–1054.
10. Furlow WL, Goldwasser B: Salvage of the eroded inflatable penile prosthesis: a new concept. *J Urol* 1987; 138:312–314.
11. Baum N, Scott FB, Suarez G: Iatrogenic chordee following insertion of inflatable penile prosthesis. *Urology* 1988; 32:442–443.
12. Bertram RA, Carson CC, Altaffer LF: Severe penile curvature after implantation of an inflatable penile prosthesis. *J Urol* 1988; 139:743–745.
13. Mulcahy JJ, Rowland RG: Tunica wedge excision to correct penile curvature associated with the inflatable penile prosthesis. *J Urol* 1987; 138:63–64.
14. Montague DK: Periprosthetic infections. *J Urol* 1987; 138:68–69.
15. Carson CC, Robertson CN: Late hematogenous infection of penile prostheses. *J Urol* 1988; 139:50–52.
16. Persky L, Luria S, Porter A, et al: *Staphyl-*

coccus epidermidis in diabetic urological patient. *J Urol* 1986; 136:466–467.
17. Bertram RA, Carson CC, Webster GD: Implantation of penile prostheses in patients impotent after priapism. *Urology* 1985; 26:325–327.
18. Gasser TC, Larsen EH, Bruskewitz RG: Penile prosthesis reimplantation. *J Urol* 1987; 137:46–47.
19. Montague DK: Penile prosthesis implantation in patients with corporeal fibrosis, in McDougal WS (ed): *Difficult Problems in Urologic Surgery.* Chicago, Yearbook Medical Publishers, 1989, pp 321–333.
20. Bour J, Steinhardt G: Penile necrosis in patients with diabetes mellitus and end stage renal disease. *J Urol* 1984; 132:560–562.
21. McClellan DS, Masih BK: Gangrene of the penis as a complication of penile prosthesis. *J Urol* 1985; 133:862–863.
22. Rossier AB, Fam BA: Indication and results of semirigid penile prostheses in spinal cord injury patients: long-term followup. *J Urol* 1984; 131:59–62.
23. Agatstein AH, Farrer JH, Raz S: Fracture of semirigid penile prosthesis: a rare complication. *J Urol* 1986; 135:376–377.
24. Tawil EA, Gregory JG: Failure of the Jonas prosthesis. *J Urol* 1986; 135:702–703.
25. Huisman TK, MacIntyre RC: Mechanical failure of OmniPhase penile prosthesis. *Urol* 1988; 31:515–516.
26. Krane RJ: OmniPhase penile prosthesis. *Semin Urol* 1986; 4:247–251.
27. Goulding FJ: Fracture of Hydroflex penile implant. *Urol* 1987; 30:490–491.
28. Stanisic TH, Dean JC, Donovan JM, et al: Clinical experience with a self-contained inflatable penile implant: the Flexi-Flate. *J Urol* 1988; 139:947–950.
29. Furlow WL, Motley RC: The inflatable penile prosthesis: clinical experience with a new controlled expansion cylinder. *J Urol* 1988; 139:945–946.
30. Mulcahy JJ: Use of CX cylinders in association with AMS700 inflatable penile prosthesis. *J Urol* 1988; 140:1420–1421.
31. Virag R: Intracavernous injection of papaverine for erectile failure (letter). *Lancet* 1982; 2:938.
32. Brindley GS: Cavernosal alpha-blockage: a new technique for investigating and treating erectile impotence. *Br J Psychiatry* 1983; 143:332–338.
33. Stief CG, Wetterauer U: Erectile responses to intracavernous papaverine and phentolamine: comparison of single and combined delivery. *J Urol* 1988; 140:1415–1416.
34. Zorgniotti AW, Lafleur RS: Auto-injection of the corpus cavernosum with a vasoactive drug combination for vasculogenic impotence. *J Urol* 1985; 133:39–41.
35. Bodner DR, Lindan R, Leffler E, et al: The application of intracavernous injection of vasoactive medications for erection in men with spinal cord injury. *J Urol* 1987; 138:310–311.
36. Sidi AA, Cameron JS, Dykstra DD, et al: Vasoactive intracavernous pharmacotherapy for the treatment of erectile impotence in men with spinal cord injury. *J Urol* 1987; 138:539–542.
37. Girdlwy FM, Bruskewitz RC, Feyzi J, et al: Intracavernous self-injection for impotence: a long-term therapeutic option? Experience in 78 patients. *J Urol* 1988; 140:972–974.
38. Nellans RE, Ellis LR, Kramer-Lwvien D: Pharmacological erection: diagnosis and treatment applications in 69 patients. *J Urol* 1987; 138:52–54.
39. Sidi AA, Cameron JS, Duffy LM, et al: Intracavernous drug-induced erections in the management of male erectile dysfunction: experience with 100 patients. *J Urol* 1986; 135:704–706.
40. Gasser TC, Roach RM, Larsen EH, et al: Intracavernous self-injection with phentolamine and papaverine for the treatment of impotence. *J Urol* 1987; 137:678–680.
41. Stief CG, Gall H, Scherb W, et al: Midterm results of autoinjection therapy for erectile impotence. *Urology* 1988; 31:483–485.
42. Watters GR, Keogh EJ, Earle CM, et al: Experience in the management of erectile dysfunction using the intracavernosal self-injection of vasoactive drugs. *J Urol* 1988; 140:1417–1419.
43. Lue TF, Hellstrom WJG, McAninch JW, et al: Priapism: a refined approach to diagnosis and treatment. *J Urol* 1986; 136:104–108.
44. Borgstrom E: Penile ulcer as complication

in self-induced erections. *Urol* 1988; 32:416–417.
45. Corriere JN, Fishman, IJ, Benson GS, et al: Development of fibrotic penile lesions secondary to the intracorporeal injection of vasoactive agents. *J Urol* 1988; 140:615–617.
46. Fuchs, ME, Brawer MK: Papaverine-induced fibrosis of the corpus cavernosum. *J Urol* 1989; 141:125.
47. Hu KN, Burks C, Christy WC: Fibrosis of tunica albuginea: complication of long-term intracavernous pharmacological self-injection. *J Urol* 1987; 138:404–405.
48. Larsen EH, Gasser TC, Bruskewitz RC: Fibrosis of corpus cavernosum after intracavernous injection of phentolamine-papaverine. *J Urol* 1987; 137:292–293.
49. Levine SB, Althof SE, Turner LA, et al: Side effects of self-administration of intracavernous papaverine and phentolamine for the treatment of impotence. *J Urol* 1989; 141:54–57.
50. Lakin ML, Montague DK: Intracavernous injection therapy in post-priapism cavernosal fibrosis. *J Urol* 1988; 140:828–829.
51. Abozeid M, Juenemann KP, Luo JA, et al: Chronic papaverine treatment: the effect of repeated injections on the simian erectile response and penile tissue. *J Urol* 1987; 138:1263–1266.
52. Reiss H: Use of prostaglandin E_1 for papaverine-failed erections. *Urology* 1989; 33:15–16.
53. Waldhauser M, Schramek P: Efficiency and side effects of prostaglandin E_1 in the treatment of erectile dysfunction. *J Urol* 1988; 140:525–527.
54. Ishii N, Watanabe H, Irisawa C, et al: Intracavernous injection of prostaglandin E_1 for the treatment of erectile impotence. *J Urol* 1989; 141:323–325.
55. Stackl W, Hasun R, Marberger M: Intracavernous injection of prostaglandin E_1 in impotent men. *J Urol* 1988; 140:66–68.
56. Lue TF: Editorial comment. *J Urol* 1989; 141:325.
57. Michal V, Kramar R, Hejhal L: Revascularization procedures of the cavernous bodies, in Zorgniotti AW, Rossi G (eds): *Vasculogenic Impotence: Proceedings of the First International Conference on Corpus Cavernosum Revascularization.* Springfield, Ill, Charles C Thomas, 1980, pp 239–255.
58. McDougal WS, Jeffery RF: Microscopic penile revascularization. *J Urol* 1983; 129:517–521.
59. MacGregor RJ, Konnack JW: Treatment of vasculogenic erectile dysfunction by direct anastomosis of inferior epigastric artery to central artery to the corpus cavernosum. *J Urol* 1982; 127:136–139.
60. Virag R: Syndrome d'érection instable par insuffisance veineuse—diagnostic et correction chirugicale à propos de 10 cas. *J Mal Vasc* 1981; 6:121–124.
61. Virag R: Revascularization of the penis, in Bennett A (ed): *Management of Male Impotence.* Baltimore, Williams & Wilkins Co, 1982, pp 219–233.
62. Bar-Moshe O, Vandendris M: Treatment of impotence due to perineal venous leakage by ligation of crura penis. *J Urol* 1988; 139:1217–1219.
63. Bennett AH, Rivard DJ, Blanc RP, et al: Reconstructive surgery for vasculogenic impotence. *J Urol* 1986; 136:599–601.
64. Lewis RW, Puyau FA, Bell DP: Another approach for vasculogenic impotence. *J Urol* 1986; 136:1210–1212.
65. Wespes E, Schulman CC: Venous leakage: surgical treatment of a curable cause of impotence. *J Urol* 1985; 133:796–798.
66. Rajfer J, Rosciszewski A, Mehringer M: Prevalence of corporeal venous leakage in impotent men. *J Urol* 1988; 140:69–71.
67. Lue TF, Hricak H, Schmidt RA, et al: Functional evaluation of penile veins by cavernosography in papaverine-induced erection. *J Urol* 1986; 135:479–482.
68. Lue TF, Hricak H, Marich KW, et al: Vasculogenic impotence evaluated by high-resolution ultrasonography and pulsed Doppler spectrum analysis. *Radiology* 1985; 155:777–781.
69. Lue TF: Personal communication.

CHAPTER 24

Complications of Penile and Scrotal Surgery and Outpatient Urologic Procedures

Charles B. Brendler, M.D.
John P. Gearhart, M.D.

PENILE SURGERY

Adult Circumcision

Adult circumcision is not a difficult procedure, but it is one of great social and psychological importance to the patient. It should not be approached casually, and should not be relegated to an unsupervised junior member of the urologic housestaff. Unlike most adult urologic operations, the cosmetic result of this operation is extremely important, and a poorly performed circumcision will leave a patient unhappy, ungrateful, and perhaps litigious.

Adult circumcision usually is performed as an outpatient procedure under local anesthesia. Local anesthetic, usually 1% lidocaine (Xylocaine), is infiltrated into the skin and subcutaneous tissue circumferentially at the base of the penis. The bottle from which the anesthetic is drawn up should be checked by the surgeon to be sure that it does not contain epinephrine. I have seen a case of skin necrosis requiring subsequent grafting at the site where 1% lidocaine containing epinephrine was inadvertently injected into the base of the penis. One must be careful in injecting the anesthetic not to injure the neurovascular bundle in the midline of the dorsum of the penis. Furthermore, one should wait at least 5 to 10 minutes after injecting the anesthetic to be sure that a complete block has been obtained. Otherwise, the patient may experience considerable discomfort during the early part of the procedure, and this painful memory may linger for some time despite an otherwise well-performed circumcision.

There are several techniques of adult circumcision, but the sleeve resection (Fig 24–1) gives the best cosmetic result. Although circumcision can be performed by making dorsal and ventral preputial slits and connecting the two incisions, the cosmetic results with this technique generally are not as good as with sleeve resection. A Gomco clamp or Plastibell device should never be used in adult circumcision, since the blood vessels are too large to control reliably with pressure. Even though hemostasis may appear adequate during surgery, the patient is likely to bleed postoperatively and develop a disfiguring hematoma. Furthermore, a clamp tends to leave gaps in apposition between

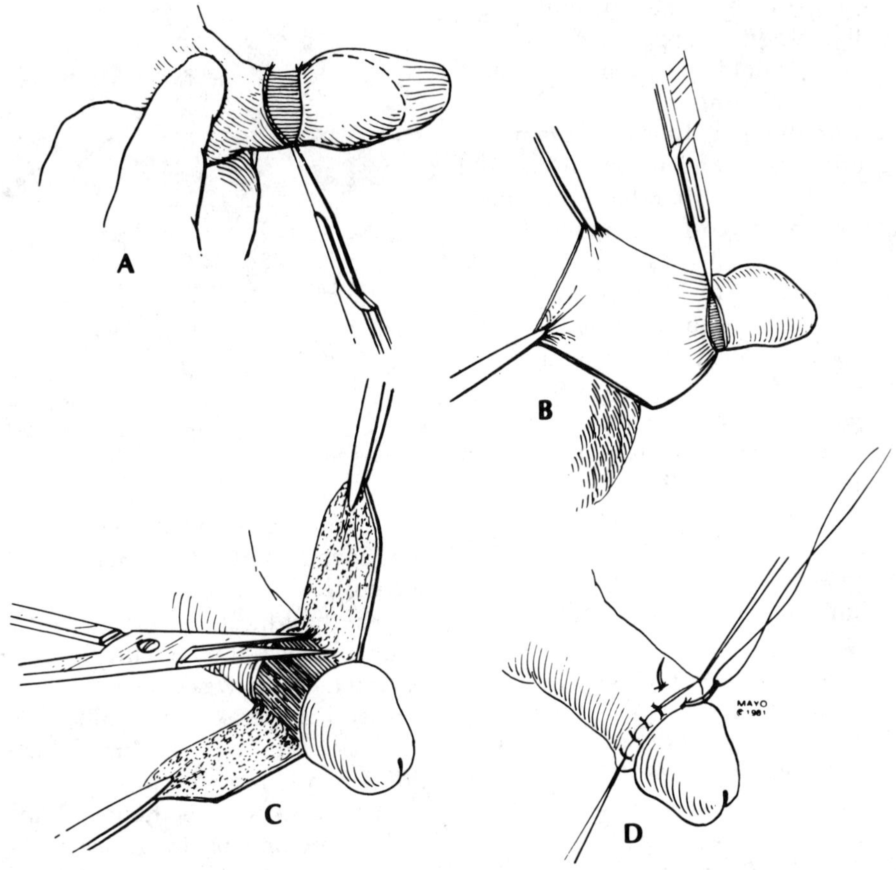

FIG 24–1.
Sleeve resection technique of circumcision. **A,** coronal junction on the skin is outlined and incised circumferentially. **B,** foreskin is retracted, and a circumferential incision is made in the mucosal skin just proximal to the coronal sulcus. **C,** sleeve of skin between the two incisions is excised. **D,** skin edges are reapproximated with interrupted absorbable sutures. (From Glenn JF (ed): *Urologic Surgery,* ed 3. JB Lippincott Co, 1983. Used by permission.)

the penile skin and the glans penis that subsequently give rise to adhesive epidermal inclusion cysts and balanoposthitis.[1]

Before beginning a circumcision, it is important to separate any adhesions between the preputial skin and the glans penis to avoid subsequent cautery or amputation injury to the glans. Following this, the proposed incision lines should be drawn on the penis with a marking pencil, noting the V of the frenulum. In planning the incision, the penis should not be stretched tautly to avoid removing too much skin.

During circumcision it is sometimes helpful to place a tourniquet around the base of the penis to control bleeding. Following skin removal, the tourniquet should be removed and every bleeding vessel controlled either with ligatures or with diathermy. The penile skin should be peeled back to look for vessels that may be hidden beneath the retracted skin edge. Hemostasis must be complete because penile skin, like scrotal skin, is very elastic, and cannot be relied on to tamponade bleeding vessels. Vessels may constrict temporarily following transection only to bleed later, and thus should be searched for meticulously.

One must be extremely careful in applying diathermy to the penis. A low-voltage current should be applied in short bursts, remembering that the current must exit through the base of the penis. A strong prolonged current may injure the dorsal neurovascular bundle with subsequent penile necrosis. Larger vessels should be controlled with fine absorbable suture. It may be worthwhile to place a saline-soaked sponge around the base of a smaller penis to help dissipate the current.[2]

Fine absorbable interrupted sutures should be used to reapproximate the skin edges following circumcision. Continuous sutures are faster, but they tend to gather the skin, giving a less satisfactory cosmetic appearance. Petroleum jelly gauze and a light pressure dressing are applied at the conclusion of the procedure. The patient is kept in the clinic for 1 hour following circumcision at which time he is examined for any bleeding. He is then discharged home with instructions not to undertake any strenuous activity for 48 hours and not to have sexual intercourse for at least 2 weeks. Spontaneous erections following circumcision may be painful and associated with recurrent bleeding, and these can be controlled by inhalation of amyl nitrite pulvules.

Paraphimosis occurs when the preputial skin becomes trapped behind the glans penis causing venous engorgement and edema of the glans. In this situation, one should first attempt to reduce the prepuce manually. This is best done by pulling the penis taut and squeezing the glans penis between the thumb and forefinger to decrease the engorgement. The thumbs are then placed on the glans penis and the preputial skin is drawn back over the glans (Fig 24–2). If manual reduction is not possible, a dorsal slit should be performed, making sure that the incision goes through the entire ring of preputial tissue in order to relieve the constriction (Fig 24–3). A formal circumcision should be done at a later date when the edema and inflammation have resolved.

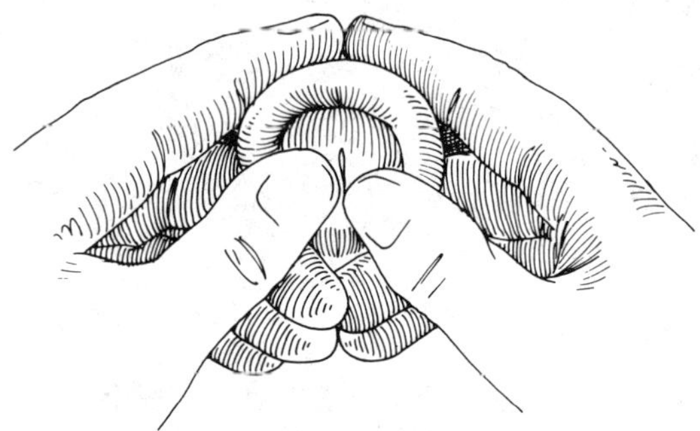

FIG 24–2.
Reduction of paraphimosis by firm compression against the glans penis. (From Glenn JF (ed): *Urologic Surgery*, ed 3. JB Lippincott Co, 1983. Used by permission.)

Urethral meatal stenosis may develop in uncircumcised men with chronic balanoposthitis. It is wise to calibrate the urethra and to perform a simultaneous urethral meatotomy at the time of circumcision when indicated.[3]

If excess skin is removed inadvertently at the time of circumcision, there are several options. If the defect is small, it should be left alone, as it will usually granulate without complications. Larger

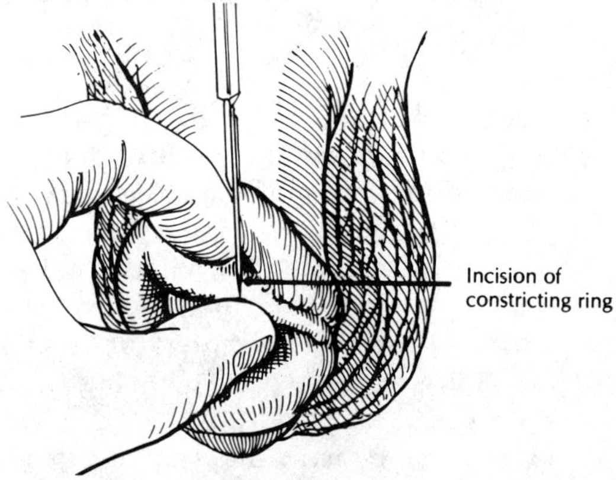

FIG 24–3.
Reduction of paraphimosis by incision of the constricting preputial ring. (From Glenn JF (ed): *Urologic Surgery*, ed 3. JB Lippincott Co, 1983. Used by permission.)

defects should be treated either by application of an immediate or delayed split-thickness skin graft.[4]

Pediatric Circumcision

The majority of pediatric circumcisions are performed using the Gomco clamp or Plastibell device. Although both are simple to use, certain basic guidelines must be followed. First, the prepuce must be completely dissected from the glans penis; a preliminary dorsal slit may aid in this dissection. Second, one must use a device of proper size; a clamp that is too small may impair penile circulation or result in injury to the glans penis, while a device that is too large may result in loss of excessive penile skin. Third, the clamp should be left in place long enough to assure adequate hemostasis and proper coaptation of the skin edges. Finally, standard electrocautery should not be used for hemostasis or to remove excess penile skin.

Any congenital anomaly involving the urethra or penile shaft should delay circumcision until a urologic evaluation has been performed. Unfortunately, we too often see infants with various degrees of hypospadias who have already undergone circumcision. These occurrences should encourage urologists to educate their fellow physicians, who perform the majority of newborn circumcisions, about the more subtle anomalies of the genitalia and their recognition. There are also hematologic contraindications to circumcision, such as Factor VIII deficiency and von Willebrand's disease. Certainly, any other major illness such as prematurity, myelomeningocele, or imperforate anus should delay circumcision.

The incidence of complications associated with pediatric circumcision ranges from 1.5% to 5.0%. These complications can be classified as (1) hemorrhagic, (2) infectious, (3) cutaneous, (4) glandular, (5) penile shaft, (6) urethral, and (7) urinary retention.

1. Hemorrhage following circumcision can occur with either of the circumcision devices, but occurs more commonly with the Gomco clamp which places total dependence for hemostasis on the crushing effect of the clamp on the wound edges.[5] Bleeding following circumcision usually stops in response to topical pressure, but occasionally a few sutures are required. Other topical measures to control postcircumcision bleeding have included the use of thrombin, absorbable gelatin sponge (Gelfoam), silver nitrate, and epinephrine. Silver nitrate should be applied carefully to avoid chemical injury. Epinephrine should be used in the same concentration as in hypospadias surgery (e.g., 1:100,000) to prevent local ischemia or systemic effects. Persistent bleeding after neonatal circumcision may be the first indication of a bleeding diathesis.

2. Most infections following circumcision are mild and easily treated with topical measures, such as wet to dry dressings and simple sitz baths. In one series, infections occurred more commonly in patients circumcised with the Plastibell device (0.72%) than with the Gomco clamp (0.14%), perhaps because of remaining devitalized tissue or because of delayed separation of the bell from the penis.[5]

3. Of all cutaneous complications, removal of excessive penile skin can be the most bothersome. If the skin loss is partial, the involved area can be allowed to epithelialize spontaneously. Larger defects are best treated with skin grafting because there is usually no loss of penile length or secondary chordee that may occur with delayed primary healing. The practice of burying the penis in the scrotum to provide skin coverage is to be condemned. Healing by secondary intention, or even by delayed skin grafting, will have cosmetic results superior to the use of scrotal skin for coverage.

The buried or concealed penis usually results from removing excessive shaft skin and leaving an excess of inner preputial epithelium. The circular wound heals and forces the penis into a submerged position beneath the pubic skin (Fig 24–4). Treatment depends on the amount of shaft skin that has been removed. Kaplan recommends a circumferential incision at the preputial ring, so that the excess inner preputial epithelium may be used in the repair.[6] This approach may obviate the need for skin grafts to provide coverage of the penile shaft.

If insufficient skin is removed, there can be contraction of the remaining preputial opening and secondary phimosis. This may cause urinary obstruction and associated acute urinary retention. If there is no contraction of the preputial opening, only a redundant foreskin will be present. This complication can usually be managed with proper hygiene, although some parents will forcefully demand recircumcision.

Another common cutaneous complication is the formation of skin bridges after circumcision. These can cause tethering of the penis, entrapment of smegma, or curvature of the penis and pain upon erection. The bridges can be small and require only simple surgical incision (Fig 24–5) or be complex and require more extensive revision. These bridges most likely originate from inadequate separation of the inner preputial epithelium from the glans at the time of circumcision.

Almost all of the above cutaneous complications can be avoided by complete dissection of the prepuce from the glans penis and enlargement of the phimotic orifice in order to keep anatomical landmarks such as the coronal sulcus in perspective. Also, by marking the skin incision at the coronal level, one can ensure excision of penile skin that will be adequate but conservative.

4. Glandular necrosis usually results from a constrictive bandage after circumcision or from the constrictive effect of an improperly sized Plastibell device.[7] Necrosis can also result from the use of epinephrine-containing solutions or from electrocautery making contact with a metal clamp. In addition to glandular necrosis, accidental laceration or amputation

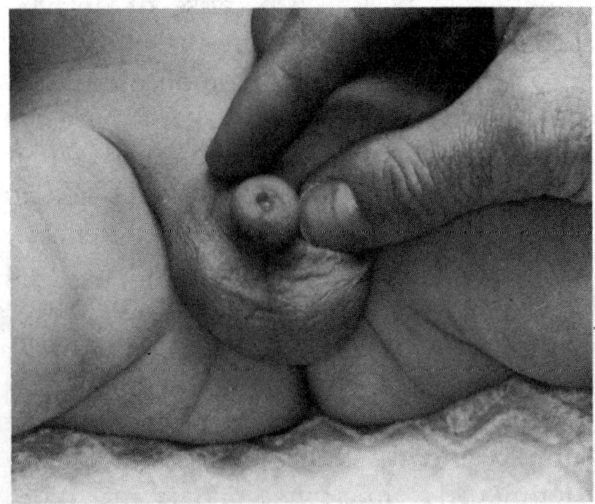

FIG 24–4.
"Concealed" penis after newborn circumcision.

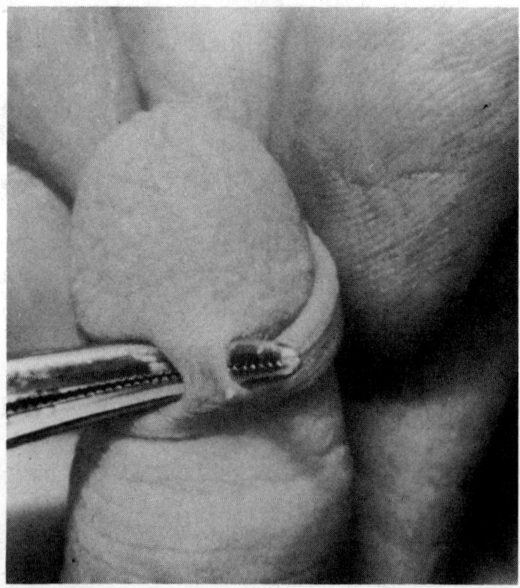

FIG 24–5.
Simple skin bridge 1 year postcircumcision. (Courtesy of Roy Witherington, M.D.)

of the glans penis during circumcision may occur from the circumcision knife. This occurs more commonly when the operator is using a blind technique, and can be prevented by proper separation of the inner surface of the prepuce from the glans and by keeping the meatus under careful scrutiny.

5. Penile shaft necrosis is usually associated with cautery-related injuries. Penile reconstruction following such injuries may be possible, but when the entire penis has been lost, changing the sex of rearing may be advisable. Additional complications involving the penile shaft include chordee and lymphedema. Chordee of the penis is usually due to dense scarring on the ventrum of the penis secondary to penile inflammation at the time of circumcision. Penile lymphedema can occur secondary to wound infection or separation and may require extensive skin and subcutaneous tissue excision prior to skin grafting to ensure a satisfactory result.

6. Urethral injury may result from laceration with the circumcision device or by careless suture placement in attempting to control bleeding. The risk of urethral injury can be minimized by using a Gomco clamp or Plastibell device of proper size and by never placing sutures blindly on the ventrum of the penis. Urethral meatitis and ulceration develop frequently following neonatal circumcision because the protective prepuce has been removed and the meatus is completely exposed to ammoniacal residues in the diapers. Meatitis and ulceration occurring in the first year of life may result in subsequent meatal stenosis.

7. Urinary retention after circumcision usually results from faulty dressing technique. Voiding usually occurs spontaneously after the dressing is removed, but improper dressing can also cause infections, glandular necrosis, and urethral fistula. If a dressing is used at all, it should be applied loosely and checked carefully after application.

Priapism

The most common complication of priapism is impotence, and this is usually a complication of the disease itself rather than of the treatment. Forty percent of men will be impotent at 1 year following treatment for priapism, but virtually 100% of men with untreated priapism will be impotent.[8] Nevertheless, it is important to explain the risk of impotence to both the patient and his family and to obtain a carefully documented consent form prior to undertaking any surgical procedure for priapism.

Most conservative measures of treating priapism such as hypotensive drugs, spinal anesthesia, and ice water enemas are ineffective and simply delay effective surgical treatment. Except for cases of priapism due to sickle cell disease which can be managed by exchange transfusion, priapism should be considered a surgical emergency. Delaying appropriate therapy increases the risk of corporal fibrosis and impotence.

Older surgical procedures for priapism involve creation of a vascular shunt between the corpus cavernosum and either the saphenous vein[9] or the corpus spongiosum.[10] Although effective, complications of corporal shunts include corporal fibrosis, shunt thrombosis requiring repeat surgery, infection, impotence, urethral fistula, and venous embolism. These formal shunting procedures have been replaced by simpler techniques that create fistulas between the corpus spongiosum of the glans penis and the distal corpora cavernosa (Fig 24–6). These techniques appear equally effective, easier to perform, and are associated with a lower risk of complications.[11, 12]

A constrictive dressing and intermittent pressure using a sphygmomanometer

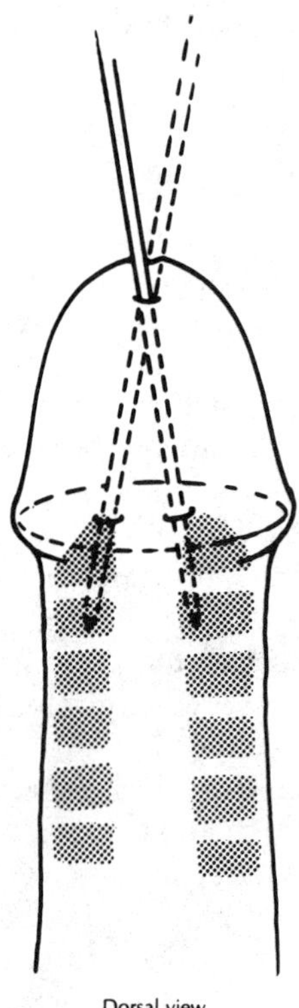

FIG 24–6.
Treatment of priapism by fenestrating the glans penis and corpora cavernosa with a biopsy needle. (From Glenn JF (ed): *Urologic Surgery*, ed 3. JB Lippincott Co, 1983. Used by permission.)

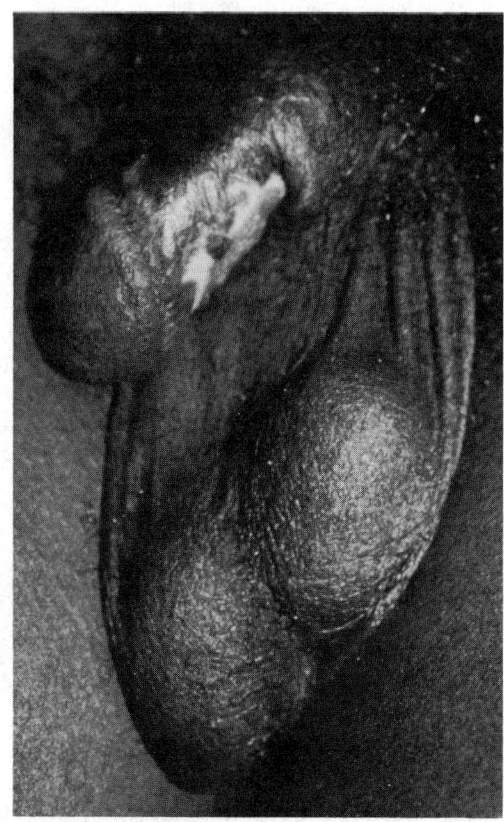

FIG 24–7.
Penile necrosis in a patient with priapism in whom constrictive dressing was applied.

are frequently applied to the penis following treatment of priapism to prevent retumescence. Excess pressure can result in significant vascular ischemia and penile necrosis (Fig 24–7). It may be preferable to tape the penis to the perineum to prevent retumescence and to avoid the use of pressure dressings altogether.

Peyronie's Disease

As with priapism, considerations regarding potency are very important in the treatment of Peyronie's disease. Most men with this condition are potent, and surgical correction is ill-advised unless the degree of penile curvature prevents adequate sexual functioning. Although surgical procedures to correct curvature (other than placement of a penile prosthesis) should not affect potency, patients should be informed of this possibility and a carefully documented informed consent obtained prior to surgery. Since Peyronie's disease frequently improves spontaneously or responds to conservative treatment with agents such as vitamin E or aminobenzoate potassium, surgery should be postponed for at least 18 months after the diagnosis is established.

Surgical options for treatment of Peyronie's disease include (1) excision of the plaque and placement of a dermal graft[13]; (2) removal of ellipses of tissue from the uninvolved corpus to straighten the penis (Nesbit procedure)[14]; and (3) placement of a penile prosthesis.[15] Although Horton and Devine have reported good results with dermal grafting, the experience of others has not been as favorable, and the procedure has not been widely adopted. When considering a Nesbit procedure the patient must be aware that by removing tissue from the normal corpus to achieve straightening, the penis will be shortened somewhat. A risk of both the dermal graft and the Nesbit procedure is injury to the dorsal neurovascular bundle which must be carefully isolated and preserved. Before inserting a penile prosthesis in a potent man with Peyronie's disease the patient must understand that he will most likely be impotent should the prosthesis subsequently have to be removed.

Penile Cancer

Partial Penectomy.—Hemorrhage is a potential concern in partial penectomy, and blood loss can be reduced greatly by applying a tourniquet or noncrushing intestinal clamp across the base of the penis prior to amputation. Following amputation, the corpora cavernosa are plicated with absorbable sutures to control bleeding prior to removal of the tourniquet or clamp.[2]

Prior to performing a partial penectomy, the tumor should be covered with a rubber glove to prevent tumor spillage. The penis should be amputated 2 to 3 cm proximal to the visible tumor margin, and the resected specimen should be sent to pathology for frozen section examination to be sure that the surgical margin is clear of tumor.[16] With this consideration in mind, one should attempt to leave as much of the penis as possible to allow the patient normal urination and sexual function. If the penile stump is inadequate for these purposes, it is preferable to transpose the urethra beneath the scrotum and to create a perineal urethrostomy. It is better to have the patient void in a sitting position than to have him drip urine over his scrotum with resultant chronic inflammation and excoriation.

The most common long-term complication of partial penectomy is urethral meatal stenosis. This can be avoided by incising the penile skin in an elliptic manner making the ventral skin edge slightly longer than the dorsal edge. The urethra and corpus spongiosum are amputated 1 cm distal to the corpora cavernosa. The urethra and corpus spongiosum are spatulated, and the ventral skin flap is then sewn to the spatulation. This creates a long elliptic suture line the opening of which terminates on the stump of the penis, thus greatly reducing the chance of subsequent stenosis (Fig 24–8).

Total Penectomy.—Hemorrhage can be considerable with total penectomy, and it is advisable to have at least 3 units of blood available. Controlled hypotensive anesthesia has been reported to greatly reduce blood loss.[2]

As with partial penectomy, the tumor should be covered with a rubber glove prior to surgery to avoid tumor spillage. Since these tumors are often necrotic and infected, administration of broad-spectrum antibiotics perioperatively is advisable. A combination of a cephalosporin and metronidazole provides effective prophylaxis against perineal flora.[2]

Penile Trauma

Skin Avulsion.—Degloving injuries of the penis usually result from industrial accidents in which the skin of the penis is caught in machinery. Skin avulsions should be grafted immediately. It is inadvisable to graft the avulsed penile skin since this may give rise to secondary infection and necrosis with delayed wound healing. It is preferable to obtain a split-thickness skin graft from another site, usually the inner thigh.[17] In cases of partial proximal skin avulsion where distal skin remains, it is best to remove the distal skin and to apply a split-thickness

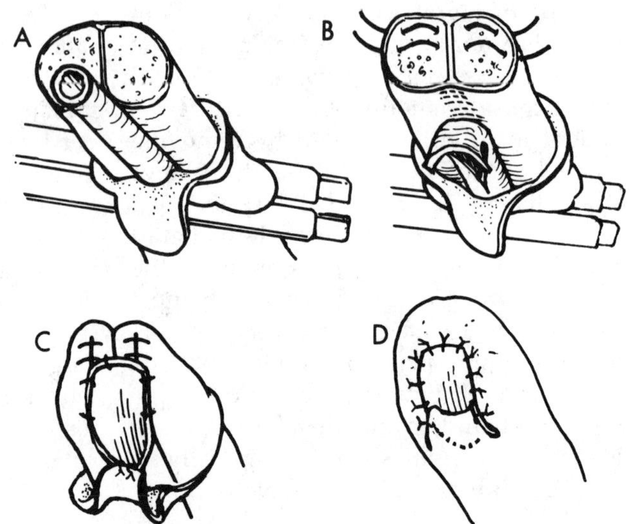

FIG 24–8.
Technique of partial penectomy. **A,** urethra is amputated 1 cm distal to where the corpora cavernosa are amputated. **B,** corpora cavernosa are plicated with 0 chromic catgut sutures. **C,** urethra is spatulated and sewn over the united corpora cavernosa. **D,** a U-shaped skin flap is used to make an elliptic anastomosis between the skin and urethra to prevent a subsequent stricture. (From Blandy JP (ed): *Operative Urology.* Oxford, Blackwell Scientific Publications, 1978. Used by permission.)

skin graft to the entire penile shaft. This is because the lymphatic drainage of the distal skin has been disrupted, and if one simply applies a skin graft proximally, the distal skin will become chronically edematous yielding a poor cosmetic result.[3]

Penile Amputation.—Penile amputation resulting from industrial accidents often cannot be repaired since the nerves and blood vessels of the corporal bodies are frequently shredded. In these situations it is probably best to reconstruct the penis using a composite graft in combination with placement of a penile prosthesis and a urethroplasty. In situations where the penis has been amputated sharply it is worthwhile to attempt penile replantation using microsurgical techniques.[18] Replantation should be attempted even if the time delay following injury is deemed excessive since there remains a slight chance for a successful result, and one loses nothing by trying. The amputated portion of the penis should be suspended in a bag of cool saline and stored on ice. The penis itself should not be placed on ice to prevent frostbite. Microsurgical technique is essential for a successful result. The blood vessels should be handled as little as possible and should not be perfused to avoid injuring smaller vessels.

The major complication of penile replantation is subsequent skin and soft tissue necrosis. Early debridement of the penile shaft is advisable since this allows earlier skin grafting. An eschar on the glans penis, however, should be left alone and not grafted since it will subsequently slough and heal spontaneously. If the deeper tissues become necrotic, one must resort to penile amputation with subsequent reconstruction using a vascularized tube graft.[19]

Penile Fractures.—A penile fracture is a rupture of the tunica albuginea of the corpus cavernosum that usually occurs during sexual activity. Penile fractures are associated with considerable bleeding and distortion of the penis. The hematoma should be drained and the corporal defect repaired as soon as possible. Conservative management with bed rest and an ice pack may give rise to a flail penis that is markedly deformed with erection. Such a deformity can be corrected by excising the weakened area of the tunica and either reapproximating the edges of the tunica or by placing a graft of either dermis or artificial material such as Dacron.[20]

SCROTAL SURGERY

General Considerations

Since the scrotum is a loose elastic sac that provides little protective tamponade, hemorrhage is a potential risk with all scrotal operations. Because the scrotum is extremely distensible, the amount of bleeding can be considerable and quite alarming to the patient expecting a rather minor operation. Significant bleeding can lead to pain, infection, and prolonged postoperative recuperation. It is thus important that all urologists be aware of general guidelines to reduce the risk of perioperative scrotal hemorrhage.

Since most of the blood vessels in the scrotum course transversely, horizontal incisions are associated with less bleeding than vertical incisions. Vascular cross-connections are numerous, however, and meticulous hemostasis is essential when incising the scrotal wall. All bleeding points should be cauterized. When closing the scrotum, it is important to incorporate both the underlying dartos muscle and the skin. This can be done in two separate layers or as a single layer using continuous absorbable suture. Simple closure of the skin alone is inadequate to prevent postoperative hemorrhage.[21]

Following scrotal surgery, it is advisable to elevate and compress the scrotum for 24 to 48 hours postoperatively to minimize edema and postoperative bleeding. This can be accomplished in several ways. The usual scrotal supporter is rather flimsy and provides very little compression. An athletic supporter housing both the penis and the scrotum is better, and a hole can be cut for the penis to allow urination with the supporter in place. Compressive dressings, which are taped to the abdomen and buttocks, are very effective but they are difficult to apply and uncomfortable for the patient when removed. A most effective means of compressing and elevating the scrotum is to suture the scrotum to the abdomen over a gauze roll (Fig 24–9).[22]

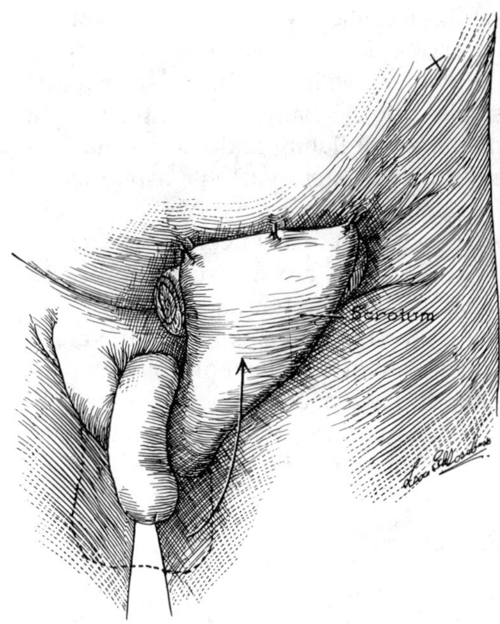

FIG 24–9.
Technique of scrotal compression by suturing the scrotum to the lower abdomen over a gauze roll.

The use of drains following scrotal surgery is controversial. Most postoperative bleeding occurs within the wall of the scrotum rather than the scrotal cavity, and therefore a drain may have little value. In addition, a drain may introduce perineal bacteria into the wound. A drain may be useful, however, during the first 24 to 48 hours to evacuate whatever blood collects in the scrotal cavity, and the risk of infection is minimal as long as the drain is removed after this time.

The management of postoperative scrotal hemorrhage requires careful observation and individualization. Since most bleeding occurs within the wall of the scrotum, reexploration is seldom necessary or helpful and may increase the risk of subsequent infection. Although the scrotum may appear markedly discolored and swollen, it is best not to reexplore unless there is an expanding hematoma. It is wiser to keep the patient at bed rest with scrotal elevation and an ice pack and to observe him for several hours. Usually the swelling will either decrease or remain stable. Occasionally, an untreated hematoma will liquify and can be managed several days later by needle aspiration.[21]

Since the scrotum is well vascularized, postoperative infection is unusual. Most infections are superficial and can be treated with simple drainage and cleansing soaks. Deep infections usually are associated with a hematoma and may require incision and drainage. If a large hematoma becomes infected, formal surgical debridement may be necessary.

Vasectomy

Vasectomy usually is performed as an outpatient procedure under local anesthesia, and, for this reason, the procedure may be initially somewhat difficult to master. One common problem is isolating the vas deferens from adjacent scrotal tissues. A towel clip is sometimes used for this purpose, but we have found it easier and less traumatic to isolate the vas between the thumb and middle finger and to deflect the testicle caudad with the index finger to put the vas on tension (Fig 24–10). Local anesthetic is then injected into the overlying skin and directly into the vas, the incision is made, and the vas isolated with an Allis clamp while still keeping the left hand in the same position so as not to lose the vas.

Since it takes about 10 ejaculations to remove all sperm from the male genital tract that are stored beyond where the vasa have been divided, patients are instructed to continue contraception for several weeks following vasectomy. At this time all patients should bring a semen sample to the clinic for examination. If the sample is azospermic, patients can discontinue contraception at that time. If sperm are still present, patients are instructed to continue contraception and to bring another sample 2 weeks later.

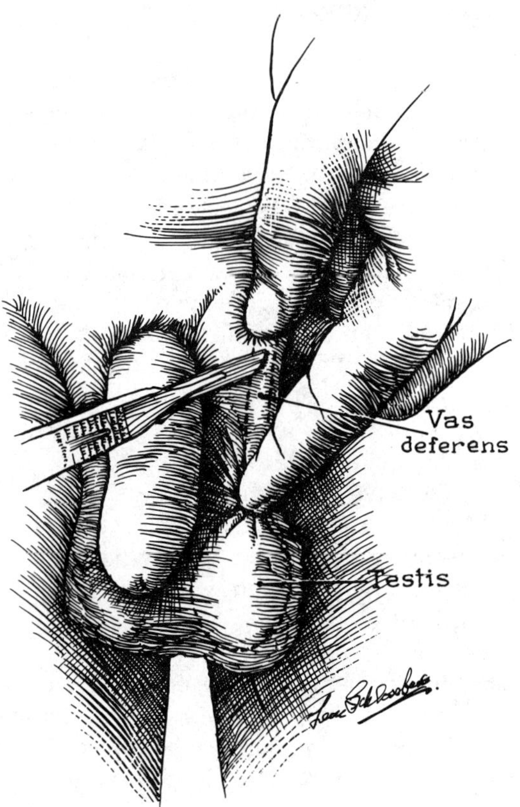

FIG 24–10.
Technique of isolating the vas deferens for vasectomy. The vas is compressed between the thumb and middle finger while keeping the testicle on stretch with the index finger.

Recanalization of the vas deferens occurs in 0% to 6% of patients.[23] The risk of recanalization can be reduced by removing a segment of the vas rather than simply ligating it, turning the ends of the vasa back on themselves, and by burying the two ends of the vas in different fascial layers. If a vasectomy must be repeated, it is best to choose a new operative site in the scrotum to avoid the fibrosis associated with the original operation.

Clinically detectable sperm granulomas occur in about 15% of patients following vasectomy and result from extravasation of seminal fluid into the perivasal tissues.[24] The incidence of sperm granulomas can be reduced by using hemoclips rather than ligatures to occlude the vasa and by lightly fulgurating the lumen of the vas with electrocautery. One should avoid excessive fulguration since this may cause necrosis of the ligated segment of the vas with subsequent sloughing of the ligature or hemoclip and possible recanalization. Most sperm granulomas cause only mild discomfort and usually resolve spontaneously. Occasionally it may be necessary to excise a persistent painful granuloma. Symptomatic granulomas associated with the epididymis may necessitate epididymectomy. After excising a granuloma, it is important to reocclude the vas completely.[21]

Nonspecific epididymitis following vasectomy usually results from epididymal engorgement. This should be treated with an anti-inflammatory agent and usually resolves rapidly. Antibiotics are unnecessary.

Sperm may escape into the circulation following vasectomy, causing formation of sperm antibodies. Although these antibodies may subsequently impair fertility following vasovasostomy, no other definite complications have been identified.[25]

Varicocelectomy

The major perioperative complication of varicocele ligation is accidental injury to the spermatic artery or to the vas deferens. The risk of injuring these structures is less if one makes the incision above the internal inguinal ring and isolates the spermatic vein in the retroperitoneum. The inguinal approach to the spermatic vein, however, may be simpler, particularly in obese or muscular patients, and modifications in the inguinal approach have reduced the risk of injury to adjacent cord structures.[26] First, the patient is positioned in a 20-degree reversed Trendelenburg position in order to distend the spermatic veins. Secondly, since the spermatic vein lies on the anterior surface of the cord, it is neither necessary nor desirable to mobilize the entire spermatic cord. If one simply dissects the branches of the vein back to where they merge near the internal inguinal ring and then ligates and divides them, there should be no risk of injuring either the spermatic artery or the vas deferens which lie posteriorly (Fig 24–11).

Epididymectomy

The major risk of epididymectomy is injury to the spermatic blood vessels. These vessels enter the testicle toward the upper pole, about two-thirds of the way up from the lower pole. The risk of vascular injury can be decreased by starting the epididymal dissection at the lower pole of

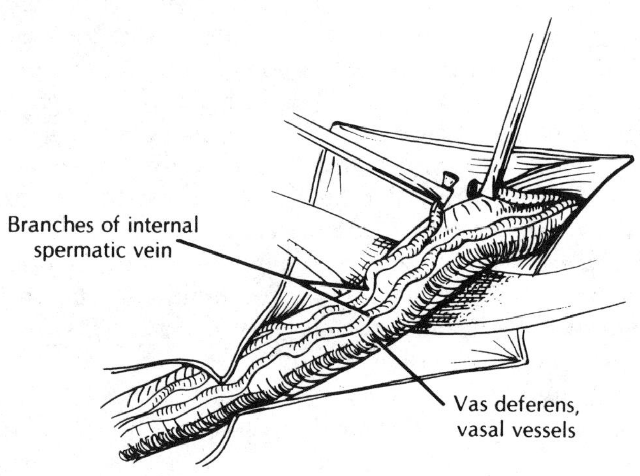

FIG 24–11.
Technique of varicocele repair. The branches of the internal spermatic vein, which lie on the anterior aspect of the spermatic cord, are ligated and divided. The internal spermatic artery and vas deferens, which lie posteriorly, are not dissected. (From Glenn JF (ed): *Urologic Surgery*, ed 3. JB Lippincott Co, 1983. Used by permission.)

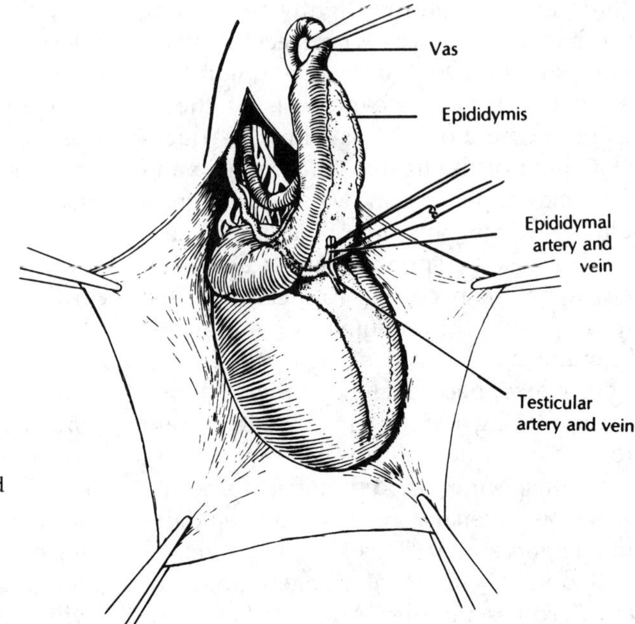

FIG 24–12.
Technique of epididymectomy. The epididymis is separated from the internal spermatic vessels. Vascular branches to the epididymis are ligated and divided carefully to preserve the testicular blood supply. (From Glenn JF (ed): *Urologic Surgery*, ed 3. JB Lippincott Co, 1983. Used by permission.)

the testicle. As the spermatic vessels are approached, the epididymal branches become obvious and can be ligated and divided, thus separating the epididymis from the vessels and allowing completion of the epididymectomy (Fig 24–12). Should the spermatic vessels be injured inadvertently, the testicle should be observed for several minutes prior to performing an orchiectomy since the testicle may survive from collateral vessels, mainly those associated with the vas deferens.

Hydrocelectomy

Most urologists find needle aspiration of a hydrocele an unsatisfactory means of treating this condition because the fluid frequently reaccumulates following aspiration. In addition, there is a risk of introducing infection within the tunica vaginalis and a risk of significant hemorrhage if the needle accidentally injures the testicle or spermatic vessels. Needle aspiration probably should be reserved for symptomatic patients who are not surgical candidates because of other health considerations.

There are several surgical techniques to correct a hydrocele. The simplest is the Lord procedure in which the hydrocele sac is opened and drained, and the redundant sac is simply plicated with absorbable sutures.[27] This technique has been reported to have fewer complications than other techniques which involve excision of the redundant sac.[28] The Lord procedure is most appropriate for thin-walled, flaccid hydroceles; it is less advisable in thick-walled, inflammatory hydroceles in which the sac should be excised. Other surgical options include formal excision of the hydrocele sac with surgical plication of the sac edges. Alternatively, one may simply open the hydrocele sac and invert it behind the spermatic cord to prevent reaccumulation of fluid, the so-called bottle technique. One should avoid wrapping the sac too tightly around the spermatic cord to prevent testicular ischemia. Following hydrocelectomy, there is usually considerable seepage of fluid into the scrotal cavity. Therefore, it is best to leave a drain brought out through a separate stab incision in the base of the scrotum for 24 to 48 hours.

Orchiectomy

The major risk of orchiectomy is hemorrhage. The spermatic vessels and vas deferens should be divided separately, and the spermatic vessels should be doubly ligated. We use a 0 chromic free ligature followed by a 2-0 chromic suture ligature. Since orchiectomy renders the scrotum empty and even more mobile, it is very easy to suture the scrotum onto the abdomen over a gauze roll following the procedure, and this provides excellent scrotal compression and elevation.

A rapidly expanding hematoma following orchiectomy signifies hemorrhage from the spermatic cord. In this situation, it is inadvisable to reopen the scrotum, as the spermatic vessels will have retracted and may be very difficult to identify and control. Rather, it is preferable to make an inguinal incision on the side of the bleeding and to interrupt the spermatic vessels in the inguinal canal.

Testicular Torsion

The most frequent complication of torsion of the spermatic cord is testicular infarction resulting from misdiagnosis. All too often, appropriate treatment is delayed because the condition is incorrectly diagnosed as epididymitis. While the two conditions may be difficult to distinguish, it should be remembered that epididymitis is uncommon in pubertal males, the time at which the incidence of testicular torsion is highest. Whenever the diagnosis is uncertain, patients should be explored immediately, since the interval between the onset of torsion and irreversible testicular necrosis is only several hours. A guiding rule is that it is far better to operate for epididymitis than to fail to operate for torsion.

A frequent concern at the time of exploration for torsion is whether or not to leave a testicle that is marginally viable. After reducing the torsion, the testicle should be wrapped in warm, moist sponges to see if it regains a normal pink color. Further information may be gained by gently incising the tunica albuginea of the testicle. The absence of arterial bleeding and liquefaction of the seminiferous tubules signifies advanced necrosis. Other signs that may be helpful include the presence of scrotal edema and bloody fluid within the tunica vaginalis, again signifying a more advanced ischemic process.[29] If there is any doubt as to the viability of the testis, it should be left behind since it may recover, and the risk of sepsis and abscess formation from leaving a nonviable testicle behind is small.

When performing an orchidopexy for torsion of the spermatic cord, the testicle should be fixed to the scrotum with at least two sutures, one at the inferior pole and one on the lateral margin, to prevent recurrent torsion. We prefer to use absorbable sutures to reduce the risk of infection; the testicle is adherent to the scrotal wall by the time the sutures dissolve.

If an orchiectomy is deemed necessary at the time of surgical exploration, placement of a testicular prosthesis should be delayed for several weeks until the wound has healed to reduce the risk of infection. A testicular prosthesis should be inserted through an inguinal incision to reduce the risk of infection and subsequent extrusion of the prosthesis.

Testicular Biopsy

Testicular biopsy can be performed safely under local anesthesia in an office setting. The incidence of pain and bleeding can be reduced by holding the testis firmly against the scrotal wall and injecting 1% lidocaine into the scrotal skin, making sure not to penetrate the tunica albuginea. An incision is then made down to the testicle and local anesthetic is applied topically on the tunica albuginea. The biopsy site is selected carefully to avoid injuring the epididymis and spermatic cord. More recently a biopsy "gun" has been utilized by some urologists.

Trauma

Scrotal Trauma.—As with penile injuries, most scrotal trauma results from the scrotum being trapped in machinery and avulsed. Unlike the penis, however, scrotal injuries seldom require subsequent skin grafting. The scrotum is extremely vascular and elastic and will regenerate completely in 6 to 8 weeks if only 20% of the scrotum is left intact.[21] Therefore, scrotal injuries are best treated initially by debridement of necrotic tissue and primary closure. If there is insufficient skin remaining after the injury, the testicles can be buried in subcutaneous pockets in the medial aspect of the thighs. The testicles should be placed above the subcutaneous fat to maintain an appropriate temperature for spermatogenesis.[30] Antibiotics are advisable even with blunt scrotal trauma because of the risk of anaerobic infections.

Testicular Trauma.—Testicular injuries should be repaired immediately since exploration yields a better chance to preserve both spermatogenic and endocrine functions. The testicle should be explored, devitalized tissue excised, and the tunica albuginea closed with absorbable suture. It is advisable to drain the scrotum for 24 to 48 hours to evacuate any hematoma. If an orchiectomy is required, it is best to delay subsequent placement of a testicular prosthesis for several weeks until complete healing has taken place and then to implant the prosthesis through a separate inguinal incision as discussed previously. If one or both testicles have been amputated traumatically, it is possible to perform testicular replantation using microsurgical techniques.[31]

OUTPATIENT UROLOGIC PROCEDURES

Cystourethroscopy

It is possible to perform cystourethroscopy in virtually all adult female and most adult males as an outpatient procedure without general or regional anesthesia. However, the urologist must explain the procedure carefully beforehand to alleviate the patient's anxiety. After cleansing the genitalia, a gel lubricant containing topical anesthetic is instilled into the urethra and left in place for at least 10 minutes prior to introducing the cystoscope. In the male, the lubricant is instilled gently into the urethra with a syringe. A soft clamp is then placed transversely on the coronal sulcus of the penis to occlude the urethra and to prevent the lubricant from escaping. In the female, the lubricant is applied to a cotton-tipped applicator which is then inserted into the urethra and left in place for 10 minutes.

The cystoscope should always be advanced gently without force to avoid injuring the urethra with resultant hemorrhage and secondary infection. In the female it is usually easier to advance the cystoscope blindly into the bladder with the obturator in place. In the male, however, it is usually easier and less traumatic to advance the cystoscope under direct vision through the urethra into the bladder. The most difficult step in male cystourethroscopy is negotiating the prostatic urethra as this is the area which is most uncomfortable for the patient. It is helpful to reassure the patient as the prostatic urethra is approached and to have him inhale and exhale deeply to help relax the pelvic floor musculature. It is sometimes recommended that patients attempt to void as the cystoscope is advanced through the prostatic urethra, but in practice this is very difficult to do. It is better to defer formal examination of the prostatic urethra until after the bladder has been examined to allow the patient to adjust to the cystoscope.

Prophylactic antibiotics are not recommended routinely prior to cystourethroscopy, but are advisable in patients whose urine is infected. A single preoperative dose of either a third-generation cephalosporin or one of the new semisynthetic penicillins appears as effective as the standard 24- to 48-hour prophylactic regimens previously recommended.[32] Patients with a history of rheumatic heart disease or patients who have prosthetic devices such as a heart valve or artificial hip should probably receive another dose of antibiotics several hours after the procedure.

Retrograde Pyelography

It is usually possible to catheterize the ureteral orifice for retrograde pyelography without using a cystoscopic bridge with an Alberran deflector. If the deflector is needed to position the ureteral catheter in the orifice, one must remember not to move the cystoscope back across the bladder neck with the deflector turned downward as this may cause significant trauma to and bleeding from the bladder neck.

When performing retrograde pyelography one should instill only 5 to 8 mL of contrast to avoid overdistention of the renal pelvis with subsequent forniceal rupture, extravasation of contrast, and flank pain. Similarly, one should never forcibly inject contrast above a point of ureteral obstruction because of the risk of subsequent sepsis. It is better to pass a whistle-tip catheter above the obstruction to ensure that appropriate drainage has been established prior to injecting contrast.

Prostatic Needle Biopsy

Prostatic needle biopsy can be accomplished safely as an outpatient procedure under local anesthesia using the perineal approach. Once again, preoperative patient reassurance along with proper local anesthetic technique will greatly reduce both anxiety and discomfort. The overlying perineal skin and soft tissues are infiltrated with 1% to 2% lidocaine using a 22-gauge spinal needle, and the anesthetic is left in place for at least 10 minutes prior to performing the biopsy. Prophylactic antibiotics are unnecessary unless the rectum is perforated with the needle. Urinary retention requiring catheter placement following prostatic biopsy is unusual. Hematuria and hematospermia occur commonly following prostatic biopsy, but usually resolve within several days and require no subsequent treatment.[33]

Transrectal needle biopsy of the prostate is associated with a significant risk of sepsis, and probably is best performed as an inpatient procedure using preoperative cleansing enemas and prophylactic antibiotics.[34] Transrectal needle aspiration of the prostate, on the other hand, can be accomplished safely with minimal morbidity as an outpatient procedure with local anesthetic and without prophylactic antibiotics.[35]

EDITORIAL COMMENT I

The authors have covered many of the most commonly performed procedures in urology. Litigation probably occurs most often following circumcision and vasectomy, since patients never expect any complications. A few other comments are listed.

There are many medical treatments for Peyronie's disease. The multiple treatments probably reflect little more than the natural history of the disease. I have sometimes injected these plaques with steroids (triamcinalone), based on previous experience with softening of keloid scars with steroid injection. If all fails, a penile prosthesis will usually rectify the problem.

In penile trauma, debridement of tissue can be less aggressive in many instances because the erectile tissue provides some vascularity for the penis as well. Secondly, sperm granuloma following vasectomy occurs more often microscopically than the 15% cited in the chapter.* Epididymectomy should not be undertaken lightly as removal of the entire epididymis will probably result in testicular atrophy even if there is no vascular impairment of the testis itself. We have studied a rat model (ACI rat) with congenital absence of the epididymis, and the testis atrophies at puberty.†

The authors have accurately addressed the complications of pediatric circumcision. In this country there are no definite indications for pediatric circumcision. A urologist in a lifetime of performing circumcisions may prevent a single case of penile cancer. The hairless preputial skin is valuable for urethral and genital reconstructions. The psychological, social, religious, and cosmetic considerations for circumcision would appear to be less significant than many of the described complications.

EDITORIAL COMMENT II

This chapter represents a combination of two earlier chapters. Increasingly, procedures are performed in an outpatient setting in an effort to reduce rising medical costs, and it has become clear that lesser procedures can be performed under local anesthesia on this basis. Although not described in this chapter, lesser hypospadias procedures and orchidopexy in the pediatric population are often performed on outpatients.

*Taxy JB, Marshall FF, Erlichman RJ: Vasectomy: Subclinical pathological changes. *Am J Surg Pathol* 1981; 5:767.

†Marshall FF, Ewing LL, Zirkin BR, et al: Testicular atrophy associated with agenesis of the epididymis in the ACI rat. *J Urol* 1982; 127:155.

REFERENCES

1. Klauber GT, Boyle J: Preputial skin-bridging. Complication of circumcision. *Urology* 1974; 3:722.
2. Blandy JP: *Operative Urology,* ed 2. Oxford, Blackwell Scientific Publications, 1986.
3. Peters PC: Complications of penile surgery, in Smith RB, Skinner DG (eds): *Complications of Urologic Surgery.* Philadelphia, WB Saunders Co, 1976, pp 408–421.
4. Klauber GT, Sant GR: Disorders of the male external genitalia, in Kelalis PP, King LR, Belman AB (eds): *Clinical Pediatric Urology,* ed 2. Philadelphia, WB Saunders Co, 1985, pp 825–863.
5. Gee WF, Ansell JS: Neonatal circumcision: A ten year overview with comparison of the Gomco clamp and the Plastibell device. *Pediatrics* 1976; 58:204.
6. Kaplan GW: Circumcision: An overview. *Curr Probl Pediatr* 1977; 7:1.
7. Sterenberg N, Golan J, Ben-Hur N: Necrosis of glans penis following neonatal circumcision. *Plast Reconstr Surg* 1981; 68:237.
8. Winter CC: Priapism, in Glenn JF (ed): *Urologic Surgery,* ed 3. Philadelphia, JB Lippincott Co, 1983, pp 803–811.
9. Grayhack JT, McCullough W, O'Conor VJ Jr, et al: Venous bypass to control priapism. *Invest Urol* 1964; 1:509.
10. Quackels R: Cure of a patient suffering from priapism by cavernospongiosa anastomosis. *Acta Urol Belg* 1964; 32:5.
11. Winter CC: Cure of idiopathic priapism. A new procedure for creating fistula between glans penis and corpora cavernosa. *Urology* 1976; 8:389.
12. Ebbehoj J: A new operation for priapism. *Scand J Plast Reconstr Surg* 1975; 8:241.
13. Devine CJ Jr, Horton CE: Surgical treatment of Peyronie's disease with a dermal graft. *J Urol* 1974; 111:44.

14. Goldstein M, Laungani G, Abrahams J, et al: Correction of adult penile curvature with a Nesbit operation. *J Urol* 1984; 131:56.
15. Raz S, deKernion JB, Kaufman JJ: Surgical treatment of Peyronie's disease: A new approach. *J Urol* 1977; 117:598.
16. Fraley EE: Penectomy and ilioinguinal lymphadenectomy, in Glenn, JF (ed): *Urologic Surgery,* ed 3. Philadelphia, JB Lippincott Co, 1983, pp 825–830.
17. Culp DA: Penoscrotal trauma, in Glenn JF (ed): *Urologic Surgery,* ed 3. Philadelphia, JB Lippincott Co, 1983, pp 813–820.
18. Heymann AD, Bell-Thompson J, Rathod DM, et al: Successful reimplantation of the penis using microvascular techniques. *J Urol* 1977; 118:879.
19. O'Brien DP III: Penile replantation, in Glenn JF (ed): *Urologic Surgery,* ed 3. Philadelphia, JB Lippincott Co, 1983, pp 821–824.
20. Nymark J, Kristensen JK: Fracture of the penis with urethal rupture. *J Urol* 1983; 129:147.
21. Dale GA: Complications of scrotal surgery, in Smith RB, Skinner DG (eds): *Complications of Urologic Surgery,* Philadelphia, WB Saunders Co, 1976, pp 395–407.
22. Orecklin J, Dale GA: A simplified form of scrotal compression dressing. Presented at meeting of American Urological Association, Western Section, 1973.
23. Hackett RE, Waterhouse K: Vasectomy—reviewed. *Am J Obstet Gynecol* 1973; 116:438.
24. Schmidt SS, Morris RR: Spermatic granuloma: The complication of vasectomy. *Fertil Steril* 1973; 24:941.
25. Fowler JE Jr, Mariano M: Immunoglobulin in seminal fluid of fertile, infertile, vasectomy and vasectomy reversal patients. *J Urol* 1983; 129:869.
26. Dubin L, Amelar RD: 986 cases of varicocelectomy: a 12 year study. *Urology* 1977; 10:446.
27. Lord PH: A bloodless operation for the radical cure of idiopathic hydrocele. *Br J Surg* 1964; 51:914.
28. Kaye K, Clayman RV, Lange PH: Outpatient hydrocele and spermatocele repair under local anesthesia. *J Urol* 1983; 130:269.
29. Harrison RH III: Testicular torsion, in Glenn JF (ed): *Urologic Surgery,* ed 3. Philadelphia, JB Lippincott Co, 1983, pp 1067–1076.
30. Culp DA, Huffman WC: Temperature determination in the thigh with regard to burying the traumatically exposed testis. *J Urol* 1956; 76:436.
31. Wacksman J, Dinner M, Straffon R: Technique of testicular autotransplantation using microvascular anastomosis. *Surg Gynecol Obstet* 1980; 150:399.
32. Childs SJ: Genitourinary surgical prophylaxis. *Infect Surg* 1983; pp 701–710.
33. Packer MG, Russo P, Fair WR: Prophylactic antibiotics and Foley catheter usage in transperineal needle biopsy of the prostate. *J Urol* 1984; 131:687.
34. Rees M, Ashby EC, Pocock RD, et al: Povidone-iodine antisepsis for transrectal prostatic biopsy. *Br Med J* 1980; 281:650.
35. Willems JS, Lowhagen T: Transrectal fine-needle aspiration biopsy for cytologic diagnosis and grading of prostatic carcinoma. *Prostate* 1981; 2:381.

CHAPTER 25

Complications of Lymph Node Dissection

John P. Donohue, M.D.

DEFINITIONS

For practical purposes, we will divide complications into major complications and minor ones. A major complication results in enough morbidity to require significant additional treatments and at least 2 more days of hospitalization. A minor complication requires little if any additional treatments and does not result in extension of hospitalization beyond 2 days. These are my own pragmatic definitions, based on the practical consequences of a complication. Complications can also be viewed in time frames, namely, acute and chronic. An acute complication develops within the immediate postoperative period, usually within the first couple of weeks, and its resolution is effected within an equally short time span. A chronic complication is one that will develop late, even after discharge, and it persists for many weeks or months or permanently. On the basis of these definitions then, we will proceed to several general observations.

GENERAL OBSERVATIONS

Avoidance is, of course, the key in any discussion of complications. The following chapter will include some technical points that may prove useful in reducing the number of complications. An important second point is the prompt recognition of complications. Finally, we must have the willingness, resolve, and ability to handle them in a forthright, prompt, and effective manner.

Lymphadenectomy in cases of urologic cancer is certainly of staging value. Therefore, it can help direct assignment of appropriate therapeutic measures. At times, it confers therapeutic benefit as well, but the value of lymphadenectomy as therapy is more difficult to demonstrate. With the exception of testis cancer, we have no strong evidence that systematic regional lymphadenectomy in association with primary tumor organ removal greatly enhances long-term survival in urologic cancers. But there is suggestive evidence, when comparing simple local organ excision to radical excision with lymphadenectomy, that such extensive surgery with lymphadenectomy seems to confer a short-term survival advantage, particularly in respect to lengthening the disease-free interval, and especially in those patients with early or low levels of nodal involvement.

Perhaps the greatest value of regional lymphadenectomy, when combined with primary organ excision for cancer, is in assessing the pathologic stage of the primary tumor. This assessment is of immediate, practical value in the selection of alternative treatment options for the patient. It also is of lasting value in subsequent analysis of data comparing treatments with different levels of disease. Hence, it permits the evaluation of a variety of interinstitutional therapeutic programs based on accurate classification of volume and extent of disease. As an outgrowth of this need, the International Union Against Cancer (IUAC) has recommended the TNM (tumor, node, metastases) classification of pathologic data, wherein extent of nodal involvement is quantified for each tumor system. Certainly the old clinical "staging" is inadequate for valid comparisons of cancer treatment programs because of the inherent understaging in descriptions lacking nodal data.

One soft-tissue cancer that seems remarkable in its curability by thorough lymphadenectomy is testis cancer. No other cancer of the urologic organ system can metastasize to multiple regional nodes, and yet among patients who have had this cancer there have been impressive survival figures with surgical resection alone. For example, with surgery alone, stage II testis cancer (regional nodes involved) is curable in the 75th percentile in stage B-I disease and at the 60th percentile in stage B-II disease with surgery alone. Naturally, the improvement in these survival figures to our current level of 98% is due to effective rescue chemotherapy with platinum-based combinations in the event of clinical relapse.[1]

RETROPERITONEAL LYMPHADENECTOMY FOR TESTIS CANCER

Complications of retroperitoneal lymphadenectomy relate to the tissues that are handled and involved in the dissection. For example, lymphatic complications include ascites and lymphocele. Vascular complications include bleeding and occasional thrombosis or inadvertent injury. Bowel complications include postoperative adhesions and ileus. Pulmonary complications involve the usual atelectasis, pneumonitis, and, occasionally, bleomycin toxic effects. Renal injuries include vascular injury, acute tubular necrosis, and ureteral injury. Finally, neural complications include infertility and paresthesias. We will consider each of these in turn (Tables 25–1 to 25–5).

Retroperitoneal lymph node dissection can be either transabdominal or thoracoabdominal.[2, 3] Each has its adherents, who have good reasons for their preference. Basically, the complication rates of the thoracoabdominal approach and the transabdominal approach are much the same.[4, 5] The purpose of lymphadenectomy in testis cancer has been twofold: first, accurate staging, and second, therapy for those who have positive nodes. The thrust of this argument must now be reconsidered in the light of increasing evidence that refinements in clinical staging will, in due course, permit those with negative *clinical* studies a high degree of confidence that they are, in fact, pathologically negative as well. At this point however, there is a 20% false-negative rate with clinical staging alone. Nonetheless, in well-controlled, tightly administered studies, those who have relapsed in clinical stage I disease for the most part have been rescued.[6, 7]

Considering its extent, retroperitoneal lymph node dissection is well tolerated. Testis cancer is usually not associated with intercurrent disease, and it occurs in vigorous, youthful men. The good cardiovascular and pulmonary status of these patients accounts substantially for the good tolerance of the procedure. Also, as a rule, only lymphatic and some sympathetic, fatty, and fascial tissues are removed. Since the gastrointestinal and genitourinary integrity is uninterrupted,

TABLE 25–1.

Retroperitoneal Lymphadenectomy for Testis Cancer: Early Postoperative Complications in 235 Patients*

Major Complications	No. of Patients	Minor Complications	No. of Patients
Pneumonitis, with empyema 1	4	Atelectasis	2
Wound infection	3	Pneumonitis, slight, focal	4
Fistula, enterocutaneous	2	Chemical pancreatitis	3
Urinoma secondary to ureteral leak	1	Ileus	2
Wound dehiscence	1	Wound infection, superficial	2
DIC, intraperitoneal hemorrhage, ascites	1	(Asthmatic) bronchospasm	1
Left renal vein thrombosis (age 4 yr)	1	Postural hypotension	1
Abscess, intraperitoneal and retroperitoneal	1	Pleural effusion	2
Sudden death, unknown cause—postoperative day 4	1	Paresthesia, hand, transient	1
		UGI bleeding	1
Septic phlebitis	1	Total in 15 patients (6% of patient group)	19
GI bleeding	1		
Brachial plexus injury	1		
Total in 13 patients (5.5% of patient group)	18		

*DIC = disseminated intravascular coagulation; GI = gastrointestinal; UGI = urinary-gastrointestinal.

there are fewer opportunities for infection or obstruction.

Extension of retroperitoneal lymph node dissection to include both suprarenal hilar zones will add to the risk by exposing renal vessels to injury and lengthening the time of operation. Earlier we reported a series of 235 patients in whom 470 suprarenal hilar units were dissected.[4] Major vessel injuries occurred in three patients, although all had a successful outcome. Segmental vascular injuries occurred in another three patients, but it was not considered practical to repair them, and the injuries resulted in no morbidity. We now realize suprahilar dissection is unnecessary in low-volume (stage IIA or B-I) disease.[8]

Risks Associated With Pretreated Patients

An emerging cohort of patients who present an exceptional challenge are patients who have completed combination therapy for bulky, advanced abdominal disease. Many of them continue with impressive retroperitoneal tumor; many have tumor extension caudad into the pelvis and cephalad in the suprahilar area, posterior mediastinum, chest, and neck. These patients are at greater risk not only for intraoperative morbidity, but also postoperative problems related to toxic effects from chemotherapy. The dramatic effects of platinum, vinblastine and bleomycin, for example, are not without a sig-

TABLE 25–2.

Intraoperative Complications

Complication	No. of Patients
Segmental branch ligation—renal artery	3
Ureteral injury	2
Main renal arterotomy, repaired	2
Renal venotomy, repaired	1
Right iliac arterotomies, replaced	1
Total no. of complications	9

TABLE 25–3.

Early Postoperative Complications

Stage	No. of Patients	
	Major Complications	Minor Complications
A (I)	2	9
B_1, B_2 (II)	5	4
B_3/C (III)	6	2
Total	13	15

TABLE 25–4.
Intraoperative Errors

Stage	No. of Patients
A (I)	2
B_1, B_2 (II)	3
B_3/C (III)	3

nificant price in toxicity. Major problems for the surgeon in these pretreated patients are pulmonary functional loss secondary to the pulmonary fibrosis due to bleomycin administration, granulocytopenia secondary to vinblastine administration, and, occasionally, renal functional loss secondary to dehydration and the use of platinum or the inadvertent use of aminoglycosides following platinum treatment. The technical demands in excising bulky tumors after the patient has undergone chemotherapy are much greater. Vascular injury is more common, and it is particularly important to avoid extended subabdominal aortic dissection in such patients. While the plane of cleavage is often easier to achieve in the subabdominal zone, the vessel wall derives its strength and resiliency in these patients from the outer layers, including the adventitia. Suture material does not hold well unless some adventitia is incorporated. In our list of complications reported earlier,[4] several dramatic vascular accidents were not included because they have been encountered only more recently. In five patients we have had to replace the aortic and/or iliac vessels intraoperatively with knitted or woven Dacron grafts. In each case, the adventitia had been stripped away and the vessel compromised so much that it was deemed unsafe or poorly functional. In one case, postoperative rupture necessitated emergency aortic grafting.

Naturally, gastrointestinal complications and pulmonary complications are higher in this group, and these have been recorded earlier. Table 25–1 delineates complications in our first 235 patients divided into class (major vs. minor) and time (early vs. late). Another group of complications involves intraoperative problems that are best classified as complications, even though they may result in no extended postoperative problems on the part of the patient (see Table 25–2).

TABLE 25–5.
RPLND* for Cancer of the Testis

Stage	No. of Patients
I	95
II	91
II and III	45 (secondary)
	4 (primary)
Total	235

*Retroperitoneal lymph node dissection.

Surgical Technique (Figs 25–1 to 25–5)

The following points of technique have proved useful in avoiding complications. Blood loss can be avoided by complete vascular dissection, prospective planned lumbar vessel ligation and division, and thorough mobilization of the great vessels. This can be achieved with the "split-and-roll" technique, which we have described previously.[1, 3] Naturally,

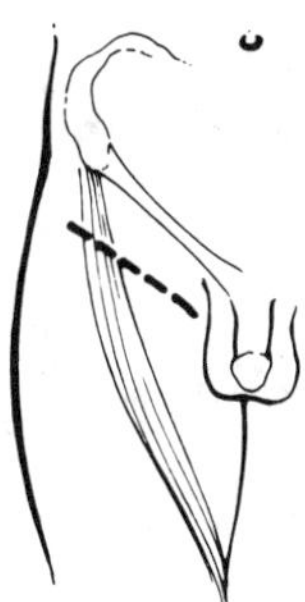

FIG 25–1.
Alternative oblique incision popularized by Baronofsky. (From Johnson DE, Ames FC: *Groin Dissection*. Chicago, Year Book Medical Publishers, 1985. Used by permission.)

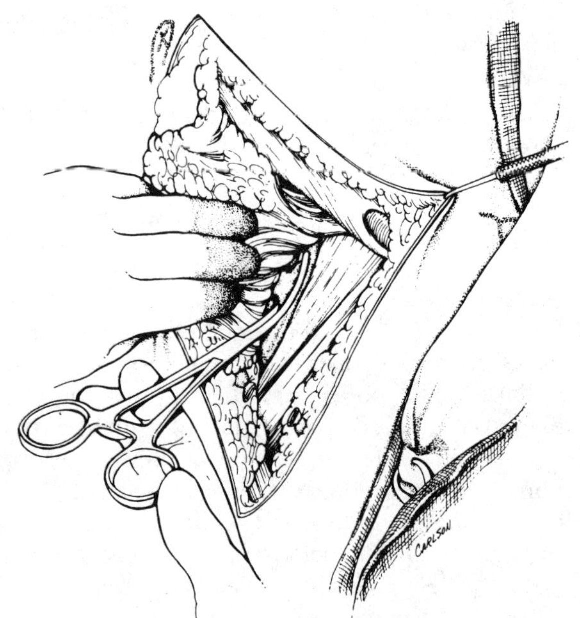

FIG 25–2.
The saphenous vein is divided at its junction with the femoral vein after the femoral vein has been partially occluded with an atraumatic vascular clamp. (From Johnson DE, Ames FC: *Groin Dissection.* Chicago, Year Book Medical Publishers, 1985. Used by permission.)

large tumors can be removed more safely after preoperative chemotherapy (i.e., chemical cytoreduction). But at times, they still have impressive dimensions after chemotherapy and require deliberate and extensive vascular mobilization using the principles of split-and-roll, thus freeing the vessels from the tumor's grasp. Also, it is safest to identify the origins of the renal vessels and dissect along these

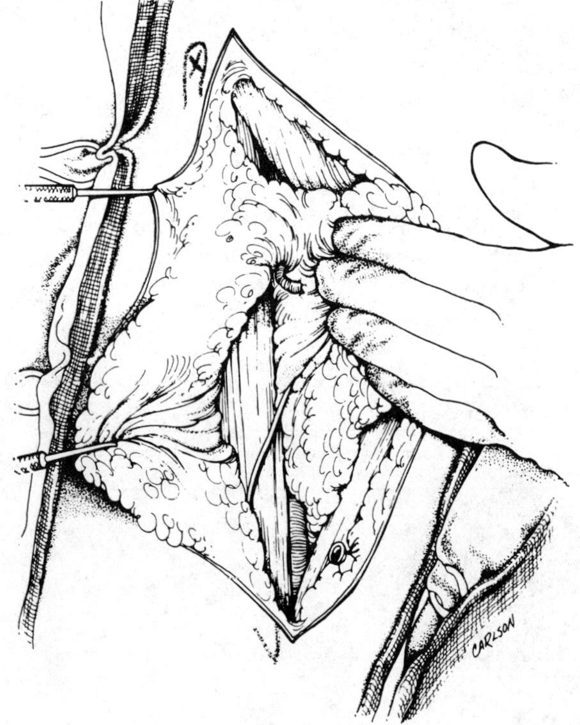

FIG 25–3.
The surgical specimen is dissected medially off the sartorius muscle together with the muscle fascia. The superficial circumflex artery and any other vessels encountered are divided between ligatures. (From Johnson DE, Ames FC: *Groin Dissection.* Chicago, Year Book Medical Publishers, 1985. Used by permission.)

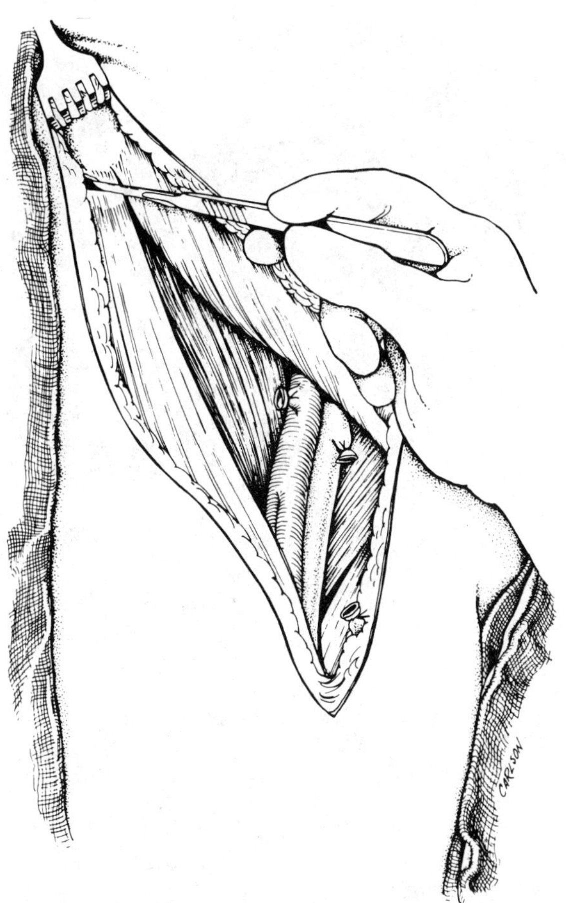

FIG 25–4.
After the surgical specimen has been removed, the sartorius muscle may be mobilized to cover the femoral vessels, if desired, by releasing its origin from the anterosuperior iliac spine with sharp dissection. (From Johnson DE, Ames FC: *Groin Dissection.* Chicago, Year Book Medical Publishers, 1985. Used by permission.)

from medial to lateral, rather than beginning in the renal hilum and dissecting medially to the great vessel origin. Branches of these vessels can be hidden in tumor masses and are much easier to recognize if one proceeds from the great vessel origin to the lateral vascular branching near the renal hilum. Mobilization of the pancreas and elevation with deep Harrington retractors has also been well described.[1, 3] As a general principle, operating at the apex of one's exposure is dangerous. Therefore, superb exposure is mandatory, and this technique of pancreatic mobilization and elevation will provide safer dissection in the suprarenal hilar area.

Also, while the ureter is normally easy to dissect from the specimen, ureteral injury will sometimes occur in the area where the gonadal vein crosses anterior to the ureter. Tenting up the specimen in the course of the dissection here may angulate the ureter and cause an inadvertent ureterotomy. Therefore, identification and separation of the ureter from adjacent structures is always appropriate. The use of a plastic wound protector and laparotomy pads helps to reduce the exposure of the wound to ambient contaminants. It is interesting that our series has a smaller infection rate than many herniorrhaphy series.

Pulmonary Complications.—Pulmonary problems in the postchemotherapy patient seem to be greatly reduced by accepting a P_{AO_2} that is subnormal but within a standard deviation of the patient's preoperative P_{AO_2} levels. The per-

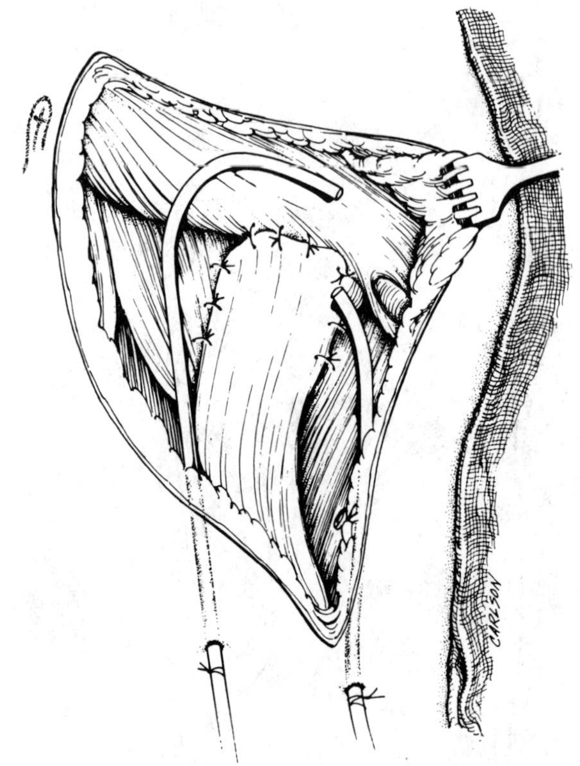

FIG 25–5.
The sartorius muscle is sutured in place over the femoral vessels. Suction catheters are placed just prior to wound closure. (From Johnson DE, Ames FC: *Groin Dissection.* Chicago, Year Book Medical Publishers, 1985. Used by permission.)

centage of inspired oxygen need not be elevated to achieve "normal" values, and the F_{IO_2} is usually around 25% intraoperatively. Another key element to avoiding pulmonary toxicity in the postchemotherapy patient is keeping the patient slightly dry. It is a mistake to overhydrate these patients in an attempt to create a large urine output during the procedure. The pulmonary vascular bed is relatively noncompliant in persons with pulmonary changes from bleomycin. Overhydration seems to be a key factor in our analysis and that of Goldinger and Schweitzer.[9] It is known that high concentrations of oxygen are damaging to pneumocytes, but the initial insult seems to be a diffusion defect caused by interstitial edema in the presence of a hypervolemic state with fixed pulmonary artery resistance. It is this interstitial edema that necessitates the raising of the inspired oxygen levels in order to get satisfactory arterial oxygenation. It is then that oxygen toxicity may supervene. Therefore, the management of a patient who has undergone previous bleomycin chemotherapy must include full pulmonary functional testing preoperatively. Also, at the time of operation, the use of the Swan-Ganz catheter will permit monitoring pulmonary artery wedge pressures. Judicious fluid replacement can keep central venous pressures and pulmonary artery pressures within a satisfactory range.

Abdominal Ascites.—Postoperative abdominal ascites is prevented by meticulous attention to clipping and/or ligature of most major lymphatics. In addition, the use of Bovie cautery in dividing these lymphatic packages may retard excessive lymph leak. Most importantly, the major contributions to the cisterna chyli and the cisterna itself should be recognized between the vena cava just caudal and posterior to the right crus of the diaphragm along the right posterolateral aspect of the aorta. The cisterna often can be visualized, dissected carefully, and ligated once or twice prior to its division below the ligature. At other times it can be safely clipped with medium or large vascular clips prior to its division. A cuff of soft lymphatic vascular tissue should be left within the clip so that it does not fall away after division.

Vascular Injury.—Venous difficulties can often be avoided by simply resecting the problematic vein, particularly if it is involved closely with the tumor. We commonly resect a segment of the vena cava below the renal veins, if necessary, to obtain adequate clearance, especially in those whose vessels have been largely replaced by tumor and who have developed excellent collaterals. The use of vascular stapling techniques here has also facilitated this maneuver. Should there be difficulty with vascular control at a foramen, usually it is best to grasp this area in an Allis clamp and oversew this area and some periosteum and/or psoas with a 2-0 silk suture ligature.

Resection of the Great Vessels During Extensive Retroperitoneal Lymphadenectomy.—While it is infrequently necessary, extensive vascular repair and/or resection is sometimes required in the course of extended postchemotherapy testis tumor dissections. While in most cases the tumor can be dissected from the great vessels with the usual split-and-roll technique, there are some occasions when the tumor actually involves the wall of the great vessel or, in the case of the venous system, invades the vessel as a tumor thrombus.

In approximately 300 postchemotherapy retroperitioneal lymphadenectomies (RPLNDs), we have had to resect the infrarenal vena cava 18 times. In most of these cases, the cava was directly involved with tumor thrombus. In the early years, we resected several cavas with active tumor thrombus from extensive retroperitoneal tumor prior to chemotherapy. In more recent years, this problem has been largely eliminated with prior chemotherapy for extensive bulky disease which has a marked cytoreductive effect. But occasionally we still have tumor thrombus in the cava either in the form of necrotic tumor covered by fibrinous thrombus and/or teratoma. In fact, on two occasions, despite salvage chemotherapy for relapsing advanced disease, active tumor with malignant elements has been found as intracaval tumor thrombus.

This operation should not be undertaken lightly as there is significant morbidity with caval resection. The morbidity is not only immediate venous congestion of the lower extremities but also continued extravasation of lymphatic tissue into a third space (I.E., retroperitoneum). In analyzing our postoperative complications, we have noted a greater frequency of abdominal ascites in patients who have had their cava resected. Therefore, abdominal ascites is an added risk factor in any patient who has the cava resected.

The technique of cava resection is relatively simple. A vessel is mobilized by dividing the various lumbar tributaries and mobilizing them as completely as possible in the infrarenal area. Usually there are several major lumbar vessels just below the level of the renal vessels and these need to be secured in order to obtain a good 360-degree clearance. Normally, we use the vascular staple clamp for this, but it can also be oversewn with any vascular suture material in a continuous suture while controlled in vascular clamps.

The distal extent of the caval resection should be as limited as possible. When possible, it is preferable to leave both iliac veins intact. This is not always possible, however, and on occasion, we have resected the venous structures below the hypogastric venous entry (i.e., at the external iliac level). This resection simply compounds lower extremity venous stasis and lymphedema which gradually reverses. The major morbidity is the risk for transient abdominal ascites in these patients, presumably secondary to massive alternative lymphatic drainage along the bodywall with leakage into a large third space created by the dissection. The absence of venous connection for lymphatic drainage is probably the culprit in such cases.

Aortic Repairs.—In this same cohort of postchemotherapy RPLND patients, we have had to use interposition aortic or tube grafts or bifurcated aortoiliac grafts in five patients. One of these was done on an emergent basis in a patient who ruptured his aorta while in the recovery room after an extended subabventitial dissection hours earlier. Fortunately, he was rescued and had a remarkably smooth postoperative course. The other four were done in a planned manner because of evident aortic involvement with tumor during the RPLND procedure itself. In each of these remaining four cases, it was apparent that the aortic wall was so heavily involved and so damaged by the tumor dissection that it would be best replaced. The decision can be made more easily if the dissection is clearly required in the subadventitial plane and the aortic wall is pale, "cheesy," and poorly controlled with suture ligature. In such patients, it is safer to simply resect the involved segment and replace it with an interposition Dacron tube graft. In each of the five cases, the patients did very well postoperatively.

Regarding technique, it is essentially the same as in aortic aneurysm repair. Care is taken to develop a safe cuff below the renal arteries, which is virtually always possible in testis tumor cases. In none of the five cases was a shunt necessary for aortic involvement in the suprarenal area. Usually, we use a running 4-0 Prolene suture to anastomose the tube graft which has been sized and preclotted. Of course the distal limb of the dissection must also be prepared at the time of the interpostion graft so as to minimize the distal ischemic time. Once again, 360-degree continuous 4-0 Prolene suture is suitable for the distal anastomosis. Care is taken to backflush the graft by removal of the distal clamps first and then under low-pressure conditions to review the integrity of the graft itself and the connections. Following this maneuver the cephalad clamp is removed. Any additional hemostasis can then be obtained at the suture line. Normally, this is unnecessary and simple digital occlusion and time is all that is needed for hemostasis. Depending on the extent of the time required, heparinization is used and then reversed with Protamine. Normally, we use one milligram per kilogram of heparin and reverse it with about two-thirds that dose of protamine. In the event of a patch graft or a relatively brief clamping, no heparinization at all is required.

Based on these experiences, it is prudent to attempt the dissection in the extra-adventitial plane whenever possible in order to avoid the need for grafting.

Spinal Cord Injuries.—While they are often asked about, we have not seen any spinal cord injuries following retroperitoneal lymphadenectomy. The spinal cord itself terminates near the level of T12, and the nutrient arteries to the spinal cord arise well above from the thoracic aorta.

Bowel and Other Gastrointestinal Complications.—Meticulous reapproximation of the mesentery of the bowel, which has been divided at its root together with the mesocolon at the time of initial mobilization, will reapproximate serous surfaces and minimize the potential for small bowel obstruction by fibrous adhesions. Placement of the viscera in a plastic bowel bag on the patient's chest also can help avoid damage to the serous surfaces of the gastrointestinal tract, which might otherwise occur if the bowel is packed with laparotomy pads over an extended period of time. It is certainly true that transabdominal lymphadenectomy produces a longer period of nasogastric tube drainage than does the thoracoabdominal approach, during which the gastrointestinal contents might be retracted into a peritoneal envelope. Aside from this complication, there is no objective difference in the incidence of gastrointestinal complications in the analysis of two major series.[4, 5]

Infertility.—Finally, infertility is a major neural complication, because removal of the sympathetic nerves causes loss of emission.[10] Comparison of several series[11–13] has led to the conclusion that the postganglionic sympathetic fibers that decussate in the preaortic area between the inferior mesenteric artery and the bifurcation of the iliac arteries are the cause of ejaculatory failure if they are divided. The preganglionic fibers leading up to the ganglia of the sympathetic chain may remain intact, but a defect persists if there has been a thorough 360-degree clearance in the low periaortic area. Several interesting clinical studies are underway both here and abroad[11–14] to shed light on this problem. Up to 70% of patients, in two series,[12, 13] are able to ejaculate if fibers in this periaortic zone are spared. Naturally, if there is gross tumor in the retroperitoneum, and if the surgeon feels the cancer-eradicating aspects of the surgery will be compromised, efforts to spare fertility are misplaced. The first priority is a cancer cure. But in those patients who appear to have completely negative tissues at exploration, it seems reasonable to preserve these low preaortic fibers, if possible.

REGIONAL LYMPHADENECTOMY FOR KIDNEY AND ADRENAL CANCER

It is difficult, if not impossible, to demonstrate any real therapeutic benefit of systematic lymphadenectomy in the treatment of adrenal and renal adenocarcinoma. Nonetheless, it is appropriate to remove the tumor en bloc within Gerota's fascia and at least the ipsilateral pericaval or periaortic lymph nodes.

Naturally, lymphatic drainage from the kidney follows venous drainage, which is quite variable and widely distributed. Many of these tumors metastasize by venous pathways, thus reducing the effectiveness of nodal dissection. The most common areas of nodal involvement are the renal hilum and near the origin of the renal vessels arising from the vena cava and aorta. Long-term studies indicate that many patients with negative nodes ultimately die of blood borne metastases. Therefore, the therapeutic impact of extended lymphadenectomy is weakened by this delayed expression of relatively common hematogenous metastases.

Several reports compare limited nephrectomy (without lymphadenectomy) to radical nephrectomy (with regional lymphadenectomy).[15] It seems those patients with stage B and C disease have early advantages through 1 to 5 years. This advantage can be extended from 5 to 10 years, according to the well-known series of Robson et al.[16] It is noteworthy, however, that 15-year data reveal an impressive drop in survival, possibly related to the delayed presentation of metastatic disease. These data reflect the biologic variability of renal cell carcinoma and the indolence in the growth rates of many of these tumors.

Surgical Technique

It is generally agreed that a regional lymphadenectomy for renal cell carcinoma is indicated for both staging and potential therapeutic purposes over the short term. The only real issue is the extent of the dissection. Most agree that at least the ipsilateral aspect of the great vessel near the tumor (cava for right-sided tumors and aorta for left-sided tumors) should be cleared of nodes from the upper to lower poles. Others, myself included, believe that the ipsilateral great vessel should be cleared 360-degrees so as to include the interaortocaval nodal group. This permits total clearance of the common shared midline lymphatics that drain both the right and left sides. Yet, one must hasten to add, we cannot demonstrate survival advantage in this group of patients, owing to small numbers and the extended surveillance required to detect delayed recurrence (Table 25–6).

Vascular injury.—The primary complications of radical lymphadenectomy for renal and adrenal tumors relate to vascular injuries. Most of these complications are related to poor exposure. While it is not the purpose of this brief review to elucidate all mechanisms of vascular injury, poor exposure accounts for most of them. The operating surgeon's insistence on clear visualization of the tissues being dissected and divided will greatly reduce vascular injury. Adequate extent of incisions and hepatic and bowel mobilization are but a few of the useful steps. A well-known injury on the right side is caused by the failure to secure the adrenal vein, which often will enter high and posterior on the cava, sometimes in conjunction with a hepatic vein. This injury is prevented by appropriate elevation of the right lobe of the liver, taping and/or retracting the cava above the level of the renal veins, and patience in dissection. Medial caval retraction and cephalad hepatic retraction are useful in the exposure process.

Arterial injuries have occurred while dissecting massive adrenal or upper pole renal tumors. Rarely, the superior mesenteric artery and/or celiac vessels may be damaged in the course of the dissection if the tumor is large enough to compress these vessels and distort the anatomy. The recognition of all anatomical landmarks is a constant requirement in such a case. In one such case, it was necessary to reconstruct the celiac artery using an au-

TABLE 25–6.

Survival Rates of Patients with Renal Cell Carcinoma (Stages A Through D) With and Without Node Dissection and Patients With Stage D With No Surgery*

		Survival Rates (%)			
Stage		1 yr	5 yr	10 yr	15 yr
Stage A:	With lymphadenectomy	100.0	67.35	50.51	
	Without lymphadenectomy	89.6	70.97	58.61	46.17
Stage B:	With lymphadenectomy	91.5	42.28		
	Without lymphadenectomy	66.7	40.44	10.49	
Stage C:	With lymphadenectomy	87.5	43.75		
	Without lymphadenectomy	56.5	25.69		
Stage D:	With lymphadenectomy	81.0	28.91		
	Without lymphadenectomy	47.7	9.12		
	No surgery	32.3	11.41	3.80	

*From the University of Texas Southwestern Medical School Affiliated Hospitals, Dallas: *Urol Clin North Am* 1980; 7:3.

togenous segment of splenic artery sewn end-to-end onto the remaining distal limb of the celiac artery.

Neurologic Complications.—The most common neurologic complication of radical nephrectomy is brachial plexus palsy. Naturally, this injury is caused by the stretching of this plexus in the placement of the patient. We take great pains in having the forearm wrapped in a blanket and taped to the ether screen, and then we check the angle of elevation of the humerus from the chest wall. If it is at a right angle and hangs freely from the ether screen, brachial plexus palsy can be avoided. Also, hyperextension of the neck aggravates brachial plexus injury.

Spinal cord injury is rare, unless it is associated with an abdominal aortic aneurysm, which is sometimes repaired in concert with this procedure.

Splenic Injury and Pancreatitis.—Splenic injury and, occasionally, pancreatitis occur from excessive retraction in a field that has not been properly prepared. Division of the splenocolic attachments and then incision of the lienophrenic attachments will allow the spleen to be elevated much more freely. In very large tumors, we sometimes continue the lienocolic division across the posterior peritoneum and up to the gastroesophageal hiatus. It is sometimes necessary to divide the short gastric vessels as well, in order to mobilize the spleen up and out of the operative field. Pancreatitis usually results through retractor injury and is best avoided by placing folded towels or laparotomy pads over the pancreas itself. The use of malleable Harrington retractors is also very helpful in avoiding this injury.

Diaphragmatic Injury.—Diaphragmatic injuries are common in extended operations for renal and adrenal cancer with or without lymphadenectomy. It is important to note that the lymph nodes in the periaortic area *below* the renal vessels are largely antereolateral. The opposite is true *above* the level of the renal vessels and the aortic hiatus of the diaphragm. There, most of the lymph nodes are posterolateral to the aorta (i.e., retrocrural). Therefore, division of the crus is sometimes necessary if the lymphadenectomy is to continue cephalad, particularly if a positive node in that area is apparent. This incision, in the crus of the diaphragm, should be closed primarily with nonabsorbable sutures. Also, a thoracoabdominal incision for this procedure involves an incision of the diaphragm in many cases. The diaphragm should be closed with interrupted suture material, and many also encourage the use of a running suture on the pleural surface to minimize transdiaphragmatic pleural effusions and future herniation. Pulmonary complications most commonly involve atelectasis and segmental or lobar collapse. The latter are avoided with appropriate ventilation and suction techniques. The former are avoided with lung inflation techniques at the conclusion of the case. It is useful to perform these maneuvers even if we do not use a chest tube and are not operating transpleurally.

Liver Injury.—Hepatic injuries may occur, particularly in the dissection of massive tumors, at the porta hepatis. If hepatic surgery is contemplated, as in the case of large right-sided tumors, a thoracoabdominal approach is encouraged, with control of the cava both above and below the diaphragm. It should be noted that cross-clamping of the cava in the chest will result in a phrenic nerve crush injury. Therefore, a tourniquet is preferable *after* dissection of the phrenic nerve off the cava.

Generally, in lymphadenectomy for renal and adrenal tumors, it is not the lymphadenectomy itself that causes complications. Most injuries relate to the removal of the primary tumor en bloc with the lymphadenectomy. Hence, they have been mentioned here, but they are discussed more fully in Chapters 9–15 regarding kidney surgery.

PELVIC LYMPHADENECTOMY FOR BLADDER AND PROSTATE CANCER

Lymphadenectomy for bladder cancer is done for much the same reason as for renal cancer. It provides data of value for pathologic staging, and it is therapeutic for some patients. While this latter point is difficult to establish on the basis of cystectomy data, Leadbetter was an early advocate of a thorough bilateral iliac lymphadenectomy in association with radical cystectomy. In his review of Leadbetter's series,[17] Dretler et al. reported in 1973 that 35 patients with positive nodes who underwent radical cystectomy for cure were followed for more than 5 years. Of these 34 patients, six (18%) survived more than 5 years. One third of the patients with involvement of only one or two nodes survived more than 5 years, whereas only 10% of those with over two nodes survived this long. Also, Reid et al.[18] reported that five of 24 patients (21%) with positive nodes survived more than 5 years; these patients belonged to a group that also had short-course preoperative radiation therapy prior to cystectomy. More recently, Skinner[19] has demonstrated a 36% five-year survival for 35 patients who had positive nodes at the time of radical cystectomy. Again, as much as this reflects meticulous lymphadenectomy, it also implies meticulous dissection on the part of the pathologist seeking nodes in the perivesical tissue during the prosection of the specimen.

On the other hand, in selected patients, cystectomy without pelvic lymphadenectomy has provided reasonably good survival data also.[20] The available data indicate that about 20% to 30% of patients who are believed to be candidates for radical cystectomy for bladder cancer will have nodal metastases if a pelvic lymphadenectomy is done with cystectomy. The incidence of positive pelvic nodes relates directly to the pathologic stage of the primary tumor (Table 25–7).[21, 22]

Those patients who benefit most from the careful pelvic lymphadenectomy en bloc with cystectomy are those with clinically undetectable micrometastases to a few nodes. It appears that as many as one third of these patients may be cured, while it is rare for those with multiple or bulky metastases to survive beyond 2 years with any sort of current therapy.

Surgical Technique

Vascular Injury.—Complications of pelvic lymphadenectomy from bladder and prostate cancer include vascular injury, acute bleeding, or delayed vascular complications, such as thrombus formation followed by pulmonary embolus. The bleeding complication is usually avoided by doing a truly radical procedure and visualizing the vessels in the course of the dissection. Most bleeding occurs because of failure to dissect and visualize the vessels. Postoperative thrombus formation remains a serious problem following any

TABLE 25–7.

Relation of Depth of Bladder Wall Invasion at Time of Cystectomy (Pathologic Stage) to Lymph Node Involvement*†

Pathologic Stage	No. of Patients	% Positive Nodes
P1 and P1S	41	5
P2	20	30
P3A	13	31
P3B	28	64
P4	8	50

*From Skinner DC: Bladder cancer, in *AUA Update Series*, lesson 39. American Urological Association, Office of Education, Houston, Texas, 1983.

†All patients received 1,600 rad preoperative radiation, and radical cystectomy and pelvic lymphadenectomy.

pelvic lymphadenectomy. Some prefer to anticoagulate these patients postoperatively, but many think it is unnecessary. Some believe it may increase complications of delayed pelvic bleeding or lymphatic accumulation.

Neurologic Injury.—Neurologic complications include an obturator nerve injury, with subsequent loss of adduction of the thigh. This complication is usually secondary to dissection of a large fixed lateral tumor. The obturator nerve is rarely injured in the course of a normal lymphadenectomy, because nodes in this area are easily separated from this firm and prominent nerve. Occasionally, the lateral femoral cutaneous and or genitofemoral nerve branches are injured in extensive dissections. The major morbidity of this injury is complaint of paresthesias in the upper thigh or groin and scrotum.

Lymphatic Injury.—A major lymphatic complication of pelvic lymphadenectomy is lymphocele. Although rare, it can be symptomatic and require drainage in many cases. Most of the time it can be managed conservatively. Some cases can be handled with ultrasonic identification, aspiration, and then replacement of a dye, such as diatrizoate (Hypaque) or tetracycline, which will irritate and scarify the pseudomembranous wall of the lymphocele and retard recurrence.

Lymphedema of the Extremities.—Lymphedema of the extremities is a major complication of pelvic lymphadenectomy, particularly if extended and followed by pelvic radiotherapy. Therefore, it is important to spare the major lymphatic trunks lateral to the iliac vessels if possible. Many feel that the split-and-roll technique can be effectively employed around the medial aspects of these vessels and the nodes drawn medially, with sparing of the adventitial lymphatics on the lateral aspects of these vessels. This maneuver can obviate lymphedema, especially if the patient is not to receive radiotherapy. It is important in the patient with prostate cancer, who may well receive external beam radiotherapy in the event a frozen section reveals nodes positive for prostatic cancer.

Bowel Injury.—Bowel injury during lymphadenectomy for bladder or prostate is rare. We have seen a retractor injury to the left colon in one patient. Pelvic abscess is, again, rare but possible, particularly if there is associated rectal injury in the course of the lymphadenectomy and cystectomy. One of the major problems with pelvic lymphadenectomy for bladder and/or prostate cancer is the relative insensitivity and sampling error involved in using frozen sections of these lymph nodes to determine the presence of cancer. A decision to proceed with prostatectomy in a man with prostate cancer depends on this report. About 9% to 10% of the time, false-negative frozen sections are reported positive on permanent sections. This deficiency will remain a chronic problem as long as human sampling and rapid review are done, as is the case with frozen sections.[23]

INGUINAL LYMPHADENECTOMY FOR PENILE CANCER

The primary spread of penile cancer is via the regional lymph nodes. Stage I tumors are confined to the glans or prepuce. Twenty percent of these patients will present with inguinal adenopathy but only 5% will actually develop delayed metastases (therefore the 5-year survival of this group of patients approaches 95% on a theoretical basis). Stage II tumors however, invade the shaft of the penis or corpora but have no clinical evidence of lymphatic or distant metastases. Twenty percent of this group are found to have microscopic lymphatic metastases and/or develop subsequent nodal disease; the estimated 5-year survival of this group is 70% to 75%. Stage III tumors are confined to the penile shaft grossly, but inguinal lymph node metastases are clinically evident. With immediate lymph node dissection, the 5-year survival in this group is 30% to 50%.[24–26]

There is considerable debate regarding the initial management of the inguinal nodes in patients with stage I and II tumors.[27, 28] Clinical evaluation of regional lymph nodes is inaccurate, yielding both false-positive and false-negative results. Approximately 20% of patients with clinically negative nodes do have occult metastases, while about 50% of those with clinically positive nodes have no tumor on histologic examination because of early inflammatory nodal change. Because of this discrepancy, most agree that, following excision of the primary penile lesion, a suitable trial of antibiotic treatment and observation is indicated before making a decision regarding inguinal lymphadenectomy. If the inguinal nodes remain clinically positive after resection of the primary tumor followed by antibiotics and a period of observation, then at least 60% of such patients will be found to have bilateral disease. In this instance, bilateral inguinal dissection should be performed. It is also recommended that if inguinal nodes are positive, the dissection should be extended to include the iliac nodes as well as inguinal nodes. On the other hand, if the inguinal nodes are negative, dissection of pelvic nodes need not be continued.

The extent of lymphadenectomy is another arbitrary area. Most believe that a subinguinal dissection of the femoral triangle is sufficient, if there is no evidence of clinically enlarged or positive nodes. Again, most surgeons operate for evidence of clinical disease after a period of observation. The subinguinal dissection is continued as a pelvic iliac nodal clearance if there is evidence of clinical disease at the time of subinguinal dissection. Because pelvic nodes are so rarely positive in the absence of positive inguinal nodes, most agree that pelvic lymphadenectomy is unnecessary in the face of the negative inguinal dissection.

Complications and morbidity of this dissection are impressive. First, the cutaneous aspects of the procedure deserve comment. Fraley and Hutchens.[29] have described a variety of options which avoid cutting into the skin fold of the groin. An incision parallel to the inguinal ligament preserves the skin flaps by staying below Camper's fascia and reflecting the skin up at the level of Scarpa's fascia, providing a rather thick skin bridge on either side. It is also important to excise any scar tissue from a previous biopsy in a generous ellipsoid. Epidermoid carcinoma is often found in such biopsy scars. Lymphadenectomy in the groin is done en bloc and has been well described.[29]

Dermal Necrosis.—The major complications are cutaneous slough of skin flaps secondary to loss of vascularity and failure to preserve subcutaneous fat with associated capillaries. Use of flourescein and a Wood's lamp will indicate nonviable tissue if the viability of a flap should be in question.

Wound Infection.—Infection of the wound is common, owing to the difficulty of achieving cleanliness in the folds of the abdomen, leg, and genitals, especially in obese patients. Meticulous surgical technique, a liberal use of antibiotics, preservation of flap vascularity, and elimination of dead space all greatly help in reducing wound infections.

Leg Lymphedema.—Leg lymphedema is common following this procedure, owing to the very thorough dissection of the lymphatic space and major tributaries along the femoral vessels and in the femoral canal. Measurement and fitting of the legs for elastic stockings and leg elevation when the patient is in bed assist in the management of this problem.

Nerve Injury.—Significant neural complications are rare, but many paresthesias are noted from injury to superficial branches of the femoral nerve, particularly in the anterior and medial aspects of the thigh and genitals.

Vascular Injury.—Vascular injuries are relatively uncommon. Saphenous venous separation at the saphenofemoral venous junction is usually uncomplicated. Occasionally, subsequent distal varicosities may develop.

A well-known vascular complication is the erosion of the femoral artery by recurrent epidermoid tumor. Usually, a thorough inguinal dissection avoids this complication and, in fact, is done for this very purpose. But occasional wound implantation or local recurrence carries this as an ominous possible complication even in the patient who has been operated on. Thorough dissection and transfer of the sartorius muscle are usually sufficient to prevent this complication.

Lymphocele and Infectious Lymphadenitis.—Two other complications related to lymphatic accumulation are lymphocele and infectious lymphadenitis. Often, tacking of the undersurface of the wound flaps to the underlying muscles and inserting a suction catheter in this area for the immediate postoperative period, together with a compression dressing when deemed advisable, prevent subcutaneous lymphocele.

Deep Vein Thrombosis.—Finally, deep vein thrombosis can sometimes occur, especially in the relatively immobile patient. While most do not recommend immobilization and elevation of the lower extremity, some do and also employ routine postoperative anticoagulation. Most feel that early mobilization is still consistent with a good result, particularly if the wound is welldressed and drained and ambulation is gradual and progressive.

EDITORIAL COMMENT I

Identified are most of the problematic areas in lymphadenectomy for urologic carcinomas. Retroperitoneal lymphadenectomy for testis tumor is changing because of the advent of chemotherapy. Many patients with massive metastatic disease with partial responses to chemotherapy are now becoming operative candidates. These patients with residual bulky lymph node metastases following chemotherapy are a difficult group of surgical patients. We, too, have had experience with aortic replacement in retroperitoneal node dissection, because often the easiest plane of dissection is between the intima and media of the aortic wall. In addition, many of these aortic walls are not strong and will not hold sutures well. An aortic vascular graft was required.

The limits of regional lymphadenectomy for renal tumors have been investigated carefully and are determined by the regional lymph node drainage of the kidney.* A periaortic dissection is satisfactory for a left-sided lymphadenectomy. On the right side, a circumvenacaval dissection with removal of interaortic vena caval nodes is more indicated on an anatomical basis. We have continued to perform lymphadenectomy primarily for possible micrometastases.

Inguinal node dissection has a high incidence of wound complications. Keeping the incision out of the groin fold and making it parallel to

*Marshall FF, Powell KC: Lymphadenectomy for renal cell carcinoma: Anatomical and therapeutic considerations. *J Urol* 1982; 128:677.

the inguinal ligament in the upper thigh will reduce these complications, along with careful attention to surgical detail.

EDITORIAL COMMENT II

Although there is increasing interest in surveillance protocols for testis tumors, I suspect there will remain subsets of patients who are at high risk and still will require retroperitoneal lymph node dissection. We have still tended to recommend retroperitoneal lymph node dissection in patients with nonseminomatous tumor for staging and possible cure.

A modified inguinal node dissection for penile cancer has been recommended by some authors with preservation of the saphenous vein and less dissection down the femoral vessels, especially if initial nodes on frozen section appear negative. Preservation of Camper's fascia with a thicker skin flap may also reduce wound complications.

REFERENCES

1. Donohue JP: Retroperitoneal lymphadenectomy, *Urologic Surgery.* in Glenn J, Boyce W (eds): Philadelphia, JB Lippincott Co, 1983.
2. Cooper JF, Leadbetter WF, Chute R: The thoracoabdominal approach for retroperitoneal gland dissection: Its application in testis tumors. *Surg Gynecol Obstet* 1950; 90:486.
3. Donohue JP: Retroperitoneal lymphadenectomy: The anterior approach including bilateral suprarenal hilar dissection. *Urol Clin North Am* 1977; 4:509.
4. Donohue JP, Rowland RG: Complications of retroperitoneal lymphadenectomy. *J Urol* 1981; 125:338.
5. Skinner DG, Melamud A, Lieskovsky G: Complications of thoracoabdominal retroperitoneal lymph node dissection. *J Urol* 1982; 127:1107.
6. Peckham M, Barrett AB, Husband SE, et al: Orchidectomy alone in testicular stage I non-seminomatous germ cell tumors. *Lancet* 1982; 2:678–680.
7. Sogani PC, Whitmore WF, Herr HW, et al: Orchiectomy alone in treatment of clinical stage I non-seminomatous germ cell tumor of the testis, abstract 362, p 194A. 1984 AUA Annual Meeting, New Orleans, May 9, 1984.
8. Donohue JP, Maynard B, Zachary M: The distribution of nodal metastases in the retroperitoneum from non-seminomatous testis cancer. *J Urol* 1982; 128:315.
9. Goldfinger PL, Schweitzer O: The hazards of anesthesia and surgery in bleomycin treated patients. *Semin Oncol* 1979; 6:121.
10. Kedia KR, Markland C, Fraley EE: Sexual function after high retroperitoneal lymphadenectomy. *Urol Clin North Am* Oct. 1977; 4:523.
11. Lange P, Narayan P, Fraley EE: Ejaculation and fertility after extended retroperitoneal lymph node dissection for testis cancer. *J Urol* 1982; 127:685–688.
12. Boedefeld E: *Transactions of the International Symposium on Testis Cancer,* Paris, October, 1984. New York, Alan R. Liss, 1984.
13. Fossa S: Personal communications, 1984.
14. Thachial JV, Jewett MAA, Rider WD: The effects of cancer and cancer therapy on male fertility: A review. *J Urol* 1981; 126:141.
15. Peters PC, Brown GL: The role of lymphadenectomy in the management of renal cell carcinoma. *Urol Clin North Am* 1980; 7:3.
16. Robson CJ, Churchill B, Anderson W: Radical nephrectomy for renal cell carcinoma. *J Urol* 1969; 101:297–301.
17. Dretler SP, Ragsdale BD, Leadbetter WF: The value of pelvic lymphadenectomy in the surgical treatment of bladder cancer. *J Urol* 1973; 109:414.
18. Reid EC, Oliver JA, Fisher IJ: Preoperative irradiation and cystectomy in 135 cases of bladder cancer. *Urology* 1976; 8:247–250.
19. Skinner DG: Management of invasive bladder cancer: A meticulous pelvic node dissection can make a difference. *J Urol* 1982; 128:34.
20. Blandy JP, England HR, Evans SJW, et al:

T-3 bladder cancer: The case for salvage cystectomy. *Br J Urol* 1980; 52:506–510.

21. Morales P, Golimbu M: The therapeutic role of pelvic lymphadenectomy in prostatic cancer. *Urol Clin North Am* 1980; 3:623–629.
22. Paulson DF: The prognostic role of lymphadenectomy in adenocarcinoma of the prostate. *Urol Clin North Am* 1980; 7:615.
23. Fowler JE Jr, Whitmore WF, Jr: The incidence and extent of pelvic lymph node metastases in apparently localized prostatic cancer. *Cancer* 1981; 12:2941.
24. Hardner CJ, Bahnalaph T, Murphy GP: Carcinoma of the penis: Analysis of therapy in 100 consecutive cases. *J Urol* 1972; 108:428.
25. de Kernion JB, Tymbuyrg P, Persky L, et al: Carcinoma of the penis. *Cancer.* 1973; 32:1256.
26. Ekstrom T, Edsmyr F: Cancer of the penis: A clinical study of 229 cases. *Acta Chir Scand* 1958; 115:25.
27. Catalona WJ: Role of lymphadenectomy in carcinoma of the penis. *Urol Clin North Am* 1980; 7:785.
28. Grabstalt H: Controversies concerning lymph node dissection for cancer of the penis. *Urol Clin North Am* 1980; 7:793–799.
29. Fraley EE, Hutchens HC: Radical ileoinguinal node dissection: The skin bridge technique: A new procedure. *J Urol* 1972; 108:279.

CHAPTER 26

Complications of Microsurgery

Jonathan P. Jarow, M.D.
Fray F. Marshall, M.D.

Microsurgical techniques are a relatively recent addition to our surgical armamentarium. Although microscopes and fine instruments have been available for many years, it was not until the development of uniformly excellent suture material of 9-0 and 10-0 nylon that sophisticated microsurgery became widespread. These sutures are now available with a variety of swaged-on needles for specialized use. Orthopedics, plastic surgery, neurosurgery, and many other disciplines use microsurgical techniques in entirely new fields of surgery using tissue transfers with both neural and vascular reconstructions.

Silber was one of the pioneers in this country in applying this technique to urology for both vasectomy reversal[1] and subsequently testicular autotransplantation.[2] More recent application to penile revascularization has been popularized by Virag[3] and others. Training in microsurgery is now a standard part of urologic residency for both clinical and laboratory use.

Visual magnification with a surgical microscope or the use of optical loupes with microsurgical techniques is also employed in pediatric urology and in small-vessel intrarenal arterial reconstructions.

COMPLICATIONS OF VASECTOMY REVERSAL

Complications of Vasectomy

Vasectomy is a simple, effective method of inducing elective male sterility. Between 250,000 and 500,000 vasectomies are performed each year in the United States.[4] Since the divorce rate approaches 50% in some areas of this country, there are a large number of potential candidates for reversal of a vasectomy at the time of later remarriage.

It has been generally recognized that vasectomy has few clinically significant complications and that vasectomy has little effect upon testicular production of androgens or sperm. On the other hand, pathologic changes have been observed at the site of vasectomy[4] and the testis.[5] Although these changes may have little effect on the hormonal or physiologic function of the individual, they may have potential implications in patients undergoing vasectomy reversal.

In the past, sperm granulomas were said to occur in a small percentage of patients undergoing a vasectomy. More recently, the resected end of the vas was studied pathologically at the time of vasectomy reversal. Forty-one percent of patients were found to have a sperm granuloma and 66% were found to have vasitis nodosa.[4] *Vasitis nodosa* was defined as proliferation of ductules originating from the vasal lumen into the surrounding vasal wall and soft tissue. This process presumably presents at a later stage as a sperm granuloma. A *sperm granuloma* was defined as an inflammatory nodule consisting of lymphocytes and histiocytes with collections of spermatozoa (Fig 26–1). These pathologic findings did not represent extravasation of spermatozoa but rather an accumulation of spermatozoa with an inflammatory response occurring within the wall of the vas itself.

When this inflammatory process occurs, it may occur throughout the length of the proximal vas as well as the epididymis. Vasal or epididymal obstruction may occur more proximally as a result of this inflammatory process. In patients who had undergone serial sectioning of the vas and the epididymis, small microgranulomas were identified in the tail of the epididymis just distal to the site of identification of spermatozoa.[5] These findings explain the presence of intravasal azoospermia observed at the time of surgery in some patients. It may also account for the higher failure rate observed in patients undergoing vasectomy reversal many years following vasectomy.

Sperm granuloma with vasitis nodosa can probably provide for recanalization of the vas so that, paradoxically, in rare instances this inflammatory process may relieve obstruction by creating an anatomical bridge between the cut ends of the vasa. In a recent study, 90% of men examined demonstrated these changes postvasectomy.[6]

The effects of vasectomy on the human testis have generally been held to be inconsequential. In some animals, such as the hamster, there can be demonstrable deleterious effects on the testis postvasectomy.[7] In the rabbit, the effects may be partly a function of time, occurring 6 to 12 months postvasectomy. In other animals, such as the rat, there have been minimal changes demonstrated. On the other hand, if the rat epididymis is occluded high in the caput, testicular atrophy will

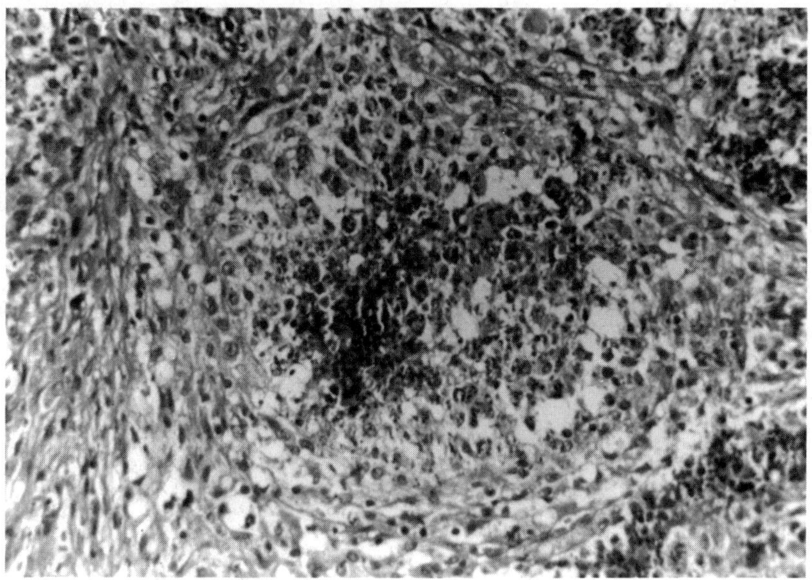

FIG 26–1.
Inflammation with spermatozoa is seen within the wall of the vas deferens.

ensue,[8] just as occurs at puberty if there is congenital absence of the epididymis in the ACI rat.[9] There have been very few reports on the changes within the human testis following vasectomy. In one controlled study significant changes, including thickening of the basal lamina and decreased Sertoli cell and spermatid counts per tubule, were observed.[10] In addition, focal interstitial fibrosis (Fig 26–2), found in almost one fourth of the patients undergoing reversal, was associated with decreased fertility despite patent surgical anastomoses. The use of this finding as a predictive parameter warrants further investigation before application due to the short follow-up period and small size of the patient group studied.

Clinically significant abnormalities in the basal serum levels of testosterone and gonadotropins have not been observed postvasectomy in man. However, a recent study by Fisch and associates[11] comparing men postvasectomy to controls has revealed subtle hormonal changes detectable by a gonadotropin-releasing hormone stimulation test.

Complications of Microsurgical Vasectomy Reversal

Anesthesia

The primary risk of microsurgical vasectomy reversal is related to the type of anesthesia used. Patients undergoing vasovasostomy may receive a local anesthetic. However, a general or regional anesthetic should be used if an epididymovasostomy is anticipated. Most pa-

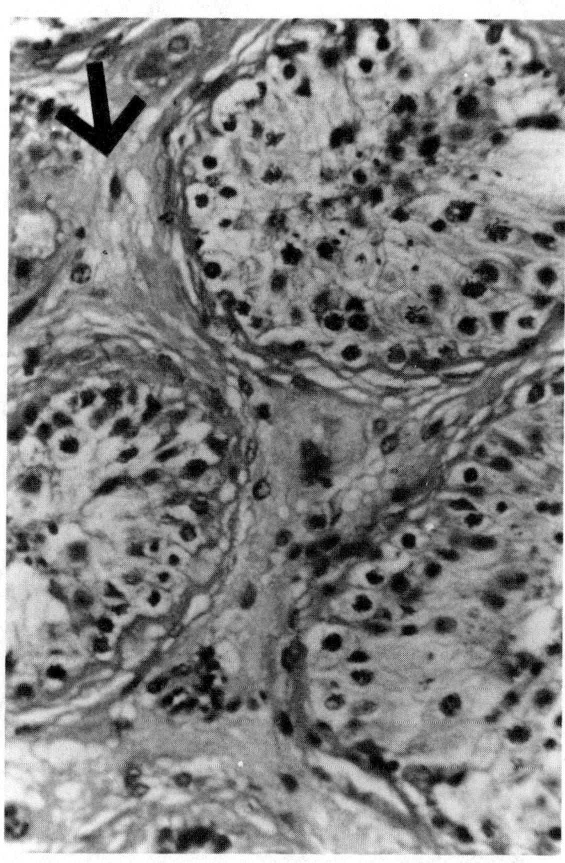

FIG 26–2.
Interstitial fibrosis is seen between the seminiferous tubules in a testis biopsy in a man having a vasectomy reversal *(arrow)*.

tients undergoing this type of surgery are good anesthetic risks. Older patients or patients with significant medical problems should be discouraged from having this operation on the basis of the risks of anesthesia. These patients are rare. There has been no significant mortality or major morbidity in several hundred microsurgical reversal cases reported. Patients have experienced mild complications, including pulmonary congestion, particularly in heavy smokers. Patients are urged not to smoke for at least 1 week before the operation. This procedure is usually performed on an outpatient basis.

Hematoma, Infection, Testicular Atrophy

The other complications that can occur with microsurgical reversal of vasectomy include the local problems related to the operation or wound. Hematoma can occur, but if the operation is done under the microscope we have found that hemostasis is usually much more accurate, and a hematoma is a rare occurrence. Bleeding vessels along the cord or vas deferens are not cauterized with the monopolar cautery. Cauterization in this area should be performed with a bipolar jeweler's forceps to reduce the amount of tissue injury. If heavy cauterization is utilized, it is conceivable that there might be injury to both the spermatic artery or vasal arterial supply. Injury to the spermatic artery may result in testicular atrophy. If there is dissection along the epididymis, dissection is careful and cauterization judicious since the testicular artery is located just below.

Because of the rugae or folds in the scrotum, a careful skin preparation is done, but routine prophylactic antibiotics are not used. Irrigation is performed with dilute polymycin and neomycin solution. Infection is a rare complication.

General Technique—Loupes, Microscope, Instruments, Suture

There are multiple aids in the performance of this surgery. Loupes of ×2 magnification with a headlamp facilitate the initial dissection. Usually a vertical lateral incision on each side of the scrotum is made over the point of previous vasectomy. The magnification and illumination facilitate the surgery. The vas can be easily seen and there is never a problem with moving the spotlight above the table. A variety of loupes are available. Some can be fitted directly into eyeglasses, and others can be mounted in a hingelike fashion over the glasses. It probably makes little difference, as long as the surgeon is comfortable with whatever glasses he uses. Occasionally, the surgeon may be tempted to use higher-power loupes; some surgeons perform the entire operation under ×4 or ×6 magnification. With the higher-power lenses the glasses become both bulkier and heavier. In addition, the field of view narrows and the surgeon and assistant may not be working in the same area at once due to tunnel vision. For that reason, higher magnification has been used with the microscope rather than higher-power loupes.

There are a number of surgical microscopes available, including those made by Zeiss or Nikon. We have been satisfied with the use of a Zeiss microscope. The simpler models may have magnification settings of ×6, ×10, ×16, ×25, and ×40. With a beam splitter, the assistant can look through the microscope at the same field. More elaborate microscopes have both a zoom lens and focus on a foot pedal, which decreases the chance of contamination during the operation. A very bright fiberoptic light system that provides more light is an important feature while operating at higher magnifications. Before commencing the surgery, the interpupillary distance is adjusted and the functioning of the microscope should be verified.

Jeweler's forceps can be obtained readily and are inexpensive. Castroviejo needle holders (nonlocking) work well. A heavy jeweler's forceps can also be used as a needle holder, although the needle is not grasped as securely. A bipolar coagulator with microforceps is necessary for hemostasis. Various clamps have been designed for approximating the free ends of the vas or epididymis, and are commercially available. However, the vas or epididymis may slip out and a traction suture approximating the adventitia on both free ends may be more helpful. Standard microscissors are used for dissection and cutting of the suture. We have usually used cut balloons to provide contrast behind the clamp and the anastomosis. A blunt-tip needle or specially designed ear irrigators can be used for irrigation.

All sutures are monofilament nylon. Sutures of 10-0 (22 μm diameter) are usually utilized for vascular anastomoses, and both 10-0 and 9-0 (35 μm) are used for microsurgical vasovasostomy. Various needles have been specifically designed for use with the vas and are available through Ethicon (Johnson & Johnson) and Sharpoint. A fairly tough needle is required to penetrate the vas and a hooked point is particularly helpful during epididymovasostomy.

General Technique

The general technique of microdissection and microanastomosis is easily learned if the surgeon takes time to study the basics of microsurgical techniques. The needle should go through the wall of the vessel or vas perpendicularly. When a tie is made, it is important that the tie be flat, and usually a surgeon's knot is used as a first throw. Generally, three knots are placed, and it is important for the knots to be square. We have performed both a standard two-layer microsurgical vasovasostomy, employing six 10-0 sutures in the mucosa, with surrounding 9-0 sutures in the muscularis. In the last 50 patients, we have placed six 9-0 sutures through the mucosa and muscularis and then placed additional muscularis sutures. The results appear to be similar with this modified two-layer anastomosis.

Microsurgical epididymovasostomies were previously performed using a specific tubule end-to-end technique. However, the circuitous course of the epididymal tubule within the epididymis led to uncertainty as to which open lumen was actually connected to the testis. The preferred technique today is an end-to-side anastomosis between the vas and epididymis. An opening in the serosa is created just proximal to the site of suspected epididymal obstruction where the tubules appear dilated. The vas is then secured to this area of the epididymis using a suture through the adventitia of the vas and epididymis. A longitudinal incision is made through the side of a specific tubule. The epididymal fluid is then examined under the microscope for sperm. If sperm are present, an end-to-side mucosal anastomosis is performed, using four interrupted 10-0 nylon sutures. The outer layer is composed of interrupted 9-0 nylon sutures between the vas deferens muscularis and epididymal serosa.

Large Gap in the Vas, Occlusion of the Vas, Intravasal Azoospermia

Occasionally a large gap in the vas is encountered at the time of microsurgical reversal when a large segment of the vas is removed. In general, it is still easy to identify both ends of the vas and achieve an adequate anastomosis, as long as both ends are dissected. In some patients, if they have had a previous herniorrhaphy, occlusion of the vas can sometimes occur within the groin. We have also encountered a patient who had had mumps orchitis and developed an atrophic testis on one side and had a herniorrhaphy on the contralateral side with occlusion of the vas. In this situation a transvasovasostomy was used with success (greater than

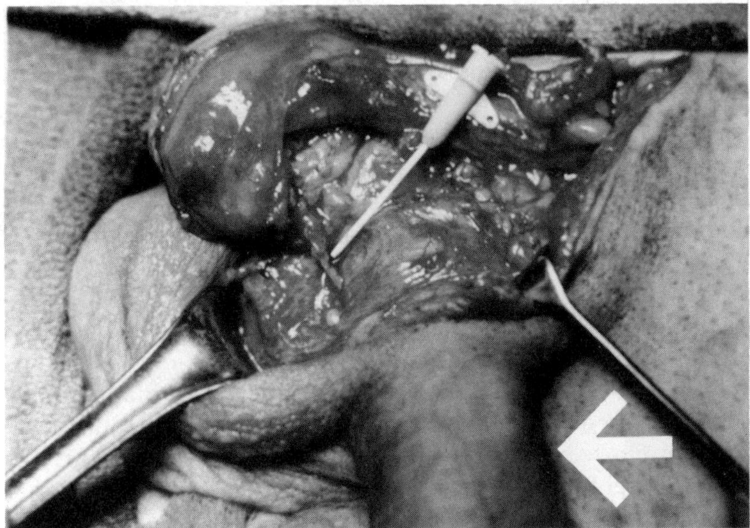

FIG 26–3.
A patient with an atrophic testis on one side and a contralateral occluded vas deferens from a herniorrhaphy required a transvasoepididymostomy. The white angiocatheter identifies the site of the anastomosis (*arrow* indicates penis).

50 million spermatazoa per milliliter, and a pregnancy). Additionally, a transvasoepididymostomy (Fig 26–3) can also be performed. It is relatively easy to perform a transvasovasostomy by bringing the vas from one side under the penis across to the other side and again employing a standard anastomosis.

On occasion, intravasal azoospermia was encountered when the proximal end of the vas was divided. We always do a touch preparation to verify the presence of vasal sperm at the time of reversal. It is sometimes helpful to dilute the specimen because the sperm may be hard to visualize within the debris. The smear can be stained to obtain better results. Intravasal azoospermia may be due to sludging, which may clear spontaneously, or to a more proximal obstruction due to a sperm granuloma. In the past, retrograde epididymograms have been used to delineate the epididymis. However, the hypertonic contrast may damage the unobstructed epididymis and cause a secondary sclerosis.

Sharlip[12] reported that almost 50% of patients with intravasal azoospermia will eventually demonstrate sperm in the ejaculate following a vasovasostomy. The vasovasostomy study group suggest that the quality of the intravasal fluid will help predict this subgroup. The significantly lower success rates with epididymovasostomy suggest that an initial vasovasostomy should be performed in most patients undergoing their first vasectomy reversal. Those patients undergoing reoperation following a failed reversal, patients with long durations of obstruction, and those patients absolutely unwilling or unable to undergo more than one procedure should have an epididymovasostomy if intravasal azoospermia is found. These issues should be discussed with the patient beforehand.

MICROVASCULAR COMPLICATIONS

General Technique

The microvascular anastomoses may be performed end-to-end or end-to-side. Microclamps are always applied. The free ends of the vessels should be matched for size and cleared of all adventitial tissue. Continuous suture is not used, because of the pursestring effect. In general, the first sutures are placed about 120 degrees apart and are left long to act as stay sutures. One side is sutured in an interrupted fashion, the stay sutures are flipped over, and the anastomosis is then completed on the opposite side. The microvascular clamps are then removed and the blood flow can be visualized. One can also use jeweler's clamps to "milk" the blood out of one segment and then release the other clamp to see if there is adequate inflow and vessel filling. If there is great discrepancy in the size of the two vessels, spatulation should be performed to allow for a satisfactory leakproof anastomosis. It is important for the surgeon to be familiar with these techniques since they are somewhat different from those used for vasectomy reversal.

Undescended Testis, Intraabdominal

The intraabdominal testis can sometimes be very difficult to place within the scrotum. The Fowler-Stephens[13] technique can be used, dividing the spermatic vessels and relying on the vasal vascular supply to the testis. Occasionally, this supply may be inadequate and, in certain instances, it may be reasonable to consider anastomosis of the epigastric vessels to the internal spermatic artery and vein.[2, 14] A midline incision is employed for exposure of the intraabdominal testis and the epigastric vessels. The intraabdominal testis can usually be identified very easily, since it is essentially an intraperitoneal organ. Vessels to the vas deferens should be preserved in a broad leaf of peritoneum during the testicular dissection. Care should be taken to identify the testicular artery before division since once divided the testicular vein has a very similar appearance. Appropriate lengths of inferior epigastric artery and vein are dissected free so that they can be turned inferiorly to the scrotum without kinking. An end-to-end anastomosis with 10-0 nylon sutures is carried out between the internal spermatic vessels and the inferior epigastric vessels. In this circumstance, the testis can usually be placed easily within the scrotum.

Penis

Penile Reimplantation.—The penis may be severed because the patient has severe psychiatric disturbances, usually schizophrenia, that led him to self-disfigurement. Occasionally there are accidents involving farm machinery or other traumatic injuries.

The organ is debrided as necessary. The urethra with the corpus spongiosum is reanastomosed with absorbable suture. The corpora cavernosa can also be reanastomosed and the deep dorsal artery, vein, and nerve can also be anastomosed with 9-0 or 10-0 nylon sutures. In such a case,[15] an essentially normal penis, with good sensation, voiding, and erection, can sometimes result.

Vascularization for Impotence.—Vasculogenic erectile impotence accounts for a major segment of patients over age 40 years with impotence. Various relatively noninvasive diagnostic tests including penile-brachial Doppler, duplex ultrasound scanning, papaverine erection test, and cavernosometry have been used to screen patients for vascular disease. Pudendal angiography may then confirm the site of vascular occlusion and cavernosography the site of venous incompetence.

Numerous microvascular procedures have been described for the treatment of impotent patients with arterial occlusion or venous leakage. These procedures have undergone evolutionary changes over the past 10 years. At this time two microvascular procedures with various minor modifications are being used regularly. These include arterialization of the dorsal vein and arterial "bypass" to the dorsal arteries.

Arterialization of the dorsal vein, described with eponyms for the various modifications, was initially intended for patients with venous incompetence. This procedure is now being applied to patients with all types of vasculogenic impotence. It is still not clear why arterialization of a penile vein should improve potency. It probably should still be viewed as an experimental procedure. The chief complications of this procedure are thrombosis of the anastomosis and hypervascularity of the glans penis. Thrombosis of the anastomosis occurs due to decreased flow and is observed early in the postoperative course in 25% of the patients followed.[3] Prophylactic measures such as heparinization, low-molecular-weight dextran, and aspirin have not significantly reduced the microvascular thrombosis rate with this type of operation. The most likely underlying etiology for this problem is the presence of competent venous valves or the high resistance of the intracorporal vascular bed. Hypervascularization of the glans was observed in 12% of the patients in one series[16] but was subsequently reduced to 3% by performing a distal ligation of the dorsal vein. Intraoperative Doppler evaluation of the glans penis may help detect and correct this problem at the time of surgery.

Most patients with atherosclerotic arterial disease have diffuse disease involving the deep arteries within the corpora. This precludes successful bypass surgery to the dorsal artery. However, those patients with a segmental proximal occlusion are excellent candidates for an end-to-side anastomosis between the inferior epigastric artery and the dorsal artery of the penis.[17] This procedure is highly successful in patients with vascular occlusions due to traumatic injuries. However, a concomitant neurogenic injury must be ruled out. The primary complication of this procedure is failure due to thrombosis of the anastomosis. Various agents have been used to prevent thrombosis, but only heparin has been shown to be effective in a controlled animal study.[18] Another complication is disruption of the anastomosis. This may be caused by too early and vigorous sexual activity and is preventable.

Renal Microvascular Surgery

Many small renal arterial branches have been surgically repaired with bench surgery.[19] Usually loupes would be employed in this circumstance rather than a microscope. We have had an experience with a donor nephrectomy in which a small polar artery was not visualized on angiography prior to renal transplantation. In this circumstance a microvascular end-to-side anastomosis has been employed, preserving 10% to 15% upper pole function. In the past this portion of the kidney was sometimes sacrificed after the vessel was ligated.

Scrotal Groin Flaps

Occasionally, with loss of tissue in the perineum, one can consider a variety of flaps, and usually a microvascular technique is not necessary. The scrotum is very elastic and provides excellent coverage in the perineum. In addition, if necessary, a musculocutaneous flap employing gracilis muscle can be used to close significant defects in the perineum, so the free-flap transfer that has been described in orthopedics has not been generally utilized in urologic management.

REFERENCES

1. Silber SJ: *Reproductive Infertility—Microsurgery in the Male and Female.* Baltimore, Williams & Wilkins Co, 1984.

2. Silber J: Microsurgery for the undescended testis. *Urol Clin North Am* 1982; 9:429.
3. Virag R: Revascularization of the penis, in Bennett AH (ed): *Management of Male Impotence.* Baltimore, Williams & Wilkins Co, 1982.
4. Taxy JB, Marshall FF, Erlichman RJ: Vasectomy: Subclinical pathologic changes. *Am J Surg Pathol* 1981; 5:767.
5. Silber SJ: Epididymal extravasation following vasectomy as a cause for failure of vasectomy reversal. *Fertil Steril* 1979; 31:309.
6. Freund MJ, Weidmann JE, Goldstein M, et al: Microrecanalization after vasectomy in man. *J Androl* 1989; 10:120.
7. Alexander NJ: Autoimmune hypospermatogenesis in vasectomized guinea pigs. *Contraception* 1973; 8:147.
8. Smith G: The effects of ligation of the vasa efferentia and vasectomy on testicular function in the adult rat. *J Endocrinol* 1962; 23:385.
9. Marshall FF, Ewing LL, Zirkin BR, et al: Testicular atrophy associated with agenesis of the epididymis in the ACI rat. *J Urol* 1982; 127:155.
10. Jarow JP, Budin R, Dym M, et al: Quantitative pathologic changes in the human testis following vasectomy: a controlled study. *N Engl J Med* 1985; 313:1252.
11. Fisch H, Laor E, Barchama N, et al: Detection of testicular endocrine abnormalities and their correlation with serum antisperm antibodies in men following vasectomy. *J Urol* 1989; 141:1129.
12. Sharlip ID: The significance of intravasal azoospermia during vasovasostomy: Answer to a surgical dilemma. *Fertil Steril* 1982; 38:496.
13. Fowler R, Stephens FD: The role of testicular vascular anatomy in the salvage of the high undescended testis. *Aust NZ J Surg* 1959; 29:92.
14. O'Brien B, Silver SJ, Rau VK, et al: Microvascular testicular transfer. *J Urol* 1976; 115:452.
15. Cohen BE, May JW Jr, Daly JSF, et al: A successful clinical reimplantation of an amputated penis by microvascular repair: Case report. *Plast Reconstr Surg* 1977; 59:276.
16. Virag R, Bennett AH, Shoukry K: Arterial and venous surgery for vasculogenic impotence: a combined French and American experience. *J Urol* 1989; 141:289A.
17. McDougal WS, Jeffery RF: Microscopic penile revascularization. *J Urol* 1983; 129:517.
18. Greenberg BM, Masem M, May JW Jr.: Therapeutic valve of intravenous heparin in microvascular surgery: An experimental vascular thrombosis study. *Plast Reconstr Surg* 1988; 82:463.
19. Novick AC: Management of intrarenal branch arterial lesions with extracorporeal microvascular reconstruction and autotransplantation. *J Urol* 1981; 126:150.

CHAPTER 27

Complications of Lasers in Urology

Terrence R. Malloy, M.D.
Alan J. Wein, M.D.

GENERAL

In the past decade lasers have become an integral part of urologic surgery. The unique property of lasers has provided advantages not previously available by standard urologic surgery.[1] The following are the salient features provided by the individual lasers in urologic conditions:

1. Tissue may be coagulated, vaporized, or incised by varying the wavelength, power, and time of application of the laser.
2. Tissue contact or traction is not required.
3. Lasers are readily adaptable in all urologic instrumentation.
4. Appropriate lasers can eliminate ureteral and renal calculi without traumatizing surrounding genitourinary structures.

As with any surgical technique, full understanding and training are necessary to properly apply lasers to the individual urologic condition. Serious complications can result when necessary precautions are not followed. Prior to discussing individual urologic system surgery, a discussion of the characteristics of each type of laser is warranted. A thorough understanding of the advantages and limitations of each laser is essential to properly utilize lasers for the appropriate pathologic condition.[2]

LASERS USED IN UROLOGIC SURGERY

In describing lasers, certain terms are used to indicate laser parameters. Table 27–1 indicates the most common indices utilized to express laser potential and effects.

Carbon Dioxide Laser.—The properties of the carbon dioxide (CO_2) laser are shown in Table 27–2. A significant characteristic is its strong absorption in tissues. Ninety-eight percent of the incident energy is absorbed in 0.01 mm of tissue, producing a cutting effect much as a surgical scalpel. The result is an incision that is relatively bloodless with a noncontact technique. Inaccessible areas can be treated.

The principal disadvantage of the CO_2 laser in urology is its inability to penetrate water. Less than 1 mm of water prevents CO_2 laser penetration to tissue, thus obliterating its effectiveness in urine or water-covered cavities. Application through urologic instruments is difficult due to the lack of a practical fiberoptic delivery sys-

TABLE 27–1.
Symbols and Units for Lasers

Term	Designation	Unit
Power	P	Watts (W)
Irradiation time	t	Seconds (s)
Energy	E=P × t	W × S=joules (J)
Irradiated area	A	cm^2
Power density	$1=\frac{P}{A}$	$\frac{W}{cm^2}$
Energy density or dose	$L=\frac{E}{A}$	$\frac{J}{cm^2}$

tem. The CO_2 laser in urology is therefore limited to cutaneous applications or to open surgery.

Argon Laser.—The argon laser has not been utilized extensively in urology. Table 27–3 lists its principal characteristics. The energy of this laser is principally absorbed by the chromogens, melanin, and hemoglobin. Tissue absorption is less than CO_2 but stronger than the neodymium:yttrium-aluminum-garnet (Nd:YAG) laser. It can be utilized through fiberoptic light guides and water does not stop its thermal effect on tissue. Intravenous administration of hematoporphyrin derivatives followed by krypton ion laser violet light photoradiation and argon laser photoradiation has produced tumoricidal effects on superficial bladder cancer and carcinoma in situ.[3, 4]

The disadvantages of the argon laser for eradication of bladder cancer is that tissue penetration is not as deep as the Nd:YAG laser. Argon photoradiation necrosis does not penetrate into the bladder muscle but produces a crater-shaped defect outlined by blackened charred material. Tissue removal increases on elevation of energy density which may ultimately result in a bladder wall perforation. The argon laser is limited to carcinoma in situ (Tis) of the bladder and superficial (T1) cancer.

Neodymium:Yttrium-Aluminum-Garnet Laser.—The Nd:YAG laser is the most widely used laser in urologic surgery. Table 27–4 outlines the salient features of the laser. Tissue penetration is highest with the Nd:YAG laser, providing excellent deep photocoagulation. It can be used in water or urine without any loss of effectiveness. The fiberoptic laser delivery system is effective through all urologic instrumentation. Excellent results

TABLE 27–2.
Properties of Carbon Dioxide Laser

1. Wavelength 10,600 nm
2. Invisible
3. Middle of infrared spectrum
4. Gas as active medium
5. 50 W
6. Strong tissue absorption
7. Scattering negligible; light energy converted into heat at tissue surface
8. Suitable for removal of tissue and for cutting at shallow depths
9. Stopped by 1 mm H_2O

TABLE 27–3.
Characteristics of Argon Laser

1. Wavelength 458–515 nm
2. Visible
3. Green light spectrum
4. Ionized argon as active medium
5. Tissue absorption less than CO_2 but stronger than Nd:YAG laser
6. Thermal action shallower than Nd:YAG laser
7. Application to indications where removal of tissue with simultaneous localized coagulation is desired

TABLE 27–4.

Features of Neodymium: Yttrium-Aluminum-Garnet (Nd: YAG) Laser

1. Wavelength 1,060 nm
2. Invisible
3. Near infrared spectrum
4. Solid state
5. 100 W
6. Optical scattering in tissue considerable; promotes uniform distribution of radiation in tissue
7. Suitable for deep thermal work, with destruction of tissue without removal
8. Slight mechanical damage to tissue surface
9. Can be used through flexible fiberoptic source
10. Can be used in water

have been obtained in treating lesions of the penis, urethra, bladder, ureters, and kidneys.

The disadvantage of the Nd: YAG laser is that specialized training is required to use the technique effectively. Unfamiliarity with the mechanics of the laser and its principles may lead to serious complications.

KTP-532 Laser.—The KTP-532 laser is a frequency-doubled Nd: YAG laser that is passed through a crystal to provide a wavelength of 532 nm (Table 27–5). This is close to the argon laser wavelength (458–515 nm). The tissue penetration is not as deep as the Nd: YAG laser but has a better cutting effect. It can be used through water and urine and has a fiberoptic delivery system. It is extremely effective in treating urethral strictures, urethral valves, and bladder neck contractures. Absorption is high in melanin so it is effective in large genital condylomas in the black population.

TABLE 27–5.

Features of KTP-532 Laser

1. Wavelength 532 nm
2. Visible green-yellow light spectrum
3. Frequency double that of Nd: YAG laser
4. 15 W
5. Can be used through flexible fiberoptic source
6. Removes tissue with simultaneous coagulation

TABLE 27–6.

Features of Pulsed Dye Laser

1. Wavelength 504 nm
2. Visible light spectrum
3. Flash lamp–tunable dye source
4. Delivered through 200-μm laser fiber
5. Will not damage ureteral wall or mucosa

Pulsed Dye Laser.—The pulsed dye laser consists of a flash lamp–pumped tunable dye laser with a wavelength of 504 nm. The pulse duration is 1 μs. Its use in destroying ureteral calculi is based on light absorption, plasma development on the stone's surface, and a repetitive acoustic shock-wave action with resultant stone fragmentation. Table 27–6 lists the principal features of the laser.

Complications are not induced by the laser shock waves since ureteral tissue and urothelium is not damaged.[5, 6] Ureteral injury is principally caused by dilatation or manipulation of ureteroscopes that traumatizes the ureteral wall.

SAFE USE OF LASERS

The safe and proper application of urologic lasers is the responsibility of the urologic surgeon and cannot be delegated to nursing personnel. The urologist must be familiar with the mechanical operations of each individual laser that he plans to utilize. Attendance at a urologic postgraduate course on lasers is mandatory prior to trying to operate with lasers. Certification in laser surgery is necessary for the protection of the patient, the hospital, and the urologist. It is also extremely beneficial that the surgeon spend time with a urologist familiar with lasers prior to attempting his initial laser surgery on his own patients.

Paramount in the safe operation of lasers in the operating room is eye protection.[7] Protective goggles are available for each laser since the individual wavelengths require lens that protect specifically against that laser wavelength. No laser should be activated without the patient and all operating room personnel wearing the correct eye protection.

Individual lasers should only be activated on tissue to be treated. The control pedal should only be under the control of the qualified surgeon. Laser beams should never be tested on drapes, sponges, or any other flammable material. Proper extinguishers should be available in the operating room in case of fire. The CO_2 laser can be stopped with water. Power to the laser should be shut off immediately if there is a suspicion of fire.

LASER APPLICATION FOR SPECIFIC UROLOGIC CONDITIONS

External Genital Condylomata (Human Papilloma Virus Infections and Benign Lesions).—Lasers have become the treatment of choice for the treatment of condylomata acuminata (genital warts). CO_2 lasers, Nd:YAG lasers and the KTP-532 laser have proved effective in numerous series.[8–10] Complications develop when lasers are not applied at the proper power setting. The CO_2 laser should not be used above 5 to 7 W on cutaneous warts. Vaporization must be precise so that deep penetration below the dermis does not occur. Damage to Buck's fascia and to the corpora cavernosa has occurred in isolated instances when the CO_2 laser has been utilized for penile condyloma.[10, 11]

The Nd:YAG and KTP-532 lasers can be applied with great safety by utilizing continuous water irrigation to cool the lesion as photoradiation is applied. Excess penetration of the dermis and underlying structures can thus be prevented.[12] The Nd:YAG laser should not be used above the 15- to 18-W range. The KTP-532 laser should only be used in the range of 5 to 8 W.

With careful application of lasers at the appropriate power setting there should be no complications with condyloma treatment. Strict adherence to power limitations will ensure excellent results.

Another major complication and disadvantage of the CO_2 laser for the treatment of condyloma acuminatum is the production of the plume (smoke) from vaporization which contains human papilloma virus (HPV) particles. Originally this smoke was felt to be biologically inactive, but Malloy and his associates have shown that the plume can contain physiologically active HPV particles.[12] When the CO_2 laser is used, protective filter masks are required for all operating personnel. Effective smoke evacuators are also necessary.

The major advantage of Nd:YAG and KTP-532 lasers over CO_2 laser application is that the condyloma can be irrigated with water while laser photoradiation is applied, thus eliminating any smoke plume and the potential inhalation of the HPV particles.

Cancer of the Penis, Urethral Carcinoma.—Lasers have been effectively utilized in treating squamous cell carcinoma of the penis. Both the CO_2 and Nd:YAG lasers have effectively treated Tis and T1 cancer of the penis. The laser therapy produces effective treatment of the primary site but careful monitoring of lymphatic metastasis must be pursued.[12, 13] Complications can be prevented by proper use of power and energy density so that forward scatter will not affect the corpora cavernosa of the penis.[14, 15]

The Nd:YAG laser can be used to treat urethral cancer, but caution must be exercised to assure complete obliteration of the lesion.[16] Periodic follow-up endoscopy is essential.

Urethral Strictures.—The KTP-532 laser has had promising results in the treatment of urethral strictures (Fig 27–1). The entire stricture can be obliterated with photoradiation (Figs 27–2 and 27–3).[17] The Nd:YAG laser photoradiation has not been as successful since it has less obliterating effect compared to the KTP-532. The complication of forward scatter is less with the KTP-532 laser wavelength since the corpora cavernosa are not affected. The power settings for the KTP-532 laser should be 9 to 13 W. Foley catheters are left to drain the bladder until urethral edema subsides.

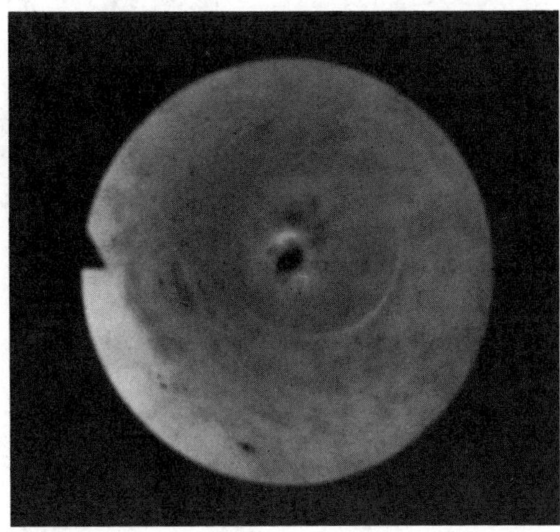

FIG 27–2.
Urethral stricture prior to laser therapy with KTP-532 laser.

Bladder Carcinoma.—The Nd:YAG laser has proved very effective in numerous series in treating superficial transitional cell carcinoma of the bladder—Tis, T0, T1, and T2.[8, 18–22] The results have been excellent with extremely low morbidity. Many patients can be treated as outpatients.[23] The major complication with the application of Nd:YAG laser photoradiation is forward scatter of energy through the bladder wall to affect intraperitoneal organs, i.e., the small and large bowel. In superficial cancers, power settings should be kept below 40 W and the laser application should not exceed 3 seconds on any one area of the tumor. With infiltrating carcinoma of the bladder, the power should not be utilized above 45 to 50 W. In patients with previous radiation to the bladder or intraperitoneal surgery, caution should be exercised since small bowel may be adherent to the bladder making it more susceptible to injury from forward scatter. After Nd:YAG laser

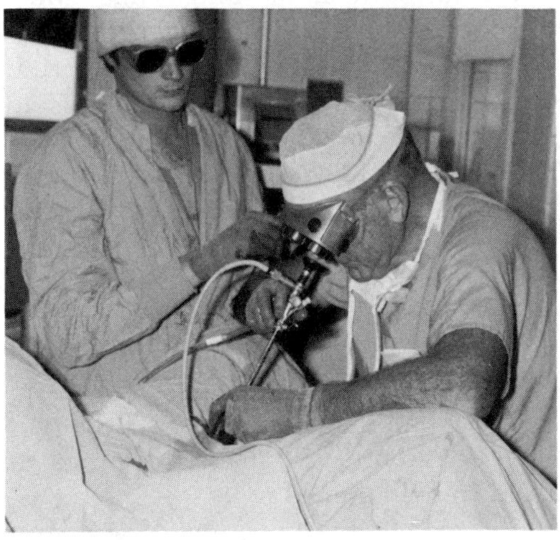

FIG 27–1.
KTP-532 laser applied to urethral stricture.

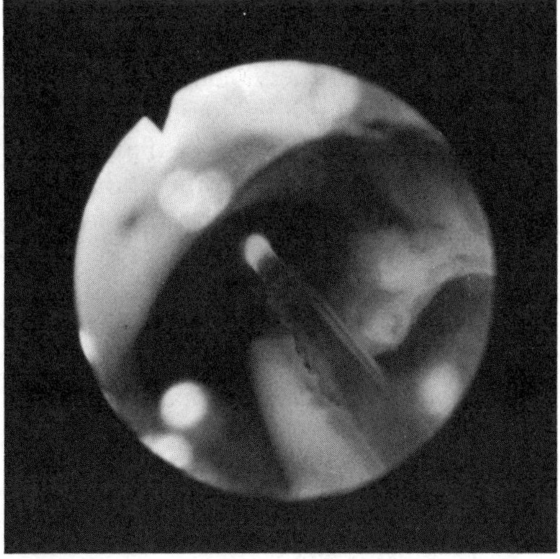

FIG 27–3.
KTP-532 laser light guide has obliterated urethral stricture.

therapy to bladder carcinoma, the patient should be maintained on clear liquids and observed from 6 to 12 hours to elicit signs of abdominal pain or peritoneal irritation. When large amounts of energy are utilized (joules), the patient should be observed for 24 hours for the potential problem of forward scatter to the intraperitoneal organs.

Photodynamic therapy for the treatment of superficial cancer has proved effective in carcinoma in situ and superficial bladder carcinoma.[4, 24] The primary problem with photodynamic therapy has been the lack of deep penetration, which limits treatment to superficial carcinoma of the bladder and carcinoma in situ. The primary complication has been skin sensitization of the patients, requiring total avoidance of sunlight for 6 to 8 weeks posttreatment.

Interstitial Cystitis.—The treatment of interstitial cystitis has met with moderate success utilizing the Nd:YAG laser. Results have been modestly successful in selected series.[25] The major complication of this form of laser therapy is forward scatter to adjacent intraperitoneal organs. These patients' bladder walls are extremely thin with many patients having experienced previous therapy, including intraperitoneal surgery. Bowel often remains adherent to the bladder, increasing the likelihood for bowel perforation and trauma induced by photoradiation thermal energy. Shanberg and Malloy reported on two cases of bowel perforation in their series of 39 patients.[25]

In utilizing the Nd:YAG laser for interstitial cystitis, power settings should not be above 25 W and a total of 25,000 J should not be exceeded. The patient should be placed in a severe lithotomy position in an effort to keep bowel off the posterior bladder wall.

Ureteral Carcinoma.—The Nd:YAG laser has been successful in treating low-grade superficial tumors of the ureter and renal pelvis. Schilling et al. reported on 10 patients treated, with only one recurrence at 14 months.[26] The major complication with this surgery is forward scatter through the thin ureteral or pelvic wall to adversely affect bowel or blood vessels. Power settings should not exceed 25 W with the time of exposure limited to 3 seconds on any one area of cancer. Obviously, injury to the ureter can also occur from ureteroscopic manipulation or the dilatation process. Stenting of the ureter with double-J stents or percutaneous nephrostomy tubes are indicated until ureteral and pelvic integrity is established.

When dealing with transitional cell tumors of the renal pelvis, the urologist must be cognizant of the position of the renal artery and vein. Forward scatter could cause serious thrombosis or perforation of these vessels if power settings are not strictly observed.

Renal Carcinoma.—Renal cell carcinoma in solitary kidneys or bilaterally impaired kidneys presents a challenge to the urologist to remove the neoplasm while preserving renal function. The Nd:YAG laser has proved to be extremely effective in decreasing renal bleeding while reducing the possibility of local recurrence.[27] When open surgical technique is utilized, the Nd:YAG laser can be applied at 35 to 40 W to the amputated surface of the kidney without fear of complications of deep thrombosis of renal vasculature. Rosemberg used the CO_2 laser effectively on various renal conditions that required surgery.[28] Percutaneous endoscopic renal Nd:YAG laser photoradiation described by Smith et al. was successful, with no major complications in nine patients.[29] Strict adherence to power is required to avoid complications.

Ureteral Calculi.—Ureteral calculi that are impacted or too large to pass through the lower one half of the ureter can be effectively obliterated utilizing an endoscopically placed pulsed dye laser. Numerous series have shown the effectiveness of this new laser technology.[30–32] Safety has been excellent as the laser will not damage ureteral tissue. Complications arise from dilatation of the ureter and/or ureteroscopic manipulation. With the introduction of the 7.2 flexible ureteroscope, dilatation is not required prior to insertion. The ureter should be intubated post-lithotomy to prevent edema and temporary colic.[33] If manipulation is a possible cause of ureteral trauma or perforation, diversion should be accomplished with a nephrostomy tube or a double-J stent for 14 to 21 days.

SUMMARY

The use of lasers in urology has become a new and vital surgical tool. Lasers have established their effectiveness in many conditions and their superiority in a few. Urologists should become familiar with the function and application of lasers. Complications can be avoided by understanding the mechanisms of the individual lasers and their proper applications. Training is essential in individual laser operations to guarantee safety for the patient and operating room personnel. This will also ensure the maximum effectiveness of the laser on the urologic condition being treated.

EDITORIAL COMMENT

Many patients ask for treatment by laser whether it be for stones, tumor, or strictures. Although it is a potentially valuable technique, the absence of tissue with the use of some lasers has been a deficiency in cancer patients. Other standard techniques, such as transurethral resection, can still be effective. On the other hand, flexible fiberoptics allows the use of lasers endoscopically, particularly in the destruction of upper tract tumors with a Nd:YAG laser or destruction of ureteral calculi with a pulsed dye laser. Photodynamic therapy has not yet received widespread acceptance. The specificity of this technique is not yet complete and new photodynamic agents will need development in the future before the technique becomes widespread. Drs. Malloy and Wein have wide experience and have summarized the complications with the use of various lasers utilized in urology.

REFERENCES

1. Malloy TR, Wein AJ: Laser technology in urology. *AUA Update Series,* lesson 27, vol 3, 1984.
2. Malloy TR, Wein AJ: Urologic neodymium YAG laser surgery. *Surg Clin North Am* 1984; 64:905.
3. Tsuchiya A, Obara N, Miwa M, et al: Hematoporphyrin derivative and laser photoradiation in the diagnosis and treatment of bladder cancer. *J Urol* 1983; 130:79.
4. Jocham D, Schmiedt E, Baumgartner R, et al: Integral laser-photodynamic treatment of multifocal bladder carcinoma photosensitized by hematoporphyrin derivatives. *Eur Urol* 1986; 12(suppl):43.
5. Dretler SP: Laser lithotripsy: A review of 20 years of research and clinical applications. *Lasers Surg Med* 1988; 8:341.
6. Segura JW, Patterson D: Use of the candela laser in the ureter. *Urol Clin North Am* 1988; 15:365.
7. Frank F, Halldorsson T: Eye-safety requirements for Nd:YAG laser application in gastroenterology, urology and neurosurgery. *Lasers Surg Med* 1984; 4:233.
8. Malloy TR, Wein AJ: Laser treatment of bladder carcinoma and genital condylomata. *Urol Clin North Am* 1987; 14:121.
9. Carpiniello VL, Malloy TR, Sedlacek TV, et al: Results of carbon dioxide laser therapy and topical 5-fluorouracil treatment for subclinical condyloma found by mag-

nified penile surface scanning. *J Urol* 1988; 140:53.
10. Stein BS: Laser treatment of condylomata acuminata. *J Urol* 1986; 136:593.
11. Schaeffer AJ: Use of CO_2 laser in urology. *Urol Clin North Am* 1986; 13:393.
12. Malloy TR, Zderic S, Carpiniello VL: Treatment of external genital lesions, in Smith J (ed): *Lasers in Urologic Surgery*, ed 2. Chicago, Year Book Medical Publishers, 1989, p 23.
13. Rosemberg SK: Lasers and squamous cell carcinoma of external genitalia. *Urology* 1986; 27:430.
14. Malloy TR, Wein AJ, Carpiniello VL: Carcinoma of penis treated with neodymium YAG laser. *Urology* 1988; 31:26.
15. Rothenberger KH: Value of the neodymium YAG laser in the therapy of penile carcinoma. *Eur Urol* 1986; 12(suppl 125).
16. Wishnow KI, Johnson DE: Effective outpatient treatment of Kaposi's sarcoma of the urethral meatus using the neodymium YAG laser. *Lasers Surg Med* 1988; 8:428.
17. Shanberg A, Baghdassarian R, Tansey L: KTP 532 laser in the treatment of urethral strictures. *Urology* 1988; 32:517.
18. McPhee MS, Arnfield MR, Tulip J, et al: Neodymium YAG laser therapy for infiltrating bladder cancer. *J Urol* 1988; 140:44.
19. Washida H, Watanabe H, Sakagami H, et al: The contact Nd:YAG laser system in the treatment of bladder cancer: a preliminary report in 48 patients. *Lasers Surg Med* 1987; 7:524.
20. Shanberg AM, Baghdassarian R, Tansey L: Use of the Nd:YAG laser in the treatment of bladder cancer. *Urology* 1987; 29:26.
21. Beisland HO, Seland P: A prospective randomized study on neodymium-YAG laser irradiation versus TUR in treatment of urinary bladder cancer. *Scand J Urol Nephrol* 1986; 20:209.
22. Hofstetter A: Treatment of urologic tumors by neodymium YAG laser. *Eur Urol* 1986; 12(suppl 21).
23. Malloy TR: Nd:YAG laser in transitional cell cancer of bladder with emphasis on outpatient potential. *Eur Urol* 1986; 12(suppl 1):25.
24. Shumaker BP, Hetzel FW: Clinical laser photodynamic therapy in the treatment of bladder carcinoma. *Photochem Photobiol* 1987; 46:899.
25. Shanberg AM, Malloy TR: Treatment of interstitial cystitis with the neodymium YAG laser. *Urology* 1987; 24:31.
26. Schilling A, Bowering R, Keiditsch E: Use of the neodymium-YAG laser in the treatment of ureteral tumors and urethral condylomata acuminata. *Eur Urol* 1986; 12(suppl 1):30.
27. Malloy TR, Schultz RE, Wein AJ, et al: Renal preservation utilizing the Nd:YAG laser. *Urology* 1986; 27:99.
28. Rosemberg SK: Some guidlines in the use of lasers in renal surgery. *Urology* 1987; 29:141.
29. Smith AD, Orihuela E, Crowley AR: Percutaneous management of renal pelvic tumors: A treatment option in selected cases. *J Urol* 1987; 137:852.
30. Watson G, Murray S, Dretler SP, et al: The pulsed dye laser for fragmenting urinary calculi. *J Urol* 1987; 138:195.
31. Teng P, Nishioka NS, Farinelli WA, et al: Microsecond-long flash photography of laser induced ablation of biliary and urinary calculi. *Lasers Surg Med* 1987; 7:394.
32. Segura JW: Pulsed dye laser for treatment of ureteral calculi. *Urol Clin North Am* 1988; 15:257.
33. Coptcoat MJ, Ison KT, Watson G, et al: Lasertripsy for ureteric stones in 120 cases: Lessons learned. *Br J Urol* 1988; 61:487.

SECTION III

Renal Complications

CHAPTER 28

Complications of Wilms' Tumor and Neuroblastoma

Stephen A. Kramer, M.D.

WILMS' TUMOR

Wilms' tumor is the most common malignant neoplasm in the urinary tract in children. More than 500 new cases occur annually in the United States.[1] This tumor occurs most often during the first 7 years of life, with a peak incidence at 3½ years. Multidisciplinary therapy, including surgical extirpation, chemotherapy, and selected radiation therapy, has produced excellent survival rates in children with localized disease and favorable histologic type (Tables 28–1 and 28–2). Although complications of treatment occur infrequently, they can lead to disastrous consequences.[2] Furthermore, as survival from Wilms' tumor continues to improve, the late adverse effects of treatment assume an increasingly important role in the refinement of tumor therapy. Most patients with Wilms' tumor are now surviving, free of disease, into adolescence and young adulthood. Each of us involved in the care of the child with Wilms' tumor must adhere to careful postoperative staging, meticulous attention to surgical detail, and judicious application of adjuvant chemotherapy and radiation therapy to avoid morbidity and mortality.

Presurgical Evaluation

Methods of Accurate Staging

Excretory Urography.—The radiologic diagnosis of Wilms' tumor is established accurately by excretory urography. Contrast material usually appears promptly in an enlarged kidney, and the pelvicaliceal system is greatly attenuated and distorted.[3] A nonfunctioning Wilms' tumor may occur in up to 10% of patients; it suggests extensive disease, with involvement of the renal pelvis or ureter, extension into the renal vein or inferior vena cava, or extrinsic obstruction of the ureteropelvic junction. Curvilinear calcification occurs in 5% to 10% of patients and is usually located peripherally.

Ultrasonography.—In determining whether an abdominal mass is solid or cystic, ultrasonography is extremely useful. This test may also be used to assess the internal consistency of Wilms' tumor and identify tumor degeneration or liquefaction.[4] Nonfunctioning Wilms' tumor usually demonstrates relatively echo-free zones and scattered internal echoes that probably represent necrotic areas within the mass. Ultrasonography appears to be the most accurate screening test in diag-

TABLE 28–1.

Current Staging of Wilms' Tumor (National Wilms' Tumor Study III)*

Stage	Description
Stage I	Tumor limited to kidney; complete excision. Capsular surface intact; no tumor rupture; no residual tumor apparent beyond margins of resection.
Stage II	Tumor extends beyond kidney but is completely excised. Regional extension of tumor; vessel infiltration; biopsy of tumor performed or local spillage of tumor confined to the flank. No residual tumor apparent at or beyond margins of excision.
Stage III	Residual nonhematogenous tumor confined to the abdomen. Lymph node involvement of hilus, periaortic chains, or site beyond; diffuse peritoneal contamination by tumor spillage or peritoneal implants of tumor; tumor extends beyond surgical margins either microscopically or macroscopically; tumor not completely removable because of local infiltration into vital structures.
Stage IV	Deposits beyond stage III, that is, lung, liver, bone, brain.
Stage V	Bilateral renal involvement at diagnosis.

*From Kramer SA, Kelalis PP: Pediatric urologic oncology, in Gillenwater JY, Grayhack JT, Howard SS, et al (eds): *Adult and Pediatric Urology*. Chicago, Year Book Medical Publishers, 1987, vol 2, pp 2001–2042. Used by permission.

nosing tumor within the inferior vena cava[5] (Fig 28–1). Interestingly, function of the kidney on excretory urography does not rule out intravenous extension and, therefore, assessment of the inferior vena cava should always be made in children with Wilms' tumor.[6] This information is extremely important in planning the proper incision and in avoiding intraoperative embolization of tumor.

Computed Tomography (CT) Scanning.—When excretory urography and ultrasonography are not diagnostic, CT scanning is useful in the differentiation of cystic from solid masses. This study may demonstrate involvement of contiguous structures and detect unsuspected contralateral Wilms' tumor (Fig 28–2). It can follow the tumor response to chemotherapy or radiation therapy and predict the surgical resectability of the tumor.[7] It is also useful in detecting small foci of thoracic or pleural metastasis. Computed tomography scanning in infants and young children often requires general anesthesia.

Magnetic Resonance Imaging.—Magnetic resonance imaging (MRI) is perhaps the most accurate and effective diagnostic method of all current imaging techniques.

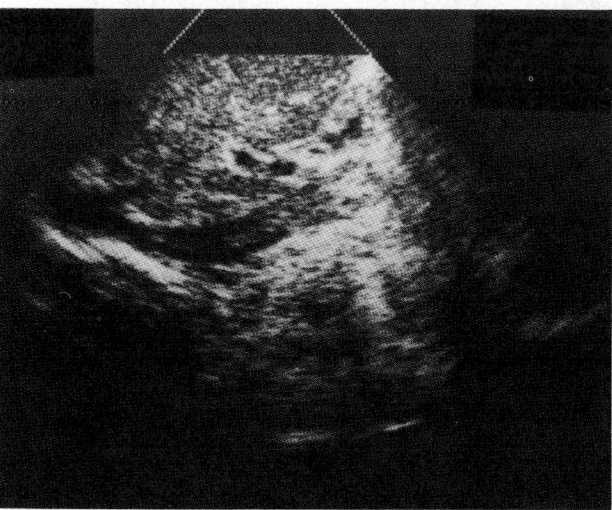

FIG 28–1.

Sagittal echogram shows free-floating intraluminal propagation of tumor thrombus within inferior vena cava. Site of attachment of thrombus to intima is at right of figure, where images blend. Other vascular structures above vena cava are normal intrahepatic vessels. Kidney tumor itself is not visible because it is off the image to right. (From D'Angio GJ, Duckett JW Jr, Belasco JB: Tumors: Upper urinary tract, in Kelalis PP, King LR, Belman AB [eds]: *Clinical Pediatric Urology*, ed 2. Philadelphia, WB Saunders Co, 1985. Used by permission.)

TABLE 28–2.
Results of the Third National Wilms' Tumor Study*†‡

Stage	Histologic Type	No. of Patients	Regimen	Survival (%) RF	Survival (%) 2-yr
I	FH	371	A + V:		
			10 wk	89	94
			6 mo	92	97
II and III	FH	380	±RT:		
			A + V, 15 mo§	83	91
			A + V + AD, 15 mo§	87	91
II	FH	187	A + V ± AD:		
			0 cGy§	91	96
			2,000 cGy§	93	97
III	FH	193	A + V ±AD:		
			1,000 cGy§	78	86
			2,000 cGy§	75	85
Any IV	Any UH	198	RT:		
			A + V + AD, 15 mo	72	81
			A + V + AD + C, 15 mo	66	76

*From Kramer SA, Kelalis PP: Pediatric urologic oncology, in Gillenwater JY, Grayhack JT, Howard SS, et al (eds): *Adult and Pediatric Urology.* Chicago, Year Book Medical Publishers, 1987, vol 2, pp 2001–2042. Used by permission

†A = actinomycin D; AD = doxorubicin; C = cyclophosphamide; FH = favorable histology; RF = relapse-free; RT = radiation therapy; UH = unfavorable histology; V = vincristine.

‡These preliminary data suggest that patients with FH stage I, II, or III disease can be treated successfully with the less intensive regimens and that better treatment is needed for patients with UH or metastasis, or both.

§Collapsed regimens from a factorial design; persistent disease at last follow-up in stage IV was scored as relapse.

This study uses magnetic fields, radiofrequency waves, and computer reconstruction to produce images that resemble x-ray CT scans but differ in information content. In children with abdominal masses, MRI has the capability of imaging in the sagittal and coronal planes, in which important additional data often are yielded. We have been particularly impressed with the ability of MRI to detect

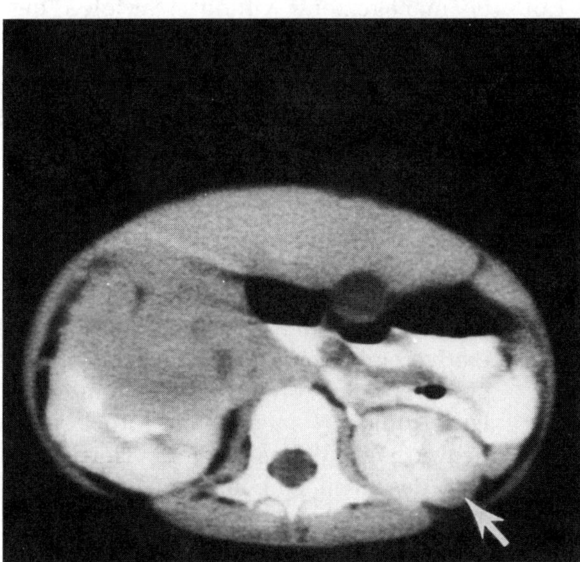

FIG 28–2.
Computed tomographic scan shows large right renal mass consistent with Wilms' tumor. Small left renal mass, not clinically detectable, is also present *(arrow)*. Diagnosis proved to be bilateral Wilms' tumor.

nodal disease and to determine whether vena caval involvement or atrial involvement is present in patients with large tumors.

Inferior Vena Cava Radiography.—In nonfunctioning or poorly functioning kidneys that are determined to be solid by CT scanning or ultrasonography or in patients with clinical signs of caval obstruction, inferior vena cava radiography is indicated. Injection of contrast material into the internal saphenous vein provides visualization of the inferior vena cava and the renal anatomy and eliminates the need for a second injection for an excretory urogram. Because of the ValSalva effect, a patient's crying can result in false-positive cavograms.[8, 9] Sedation often prevents this problem. It is important to know whether a thrombus extends below the diaphragm, into the supradiaphragmatic portion of the inferior vena cava, or into the right atrium.[10] When the cavogram shows complete obstruction, the cephalad extension of the tumor thrombus must be defined by superior vena cava radiography with catheterization of the right side of the heart.[11, 12]

Angiography.—Although used infrequently today in the evaluation of abdominal masses in children, angiography can help determine the extent of disease in patients with bilateral Wilms' tumor and with Wilms' tumor occurring in horseshoe kidneys.[13] The National Wilms' Tumor Study recommends arteriography if (1) the mass is not clearly intrarenal, (2) the lesion is small and cannot be assessed accurately by ultrasonography or CT scanning, (3) tumors are bilateral and heminephrectomy is being considered, and (4) nonvisualization of the kidney cannot be assessed adequately by other methods.[14] Angiography is also helpful in evaluating the extent of liver metastases or direct extension of tumor into other organs.

Other Tests.—Chest roentgenography with frontal and lateral views is essential, because the thorax is the most common site for metastatic disease. Computed tomography scanning of the chest is extremely useful for detecting small metastatic lesions not visible on routine roentgenograms. In patients with hematuria and a nonfunctioning kidney, retrograde pyelography is useful in assessing ureteral metastases and caliceal invasion that would indicate the need for en bloc nephroureterectomy.[15] This study is also indicated in patients with postnephrectomy hematuria to rule out vesical or ureteral metastases from Wilms' tumor.

Needle Biopsy

In patients with suspected massive Wilms' tumor on preoperative evaluation, percutaneous fine-needle aspiration can be accomplished to establish the diagnosis. Primary cytoreductive chemotherapy can then be instituted before exploratory celiotomy. Early experience with this technique indicates that it is safe, reproducible, and reliable as an alternative method of establishing a pathologic diagnosis in children with presumed neoplastic disease.[16] Confirmation of malignancy and identification of the cell type allow appropriate preoperative chemotherapeutic management without fear of a mistaken diagnosis and rule out the possibility of benign disease.

Adjuvant Measures

Inoperable primary tumor may require preoperative treatment to effect surgical extirpation.

Angiographic Embolization.—Preoperative embolization of Wilms' tumor has been reported to allow easier removal of large tumors.[17] In patients with large or hemorrhagic Wilms' tumors, Harrison et al.[18] described embolization of the renal artery with gelfoam particles before nephrectomy. This maneuver tends to reduce vascularity, shrinks the bulk of the tumor by emptying the vascular spaces, and may reduce the incidence of tumor spillage into the renal vein during surgical manipulation.

Preoperative Chemotherapy.—In selected children with surgically unresectable Wilms' tumor proved by biopsy, preoperative chemotherapy has been shown to reduce the size of the mass and to allow partial or total nephrectomy.[19, 20]

Preoperative Radiation Therapy.—Most Wilms' tumors are radiosensitive, and adjunctive radiation therapy, both preoperative and postoperative, has produced significant improvement in relapse-free survival. In selected children, preoperative irradiation reduces the size of large tumors, decreases the incidence of intraoperative rupture of the tumor, and makes excision less hazardous.[14]

Surgical Technique—Prevention of Complications

Preoperative Preparation of the Patient.—All intravenous access should be established through the neck and upper extremities to permit adequate fluid replacement in case of extensive blood loss or caval resection. It is particularly important to avoid placement of infusion lines in the lower extremities, because manipulation of the inferior vena cava during surgery will adversely affect fluid replacement or blood transfusion. Only children in whom an intestinal resection appears likely need undergo preoperative bowel preparation. In equivocal cases, the 24-hour GoLytely preparation can be administered easily and effectively without complication.

Type of Incision.—Surgical extirpation remains the cornerstone of therapy for all children with Wilms' tumor.[14, 21–24] The child is placed in the supine position and then rotated 45 degrees with the involved side up (Fig 28–3). It is important to make a generous transperitoneal incision to afford maximal exposure and prevent intraoperative spillage of tumor.[22] A transverse transperitoneal incision with division of the ipsilateral rectus muscle affords adequate exposure. A formal thoracoabdominal incision is rarely needed; however, this approach may be used for very large tumors involving the upper pole and for excision of ipsilateral pulmonary metastatic lesions. A supine subcostal modification of the thoracoabdominal incision provides equally good exposure in selected patients.[25] When the peritoneal cavity is opened, the extent of tumor should be assessed, the liver inspected, and the periaortic area and vena cava palpated to determine whether primary excision should be done. The flank approach should never be used for children with Wilms' tumor, because adequate staging cannot be done; the abdomen, contralateral kidney, and lymph nodes cannot be assessed accurately; and there is an increased likelihood of tumor spillage.[2, 22, 26]

Contralateral Kidney.—The 5.4% incidence of bilateral Wilms' tumor makes it imperative that the contralateral kidney be explored before the Wilms' tumor is dissected.[14] Gerota's fascia should be opened, and the contralateral kidney should be mobilized from its perirenal fat and fascia to allow thorough inspection and palpation of both anterior and posterior surfaces. Any suspicious lesion or lesions should be biopsied, and the site or sites should be marked with titanium clips. Bilateral Wilms' tumor alters the surgical approach significantly (see below), so the status of the contralateral kidney must be determined *before* nephrectomy.

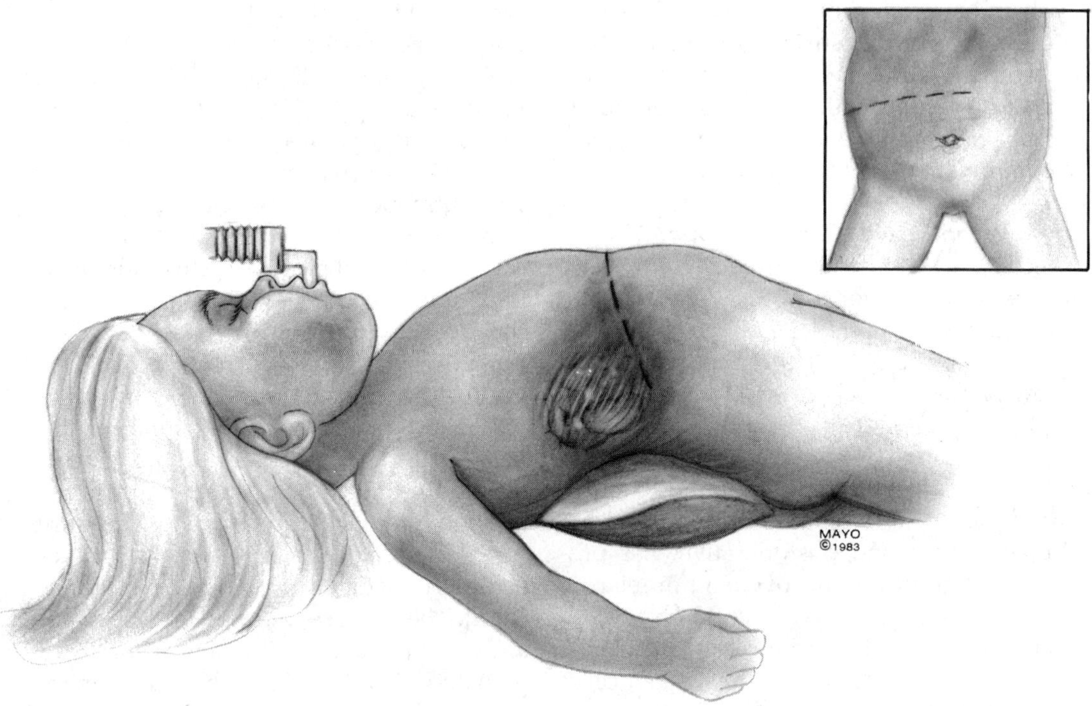

FIG 28–3.
Generous transabdominal incision provides adequate exposure for removal of large Wilms' tumor in children. (From Gilchrist GS, Telander RL: Adrenal medulla and sympathetic chain, in Kelalis PP, King LR, Belman AB [eds]: *Clinical Pediatric Urology,* ed 2. Philadelphia, WB Saunders Co, 1985, vol 2. Used by permission.)

Mobilization of Colon.—The colon is mobilized from the anterior surface of the kidney by incising the white line of Toldt. The colon is reflected medially, with care being taken to preserve all mesenteric vascular supply.

Ligation of Renal Pedicle.—The renal vein is often splayed over the tumor and must be handled with extreme caution. Although early ligation of the renal vein does not appear to have an appreciable effect on the patient's survival, it is important to separately ligate the renal vein and artery early to avoid tumor manipulation and possible dissemination. The surgeon should isolate and ligate the renal artery first, to avoid increased venous pressure within the tumor, which may predispose to dissemination or rupture of the tumor.

Surgical Extirpation.—Complete surgical extirpation implies removal of the perirenal fascia, adrenal gland (with upper pole tumors), and tumor without the opening of Gerota's fascia. Recent evidence, however, suggests that simple nephrectomy is associated with similarly good survival rates. Tumors that have grown into the surrounding structures are removed in continuity if possible. This resection can include a segment of the colon, segment of the spleen, tail of the pancreas, portion of the stomach, segment of the diphragm, or part of the psoas muscle.[2] However, heroic surgical efforts to remove all tumor are not necessary; leaving small amounts of tumor behind has not been associated with more frequent abdominal recurrences or a decrease in survival.[22] A nonresectable tumor should be identified with titanium clips to allow accurate delineation for postoperative radiation therapy. These clips are radiopaque and, unlike metallic clips, do not scatter the beam during postoperative CT scanning. Chemotherapy and radiation therapy are then administered. Second-look procedures are accomplished thereafter for excision of residual disease (Fig 28–4). Bench surgery has been performed, but it should be reserved for highly selected cases.[27, 28]

Caval Extension of Tumor.—Wilms' tumor extends into the inferior vena cava in approximately 6% of cases and may be clinically asymptomatic in more than 50%.[6, 6a] Involvement of the renal vein or inferior vena cava by tumor does not adversely affect the prognosis if treatment is appropriate.[22] The renal vein and vena cava should be palpated carefully for intraluminal tumor. The surgeon should be thoroughly familiar with the anatomy of the normal collateral circulation of the renal veins and inferior vena cava as well as the pathophysiology of caval or renal vein obstruction[6] (Fig 28–5).

Tumor thrombus within the vena cava can be (1) free-floating, (2) adherent to the wall of the inferior vena cava, (3) infiltrating the wall of the inferior vena cava, or (4) extending into the right atrium. In patients with *free-floating tumor thrombus,* vasculature is controlled by the placing of vessel loops or clamps proximally and distally on the vena cava and around the contralateral renal vein. Once vascular control is established, a cavotomy is performed and the tumor is extracted. The procedure should be done with the pa-

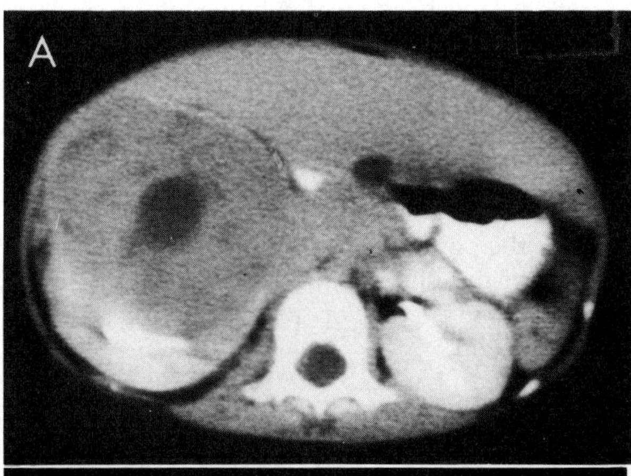

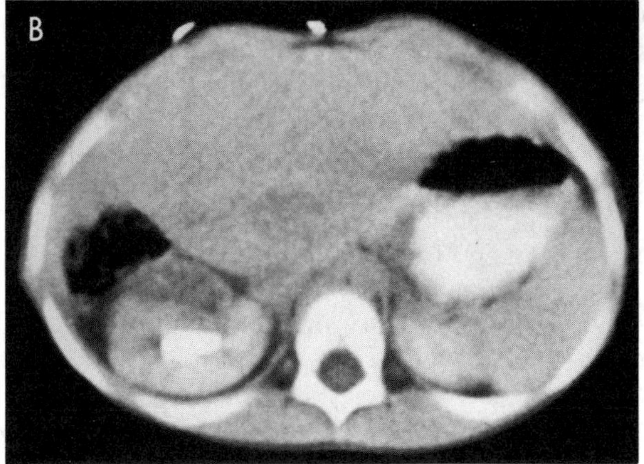

FIG 28–4.
Computed tomographic scans. **A,** large solid right renal mass proved on biopsy to be Wilms' tumor. **B,** after cytoreductive chemotherapy and radiation therapy, right renal mass is much smaller. Patient underwent successful right heminephrectomy, with excision of all tumor.

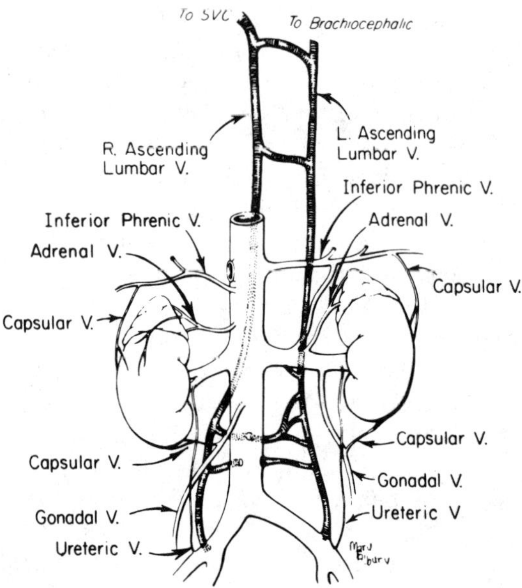

FIG 28–5.
Normal collateral circulation of renal veins and inferior vena cava. (From Clayman RV Jr, Gonzalez R, Fraley EE: *J Urol* 1980; 123:157–163. Used by permission.)

tient in the Trendelenburg position to avoid air embolus.

Tumor thrombus adherent to the wall of the inferior vena cava can be extracted by the Fogarty or Foley balloon catheter. After proper vascular control has been secured, either one of these catheters is placed into the vena cava, and the intracaval thrombus is extracted through the venotomy site. After recovery of thrombus, the inferior vena cava is flushed with saline, the contents are aspirated, and the vena cava is refilled with blood after release of the contralateral renal vein clamp and distal inferior vena caval clamp initially to displace intraluminal air. The venotomy is then closed with running 5-0 Prolene sutures.

In patients with retrohepatic extension of tumor into the inferior vena cava, the liver must be released by division of the triangular, coronary, and falciform ligaments. This technique involves systematic clamping of the superior mesenteric artery, porta hepatis, distal portion of the inferior vena cava, contralateral renal vein, and then the proximal portion of the inferior vena cava before suprahepatic clamping of the inferior vena cava (Pringle maneuver). This technique is important in decreasing hemorrhage and sequestration of blood in the liver.

Infiltration of the wall of the inferior vena cava by tumor thrombus often requires resection of the vena cava. The left renal vein usually has adequate collateralization from the adrenal, phrenic, gonadal, and lumbar vessels.[29] In right-sided Wilms' tumor, resection of the vena cava may be appropriate only if adequate collateralization can be demonstrated to the left kidney.

If pressures in the occluded contralateral renal vein are increased after nephrectomy and caval resection, the renal vein must be reanastomosed to another vein to establish adequate drainage. In cases of right nephrectomy, the left renal vein can be anastomosed to the splenic vein or reanastomosed to the inferior vena cava with an interposition vein graft or Dacron graft. In cases of left nephrectomy, the right renal vein can be anastomosed to the portal vein[30] or to the superior portion of the divided inferior vena cava through a vein graft or prosthetic interposition graft.

In patients with *endocardiac extension of tumor,* a sternal splitting and midline abdominal incision or a combined median sternotomy and thoracoabdominal approach provides excellent exposure of the right atrium and intrapericardial portion of the inferior vena cava.[5] Extracorporeal circulation is required in these situations, and it is necessary that a combined approach with a cardiac surgeon be undertaken. Tumor that has extended into the atrium can be removed directly by the thoracic team, and thrombus in the inferior vena cava can be removed by a Fogarty or Foley balloon catheter passed up through a venotomy in the abdominal vena cava.

Lymphadenectomy.—The presence or absence of lymph node metastasis is of major importance in determining relapse-free survival; thus, patients should undergo regional lymphadenectomy with selective sampling of suspicious nodes.[3] There is no evidence, however, that lymph node resection alters the outcome in patients with Wilms' tumor; therefore, formal and aggressive lymph node dissection is neither warranted nor recommended.

Bilateral Wilms' Tumor.—The incidence of synchronous bilateral Wilms' tumors ranges from 4.4%[31] to 7%.[32] In approximately one third of patients, bilateral Wilms' tumors have not been recognized before surgical exploration.[33] This fact emphasizes the need for visual inspection and palpation of both kidneys intraoperatively. The third National Wilms' Tumor Study group established guidelines based on histologic type of neoplasm for bilateral Wilms' tumors. In patients with favorable histologic patterns, the bilateral tumors are biopsied and lymph node sampling is accomplished. Chemotherapy is administered postoperatively, with the drug regimen and interval determined by the most advanced stage of disease. Second- and third-look procedures follow adjunctive chemotherapy with attempts at maximal conservation of renal parenchyma by either excisional biopsies or partial nephrectomies. In patients with bilateral Wilms' tumor and unfavorable histologic patterns, the diagnosis is established initially by renal biopsies, and postoperative chemotherapy is administered with actinomycin D, vincristine, and doxorubicin for 15 months; a dose of 1,500 rad is directed to the flank. During a second-look procedure, nephrectomy or bilateral nephrectomy is indicated if there is any chance that more conservative measures will not remove all tumor.

Horseshoe Kidney.—There is an increased incidence of Wilms' tumor in children with horseshoe kidney.[34, 35] The treatment of choice is ipsilateral nephrectomy with removal of the isthmus. If tumor arises in the isthmus itself, surgery involves isthmusectomy with resection of both lower poles.

Specific Complications

Vascular

Arterial.—Iatrogenic injury to the aorta or its major branches during nephrectomy for Wilms' tumor has been reported rarely. These catastrophic injuries have most often been identified intraoperatively and repaired by primary reanastomosis or with an interpositional hypogastric artery graft. Four patients in the third National Wilms' Tumor Study had superior mesenteric artery injuries intraoperatively.[36] In three of them, gastrointestinal complications did not develop postoperatively, whereas the fourth patient required small bowel resection and eventually died in the perioperative period. In particularly large tumors, one or both contralateral renal vessels may be ligated mistakenly. One should avoid these serious errors by identifying the aorta and vena cava and, if necessary, the contralateral renal artery and vein before ligating and dividing the vessels to the involved kidney. In young patients, the inferior mesenteric artery can usually be divided, if necessary, with impunity. It is important, however, to ligate this artery close to the aorta to preserve the marginal artery of Drummond.

Venous.—In adults, ligation of the left renal vein is safe if there are adequate venous collaterals from the adrenal, inferior phrenic, gonadal, lumbar, and retroaortic venous plexuses.[37] In children, however, the experience with left renal vein ligation is limited.[38] Miedema and

Stubenbord[39] reported that a 10-month-old boy had complete renal failure and later died after left renal vein ligation in association with right nephrectomy for Wilms' tumor. At least three cases of renal dysfunction after left renal vein ligation have been reported, and one required dialysis.[38, 40–42] Revascularization procedures, often required, usually involve primary reanastomosis of the left renal vein to the inferior vena cava. During revascularization, it is most important to continue adequate hydration and perhaps heparinization intraoperatively and postoperatively.

Extension of Wilms' tumor through the inferior vena cava into the heart presents a technical challenge to the surgeon and has been associated with significant morbidity.[43]

Caval extension of tumor must be approached cautiously, because patients who undergo cavotomy are at risk for air embolus. This complication can be prevented if the patient is placed in the Trendelenburg position before the inferior vena cava is opened and if air is aspirated with refilling of blood before closure of the venotomy (see above).

Tumor thrombus with extension into and obstruction of the inferior vena cava and hepatic veins may produce an acute Budd-Chiari syndrome. Primary chemotherapy followed by successful excision of the tumor and tumor thrombus with cardiopulmonary bypass has been reported.[44]

Potentially fatal intraoperative tumor embolization to the pulmonary artery may occur in patients with endocardiac extension of tumor. This complication should be prevented by a thorough and detailed preoperative evaluation that determines the extent of the tumor thrombus.

In a recent review of 15 patients from the second National Wilms' Tumor Study who had intraatrial tumor thrombus, 11 had operative complications. Major intraoperative hemorrhage occurred in 6 patients, and tumor embolization occurred in 2.[43] Removal of a tumor thrombus extending into the heart requires a combined approach with a cardiac surgeon and extracorporeal circulation. A midline abdominal incision allows extension into a median sternotomy and avoids abdominal wall collaterals. The contralateral kidney is explored first. The affected tumorous kidney is then mobilized and resected before heparinization for cardiopulmonary bypass. After nephrectomy, the patient is heparinized and cardiopulmonary bypass is begun. Circulatory arrest, hypothermia, and total exsanguination allow removal of the inferior vena caval thrombus and atrial thrombus in a bloodless field.

Adjacent Organs

Bowel.—Wilms' tumor occasionally invades the bowel wall and necessitates resection of part of the small or large intestine. Identification and preservation of all the mesenteric blood supply are mandatory to avoid ischemic necrosis. This situation can be compounded if radiation therapy is required postoperatively, causing further diminution of the vascular supply and radiation colitis.

Liver.—Wilms' tumor arising from the right kidney may extend into the liver and form a dense pseudocapsule secondary to adhesions of the affected kidney to the liver itself. This extension is often removable without the need for partial hepatectomy. Extension into the liver itself is rare, and it is most unusual that extended hepatic resection is required for metastatic disease confined to the liver. In both situations, careful mobilization of the liver is mandatory to avoid brisk and extensive bleeding from the short hepatic veins.

The most frequent hepatic complications of Wilms' tumor treatment occur within 2 months after completion of abdominal radiation therapy, particularly in right-sided disease, and consist of transient hepatomegaly, ascites, and mild elevation of the serum transaminase value.[45] Late complications in long-term survivors of Wilms' tumor include portal hypertension after irradiation injury.[46, 47] Barnard et al.[48] reported on a patient with noncirrhotic portal fibrosis after therapy for Wilms' tumor. These authors recommended that survivors of Wilms' tumor be periodically reassessed for evidence of liver dysfunction and portal hypertension.[48]

Pancreas.—Cutaneous pancreatic fistulas may occur as a result of injury to the pancreas at the time of left nephrectomy. Furthermore, resection of the tail of the pancreas may be necessary to allow en bloc removal of the tumor. In this situation, it is essential that the cut end of the pancreas be carefully oversewn with a running locked silk suture to avoid pancreatic fistulas.[49, 50]

Spleen.—Wilms' tumor rarely involves the spleen, and it is usually possible to dissect off the spleen by elevating it superiorly and anteriorly. Splenectomy is usually the result of iatrogenic injury during retraction. Splenic laceration can most often be prevented by use of a well-padded Deaver retractor and judicious retraction in the left upper quadrant. Young children are at increased risk for sepsis and death from pneumococcal infection after splenectomy.[51] It is important, therefore, that every attempt be made to preserve the spleen by either partial or subtotal splenectomy.[52]

Diaphragm.—When the tumor extends into the diaphragm, the diaphragm can usually be resected and closed primarily. In selected patients with large defects, Marlex mesh has been used successfully.

Cisterna Chyli.—Chylous ascites may be caused by inadvertent disruption of the cisterna chyli during nephrectomy and lymph node dissection.[53] Electrocauterization is inadequate to seal the lymphatic vessels, and the treatment of choice is ligation of the cisterna chyli.[2] Ascites usually resolves spontaneously but may require several paracenteses.

Adrenal Gland.—The adrenal gland is usually removed en bloc with upper pole lesions. It is important to preserve at least one adrenal gland during resection of bilateral upper pole tumors. Inadvertent bilateral adrenalectomy during excision of bilateral Wilms' tumors produces a hypotensive crisis postoperatively and necessitates long-term mineralocorticoid and glucocorticoid supplementation.

Lung.—Pulmonary nodules can be managed with wedge excision of gross tumor if involvement is ipsilateral. In patients with bilateral pulmonary tumors, thoracotomy is deferred, both lung fields are irradiated preoperatively, and residual tumor is excised at a second-look procedure. Patients undergoing pulmonary resection of metastatic lesions must be monitored for atelectasis or pneumothorax postoperatively.

Whole-lung irradiation is associated with immunosuppression. Diffuse interstitial pneumonitis was reported in 13% of patients with stage IV disease in the third National Wilms' Tumor Study.[54] Each patient had undergone whole-lung-field irradiation. The cause of the pneumonia was *Pneumocystis carinii* in 3 patients, varicella in 1 patient, and unknown in 15 patients. Diffuse interstitial pneumonitis that develops within the first 3 months after pulmonary irradiation should not be classified as "radiation pneumonitis" until a complete evaluation to rule out an infectious agent has been undertaken. Immunofluorescent staining with a monoclonal antibody, bronchoalveolar lavage, or open lung biopsy may be necessary to determine the specific cause of the pneumonitis.[54]

Brain

Intracranial metastasis from Wilms' tumor occurs rarely and almost exclusively with sarcomatoid Wilms' tumor. Spontaneous intracranial hematoma is an unusual clinical presentation of brain metastasis.[55] Metastatic Wilms' tumor to the brain with cerebral hemorrhage, loss of consciousness, and convulsions has been reported in the absence of pulmonary metastasis.[56]

Kidney

The occurrence of renal disease after treatment may be related to a delayed effect of the tumor treatment or an intrinsic abnormality of the kidney related to the tumor process. Glomerular disease, either focal glomerulosclerosis or membranoproliferative glomerulonephritis, may be present at the time the Wilms' tumor is first detected or may develop in the remaining kidney after successful treatment of Wilms' tumor.[57–59] The kidney that remains after nephrectomy may be at risk for hemodynamic injury caused by progressive glomerular damage from hyperfiltration, an adaptive mechanism of compensatory hypertrophy after nephrectomy.[59, 60]

In a long-term follow-up of 22 patients with solitary kidneys who had undergone nephrectomy for Wilms' tumor, Kramer and Ritchey[61] found only minimal increases of serum creatinine concentration and proteinuria. Hypertension, radiographic evidence of pyelonephritic scarring, obstructive uropathy, or calculi did not develop in any of the patients.

The combined occurrence of glomerular disease, proteinuria, genital anomalies, and Wilms' tumor has been described by Drash et al.[62] The nephrotic syndrome and renal insufficiency may develop if the patient survives beyond early infancy.

Urinary extravasation may occur after partial nephrectomy, isthmusectomy for horseshoe kidney, or inadvertent injury to the ureter. Urinary extravasation can be handled effectively with drainage and stenting. Percutaneous placement of nephrostomy tubes and ureteral stents has obviated reexploration in most patients.

Miscellaneous

Wilms' tumor is one of the malignant lesions associated with acquired von Willebrand's disease.[63] Patients with Wilms' tumor who have excessive bruising on presentation should be evaluated for acquired von Willebrand's disease, since at least two cases with this association have been reported.[63, 64] Coagulation abnormalities usually resolve after treatment of the malignant renal tumors.

The combination of Wilms' tumor and consumption coagulopathy is rare but has been associated with venous thrombosis and death.[65] Removal of the tumor may result in return of clotting factors to normal and clinical improvement of the patient.[66, 67]

As increase in serum calcium concentration has been reported in patients who have malignant rhabdoid tumors of the kidneys without skeletal metastasis.[68] Hypercalcemia may be related to increased N-terminal parathormone serum levels before nephrectomy.[69] Complete disappearance of hypercalcemia after surgery confirms that a humoral factor from the tumor was responsible for the increase in serum calcium levels.[68]

Spillage of Tumor

Meticulous surgical technique is mandatory, because spillage of tumor results in an increased incidence of abdominal recurrence and higher mortality.[22] Thus, the tumor must be handled gently, and excess manipulation must be avoided.

Careful control of the venous outflow is essential. Once the renal pedicle, particularly the renal artery, has been ligated, the tumor tends to become quite soft and is much more likely to rupture. Local spillage of tumor confined to the flank is stage II disease; diffuse peritoneal contamination by tumor spillage is stage III. Thus, even minimal spillage of tumor requires more extensive chemotherapy and radiation therapy postoperatively and places the patient at risk for potential side effects of adjuvant therapy.

Sequelae of Therapy

Acute Toxicity

Bone marrow toxicity and hepatic toxicity are the most frequent acute complications after treatment of children with Wilms' tumor.[14] Bone marrow suppression occurs most commonly in the earliest months of treatment in patients undergoing both chemotherapy and radiation therapy. Acute toxicities in the liver, kidney, or lungs are rarely severe enough for one to discontinue chemotherapy despite the ability of actinomycin D and doxorubicin to reactivate latent radiation damage.

Late Toxicity

The Late Effects Study Group found that 28% of survivors had appreciable sequelae at 5-year follow-up. The most common among these were infections due to absent spleens (previous splenectomy), renal failure, severe scoliosis, and bowel obstruction. Thirty percent of children had some degree of clinically significant musculoskeletal abnormality after irradiation. The most common side effect of radiation therapy is scoliosis with or without kyphosis.[70] Up to 73% of children who have received radiation therapy for Wilms' tumor have had some disturbance of growth within the treatment field.

Second malignant neoplasms can develop in survivors of Wilms' tumor. Most of these occur in irradiated areas. The predominant tumors have been soft-tissue sarcomas, bone tumors, leukemia, and lymphomas.[71]

NEUROBLASTOMA

Neuroblastoma, the most common solid tumor of infancy and childhood, accounts for approximately 50% of all neonatal malignancies. The tumor occurs in about 1 of every 10,000 live births.[72] The peak age at presentation is 1½ years. Age at the time of diagnosis remains the single most important factor influencing prognosis in patients with neuroblastoma[73, 74] (Fig 28–6). Although several other childhood cancers have shown excellent response rates to multidisciplinary therapy, the treatment and prognosis for neuroblastoma have remained disappointing over the past several years. Despite a trial of several chemotherapeutic agents, with and without radiation therapy, the 2-year survivorship for patients with neuroblastoma remains approximately 20% overall (Tables 28–3 and 28–4).

The widespread use of prenatal ultrasonography in the detection of fetal abnormalities has allowed earlier detection of neuroblastoma in utero. Fetoplacental anasarca secondary to fetal neuroblastoma

TABLE 28–3.
Staging of Neuroblastoma*

Stage	Description
Stage I	Tumor limited to organ of origin
Stage II	Regional spread that does not cross the midline
Stage III	Tumors extending across the midline
Stage IV	Distant metastases
Stage IV-S	Small primary tumor and metastases limited to liver or skin or bone marrow without radiographic evidence of bone metastasis

*From Kramer SA, Kelalis PP: Pediatric urologic oncology, in Gillenwater JY, Grayhack JT, Howard SS, et al (eds): *Adult and Pediatric Urology.* Chicago, Year Book Medical Publishers, 1987, vol 2, pp 2001–2042. Used by permission.

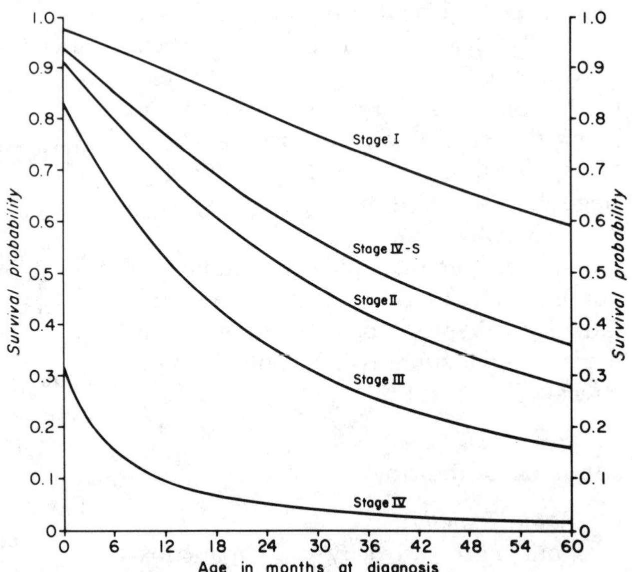

FIG 28–6.
Probability of survival by stage and age in months at diagnosis for patients free of disease for 2 years; 246 patients were analyzed. (From Breslow N, McCann B: *Cancer Res* 1971; 31:2098–2103. Used by permission.)

has been diagnosed by prenatal ultrasonography.[75]

Presurgical Evaluation

Methods of Accurate Staging

Most patients with neuroblastoma are first seen because of an abdominal mass, which is usually fixed and nodular and often extends across the midline. Sudden enlargement of the mass may be secondary to hemorrhage within the tumor.

TABLE 28–4.
Number of Patients with Neuroblastoma Surviving 2 Years by Age and Stage at Diagnosis*†

	Stage					
Age (yr)	I	II	III	IV	IV-S	%
<1	12/14	10/11	5/8	5/15	14/21	67
1–2	4/4	3/5	4/7	2/33	0/0	26
>2	6/8	2/5	0/10	12/81	1/1	20
Total, %	85	71	36	15	68	

*From Duckett JW: Neuroblastoma, in Glenn JF (ed): *Urologic Surgery*, ed 3. Philadelphia, JB Lippincott Co, 1983, pp 55–61. Used by permission.
†The population consists of 223 patients in whom the diagnosis was made between February 1942 and December 1978. Data are from the Tumor Registry, Children's Hospital of Philadelphia, March 1981.

Neonatal neuroblastoma may rupture during delivery and produce significant intraabdominal bleeding, renal failure, and death.[76] The first sign of illness may be due to widespread disease, which causes weight loss, irritability, fever, anemia, and bone pain from skeletal metastases.

Excretory Urography.—The radiologic diagnosis of neuroblastoma is suggested by excretory urography. The kidney, ureter, and bladder examination shows stippled calcification in 50% to 65% of patients and peripheral calcification in approximately 10%. The tumor most often displaces the kidney inferiorly and laterally, creating a "drooping lily" appearance.[77] Lateral films are helpful in showing anterior displacement of the tumor. A paraureteral tumor may displace one ureter laterally and cause ureteral compression with hydronephrosis or may simulate a ureteropelvic junction obstruction. Upward and lateral displacement of the lower pole of the kidney suggests that the tumor is arising in the lumbar sympathetic chain. Infrequently, the tumor invades the renal parenchyma, creating caliceal distortion and making differentiation from Wilms' tumor very difficult.

Ultrasonography.—As an initial screening procedure, ultrasonography is helpful in distinguishing between solid and cystic masses and in defining the organ or structure of tumor origin. Ultrasonography cannot readily detect tumor extension into the mediastinum and lacks the precision of CT scanning in defining anatomical relationships.

Computed Tomographic Scanning.—For the detection and delineation of primary neuroblastoma and recurrent tumor, CT is extremely sensitive.[78] Serial scanning provides a method of monitoring the response to therapy in inoperable cases and in assisting the surgeon in evaluating the feasibility of delayed excision after chemotherapy or radiation therapy. In infants and young children, sedation and occasionally general anesthesia are required to obtain satisfactory studies.

Magnetic Resonance Imaging.—Magnetic resonance imaging is proving extremely useful for the initial diagnosis, confirmation, or exclusion of extradural tumor extension and determination of the extent of disease in patients with neuroblastoma. This study is particularly helpful in demonstrating vascular displacement or encasement by tumor. As it is with Wilms' tumor, MRI appears to be the best imaging technique for characterizing the tumor and following the response of tumor to chemotherapy or radiation therapy.

Radionuclide Bone Scanning.—This test should be used as the screening procedure of choice in children thought to have skeletal metastasis. *Radiologic bone surveys* reveal lytic or blastic skeletal metastases and help confirm the diagnosis of neuroblastoma.

Bone Marrow Aspiration and Biopsy.—Before surgery in all children with suspected neuroblastoma, bone marrow aspiration and biopsy should be performed. Up to 70% of children may have evidence of bone marrow involvement that does not necessarily correlate with radiologic evidence of skeletal metastases.[79]

Tumor Markers.—Vanillylmandelic acid and homovanillic acid are tumor markers that are by-products of catecholamine metabolism that are most often measured clinically. One or more of these tumor markers is elevated at the time of diagnosis in up to 90% of patients with neuroblastoma.[80] Measurement of these urinary metabolites is valuable not only for diagnosis but also for following tumor activity during and after therapy.[81]

Needle Biopsy

In patients with suspected massive neuroblastoma on preoperative evaluation, percutaneous fine-needle aspiration can be accomplished to establish the diagnosis.[16] Cytoreductive chemotherapy and radiation therapy may then be begun before exploratory laparotomy, as described under Wilms' Tumor.

Surgical Technique—Prevention of Complications

Preoperative Preparation of the Patient.—Anemia and any metabolic abnormalities should be corrected preoperatively. Hypertension occurs in approximately 5% of children and should also be controlled before surgery. All intravenous access should be established through the neck and upper extremities to permit adequate fluid replacement. Patients with neuroblastoma do not routinely require preoperative bowel preparation.

The operative principles for the treatment of abdominal neuroblastoma are similar to those recommended for Wilms' tumor. Neuroblastoma in the abdomen usually arises from the adrenal gland but may arise from the sympathetic chain or the organs of Zuckerkandl. The surgeon should evaluate carefully the feasibility of complete surgical extirpation of the tumor, because surgical resection is still the most successful means of curing localized disease.[82]

Localized and mobile adrenal lesions that do not invade the surrounding structures can be resected without nephrectomy. Neuroblastoma rarely invades the renal parenchyma, but it may be so adherent to the renal hilum and vessels that nephrectomy is necessary to remove the primary tumor completely. The surgeon should excise as much tumor as is safely possible and accomplish a regional lymphadenectomy for staging. Duckett and Koop[83, 84] demonstrated that partial resection or debulking of neuroblastoma is beneficial even when total extirpation is not possible. However, resection of intestine and abdominal organs is not included in an en bloc excision, because survival is not enhanced.[85]

Abdominal neuroblastoma is often extensive and may involve vital organs such as the portal structures and celiac axis. Large tumors are more hemorrhagic, and attempted resection may result in uncontrolled bleeding and death. If the tumor is deemed unresectable, it should be biopsied; the margins are marked with titanium clips, and the abdomen is closed. The tumor should then be treated with chemotherapy or radiation therapy (or both) to decrease its size and vascularity. Two to 3 months thereafter, when the primary tumor is often much less vascular and smaller and is more likely to be resectable, a second-look procedure is done.[86, 87] Interestingly, about 50% of neuroblastomas can be completely resected during second-look procedures; thus, the tumor is converted to stage I or II disease.[26, 82, 88]

"Spoon-out" Procedure.—Neuroblastoma is a pseudoencapsulated tumor, and at times it is possible to open the pseudocapsule to a limited extent and "spoon out" the gelatinous contents.[83] This technique should be carefully controlled; a small incision is made into the pseudocapsule and is brought down into the tumor through the relatively solid cortex and into the inner necrotic mass. If brisk bleeding is encountered, the pseudocapsule and cortex should be sutured together to confine the hemorrhage. A long, sweeping incision through the pseudocapsule often produces uncontrollable bleeding.

Metastatic Disease.—In patients with metastatic disease radiographically, the diagnosis should be established by lymph node biopsy or bone marrow biopsy only. Exploratory celiotomy should be deferred until after chemotherapy and radiation therapy.

Children with stage IV-S disease probably require little or no therapy. Most of these children are younger than 1 year and have a high spontaneous cure rate. The diagnosis is established by bone marrow biopsy, liver biopsy, or biopsy of a subcutaneous nodule. Surgical exploration is indicated only if resection of the primary tumor is deemed clinically feasible. Recent data indicate that radiation therapy or chemotherapy should be withheld unless there is evidence of disease progression over a period of observation.[89] Occasionally, patients with stage IV-S disease have rapid expansion of the liver with metastases, so that respiration is compromised. In this subgroup of children, an artificial hernia can be created for the abdominal cavity by the sewing of a piece of Dacron faced with Silastic to the edges of the abdominal incision.[83, 90] Hepatomegaly usually responds adequately to radiation therapy.

Specific Complications

Surgery is technically much more difficult for neuroblastoma than for Wilms' tumor. Venous drainage varies more, and neuroblastoma tends to spread by direct invasion into surrounding structures. Metastases are evident in 60% to 90% of patients at the time of presentation.[73, 84] Dissemination of tumor occurs early in the regional lymph nodes, liver, and bone and later in the lungs and brain. Many of the potential complications in children undergoing exploratory celiotomy for neuroblastoma are similar to those described under the discussion of Wilms' Tumor. Injuries to specific organs—for example, liver and pancreas—occur more frequently during dissection for neuroblastoma than for Wilms' tumor, and these will be discussed in further detail in this section.

Vessels.—Large tumors may encompass the abdominal viscera, and major vessels may be ligated inadvertently. It is very important to ligate the vessels initially near the inferior vena cava and aorta to prevent extensive bleeding during mobilization of the tumor.

Severe arterial hypertension may be associated with neuroblastoma and require continuous phentolamine perfusion to permit early surgical intervention while preventing intraoperative and postoperative hypertension.[91] Autonomic dysreflexia reported in a paraplegic patient was presumably from the synergistic effect of circulating catecholamines from the tumor and the disruption of autonomic pathways secondary to metastatic myelopathy.[92]

Bowel.—Patients undergoing exploratory celiotomy are at risk for bowel obstruction from either postoperative adhesions or intussusception. Abdominal distention secondary to a large neuroblastoma often makes abdominal closure difficult and may be associated with evisceration or dehiscence postoperatively.

Neuroblastomas are known to cause chronic diarrhea secondary to poorly understood mechanisms of neurohumoral effects on bowel motility and secretions. Metastatic neuroblastoma may result in intractable diarrhea from secretion of vasoactive intestinal peptide.[93] Neuroblastomas may cause intestinal lymphangiectasia and protein-losing enteropathy by blocking lymphatic vessels.[94]

Liver.—Invasion of the liver by neuroblastoma may necessitate partial hepatectomy. In situations in which hepatic resection is contemplated, the surgeon must carefully mobilize the triangular and coronary ligaments to prevent brisk and extensive bleeding from the short hepatic veins.

Pancreas.—Invasion of the pancreas may require resection of the tail of the pancreas to allow en bloc removal of the tumor. The cut end of the pancreas must be carefully oversewn with a running lock silk suture to avoid pancreatic fistula. Injury to the main pancreatic duct or to any of the smaller tributaries may result in pancreatic fistula, abscess, or pseudocyst. Even though the pancreas is repaired and drained at the time of injury, a fistula may develop.[49] If the pancreas is injured and the main duct transected, the proximal duct should be ligated with nonabsorbable suture. The cut surface of the gland should be closed with nonabsorbable horizontal mattress sutures. If trauma to the gland has been only minimal, without disruption of the duct system, simple surgical repair and drainage are indicated.[50] The pancreatic bed should be drained with soft sump tubes to closed suction. Generalized peritonitis usually develops in patients in whom the injury is not observed intraoperatively and in whom no drain has been left. When drains have been left, the diagnosis can be suspected by persistent drainage and a sinogram demonstrating communication with the pancreas and can be confirmed by elevation of amylase and bicarbonate in the abdominal fluid. Treatment is expectant, and most fistulas close spontaneously with adequate drainage.[50] In cases of persistent drainage, hyperalimentation may be necessary. Rarely, excision of the fistulous tract and Roux-en-Y loop pancreaticojejunostomy are necessary.

Adrenal gland.—In patients undergoing right adrenalectomy, the short adrenal veins, which come directly off the inferior vena cava, are at risk for rupture. Attempted ligation of these small vessels is difficult, and sutures often come loose. Meticulous control of the adrenal veins is best achieved by application of silver clips before division of the vessels.

Central Nervous System.— Although neuroblastoma is diagnosed with spinal cord compression in only 1% to 4% of cases, extraneural neuroblastoma is one of the most common causes of spinal cord compression and accounts for 12% to 30% of pediatric spinal tumors.[95] Neuroblastoma may be accompanied by acute cerebellar encephalopathy associated with opsoclonus, polymyoclonus, and irritability.[96]

EDITORIAL COMMENT I

This excellent chapter indicates how to avoid complications with Wilms' tumor and neuroblastoma patients. It should be emphasized that Wilms' tumor is not handled in the same fashion as adult renal cell adenocarcinomas. Adjuvant chemotherapy or radiation therapy has markedly improved survival. In general, if a nephrectomy is being considered, a radical nephrectomy is performed rather than a simple nephrectomy. The Wilms' tumor and tumor thrombus is often quite gelatinous, and the use of the Fogarty or Foley catheters for removal of tumor thrombus should be done with extraordinary care so that embolization does not occur. In general, we would consider use of cardiopulmonary bypass, even with hypothermia and cardiac arrest, if there is involvement of the suprahepatic vena cava.*†

EDITORIAL COMMENT II

The treatment for Wilms' tumor has become so effective with combination surgery, chemotherapy, and radiation that the focus is increasingly on the complications of these treatments. Neuroblastoma, on the other hand, has remained somewhat resistant to treatment but the complications in the management of both of these neoplasms remain significant. This chapter has been extensively updated and more than 30 new references have been added.

REFERENCES

1. Young JL Jr, Miller RW: Incidence of malignant tumors in U.S. children. *J Pediatr* 1975; 86:254–258.
2. Ehrlich RM: Complications of Wilms' tumor surgery. *Urol Clin North Am* 1983; 10:399–406, Aug.
3. Kramer SA, Kelalis PP: Wilms' tumor 1984. *AUA Update Series,* lesson 18, vol 3, 1984, pp 1–8.
4. Gates GF, Miller JH, Stanley P: Necrosis of Wilms' tumors. *J Urol* 1980; 123:916–920.

*Theman T, Williams WG, Simpson JS, et al: Tumor invasion of the upper inferior vena cava: The use of profound hypothermia and circulation arrest as a surgical adjunct. *J Pediatr Surg* 1978; 13:331.

†Marshall FF, Reitz BA, Diamond DA: A new technique for management of renal cell carcinoma involving the right atrium: Hypothermia and cardiac arrest. *J Urol* 1984; 131:103.

5. Luck SR, DeLeon S, Shkolnik A, et al: Intracardiac Wilms' tumor: Diagnosis and management. *J Pediatr Surg* 1982; 17:551–554.
6. Gonzalez R, Clayman RV, Sheldon CA: Management of intravascular nephroblastoma to avoid complications. *Urol Clin North Am* 1983; 10:407–415.

6a. Ritchey ML, Kelalis PP, Breslow N, et al: Intracaval and atrial involvement with neuroblastoma: Review of National Wilms' Tumor Study–3. *J Urol* 1988; 140:1113–1118.

7. Cohen MD, Weber T, Smith JA, et al: The role of computerized tomography in the diagnosis and management of patients with bilateral Wilms' tumor. *J Urol* 1983; 130:1160–1162.
8. Berdon WE, Baker DH, Santulli TV: Factors producing spurious obstruction of the inferior vena cava in infants and children with abdominal tumors. *Radiology* 1967; 88:111–116.
9. Tucker AS: The roentgen diagnosis of abdominal masses in children: Intravenous urography vs. inferior venacavagraphy. *Am J Roentgenol* 1965; 95:76–90.
10. Slovis TL, Cushing B, Reilly BJ, et al: Wilms' tumor to the heart: Clinical and radiographic evaluation. *AJR* 1978; 131:263–266.
11. Schullinger JN, Santulli TV, Casarella WJ, et al: Wilms' tumor: The role of right heart angiography in the management of selected cases. *Ann Surg* 1977; 185:451–455.
12. Grosfeld JL, Weber TR: Surgical considerations in the treatment of Wilms' tumor, in Gonzalez-Crussi F (ed): *Wilms' Tumor (Nephroblastoma) and Related Renal Neoplasms of Childhood.* Boca Raton, Fla, CRC Press, 1984, pp 263–283.
13. Katzen BT, Markowitz M: Angiographic manifestations of bilateral Wilms' tumor. *Am J Roentgenol* 1976; 126:802–806.
14. D'Angio GJ, Duckett JW Jr, Belasco JB: Tumors: Upper urinary tract, in Kelalis PP, King LR, Belman AB (eds): *Clinical Pediatric Urology,* ed. 2. Philadelphia, WB Saunders Co, 1985, vol 2, pp 1157–1188.
15. Stevens PS, Eckstein HB: Ureteral metastasis from Wilms' tumor. *J Urol* 1976; 115:467–468.
16. Ehrlich RM: Percutaneous fine needle aspiration to identify malignancy in children (abstract). Presented at the American Academy of Pediatrics, Chicago, Sept 15–20, 1984.
17. Danis RK, Wolverson MK, Graviss ER, et al: Preoperative embolization of Wilms' tumors. *Am J Dis Child* 1979; 133:503–506.
18. Harrison MR, de Lorimier AA, Boswell WO: Preoperative angiographic embolization for large hemorrhagic Wilms' tumor. *J Pediatr Surg* 1978; 13:757–758.
19. Broecker BH, Perlmutter AD: Management of unresectable Wilms' tumor. *Urology* 1984; 24:170–174.
20. Bracken RB, Sutow WW, Jaffe N, et al: Preoperative chemotherapy for Wilms' tumor. *Urology* 1982;19:55–60.
21. Kramer SA: Pediatric urologic oncology. *Urol Clin North Am* 1985; 12:31–42.
22. Leape LL, Breslow NE, Bishop HC: The surgical treatment of Wilms' tumor: Results of the National Wilms' Tumor Study. *Ann Surg* 1978; 187:351–356.
23. Woodard JR: Wilms' tumor, in Glenn JF (ed): *Urologic Surgery,* ed 3. Philadelphia, JB Lippincott, Co, 1983, pp 105–121.
24. Kelalis PP: Tumors of the urinary tract. *Int Perspect Urol* 1987; 14:318–329.
25. Cole AT, Fried FA, Bissada NK: The supine subcostal modification of the thoraco-abdominal incision. *J Urol* 1974; 112:168–171.
26. Grosfeld JL, Ballantine TVN, Baehner RL: Experience with "second-look" operations in pediatric solid tumors. *J Pediatr Surg* 1978; 13:275–280.
27. Anderson KD, Altman RP: Selective resection of malignant tumors using bench surgical techniques. *J Pediatr Surg* 1976; 11:881–882.
28. Lilly JR, Pfister RR, Putnam CW, et al: Bench surgery and renal autotransplantation in the pediatric patient. *J Pediatr Surg* 1975; 10:623–630.
29. Duckett JW Jr, Lifland JH, Peters PC: Resection of the inferior vena cava for adjacent malignant diseases. *Surg Gynecol Obstet* 1973; 136:711–716.
30. McCullough DL, Gittes RF: Vena cava resection for renal cell carcinoma. *J Urol* 1974; 112:162–167.
31. Breslow NE, Beckwith JB: Epidemiological features of Wilms' tumor: Results of the

National Wilms' Tumor Study. *J Natl Cancer Inst* 1982; 68:429–436.

32. Wasiljew BK, Besser A, Raffensperger J: Treatment of bilateral Wilms' tumors—a 22-yr experience. *J Pediatr Surg* 1982; 17:265–268.
33. Ehrlich RM, Bloomberg SD, Gyepes MT, et al: Wilms' tumor, misdiagnosed preoperatively: A review of 19 National Wilms' Tumor Study I cases. *J Urol* 1979; 122:790–792.
34. Shashikumar VL, Somers LA, Pilling GP IV, et al: Wilms' tumor in the horseshoe kidney. *J Pediatr Surg* 1974; 9:185–189.
35. Mesrobian H-GJ, Kelalis PP, Hrabovsky E, et al: Wilms' tumor in horseshoe kidneys: A report from the National Wilms' Tumor Study. *J Urol* 1985; 133:1002–1003.
36. Ritchey ML, Lally KP, Kelalis PP: Superior mesenteric artery injuries during nephrectomy for Wilms' tumor. *J Urol*, in press.
37. Erlik D, Barzilai A, Shramek A: Renal function after left renal vein ligation. *J Urol* 1965; 93:540–544.
38. Pathak IC: Survival after right nephrectomy, excision of infrahepatic vena cava and ligation of left renal vein: A case report. *J Urol* 1971; 106:599–602.
39. Miedema BW, Stubenbord WT: Irreversible renal failure following right nephrectomy and left renal vein ligation. *J Urol* 1984; 132:335–336.
40. Tucci P, Diagonale AM, Visani S, et al: Renal vein ligation in absence of vena caval obstruction. *Urology* 1980; 15:397–400.
41. Sarti L: Total prosthetic transplantation of the inferior vena cava with venous drainage restoration of the one remaining kidney on the graft, successfully performed on a child with Wilms' tumor. *Surgery* 1970; 67:851–855.
42. Kramer SA: Unpublished data.
43. Nakayama DK, deLorimier AA, O'Neill JA Jr, et al: Intracardiac extension of Wilms' tumor: A report of the National Wilms' Tumor Study. *Ann Surg* 1986; 195:693–697.
44. Schraut WH, Chilcote RR: Metastatic Wilms' tumor causing acute hepatic-vein occlusion (Budd-Chiari syndrome). *Gastroenterology* 1985; 88:576–579.
45. Thomas PRM, Tefft M, D'Angio GJ, et al: Acute toxicities associated with radiation in the Second National Wilms' Tumor Study. *J Clin Oncol* 1988; 6:1694–1698.
46. Roback SA, Nesbit ME Jr, Sharp HL, et al: Portal hypertension following surgery, x-radiation, and actinomycin D therapy of nephroblastoma. *J Pediatr* 1971; 78:1031–1034.
47. Thomas PRM, Griffith KD, Fineberg BB, et al: Late effects of treatment for Wilms' tumor. *Int J Radiat Oncol Biol Phys* 1983; 9:651–657.
48. Barnard JA, Marshall GS, Neblett WW, et al: Noncirrhotic portal fibrosis with Wilms' tumor therapy. *Gastroenterology* 1986; 90:1054–1056.
49. Spirnak JP, Resnick MI, Persky L: Cutaneous pancreatic fistula as a complication of left nephrectomy. *J Urol* 1984; 132:329–330.
50. Werschky LR, Jordan GL Jr: Surgical management of traumatic injuries to the pancreas. *Am J Surg* 1968; 116:768–772.
51. Austrian R: The assessment of pneumococcal vaccine (editorial). *N Engl J Med* 1980; 303:578–580.
52. Dixon JA, Miller F, McCloskey D, et al: Anatomy and techniques in segmental splenectomy. *Surg Gynecol Obstet* 1980; 150:516–520.
53. Hertz J, Shapiro SR, Konrad P, et al: Chylous ascites following retroperitoneal lymphadenectomy: Report of 2 cases with guidelines for diagnosis and treatment. *Cancer* 1978; 42:349–352.
54. Green DM, Finklestein JZ, Tefft ME, et al: Diffuse interstitial pneumonitis after pulmonary irradiation for metastatic Wilms' tumor: A report from the National Wilms' Tumor Study. *Cancer* 1989; 63:450–453.
55. Ramsay NKC, Dehner LP, Coccia PF, et al: Acute hemorrhage into Wilms' tumor: A cause of rapidly developing abdominal mass with hypertension, anemia, and fever. *J Pediatr* 1977; 91:763–765.
56. Takamiya Y, Toya S, Otani M, et al: Wilms' tumor with intracranial metastases presenting with intracranial hemorrhage. *Child's Nervous System* 1985; 1:291–294.
57. Welch TR, McAdams AJ: Focal glomerulosclerosis as a late sequela of Wilms' tumor. *J Pediatr* 1986; 108:105–109.

58. Scully RE, Mark EJ, McNeely BU: Case records of the Massachusetts General Hospital: Case 17-1985: Presentation of case. *N Engl J Med* 1985; 312:1111–1119.
59. Zucchelli P, Cagnoli L, Casanova S, et al: Focal glomerulosclerosis in patients with unilateral nephrectomy. *Kidney Int* 1983; 24:649–655.
60. Brenner BM (principal discussant): Hemodynamically mediated glomerular injury and the progressive nature of kidney disease (Nephrology Forum). *Kidney Int* 1983; 23:647–655.
61. Kramer SA, Ritchey ML: The solitary kidney: Part 1. *Dial Pediatr Urol* 1988; 11(No. 1):1–8.
62. Drash A, Sherman F, Hartmann WH, et al: A syndrome of pseudohermaphroditism, Wilms' tumor, hypertension, and degenerative renal disease. *J Pediatr* 1970; 76:585–593.
63. Scott JP, Montgomery RR, Tubergn DG, et al: Acquired von Willebrand's disease in association with Wilms' tumor: Regression following treatment. *Blood* 1981; 58:665–669.
64. Noronha PA, Hruby MA, Maurer HS: Acquired von Willebrand disease in a patient with Wilms' tumor. *J Pediatr* 1979; 95:997–999.
65. Wang AH, Gibbons ISE, Nedwich A, et al: Wilms' tumor associated with venous thrombosis and consumption coagulopathy. *Am J Dis Child* 1972; 123:599–601.
66. Peterson NE, Galloway B: Wilms' tumor with consumption coagulopathy. *Urology* 1982; 19:74–77.
67. Procianoy RS, Giacomini CB, Mattos TC, et al: Congenital Wilms' tumor associated with consumption coagulopathy and hyperbilirubinemia. *J Pediatr Surg* 1986; 21:993–994.
68. LeBlanc A, Caillaud JM, Hartmann O, et al: Hypercalcemia preferentially occurs in unusual forms of childhood non-Hodgkin's lymphoma, rhabdomyosarcoma, and Wilms' tumor: A study of 11 cases. *Cancer* 1984; 54:2132–2136.
69. Rousseau-Merck MF, Boccon-Gibod L, Nogues C, et al: An original hypercalcemic infantile renal tumor without bone metastasis: Heterotransplantation to nude mice: Report of two cases. *Cancer* 1982; 50:85–93.
70. Kramer SA, Kelalis PP: Pediatric urologic oncology, in Gillenwater JY, Grayhack JT, Howard SS, et al (eds): *Adult and Pediatric Urology.* Chicago, Year Book Medical Publishers, 1987, vol 2 pp 2001–2042.
71. Meadows AT, Baum E, Fossati-Bellani F, et al: Second malignant neoplasms in children: An update from the Late Effects Study Group. *J Clin Oncol* 1985; 3:532–538.
72. Breslow N, McCann B: Statistical estimation of prognosis for children with neuroblastoma. *Cancer Res* 1971; 31:2098–2103.
73. Koop CE, Hernandez JR: Neuroblastoma: Experience with 100 cases in children. *Surgery* 1964; 56:726–733.
74. Priebe CJ Jr, Clatworthy HW Jr: Neuroblastoma: Evaluation of the treatment of 90 children. *Arch Surg* 1967; 95:538–545.
75. Hainaut F, Bouton JM, Plot C, et al: Anasarque foeto-placentaire secondaire à un neuroblastome. Diagnostic prénatal (English abstract). *J Gynecol Obstet Biol Reprod (Paris)* 1987; 16:367–372.
76. Angerpointner TA: Ein Fall von geburtstraumatisch rupturiertem, kongenitalem Neuroblastom (English abstract). *Monatsschr Kinderheilkd* 1985; 133:241–242.
77. Kramer SA, Bradford WD, Anderson EE: Bilateral adrenal neuroblastoma. *Cancer* 1980; 45:2208–2212.
78. Stark DD, Brasch RC, Moss AA, et al: Recurrent neuroblastoma: The role of CT and alternative imaging tests. *Radiology* 1983; 148:107–112.
79. Finklestein JZ, Ekert H, Isaacs H Jr, et al: Bone marrow metastases in children with solid tumors. *Am J Dis Child* 1970; 119: 49–52.
80. Williams CM, Greer M: Homovanillic acid and vanilmandelic acid in diagnosis of neuroblastoma. *JAMA* 1963; 183:836–840.
81. Liebner EJ, Rosenthal IM: Serial catecholamines in the radiation management of children with neuroblastoma. *Cancer* 1973; 32:623–633.
82. Exelby PR: Retroperitoneal malignant tumors: Wilms' tumor and neuroblastoma. *Surg Clin North Am* 1981; 61:1219–1237.
83. Duckett JW: Neuroblastoma, in Glenn JF

(ed): *Urologic Surgery*, ed 3. Philadelphia, JB Lippincott Co, 1983, pp 55–61.

84. Duckett JW, Koop CE: Neuroblastoma. *Urol Clin North Am* 1977; 4:285–295.
85. Gilchrist GS, Telander RL: Adrenal medulla and sympathetic chain, in Kelalis PP, King LR, Belman AB (eds): *Clinical Pediatric Urology*, ed 2. Philadelphia, WB Saunders Co, 1985, vol 2, pp 1252–1271.
86. Koop CE: The role of surgery in resectable, nonresectable, and metastatic neuroblastoma. *JAMA* 1968; 205:157–158.
87. Koop CE, Kiesewetter WB, Horn RC: Neuroblastoma in childhood: An evaluation of surgical management. *Pediatrics* 1955; 16:652–657.
88. Smith EI, Krous HF, Tunell WP, et al.: The impact of chemotherapy and radiation therapy on secondary operations for neuroblastoma. *Ann Surg* 1980; 191:561–568.
89. Schwartz AD, Dadash-Zadeh M, Lee H, et al: Spontaneous regression of disseminated neuroblastoma. *J Pediatr* 1974; 85:760–763.
90. Schnaufer L, Koop CE: Silastic abdominal patch for temporary hepatomegaly in stage IV-S neuroblastoma. *J Pediatr Surg* 1975; 10:73–75.
91. Champoux L, Gauthier M: Phentolamine en perfusion continue dans le traitement d'une hypertension arterielle sévère associée à un neuroblastome. *Can Anaesth Soc J* 1984; 31:206–209.
92. Wright KC, Agre JC, Wilson BC, et al: Autonomic dysreflexia in a paraplegic man with catecholamine-secreting neuroblastoma. *Arch Phys Med Rehabil* 1986; 67:566–567.
93. Tiedemann K, Pritchard J, Long R, et al: Intractable diarrhoea in a patient with vasoactive intestinal peptide-secreting neuroblastoma: Attempted control by somatostatin. *Eur J Pediatr* 1981; 137:217–219.
94. Gerdes JS, Katz AJ: Neuroblastoma appearing as protein-losing enteropathy. *Am J Dis Child* 1982; 136:1024–1025.
95. Punt J, Pritchard J, Pincott JR, et al: Neuroblastoma: A review of 21 cases presenting with spinal cord compression. *Cancer* 1980; 45:3095–3101.
96. Telander RL, Smithson WA, Groover RV: Clinical outcome in children with acute cerebellar encephalopathy and neuroblastoma. *J Pediatr Surg* 1989; 24:11–14.

CHAPTER 29

Complications of Antenatal Intervention

Mark F. Bellinger, M.D.

A dramatic evolution has occurred which will have a profound impact on the urologic care of infants and children and will undoubtedly alter many concepts basic to our current understanding of congenital urinary tract anomalies: The fetus has become a patient. In the early 1960s, studies on Rh immunization led to invasive therapy by intrauterine transfusion and the first concepts of fetal-maternal medicine.[1] Subsequently, successful amniocentesis is used routinely as a screen for genetic disease.[2] The most controversial phase of fetal evaluation and therapy has occurred during the past 5 years and has coincided with major technical advances in the field of diagnostic obstetric ultrasound. Sonography has not only allowed the detection of fetal urinary tract dilatation, but it is currently the basis for perinatal therapy, including percutaneous procedures. An assessment of the complications of antenatal intervention must include a consideration of the pitfalls in our current ability to evaluate fetal urinary tract disease.

ULTRASOUND EXAMINATION OF THE FETUS

Since the report by Garrett et al.[3] in 1970 documenting fetal polycystic kidney disease, the detection of fetal urinary tract dilatation has become commonplace. Diagnostic ultrasound imaging relies upon differences in tissue density rather than upon contrast agents, and the fluid-filled urinary tract provides an excellent subject for study (Figs 29–1 and 29–2). Cystic lesions as small as 2.0 mm may be visualized.[4] The urine-filled bladder may be documented early in the third month of gestation, and normal kidneys can be identified in a large number of fetuses at 12 to 14 weeks, while 50% to 70% of kidneys are visible at 15 to 17 weeks, and nearly all are visible by 18 to 20 weeks gestation.[5] Clearly, dilated kidneys may be visible early in gestation.[6]

Fetal urinary tract dilatation may be detected during evaluation of gestational age, during screening examination of a pregnancy at risk for congenital fetal anomalies, or by serendipity. Complete ultrasound study of the fetus with a documented or suspected urinary tract abnormality is a detailed, painstaking examination, including assessment of placental location and consistency, total intrauterine volume, and, especially, determination of amnionic fluid volume. Although a direct cause-effect relationship between severe renal anomalies, oligohydramnios, and pulmonary hypoplasia is uncertain, their coexistence is commonly appreciated.[7] Complete fetal examination includes cranial imaging and determination of biparietal diameter, cardiac examination and as-

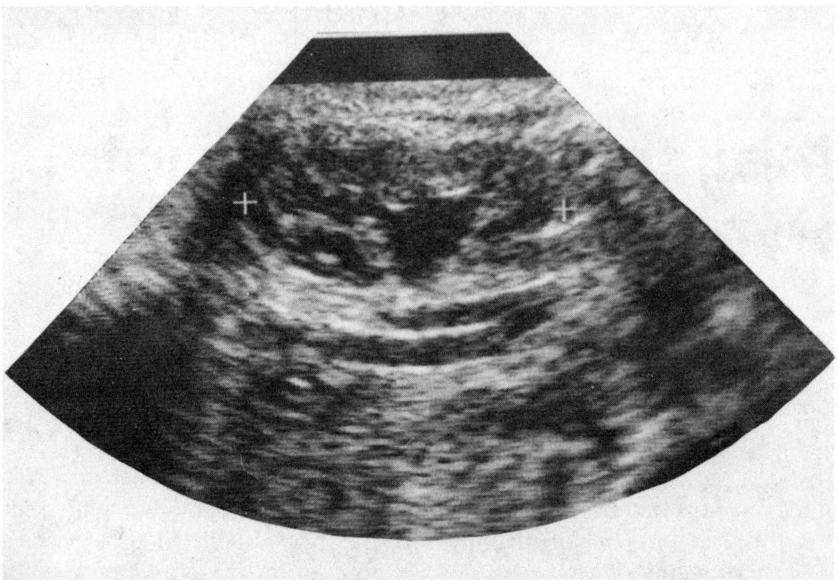

FIG 29–1.
Longitudinal scan of a normal kidney with mild prominence of the renal pelvis at 30 weeks' gestation.

sessment of thoracic volume, measurement of abdominal circumference, examination of the spine for dysraphism, assessment of femur length and limb development, examination of external genitalia, and sex determination. Such comprehensive examinations are important in light of the spectrum of lesions (i.e., VATER,[8] VACTERL[9]) that may be associated with congenital renal anomalies. Kid-

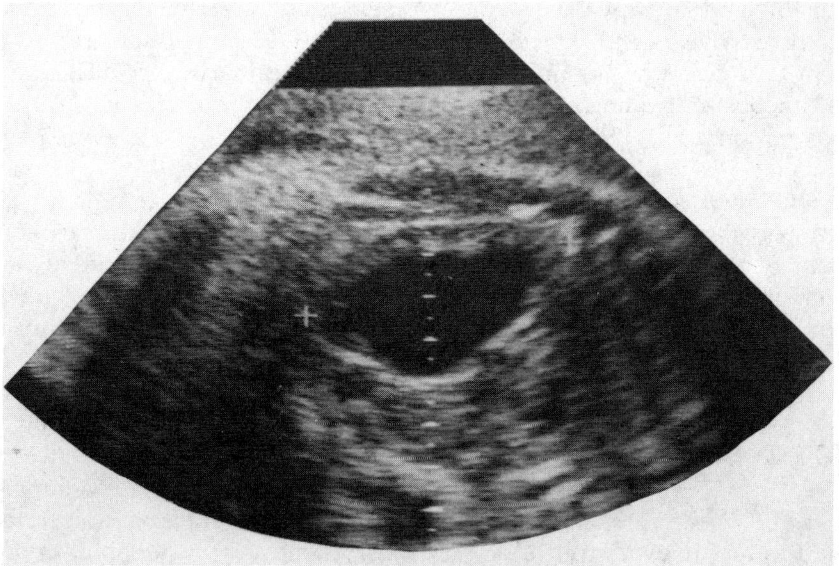

FIG 29–2.
Marked left fetal hydronephrosis at 34 weeks, longitudinal scan. Note thinned renal cortex.

ney size must be documented. Grannum and colleagues have tabulated fetal kidney circumference abdominal circumference (KC/AC) ratios, which have a small range of normal (0.27–0.30) during gestation and are designed to correct for differences in fetal size.[10] While the detection of cystic change or hydronephrosis is important, it is most critical to determine whether the abnormality is unilateral or bilateral, since this will have a great impact on considerations of therapy.[11] In addition to documentation of gross dilatation, high-resolution ultrasound offers the ability to assess renal parenchymal echogenicity. Although somewhat subjective, the finding of increased echogenicity should raise concern about parenchymal dysplasia (Fig 29–3).[12]

Pitfalls of Fetal Urinary Tract Sonography

Ultrasound imaging is a tomographic technique, displaying slices of the subject in a plane determined by the position and orientation of the transducer. As such, it is a highly subjective, extremely operator-dependent examination with many potential pitfalls. Examination of the fetus further challenges the observer's ability in both performance and interpretation, since fetal motion requires constant reorientation to maximize accuracy and minimize artifact. Real-time imaging, particularly advantageous in fetal examinations, enables rapid reassessment of fetal position, the ability to observe fetal voiding, and videotape recording for review. Advanced technology has put high-resolution machines into the hands of many less-experienced observers, who frequently are the first to detect a cystic mass in the fetal abdomen. The urologist consulted for evaluation of a fetal urinary anomaly must thus keep in mind four basic tenets of fetal ultrasound: (1) the declaration of normal or abnormal fetal anatomy requires at least two confirming studies, (2) fetal ultrasonography demands a trained observer knowledgeable in the multiplicity of fetal and pediatric anomalies, (3) ultrasound provides

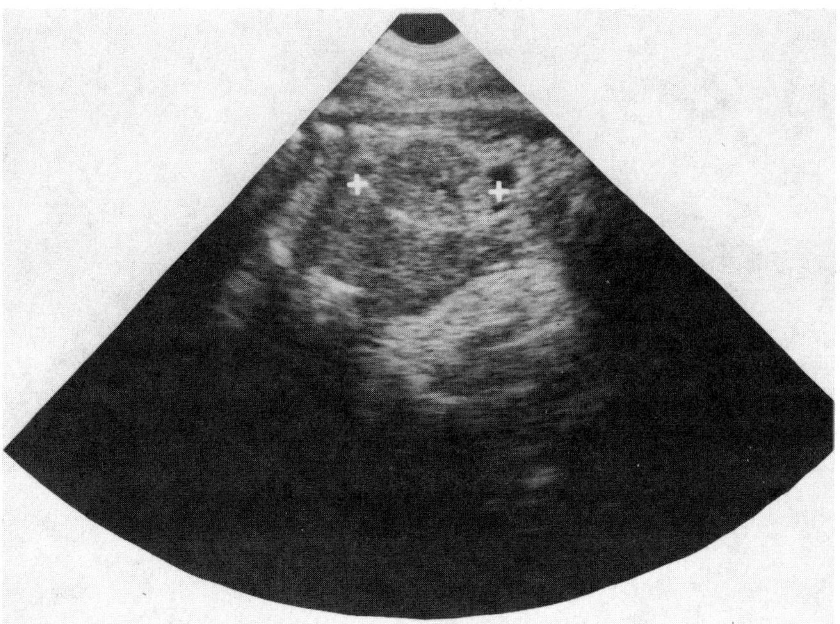

FIG 29–3.
Longitudinal scan of small, echogenic fetal kidney (marked by *plus signs*). Diagnosis: renal dysplasia.

only anatomical, not functional, information, and (4) there is no substitute for being present at the time of the examination.

Evaluation of bladder function is extremely important. The human fetus voids frequently, and ultrasound-based parameters have been suggested to determine hourly fetal urine output.[13] In the assessment of bladder function, several concepts are important to recall: (1) serial studies are necessary to document both that the bladder fills and that it can empty; (2) upper urinary tract dilatation postnatally, as antenatally, may occur secondary to bladder distention, and reevaluation after voiding is extremely important; (3) severe vesicoureteric reflux (VUR) may give a false impression of abnormal bladder emptying; and (4) although bladder distention is the most common cause of a cystic mass in the lower fetal abdomen, ureterocele, anterior meningocele, hydrocolpos, bowel duplication cysts, and cystic sacrococcygeal teratoma have been reported to have similar sonographic characteristics (Fig 29–4).[4, 14]

It should be evident that the interpretation of fetal urinary tract dilatation as determined by ultrasound involves an educated differential diagnosis at best. Ureteropelvic junction obstruction, ureteral duplication with ureterocele, and other commonplace lesions can be diagnosed with some accuracy based upon sonographic appearance and statistical considerations. We have been impressed, however, that in severe bladder dilatation with bilateral hydroureteronephrosis, differential diagnosis is difficult and often hampered by the presence of combined lesions (i.e., reflux with ureteropelvic junction obstruction) (Fig 29–5).

Complications of Ultrasound Examination

The most common complication of diagnostic fetal ultrasound is improper diagnosis, leading to misguided parental counseling and unnecessary diagnostic or therapeutic intervention. As noted above, many pitfalls inherent in fetal ultrasound

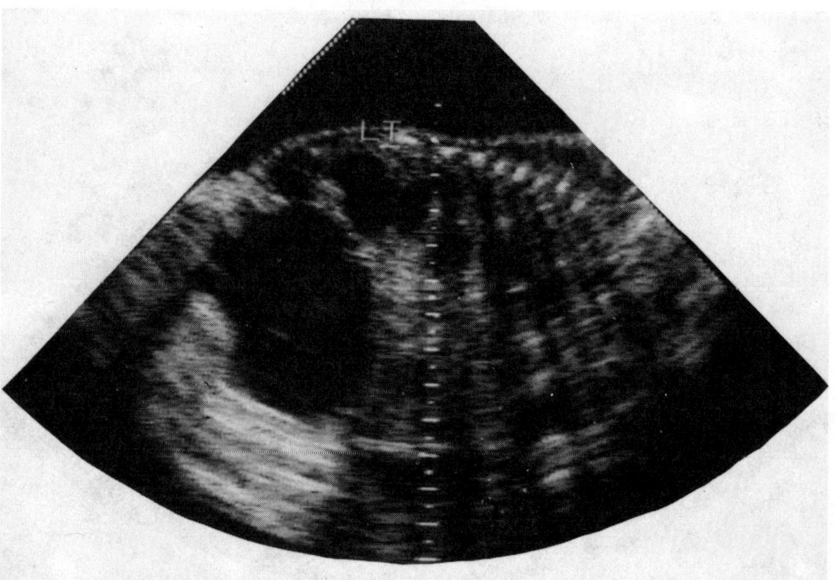

FIG 29–4.
Cystic sacrococcygeal teratoma in a twin fetus, sagittal scan, spine upward. Cystic mass near spine (*LT*) is tumor. Large cystic lesion thought to be bladder is extension of cystic tumor into abdomen.

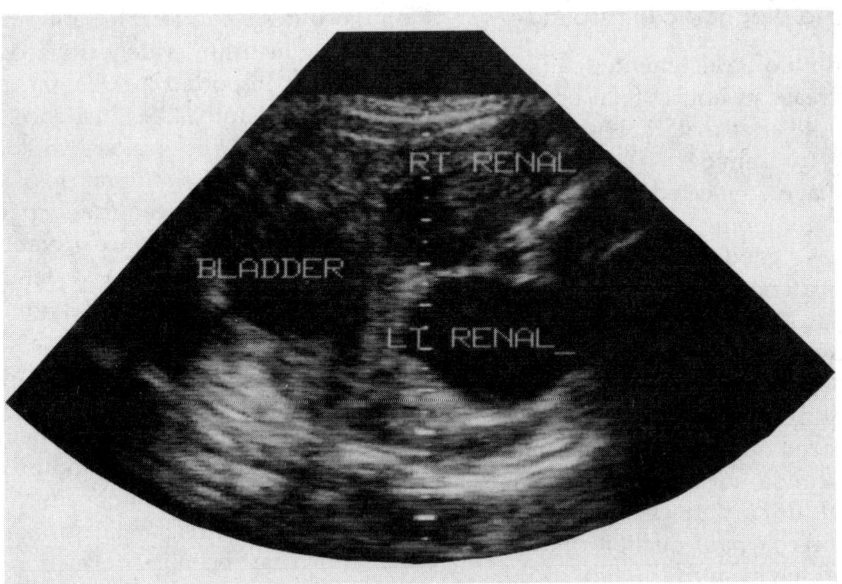

FIG 29–5.
Coronal scan of male fetus with large bladder and bilateral hydroureteronephrosis, thought to be posterior urethral valves. Postnatal evaluation revealed massive bilateral vesicoureteric reflux and right secondary ureteropelvic junction obstruction.

hamper diagnosis. Even when the portrayal of fetal anatomy is accurate, the extreme distensibility of the fetal and infant urinary tract, together with the variable configurations that a single entity may assume (i.e., bladder and upper tract changes secondary to posterior urethral valves), may hamper diagnosis.[15] In addition, transient fetal hydronephrosis is known to occur, although its etiologies are poorly understood.[16]

Ultrasound is high-frequency mechanical energy that causes oscillation of tissue molecules. Although sound reflected back to the transducer produces an image, some energy is absorbed as heat. Biologic effects of ultrasound may be due to heat or cavitation (violent collapse of air bubbles resulting in heat and shock waves).[17] Exposure of pregnant rats to high-intensity sound causes fetal weight reduction and increased fetal loss. Long-term exposure of mice gonads to ultrasound produces sterility.[18] In the human, the long-term and cumulative effects of diagnostic fetal ultrasound are poorly understood. Wilson and Waterhouse[19] studied the maternal histories of 1,731 children who died with cancer and 1,731 controls and found no evidence that fetal ultrasound increased subsequent risk of childhood cancer or leukemia. In a similar epidemiologic study, Cartwright et al.[20] came to identical conclusions. The lack of data on the long-term effects of ultrasound on the fetus has led a recent consensus conference to recommend that ultrasound examination during pregnancy be performed for specific medical indications only and not for routine screening.[21] When studies are performed, documentation of cumulative exposure is important, and all patients must be counseled about possible consequences to the fetus of ultrasound exposure. An unstudied effect of prenatal diagnosis is the alteration in traditional maternal-fetal bonding that may occur during the process of in utero diagnosis.[22] Currently, a prospective study is underway at the University of Manitoba to assess the long-term risk of fetal ultrasound examination.[17]

Adjuncts to Diagnostic Ultrasound

Wladimiroff documented an 80% to 150% increase in hourly fetal urinary production rate after maternal administration of 60 mg furosemide.[23] Harrison and colleagues have advocated this test as helpful in determining whether fetal renal function is "good" or "bad" in the presence of bilateral hydronephrosis or hydronephrosis of a solitary kidney.[24] Results have proved useful in cases of bilateral renal agenesis and in cases of severe bilateral renal dysplasia where no bladder can be visualized on repeated examination after furosemide administration. However, in partial urinary tract obstruction, the production of poor-quality dilute urine may continue even in the face of poor renal function, leaving the examiner with a false sense of security.[25] The furosemide stimulation test has extremely limited usefulness and should not be considered an indicator of adequate fetal renal function.

Percutaneous aspiration of fetal urinary structures may have promise as an indicator of fetal renal function. If aspiration is followed by refilling with urine, urine production is documented.[24, 26] As with the furosemide test, this does not indicate functional capacity, however. Recently, Glick and colleagues described their initial analysis of fetal bladder aspiration in a small number of fetuses. Their data suggest that urine from "good" kidneys demonstrates a lower sodium content and lower osmolality than urine from "bad" kidneys.[27]

FETAL URINARY TRACT INTERVENTION

Percutaneous Techniques

Percutaneous drainage of fetal hydronephrosis may be accomplished by needle aspiration or placement of an internal or external shunt catheter.[24, 28–30] Percutaneous needle aspiration of fetal urinary structures is similar to the techniques of amniocentesis and fetal intrauterine transfusion, which are widely utilized. Farahani et al.[31] reported a 0.8% incidence of bloody taps and 0.9% incidence of fetal loss within 8 weeks after amniocentesis compared to 0.53% normal loss in 2,100 consecutive amniocenteses performed with ultrasound guidance. Ryan et al.[32] reported a 1.7% incidence of fetal loss in 291 cases, associated with fetal or umbilical cord trauma and bleeding. Cromie[33] documented penetrating renal trauma of the fetus secondary to amniocentesis, and others have reported subdural hematoma, splenic laceration, pneumothorax, cardiac trauma, and cardiac tamponade.[34]

Although direct fetal urinary tract puncture has been performed relatively infrequently, the hazards of a similar procedure, intrauterine fetal transfusion, are well documented. Maternal complications are rare, the most common being sepsis, which occurs in less than 1% of cases. Fetal risks are much greater. Prior to routine ultrasound guidance, fetal mortality was 6% to 24%, primarily due to cardiac tamponade or exsanguination from umbilical or fetal vascular trauma. With ultrasound guidance, fetal risk is lower, 3.6% to 9.3% in recently reported series.[35]

Harrison has developed a system for percutaneous placement of indwelling fetal-amnionic shunt catheters.[36] In his early experience, three fetuses had shunt placement in late gestation for bilateral hydroureteronephrosis and bladder distention. One fetus died of pulmonary hypoplasia and two survived.[16] Recently, Manning[37] updated the International Fetal Surgery Report in which 52 cases of chronic vesicoamnionic shunt were summarized. In 3 of 52, a single shunt was successful in decompressing fetal hydronephrosis, but, in general, multiple shunt placements were necessary to provide continued fetal urinary tract decompression. Approximately 7% of fetal mortalities were associated directly with the shunting procedure.[37] Glick et al. have reported an unacceptable incidence of chorioamnionitis and fetal loss associated with chronic catheterization.[27]

Fetal Surgery for Hydronephrosis

Although fetal surgery has been well documented in animals, the ability to perform primate hysterotomy required the development of coordinated anesthetic and tocolytic techniques.[38] Isolated reports of fetal vesicostomy and ureterostomy in late gestation have been reported without maternal or fetal loss.[39] These techniques would seem to carry higher maternal and fetal risks than percutaneous shunt procedures and require the experience and approach that few centers in the world can offer.

Efficacy of Antenatal Intervention

The aim of antenatal intervention in fetal hydronephrosis is to stabilize renal function and prevent the progression of renal damage during the remainder of gestation. At the outset, it must be stated that a determination of the efficacy of prenatal intervention is hampered by limited knowledge of the natural history of fetal hydronephrosis, by the varied causes of hydronephrosis, and by the variable pathology and radiographic configuration that any single lesion may assume.[40, 41] Limited understanding of the embryologic events that result in urinary obstruction and, in particular, the relationship between obstruction, ureteral bud anomalies, and renal dysplasia restricts our ability to determine which situations might benefit maximally from antenatal urinary diversion.[42, 43] It is appreciated, however, that infants with unilateral hydronephrosis in general have adequate renal function and are not in danger of pulmonary hypoplasia.[11, 44] Bilateral hydronephrosis is worrisome, but Hellstrom and colleagues reported the data on 13 fetuses with bilateral hydronephrosis and normal amnionic fluid, of which 5 had spontaneous resolution before birth, and 7 of the 8 with persistent hydronephrosis survived with normal renal function after postnatal correction.[45]

Harrison et al. have reported on the management of 26 cases of fetal hydronephrosis.[16, 36] Three resolved spontaneously before birth. Eight with evidence of poor function in utero all failed to survive. Of nine fetuses subject to in utero decompression or early delivery, three died and six survived, one with renal failure. All who survived had late intervention (after 30 weeks). Manning's data from the International Fetal Surgery Report associated 7% of fetal mortality directly with the shunting procedure. Twenty-nine of 52 fetuses subject to intervention died, 6 as stillbirth (2 with associated anomalies), and 23 as neonates (2 from associated anomalies, 20 from pulmonary hypoplasia, and 1 from renal failure). Of extreme importance is the analysis of outcome: there was no obvious relationship between gestational age at diagnosis and subsequent outcome, nor between gestational age at intervention and outcome (0% survival with intervention at 22–24 weeks and 86% survival with intervention at 26–28 weeks). Thus, earlier detection and treatment did not appear to improve survival. It is unknown whether late gestational intervention influenced postnatal renal function.[37] Sholder et al. assessed 18 fetuses diagnosed with antenatal hydronephrosis and found that only 12 (66%) of the antenatal diagnoses corresponded to postnatal diagnoses. Of 6 fetuses with bilateral hydroureteronephrosis and oligohydramnios who underwent percutaneous catheter placement, 1 died of a catheter-related complication and no fetus had any recognized benefit from antenatal intervention.[46] Such figures are sobering. It is apparent that our current understanding of the natural history of fetal hydronephrosis does not allow us to determine ration-

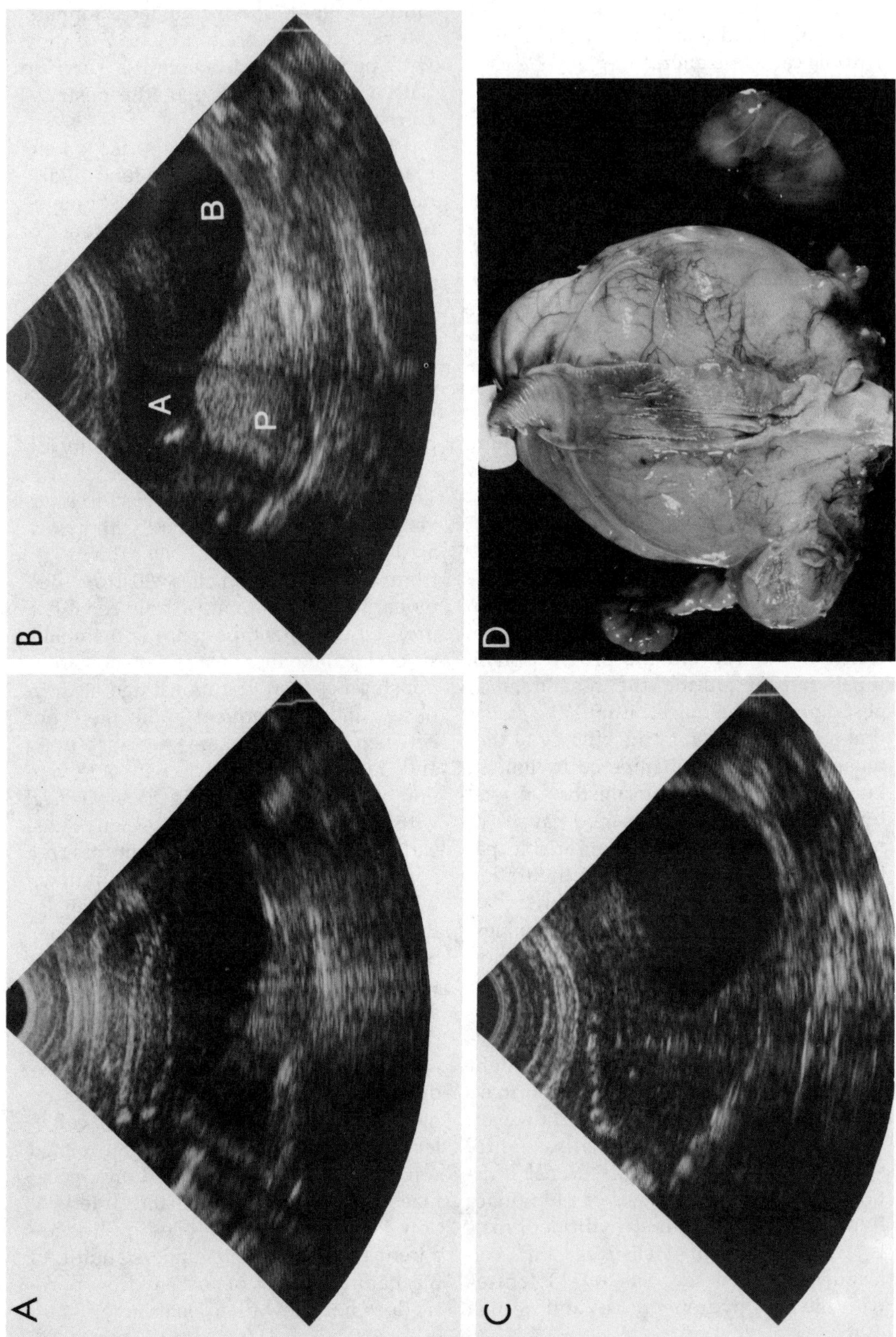
A
B
A
P
B
C
D

ally which fetuses, if any, may benefit from prenatal decompression (Fig 29–6).[47] It would seem that late gestational intervention or early delivery risks pulmonary complications at a stage when renal functional capacity is beyond influence.[48, 49] The hope that earlier intervention might prove beneficial has been thwarted by renal dysplasia and irreversible parenchymal disorganization in many cases.[50] The risks of intervention must be weighed against such data. Mandell et al. have demonstrated preservation of renal function when reconstructive surgery is performed in the neonatal period in unilateral hydronephrosis.[44] Our experience supports this conservative approach in the vast majority of instances of fetal urinary tract dilatation. It appears that the factors inherent in the embryogenesis and natural history of the obstruction will likely determine the outcome of renal function with or without intervention. Research currently in progress seeks to increase our knowledge about the natural history of fetal hydronephrosis and investigate the possibility of isolating a marker of fetal renal maturity and function. Even with the availability of such an assessment of fetal well-being, antenatal intervention is an extremely hazardous experimental procedure that should be carried out in a very few well-equipped centers that have the ability to study both clinically and experimentally the natural history of fetal hydronephrosis and the efficacy of prenatal decompression in improving postnatal renal function.

EDITORIAL COMMENT I

Antenatal intervention, especially for hydronephrosis, has great emotional appeal but very few practical indications at the present time. The urinary tract in the fetus is essentially formed by the end of the first month of gestation. It is not until 3 to 4 months that kidneys can be identified sonographically. The major renal problems of dysplasia are irreversible at that time. Even "hydronephrosis" has been seen in utero, but after birth the urinary tract appears normal on sonography and radiography. In addition, there can be significant fetal injury and death with intervention. For these reasons, there appear to be very few indications at the present time for direct intervention, because the intervention cannot be performed early enough to correct most anomalies and is of only questionable benefit. If performed in the last trimester, it is associated with significant risk.

EDITORIAL COMMENT II

Although many urologists, pediatric surgeons, and radiologists have an interventional orientation, it is still apparent that the risks of fetal intervention are very significant and the newborn should be reevaluated for appropriate diagnosis and management. Some "abnormalities" have resolved on neonatal reevaluation without any intervention.

FIG 29–6.

A, sagittal scan of 15-week fetus, spine upward, with large (9 × 8 × 9 cm) cystic abdominal mass. **B,** repeated scan at 18 weeks. *P* = placenta; *B* = fetal bladder; *A* = markedly diminished amnionic fluid. Bladder-amnionic shunt inserted with return of amnionic fluid volume to normal. **C,** shunt malfunction at 22 weeks. Sagittal scan, thorax left, huge bladder right with diminished amnionic fluid. **D,** shunt reinsertion at 24 weeks associated with fetal death. Catheter had migrated out of bladder. Autopsy revealed bilateral hydronephrosis without dysplasia, large bladder with imperforate anus. Lung development normal.

REFERENCES

1. Liley AW: Intra-uterine transfusion of foetus in haemolytic disease. *Br Med J* 1963; 2:1107.
2. Young SR, Wade RV, Watt GW, et al: The results of one thousand consecutive prenatal diagnoses. *Am J Obstet Gynecol* 1983; 147:181.
3. Garrett WJ, Grunwald G, Robinson DE: Prenatal diagnosis of fetal polycystic kidney by ultrasound. *Aust NZ J Obstet Gynaecol* 1970; 10:7.
4. Fourcroy JL, Blei CL, Glassman LM, et al: Prenatal diagnosis by ultrasonography of genitourinary anomalies. *Urology* 1983; 22:223.
5. Lawson TL, Foley WD, Berland LL, et al: Ultrasonic evaluation of fetal kidneys. *Radiology* 1981; 138:153.
6. Hadlock FP, Deter RL, Carpenter R, et al: Sonography of fetal urinary tract anomalies. *AJR* 1981; 137:261.
7. Thomas IT, Smith DW: Oligohydramnios, cause of the non-renal features of Potter's syndrome, including pulmonary hypoplasia. *J Pediatr* 1974; 84:811.
8. Quan L, Smith DW: The VATER association—vertebral defects, anal atresia, TE fistula with esophageal atresia, radial and renal dysplasia: A spectrum of associated defects. *J Pediatr* 1973; 82:104.
9. Heyman MB, Berquist WE, Fonkalsrud EW., et al: Esophageal muscular ring and the VACTERL association: A case report. *Pediatrics* 1981; 67:683.
10. Grannum P, Bracken M, Silverman R, et al: Assessment of fetal kidney size in normal gestation by comparison of ratio of kidney circumference to abdominal circumference. *Am J Obstet Gynecol* 1980; 136:249.
11. Kramer SA: Current status of fetal intervention for congenital hydronephrosis. *J Urol* 1983; 130:641.
12. Mahony BS, Filly RA, Callen PW, et al: Fetal renal dysplasia; Sonographic evaluation. *Radiology* 1984; 152:143.
13. Wladimiroff JW, Campbell S: Fetal urine-production rates in normal and complicated pregnancy. *Lancet* 1974; 1:151.
14. Hill LM, Breckle R, Gehrking WC: The prenatal detection of congenital malformations by ultrasonography. *Mayo Clin Proc* 1983; 58:805.
15. Diament MJ, Fine RN, Ehrlich R, et al: Fetal hydronephrosis; Problems in diagnosis and management. *J Pediatr* 1983; 103:435.
16. Harrison MR, Golbus MS, Filly RA, et al: Management of the fetus with congenital hydronephrosis. *J Pediatr Surg* 1982; 17:728.
17. Manning FA, Lange IR, Morrison I, et al: Treatment of the fetus in utero: Evolving concepts. *Clin Obstet Gynecol* 1984; 27:378.
18. Ultrasound in industry and medicine. *Reprod Toxicol Newsletter* 1984; 3:17.
19. Wilson LM, Waterhouse JA: Obstetric ultrasound and childhood malignancies. *Lancet* 1984; 2:997.
20. Cartwright RA, McKinney PA, Hopton PA, et al: Ultrasound examinations in pregnancy and childhood cancer. *Lancet* 1984; 2:999.
21. The use of diagnostic ultrasound during pregnancy. *JAMA* 1984; 252:669.
22. Fletcher JC, Evans MI: Maternal bonding in early fetal ultrasound examinations. *N Engl J Med* 1983; 308:392.
23. Wladimiroff JW: Effect of furosemide on fetal urine production. *Br J Obstet Gynaecol* 1973; 80:680.
24. Harrison MR, Filly RA, Parer JT: Management of the fetus with a urinary tract malformation. *JAMA* 1981; 246:635.
25. Diamond DA, Sanders R, Jeffs RD: Fetal hydronephrosis; Considerations regarding urological intervention. *J Urol* 1984; 131:1155.
26. Weinstein L, Anderson CF, Finley PR, et al: The in utero management of urinary outflow tract obstruction. *J Clin Ultrasound* 1982; 10:465.
27. Glick PL, Harrison MR, Adzick NS, et al: Management of the fetus with congenital hydronephrosis II; Diagnostic assessment and selection for treatment. *J Pediatr Surg* 1985; 20:376.
28. Golbus MS, Harrison MR, Filly RA, et al: In utero treatment of urinary tract obstruction. *Am J Obstet Gynecol* 1982; 142:383.
29. Manning FA, Harman CR, Lange IR, et al: Antepartum chronic fetal vesicoamnionic shunts for obstructive uropathy: A

report of two cases. *Am J Obstet Gynecol* 1983; 145:819.

30. Shaler E, Weiner E, Feldman E, et al: External bladder—Amniotic fluid shunt for fetal urinary tract obstruction. *Obstet Gynecol* 1984; 63(suppl):315.
31. Farahani G, Goldman MA, Davis JG, et al: Use of the ultrasound aspiration transducer in midtrimester amniocentesis. *J Reprod Med* 1984; 29:227.
32. Ryan GT, Ivy GR, Pearson JW: Fetal bleeding as a major hazard of amniocentesis. *Obstet Gynecol* 1972; 40:702.
33. Cromie WJ, Bates RD, Duckett JW: Penetrating renal trauma in the neonate. *J Urol* 1978; 119:259.
34. Galle PC, Meis PJ: Complications of amniocentesis. *J Reprod Med* 1982; 27:149.
35. Larkin RM, Knochel JQ, Lee TG: Intrauterine transfusions; New techniques and results. *Clin Obstet Gynecol* 1982; 25:303.
36. Harrison MR, Golbus MS, Filly RA: *The Unborn Patient; Prenatal Diagnosis and Treatment*. New York, Grune & Stratton, 1984.
37. Manning FA: Unpublished data, 1984.
38. Harrison MR, Anderson J, Rosen MA, et al: Fetal surgery in the primate I: Anesthetic, surgical and tocolytic management to maximize fetal-neonatal survival. *J Pediatr Surg* 1982; 17:115.
39. Harrison MR, Golbus MS, Filly RA, et al: Fetal surgery for congenital hydronephrosis. *N Engl J Med* 1982; 306:591.
40. Glazer GM, Filly RA, Callen PW: The varied sonographic appearance of the urinary tract in the fetus and newborn with urethral obstruction. *Radiology* 1982; 144:563.
41. Gruenwald SM, Crocker EF, Walker AG, et al: Antenatal diagnosis of urinary tract abnormalities: Correlation of ultrasound appearance with postnatal diagnosis. *Am J Obstet Gynecol* 1984; 148:278.
42. Berkowitz RL, Glickman MG, Smith GJW, et al: Fetal urinary tract obstruction; What is the role of surgical intervention in utero? *Am J Obstet Gynecol* 1982; 144:367.
43. Mackie GG, Stephens FD: Duplex kidneys; A correlation of renal dysplasia with position of the ureteral orifice. *J Urol* 1975; 114:274.
44. Mandell J, Kinard HW, Mittelstaedt CA, et al: Prenatal diagnosis of unilateral hydronephrosis with early postnatal reconstruction. *J Urol* 1984; 132:303.
45. Hellstrom MJG, Kogan BA, Jeffrey RB Jr, et al: The natural history of prenatal hydronephrosis with normal amounts of amniotic fluid. *J Urol* 1984; 132:947.
46. Sholder AJ, Maizels M, Depp R, et al: Caution in antenatal intervention. *J Urol* 1988; 139:1026.
47. McFayden IR: Obstruction of the fetal urinary tract; A role for surgical intervention in utero? *Br Med J* 1984; 288:459.
48. Blane CB, Koff SA, Bowerman RA, et al: Non-obstructive fetal hydronephrosis; Sonographic recognition and therapeutic implications. *Radiology* 1983; 147:95.
49. McFayden IR, Wigglesworth JS, Dillon MJ: Fetal urinary tract obstruction: Is active intervention before delivery indicated? *Br J Obstet Gynaecol* 1983; 90:342.
50. Bellinger MF, Comstock CH, Grosso D, et al: Fetal posterior urethral valves and renal dysplasia at 15 weeks gestational age. *J Urol* 1983; 129:1238.

SECTION IV

Complications of Ureteral and Vesical Surgery

CHAPTER 30

Complications of Cutaneous Vesicostomy and Ureterostomy

H. Norman Noe, M.D.

In recent years, urinary diversion has been used less frequently as a method of management for many urologic conditions encountered in children. Improved techniques, better instrumentation, and more efficient approaches to management have evolved, resulting in initial correction or primary reconstruction of the underlying abnormalities, even in infants. Permanent urinary diversion has certainly been avoided when possible as poor long-term results have accumulated. Temporary diversion still retains a useful place in pediatric urology but has been used with decreasing, frequency. This chapter will deal solely with the complications of temporary diversion, since permanent diversion is discussed elsewhere in the text (see Chap. 16, complications of urinary diversion).

Intubated diversion is mentioned only for completeness. The chronic infections with progressive hydronephrosis associated with intubated diversion lead to renal and life-threatening problems in children that are intolerable. It is no longer a recommended form of diversion in children other than for very short-term purposes or in emergency situations. It is for the above-mentioned reasons that tubeless diversion has been used whenever temporary diversion is indicated. The two major forms of temporary diversion that can be used for short or extended periods in children are cutaneous vesicostomy and ureterostomy. These techniques are especially applicable when extended periods of diversion are necessary. The procedures are discussed in regard to their indications and the prevention and management of complications.

VESICOSTOMY

Vesicostomy was advocated by Blocksom in 1957.[1] The procedure was subsequently modified and advocated by some for use as a means of permanent diversion.[2–4] This technique to provide permanent diversion caused dissatisfaction primarily when used for adults, in whom skin flaps were used to construct the vesicostomy. The hair contained in the skin flaps led to encrustation, stone formation, and resistant urinary tract infections. Also, the inability to fit the vesicostomy with an appropriate collection device ultimately led most centers to avoid it as a means of permanent diversion.

The overall experience with vesicostomy led to application of this technique as a method of temporary diversion in children. The hair associated with the skin flaps is not a problem in children. Additionally, no collection device is needed, since these children wear diapers as their means of collection. Experience has grown in the use of vesicostomy as temporary diversion in children, and it appears that the Blocksom technique has gained the most popularity.[5-16] The advantages of this technique are that it is a quick, tubeless, and readily reversible method of urinary diversion which, in the more abdominally-positioned bladder of the child, is easy to perform. The use of skin flaps requires a more extensive procedure and seems to offer little advantage, particularly in the younger child. A major advantage of vesicostomy is that, when successful, it prevents the need for higher diversion and thus a more complex reconstruction at a later date.

Indications and General Considerations

The most common conditions that have been managed by vesicostomy are shown in Table 30–1. In general, the purpose is to decompress the urinary system at the bladder level and, by its tubeless nature, diminish the chance of urinary tract infection. Although many of the conditions shown in Table 30–1 are managed by primary definitive surgical correction, there are clinical instances in which a small and septic or uremic infant would be more safely managed after a period of diversion and resultant clinical improvement. Vesicostomy has had its widest application in the management of the neurogenic bladder with or without reflux. Infravesical obstruction due to many causes has responded well to the use of vesicostomy with definitive correction carried out at a later date. Although primary reflux is best managed by reconstruction, the septic neonate, in some instances, may be best served by a temporary tubeless diversion that can allow restoration of ureteral function and muscular tone. This may prevent the need for ureteral tailoring at the time of reimplantation.

TABLE 30–1.
Conditions Managed by Vesicostomy

Conditions Managed by Vesicostomy
Neurogenic vesical dysfunction
Vesicoureteral reflux
Urethral valves
Prune belly syndrome
Ureterocele
Cloacal and urogenital sinus anomalies
Urethral trauma
Pelvic tumors

Some idea as to the effectiveness of vesicostomy can be obtained preoperatively by studies taken when drainage has been established by bladder catheterization. A simple drainage film with the catheter indwelling following a cystogram on a child with severe reflux or valves can show whether the upper urinary system is decompressed. Likewise, renal ultrasound or renal scan with the bladder decompressed can also provide needed information in this regard. The measurement of renal function and urinary output during a period of bladder catheterization can also add helpful information about the effectiveness of drainage by vesicostomy.

Technical Aspects

The overall complication rate associated with vesicostomy is quite low, and, of equal importance, when encountered, it is usually easy to manage. As with any complication of a surgical procedure, the anticipation of potential difficulties and their prevention provides the best type of management. Attention to some areas of technical detail at the time of surgery can be most helpful in this regard. The technique of cutaneous vesicostomy most widely used is that described and popularized by Duckett.[5] A 2-cm incision is made transversely approximately halfway between the umbilicus and the symphysis over the dome of the bladder. Distension of the bladder via catheter at the operating table is helpful in planning the actual site of cystotomy, which should be as cephalad as possible on the bladder dome. This is especially important in a large, redundant bladder, since it helps to immobilize the dome, provide optimum drainage, and minimize prolapse. Attempts should be made to stay extraperitoneal in the dissection, and if the bladder is redundant, it has been advised that the bladder be tacked to the fascia both superiorly and inferiorly to minimize the possibility of prolapse.[14]

Complications

Failure to Decompress the Upper Urinary System.—It is usually easy to determine if vesicostomy will be successful in the decompression of the upper urinary system by observation and studies during a period of catheter drainage. If hydronephrosis diminishes with the bladder decompressed, particularly if renal function improves, it is reasonable to assume that vesicostomy will prove useful as a technique of diversion (Fig 30–1). Early in the use of vesicostomy, it was feared that obstruction would occur at the ureterovesical junction caused by a thick-walled bladder. This obstruction infrequently occurs. Some children have transient edema, inflammation, detrusor spasm, or a combination of such factors which can produce increasing obstruction of the upper urinary system at the ureterovesical junction.[17] This phenomenon can be managed by short-term drainage with percutaneous nephrostomy or ureteral stent. If the obstruction reverses, then vesicostomy can be allowed to provide decompression and the intubated diversion discontinued. If continued obstruction of the upper urinary tracts is on the basis of ureteral tor-

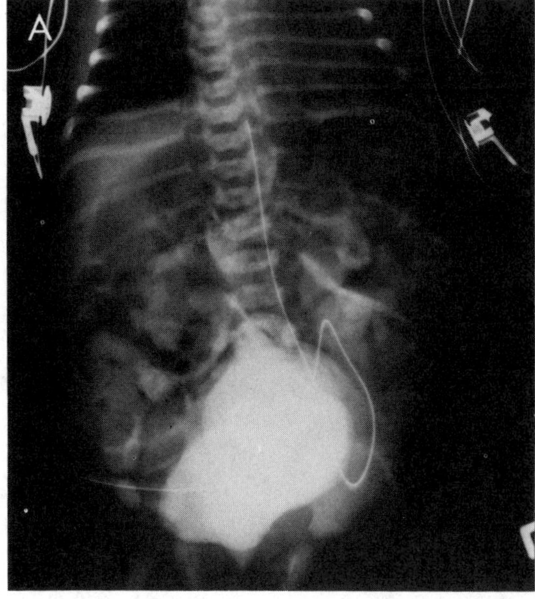

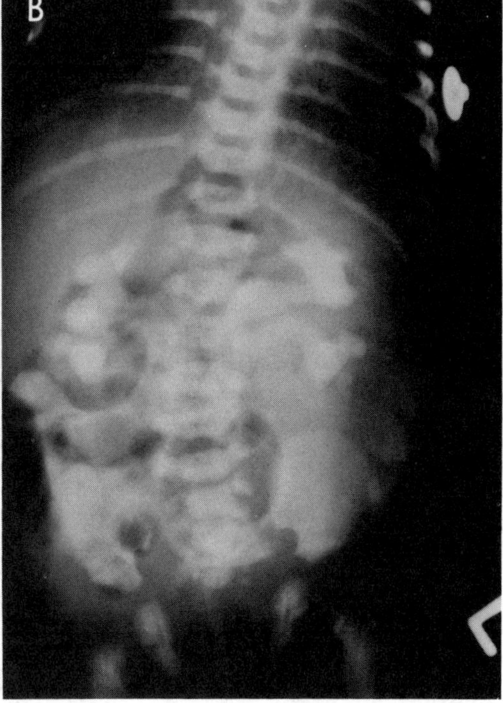

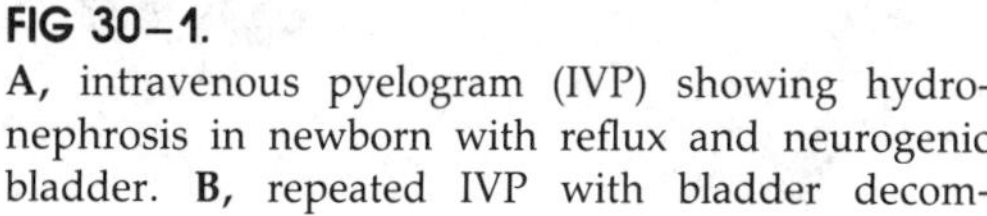

FIG 30–1.
A, intravenous pyelogram (IVP) showing hydronephrosis in newborn with reflux and neurogenic bladder. **B,** repeated IVP with bladder decompressed, showing also good decompression of the upper tracts.

tuosity, extreme dilatation, ureteral atony, or actual ureterovesical obstruction, loop cutaneous ureterostomy would be necessary to establish a more efficient form of temporary drainage.

Prolapse.—Prolapse, in many series, appears to be the most common complication encountered with vesicostomy (Fig 30–2). Points of technique important in minimizing the chance of prolapse include placing the incision in the bladder as cephalad on the dome as possible. With a large, redundant bladder, the most cephalad portion may actually be above the urachal remnant. Immobilizing the dome can prevent prolapse of the posterior wall of the bladder through the stoma. Fixation of the bladder wall superiorly and inferiorly to the inferior surface of the fascia can be helpful in immobilizing the bladder dome. Placing the incision beneath the bladder dome, in addition to inviting prolapse, may allow obstruction of the stoma and prevent its ability to drain the urinary system adequately. If a question remains as to the exact location of the most cephalad portion of the bladder, this area can be estimated by filling the bladder per catheter at the time of surgery. Keeping the skin and fascial incision to approximately 2 to 2½ cm also assures that the stoma is of proper size. It is obvious that a stoma that is too large predisposes to prolapse.

Correction of prolapse consists of revising the stoma, placing the opening in the bladder in the most cephalad portion of the dome, and narrowing any fascial enlargement that exists.

Eversion of the mucosa is frequently seen but does not represent true prolapse.

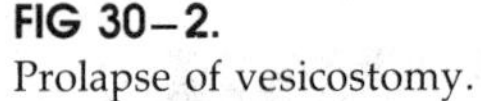

FIG 30–2.
Prolapse of vesicostomy.

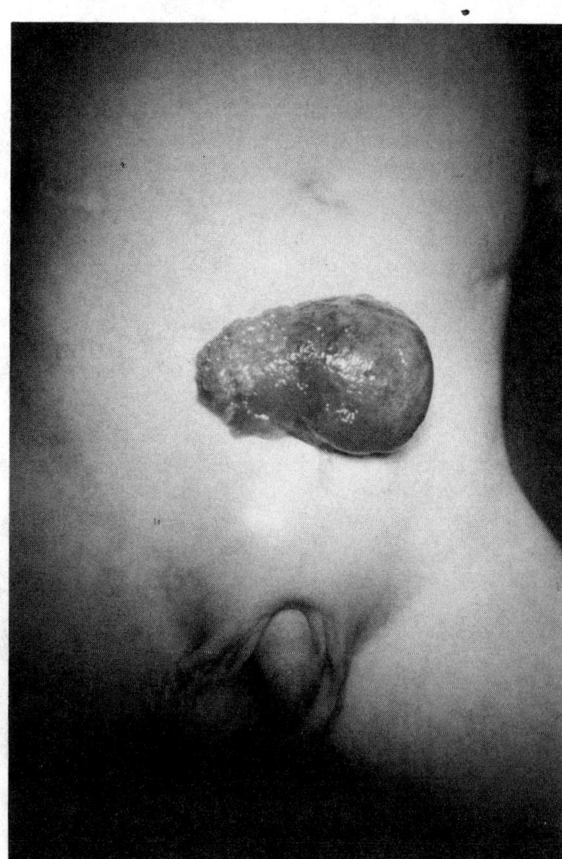

It is common to see mucosal changes such as squamous metaplasia over the exposed bladder, but this tissue is removed at the time of vesicostomy closure and appears to be of no long-term consequence.

Stenosis.—Stenosis can be difficult to define in a child with a vesicostomy. A stoma that appears large initially may diminish in size as the child grows but continues to serve to decompress the bladder satisfactorily. It must be remembered that the purpose of vesicostomy is to provide a low-pressure system with adequate drainage of the bladder. An opening that appears narrow can continue to keep the bladder decompressed and not represent a true stenosis. A stenosis would then, most likely, be associated with large residuals, continued or increasing upper tract distension, or increasing bladder pressures as measured urodynamically. In my experience, stenosis has most frequently occurred in thickened bladders, particularly in otherwise neurologically normal children with normal abdominal muscular function. Growth and tension at the anastomosis can serve to narrow the stoma and diminish its drainage capacity. Severe dermatitis can lead to increased scarring at the stoma site and also serve to narrow the opening. When encountered, this complication can be best managed by simple stomal revision, enlarging the fascial opening and assuring that the bladder is under no tension and that the mucosa is properly everted. Postoperative dilatation of the stoma using a gloved finger can be helpful in maintaining adequate caliber, but this is not done routinely. This procedure is reserved for the situations in which it is thought that stenosis is likely to be developing.

Urinary Tract Infection.—Periodic bacteriuria in patients with vesicostomy can be demonstrated in a large percentage of patients. Chemoprophylaxis can be used in these instances, but resistant organisms can persist in the urine, causing clinically significant urinary tract infections. Culture validity can be assured by using either percutaneous aspiration of bladder urine, urethral catheterization, or double-lumen catheterization of the stoma as the procedure for urine collection. A single urine culture that is positive should be repeated to rule out contamination and to insure accuracy as a treatment guide in a symptomatic patient. If symptomatic infections continue to be problematic despite prophylaxis, reconstruction and closure of the vesicostomy are undertaken at the earliest possible time. It must be remembered that when infections are encountered, residual urine, a poorly functioning stoma, stomal stenosis, or stones should be suspected, and, if possible, a correction of any underlying abnormality should be performed to allow retention of the vesicostomy for a longer period of time if necessary. In a series of 35 patients I have treated, 6 had urinary tract infections, with all patients having urethral valves with upper tract dilatation and tortuosity, suggesting that stasis does play a role in predisposition to clinically significant urinary tract infections.

Dermatitis.—Dermatitis is commonly seen in children with vesicostomy. It is usually transient and treated with the appropriate antifungal or anti-inflammatory agent. Urinary acidification and the use of protective agents around the stoma can be helpful as preventive measures. If persistent and severe, such dermatitis has been noted to result in stomal stenosis, but this is not seen routinely.

Stones.—Stone formation has been reported, but usually in conjunction with urinary tract infections. If small, the stones can simply be grasped and removed through the stoma or crushed and evacuated by irrigation. Any associated infection should be controlled with antibiotics. Stone formation has been observed

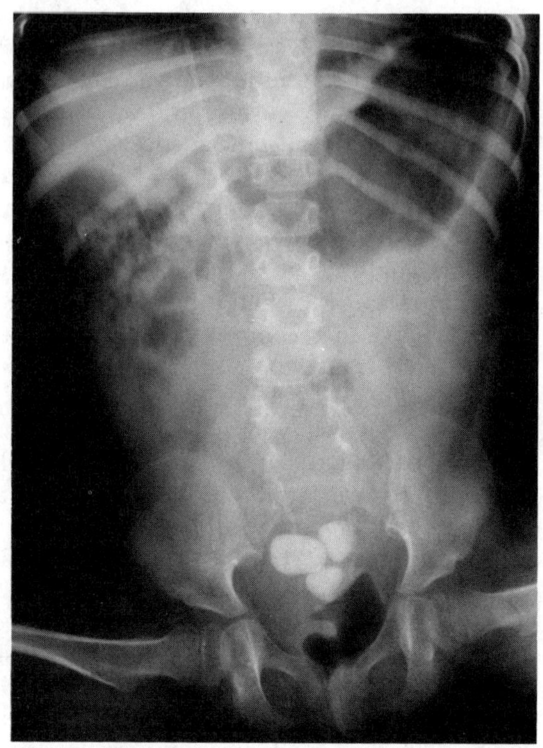

FIG 30–3.
Bladder stones with recurrent resistant infections after vesicostomy closure.

even after vesicostomy closure, and if resistant infections continue to persist, stone formation should be suspected (Fig 30–3).

Miscellaneous or Associated Conditions.—Parastomal hernia can be present with prolapse and is usually managed by appropriate stomal revision.

Urethral incontinence is of little concern in children, since the majority of those with vesicostomy are in diapers. Incontinence could theoretically be important in the older child, but, in most instances, reconstruction will be accomplished before they reach the age of social concern.

Urethral stricture has been observed in children who have had valves fulgurated or have had other urethral procedures performed at the time vesicostomy was first established. This results in the so-called "dry" urethra, and for this reason definitive valve ablation is usually delayed until the vesicostomy is closed. Vesicostomy has been offered as a means to prevent postvalve strictures in children by waiting until they grow large enough so that the valves can be resected without excessive urethral trauma in the older, larger child.[18]

The fear of diminished bladder capacity that would affect definitive reconstructive procedures has been unfounded. Bladder capacity has been observed to decrease only in children with prior severe infections or periods of intubated diversion leading to fibrosis of the bladder. A period of temporary drainage by vesicostomy can actually facilitate reconstruction by allowing bladder thickening to diminish and dilated ureters to return to a more normal caliber. This can actually prevent the need to tailor such ureters and provide a bladder that is more favorable for surgical success.

URETEROSTOMY

Ureterostomy, once a popular form of supravesical diversion, has been used less frequently in most centers as the trend against diversion in children continues. There remain instances in which tubeless diversion at a high level is still valuable.

Intubated ureterostomy is periodically advocated as a temporary form of diversion in various reconstructive procedures in children. The advantage is its nonoperative reversibility and the provision of continued access to the upper urinary system for appropriate interval studies. The use of intubated ureterostomy for other than very short periods is limited by the problems inherent with foreign bodies and associated infection. This technique continues to see limited application.

The two major forms of tubeless diversion above the bladder level are loop cutaneous ureterostomy and end cutaneous ureterostomy. Both techniques are well described in standard urologic texts. Loop ureterostomy was first popularized by Johnston.[19] The ease of performance and its reliability in providing drainage of the kidney allowed it to be applied to the small, azotemic, and critically ill infant or neonate as a temporizing procedure. Experience has accumulated at several centers[20–27] that has proven this to be a safe and reliable technique, but it carries with it certain disadvantages, including problems encountered in reconstruction of the urinary tract at a later time.

The use of the terminal ureter as a means of diversion in the form of end cutaneous ureterostomy can be a temporizing procedure, but it has more often been advocated as a form of permanent urinary diversion. The technical aspects of this procedure are quite different from that of loop cutaneous ureterostomy and the complications include stomal difficulties similar to those seen with other forms of permanent diversion.

Loop Ureterostomy

Loop ureterostomy has as its major advantage its ease of performance, reliability of upper tract drainage, and lack of disturbance of the distal ureter. Proper patient selection is essential to ensure the success of this technique. An absolute prerequisite for the application of this technique is that a dilated and tortuous ureter be present. This technique can be applied in any situation where distal obstruction exists and lower diversion or primary reconstruction is deemed ineffective or inadvisable. The dissection of the ureter in the exteriorized loop should be minimized, with particular attention paid to preserving the ureteral vasculature within the adventitia. Since the blood supply of the ureter is regional, preservation of the vasculature can be especially important in the reconstructive phases. The stoma is placed within a small subcostal or anterior subcostal incision and should be under no tension, nor should the fascia be closed behind the stoma, which could be a contributing factor to stomal stenosis. The loop to be exteriorized should be as near the ureteropelvic junction as possible to avoid ureteral kinking, which can obstruct drainage of the proximal portion of the ureter. Tension or damage to the ureteropelvic junction should be avoided, likewise, to prevent future obstruction. Dissection should remain retroperitoneal, and if a question exists as to the differentiation of the ureter from the bowel, aspiration of urine using a small-bore needle can confirm the identity of the ureter. The stoma is created by sewing the ureteral margins flush with the skin in the anticipation of diaper dressings as collection devices instead of the usual stomal appliances.

Modification of the loop cutaneous ureterostomy consists of either a Y-type ureterostomy or ring ureterostomy.[28, 29] The advantage of these modified techniques is the preservation of ureteral continuity and continued flow of urine into the bladder to prevent bladder defunctionalization. The fear of bladder contraction secondary to bladder defunctionalization has been more a theoretical than a practical consideration. Bladder contraction usually occurs only in cases in which supravesical diversion has occurred with severe bladder infection, leading to fibrosis of the detrusor. In this latter instance, one of these modified techniques could be particularly useful. The disadvantage of these modified techniques is the greater dissection required and the additional time consumed in the performance of the procedure, which, in a sick infant, may be undesirable.

Complications

Acute.—The most serious immediate complications of this procedure would be ureteral tissue loss or slough. Prevention of this complication is dependent on attention to detail and dissection that preserves ureteral adventitia and blood supply. Stomal bleeding can occur in the immediate postoperative period, but it is usually easily managed by local measures. Entry into the bowel is a possibility, but identification by aspiration of the ureter can be helpful in avoiding this undesirable result. Failure to drain the upper urinary system is caused by poor selection of the ureteral loop to be exteriorized, usually leading to kinking or obstruction proximally. If the stoma has to be catheterized for drainage, it should be revised if the ureterostomy is to remain in place for an extended period. Catheterization of the proximal limb of the ureterostomy at the time of surgery can assure that there is adequate drainage and minimizes the chance of encountering proximal obstruction in the immediate postoperative period.

Late.—Delayed complications and management problems are primarily those related to stomal irritation. Urinary acidification and appropriate local antiinflammatory, antibacterial, or antifungal measures are usually helpful in this regard. Bacilluria does occur, but if drainage has been properly established, the number of episodes of clinically significant pyelonephritis are minimal. It is possible that, with long-term diversion by cutaneous ureterostomy, continued infection can lead to ureteral scarring with loss of peristalsis. This loss can be especially important in the problems associated with reconstruction. Stenosis is an unusual complication of loop cutaneous ureterostomy because of the large caliber of the ureter. It can occur, however, if tension is present at the ureteral stoma or if continued infection is present and irritation occurs at the stomal site. In those patients in whom the ureterostomy has remained in place for an extended period of time, body growth, with increasing abdominal wall thickness and subcutaneous fat, has been associated with increasing stenosis of these ureteral stomas with time. The formation of stones within the urinary system has been observed in children diverted by ureterostomy, as with other forms of diversion (Fig 30–4).

Although not an immediate or late complication of ureterostomy, a significant problem associated with the use of this form of diversion is that encountered in urinary reconstruction. In selected cases, simple closure of the ureterostomy is all that is required. Dissection and freeing of the proximal and distal limbs of the exteriorized loop of ureter and resection and primary ureteral reanastomosis are usually sufficient. In those instances in which distal reconstructive procedures are required, the problem can become more complex. Controversy still exists as to whether a staged or single-procedure reconstruction is best performed in a child with loop ureterostomy.[30–32] Regardless of the reconstruction technique, strict attention to detail and preservation of re-

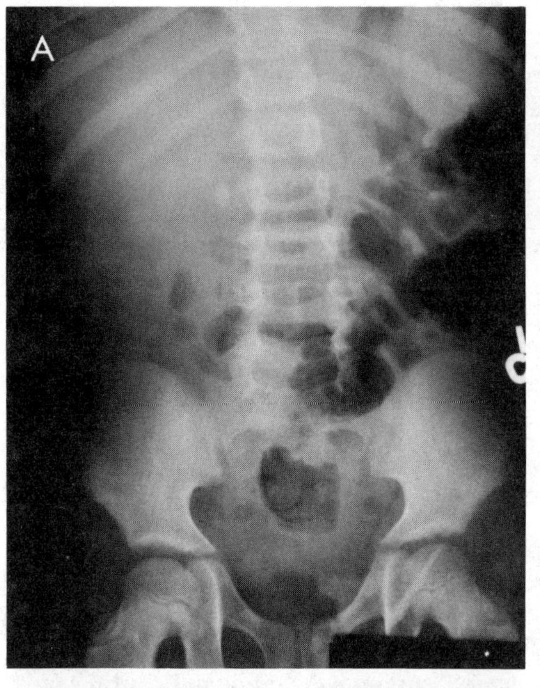

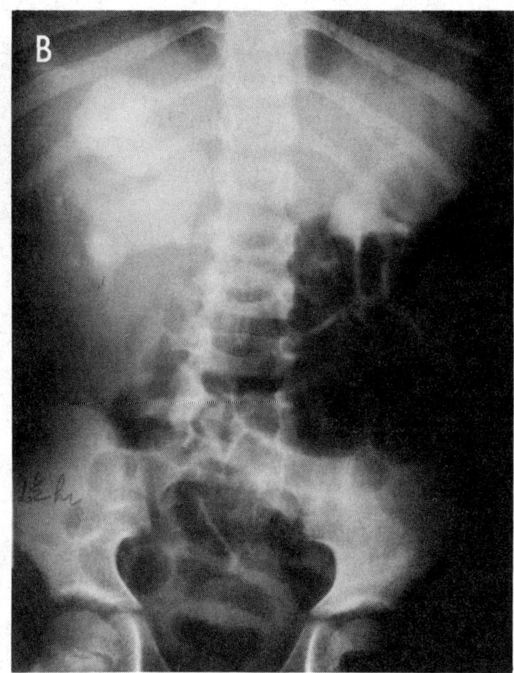

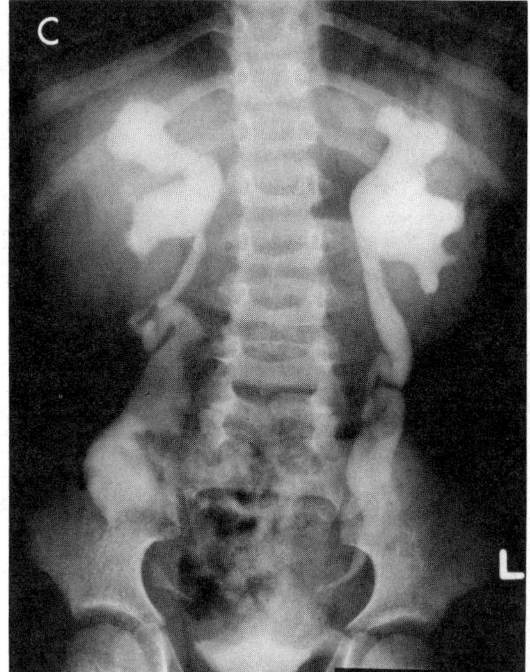

FIG 30–4.
A, plain roentgenogram showing right renal stone in a patient with prune belly syndrome and loop ureterostomies. **B,** intravenous pyelogram (IVP) showing stone obstructing ureteropelvic junction. **C,** IVP after undiversion and stone removal.

gional blood supply to the ureter are essential to the success of the procedure. It would seem prudent to perform staged reconstruction if there is a question of the degree of distal ureteral dissection required in the reconstruction.

End Cutaneous Ureterostomy

End cutaneous ureterostomy requires use of the terminal or distal portion of the proximal ureter after the ureter has been transected distally. It is not recommended as a form of temporary diversion and has been advocated in the past more for diversion that could be permanent. This technique also requires that a dilated, somewhat tortuous ureter be present. End cutaneous ureterostomy can be performed through a single lower abdominal incision, with the stoma best placed to one side of the midline. As with any form of potentially permanent diversion, stoma formation and site selection are of greatest importance. In most cases, the dissection can remain retroperitoneal, but some prefer to go inside the peritoneum to assure the most direct line of access of the ureter to the skin. Some advocate combining transureteroureterostomy with a single ureteral stoma, using the skin flap technique to improve stomal construction.[33] Others prefer bringing both ureters to the skin and constructing the stoma in a butterfly fashion.[34] As with loop ureterostomy, failure to respect the ureteral blood supply can lead to ureteral slough and stenosis. If the ureter has not been sufficiently straightened and the stoma is not dependent, failure to drain the upper urinary systems can occur more frequently than with the higher loop diversion.

The greatest problems in the use of this technique seem to center around the stoma and appliance failure. Stomal irritation with encrustation and stenosis can be minimized by proper placement and construction of the stoma at the time of the initial surgery. Acidifying the urine and assuring the appliance with a proper face plate configuration is helpful in stomal management. Local measures, as with other forms of stomal irritation, can also be helpful (Fig 30–5).

Peritoneal adhesions, with resultant

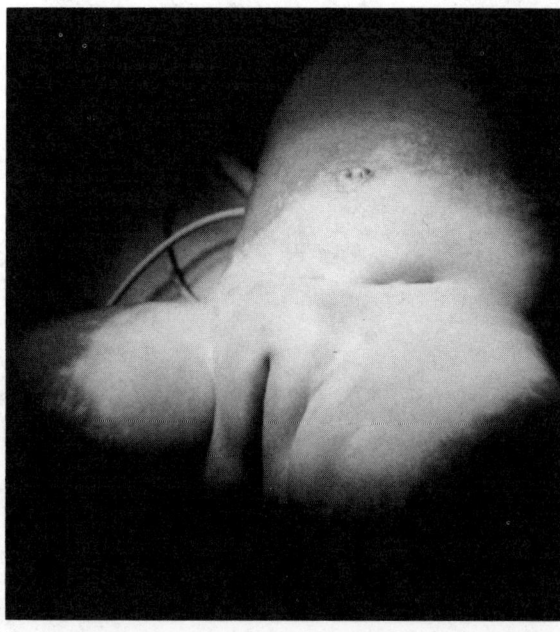

FIG 30–5.
Stomal irritation and marked pigment loss of surrounding skin at ureterostomy site.

intestinal obstruction, is possible if intraperitoneal dissection is performed. Bacilluria with recurrent pyelonephritis and possible stone formation is, likewise, a known complication of this form of diversion. Long-term diversion by this technique can ultimately lead to ureteral tissue changes and dysfunction, which can be undesirable, since they might affect reconstruction efforts.

OTHER FORMS OF HIGH DIVERSION

Cutaneous pyelostomy has been advocated, and it appears to be accompanied by the same complications that afflict loop cutaneous ureterostomy. One unusual complication has been herniation of the cutaneous pyelostomy and of the kidney itself, which appears to be related to renal dysplasia and the size of stoma formation.[35] If cutaneous pyelostomy is used for diversion, and renal pelvic volume decreases, reconstruction could require the use of a dismembered pyeloplasty and upper ureteral dissection in association with required lower ureteral dissection and reconstruction.

Terminal loop cutaneous ureterostomy has been used when it is necessary to divert a patient with normal caliber ureters.[36] By bringing the terminal ureter subcutaneously, the distal segment undergoes neovascularization and decreases the chance that stomal stenosis will be encountered with the exteriorized normal ureter. This technique would seem to have a very limited place in the management of obstructive problems in children.

EDITORIAL COMMENT

As Dr. Noe indicates, there are fewer indications for cutaneous vesicostomy and ureterostomy because urologists now tend to utilize primary reconstruction. I have utilized temporary vesicostomy for a neonatal prune belly syndrome when significant respiratory problems were present. I have also utilized a cutaneous pyelostomy for a pyonephrosis in a newborn and then reoperated at 4 to 6 months and performed a standard pyeloplasty. A loop ureterostomy often makes a later reconstruction more difficult and hazardous, so it should be considered with great caution.

REFERENCES

1. Blocksom B: Bladder pouch for prolonged tubeless cystostomy. *J Urol* 1957; 78:398.
2. Lapides J, Ajenian EP, Lichtwardt JR: Cutaneous vesicostomy. *J Urol* 1960; 84:609.
3. Ross G Jr, Michener FR, Brady C Jr, et al: Cutaneous vesicostomy: A review of 36 cases. *J Urol* 1965; 94:402.
4. Paquin AJ Jr, Howard RS, Gillenwater JY: Cutaneous vesicostomy: A modification of a technique. *J Urol* 1968; 99:270.
5. Duckett JW JR: Cutaneous vesicostomy in childhood: The Blocksom technique. *Urol Clin North Am* 1974; 1:485.
6. Ireland GW, Geist RW: Difficulties with vesicostomies in 15 children with meningomyelocele. *J Urol* 1970; 103:341.
7. Karafin L, Kendall AR: Vesicostomy in the management of neurogenic bladder disease secondary to meningomyelocele in children. *J Urol* 1966; 96:723.
8. Bell TE, Hoddin AO, Evans AT: Tubeless cystostomy in children. *J Urol* 1968; 100:459.
9. Belman AB, King LR: Vesicostomy—Useful means of reversible urinary diversion in selected infants. *Urology* 1973; 1:208.
10. Lytton B, Weiss RM: Cutaneous vesicostomy for temporary urinary diversion in infants. *J Urol* 1971; 105:888.
11. Allen TD: Vesicostomy for the temporary diversion of the urine in small children. *J Urol* 1980; 123:929.
12. Mandell J, Bauer SB, Colodny AH, et al: Cutaneous vesicostomy in infancy. *J Urol* 1981; 26:92.
13. Bruce RR, Gonzales ET Jr: Cutaneous

vesicostomy: A useful form of temporary diversion in children. *J Urol* 1980; 123:927.
14. Cohen JS, Harbach LB, Kaplan GW: Cutaneous vesicostomy for temporary urinary diversion in infants with neurogenic bladder dysfunction. *J Urol* 1978; 119:120.
15. Snyder HM III, Kalichman MA, Charney E, et al: Vesicostomy for neurogenic bladder with spina bifida: Follow-up. *J Urol* 1983; 130:724.
16. Noe, HN, Jerkins GR: Cutaneous vesicostomy experience in infants and children. *J Urol* 1985; 134:301.
17. Noe HN, Jerkins GR: Oliguria and renal failure following decompression of the bladder in children with posterior urethral valves. *J Urol* 1983; 129:595.
18. Myers DA, Walker RD III: Prevention of urethral strictures in the management of posterior urethral valves. *J Urol* 1981; 126:655.
19. Johnston JH: Temporary cutaneous ureterostomy in the treatment of advanced congenital urinary obstruction. *Arch Dis Child* 1963; 38:161.
20. Williams DI, Rabinovitch MM: Cutaneous ureterostomy for the grossly dilated ureter of childhood. *Br J Urol* 1967; 39:696.
21. Perlmutter AD, Tank ES: Loop cutaneous ureterostomy in infancy. *J Urol* 1968; 99:559.
22. Perlmutter AD, Patil J: Loop cutaneous ureterostomy in infants and young children: Late results in 32 cases. *J Urol* 1972; 107:655.
23. Rabinowitz R, Barken M, Schillinger JF, et al: Surgical treatment of the massively dilated ureter in children. Part I: Management by cutaneous ureterostomy. *J Urol* 1977; 117:658.
24. Hendren HW: Complications of ureterostomy. *J Urol* 1978; 120:269.
25. Retik AB, Perlmutter AD: Temporary urinary diversion in infants and young children, in Harrison JH, Gittes RF, Perlmutter AD, et al: *Campbell's Urology*, ed 4. Philadelphia, WB Saunders Co, 1979.
26. Feminella JG Jr, Lattimer JK: A retrospective analysis of 70 cases of cutaneous ureterostomy. J Urol 1971; 106:538.
27. Sadlowski RW, Belman AB, Filmer RB, et al: Followup of cutaneous ureterostomy in children. *J Urol* 1978; 119:116.
28. Sober I: Pelvioureterostomy-en-Y. *J Urol* 1972; 107:473.
29. Cromie WJ, Williams DI: "Ring" ureterostomy. *Br J Urol* 1975; 47:789.
30. Duckett JW Jr: Anomalies of the urethra, in Harrison JH, Gittes RF, Perlmutter AD, et. al.: *Campbell's Urology*, ed 4. Philadelphia, WB Saunders Co, 1979.
31. Dwoskin JY: Management of the massively dilated urinary tract in infants by temporary diversion and single-stage reconstruction. *Urol Clin North Am* 1974; 1:515.
32. Novak ME, Gonzales ET: Single stage reconstruction of urinary tract after loop cutaneous ureterostomy. *Urology* 1979; 11:134.
33. Straffon RA, Kyle K, Corvalan J: Techniques of cutaneous ureterostomy and results in 51 patients. *J Urol* 1970; 103:138.
34. Lapides J: Butterfly cutaneous ureterostomy. *J Urol* 1962; 88:735.
35. Francis DR, Bucy JG: Inside-out kidney: An unusual complication of cutaneous pyelostomy. *J Urol* 1974; 112:514.
36. Amin M, Clark R, Hoverton LW, et al: Terminal loop cutaneous ureterostomy: An experimental study and its clinical application. *J Urol* 1977; 118:383.

CHAPTER 31

Complications of Reimplantation and Ureterocele Surgery

Richard C. Rink, M.D.
Michael E. Mitchell, M.D.

Surgery to correct "routine" vesicoureteral reflux in most centers today has reached success that is unparalleled by other major operative procedures, yet the majority of patients are managed nonoperatively. It is for this reason that prior to discussion of any *surgical* complications and their prevention we must first examine complications of *nonsurgical* therapy. Several factors have led to the medical management of vesicoureteral reflux but seldom are the complications of this choice discussed.

NONSURGICAL COMPLICATIONS

Normand and Smellie followed the course of children with reflux for 9 to 15 years. In those without ureteral dilatation, 80% had spontaneous resolution of their reflux. However, in those children with dilated ureters, resolution was noted in only 41%.[1] In the patients without primary bladder pathology or bladder outlet obstruction, new renal scarring or the extension of established scars has been satisfactorily documented *only* in those with infection.[2] The cornerstone of medical management therefore is the ability to properly select patients without bladder and urethral dysfunction and to keep the patient infection-free with continuous low-dose antibiotics. Normand and Smellie, using chronic prophylactic antibiotic therapy, noted an infection rate of approximately 4.5% per year.[1] Although this represents a small group of patients, they are at risk for upper tract infection and its sequelae. Some authors believe that the water hammer effect of reflux may have a deleterious result on renal function and growth without infection, but this effect generally occurs only with very high intravesical pressures. Renal growth and function are generally not impaired if the bladder pressure is normal and the child remains free of infection.[3] However, there may be a decrease in renal growth following a renal infection.[4]

Assumptions and Risks of Medical Management

The risks for medical complications relate to (1) patient compliance with the medical program, (2) long-term, drug-related side effects, (3) persistent reflux, (4) renal scarring, and (5) recurrent infection.

Medical therapy is totally dependent on patient and family compliance. Compliance rates in the best of hands have been greater than 90%.[1] Noncompliant patients are untreated and at significant risk for infection and renal scarring. The potential for complications from long-term drug therapy must be weighed carefully in every patient. The side effects of any medication taken chronically are to be anticipated. Development of drug allergies has most commonly resulted in failure of medical management in our experience. Gastrointestinal and emotional reactions to Trimethoprim/Sulfa and Nitrofurantoin are not uncommon, and severe reactions such as blood dyscrasias and interstitial pneumonitis have been reported.[5–7] Furthermore, the long-term implications of chronic antibiotic therapy have not been clearly defined, and it is hoped that it will not prove to be more significant than the risks of nontreated reflux.

The basic assumptions of medical management are that infection can be prevented with chronic antibiotic therapy and that reflux spontaneously resolves with time. The efficacy of antibiotic therapy, though not without its problems, has been clearly proved when properly applied. What is to be done, however, with that group of teenage and young adult patients who have persistent reflux after chronic antibiotic therapy? Although Ransley[8] warns against the temptation to surgically correct reflux at maturity due to its benignity, Libertino[9] believes adult reflux should be treated surgically. The implication of reflux in the adult, particularly during pregnancy, is not clear.

Hypertension is now known to have a close association with pyelonephritis and renal scarring.[10] The incidence has been shown to increase with advancing age. In patients with bilateral renal scarring, hypertension has been noted to develop in 18% with long-term follow-up, whereas hypertension will occur in 11.3% if scarring is unilateral.[11] Unfortunately, treatment of reflux is often initiated after scarring has occurred. Medical management can clearly prevent new scarring. However, medical therapy (and antireflux surgery) probably do not change the potential for hypertension to develop in those patients with renal scarring, although further study is required.[2, 12, 13] Chronic follow-up to check for hypertension is mandatory in all patients with renal scarring with or without resolution of reflux.

Clinical Grouping of Patients

Persistent infection is the most common complication of medical management of reflux. To us, the single most important factor in preventing infection is the proper clinical grouping of patients with reflux. Children with neurogenic bladder (group 1), bladder outflow obstruction (group 2), voiding dysfunction (group 3), or massive vesicoureteral reflux (group 4), and neonates with severe reflux (group 5), are different from otherwise normal children with primary reflux who happen to contract a urinary tract infection (group 6). It is incumbent upon the physician to recognize these six groupings. Routine medical management alone for patients who fall into the first four groups is apt to result in failure, whereas the child in group 6 with antibiotic therapy has a good potential for spontaneous resolution of reflux and cessation of infection. Treatment in the first five groupings must be directed at the primary problem, that is, treatment of the neurogenic bladder, correction of bladder outflow obstruction, management of the voiding dysfunction, or surgical correction of reflux itself.

The overwhelming majority of patients with vesicoureteral reflux are first identified after a urinary tract infection in early childhood. However, with increased maternal ultrasonography, many neonates are identified with significant vesicoureteral reflux *prior* to any infection event. These patients are a special high-risk group that potentially can be protected from any renal injury (i.e., suffering from the "Big Bang"[14]). To allow these neonates to grow without correction of their reflux places a tremendous burden and responsibility on medical therapy, since any breakthrough infection has great potential to result in renal scarring. Certainly the potential surgical complications, obstruction in particular, are greater when dealing with the neonate's ureters and bladder, but in most pediatric urologic centers these risks are acceptable. Generally, we are in favor of surgical correction in these children.

A difficult group of otherwise "normal" children with vesicoureteral reflux who are at high risk for failure of medical management are those who present the triad of infection, reflux, and wetting. Their infections are often refractory to standard medical management. Often bacteriuria occurs during antibiotic therapy, and these organisms are often resistant to commonly used antibiotics. In fact, as a tertiary referral center, these children comprise our largest group of reflux patients. Unfortunately, they represent an overlap of two problems: (1) voiding dysfunction with recurrent infection and (2) reflux. The latter sometimes is even causally related to the former. Now it is appreciated that treatment of the voiding dysfunction may eliminate infection and even the need for antireflux surgery. In those that ultimately do require surgery, aggressive treatment of the voiding dysfunction will maximize the chance for success. These patients often do well on anticholinergic therapy but often also require extensive voiding reconditioning to insure regular complete bladder emptying.

Koff has noted that most children making the transition from infantile to adult voiding patterns will transiently have incoordination of sphincter and detrusor.[15] As a group, these children usually do well until the time of toilet training. Two populations have been identified by Koff. Those children with persistent uninhibited contractions during bladder filling will voluntarily constrict their sphincter to maintain control. This generates high intravesical pressures, which may be associated with infection and reflux. Symptomatically, most have frequency and wetting and display Vincent's curtsy. Reflux has been noted to occur in 50% of patients with uninhibited contractions. Resolution of reflux occurs in 42% with downgrading of reflux to Grade I in another 16% after treatment consisting of anticholinergics, frequent voidings, and fluid restriction.[15]

A second grouping of these "normal" children with voiding dysfunction have sphincter-detrusor incoordination during bladder emptying.[15] In our experience these children are almost all female and display incomplete bladder emptying. They usually can be successfully treated at home with *vigorous* efforts to modify voiding behavior. These patients often respond to frequent, timed voidings (every two hours) and efforts to insure complete bladder emptying. Rarely, this dysfunction may be quite severe, with associated fecal incontinence and social unrest. These patients may require short-term, intermittent clean catheterization, behavior modification, or biofeedback. We are impressed by the resolution of reflux, infection, and wetting if the voiding dysfunction is corrected. These are also the children who persist with urinary tract infections after surgical correction of reflux.

SURGICAL COMPLICATIONS

The Nondilated Ureter

Many surgical techniques are popular today and all have good results if done correctly. Several factors are important for a successful antireflux procedure, but the single most important thing, no matter what the procedure, is providing good detrusor muscle backing for the ureter in its submucosal tunnel. In general, the tunnel length-to-ureteral diameter ratio should be 5:1, but a tunnel length of 1.5–3.0 cm in a nondilated ureter is satisfactory.[16] As Hendren has stressed, avoidance of handling the ureter with forceps is imperative.[17] Other important technical aspects of antireflux surgery include (1) a tension-free anastomosis, (2) preservation of ureteral blood supply, (3) good ureteral fixation, (4) adequate closure of the hiatus, (5) placement of the hiatus in the immobile bladder base, and (6) avoidance of ureteral angulation.

Risks of Routine Reimplantation (Mechanical Factors; Fig 31–1).—Although risks are minimal today for children undergoing surgery, antireflux surgery is not totally without problems. Reflux postoperatively can be either persistent, that is, there can be continued reflux of the operated ureter, or new (contralateral nonoperated) reflux. Ipsilateral persistent reflux has been blamed on the new orifice being too lateral and the submucosal tunnel too short (Fig 31–2).[17] Gibbons and Gonzales found this reflux to be generally a lower grade, with a good chance for spontaneous resolution.[16] In Hendren's review of 1,259 reimplantations of nondilated ureters by the intravesical or combined technique, only 15 ureters (1%) refluxed postoperatively and seven of these did not require reoperation.[17] Delayed reflux following an initial successful outcome has been described.[11, 18]

Carpentier et al.[19] compared 100 Politano-Leadbetter reimplantations with 100 Cohen reimplantations and found persistent reflux in 9% of the former and 3% of the latter. Although this represents a sig-

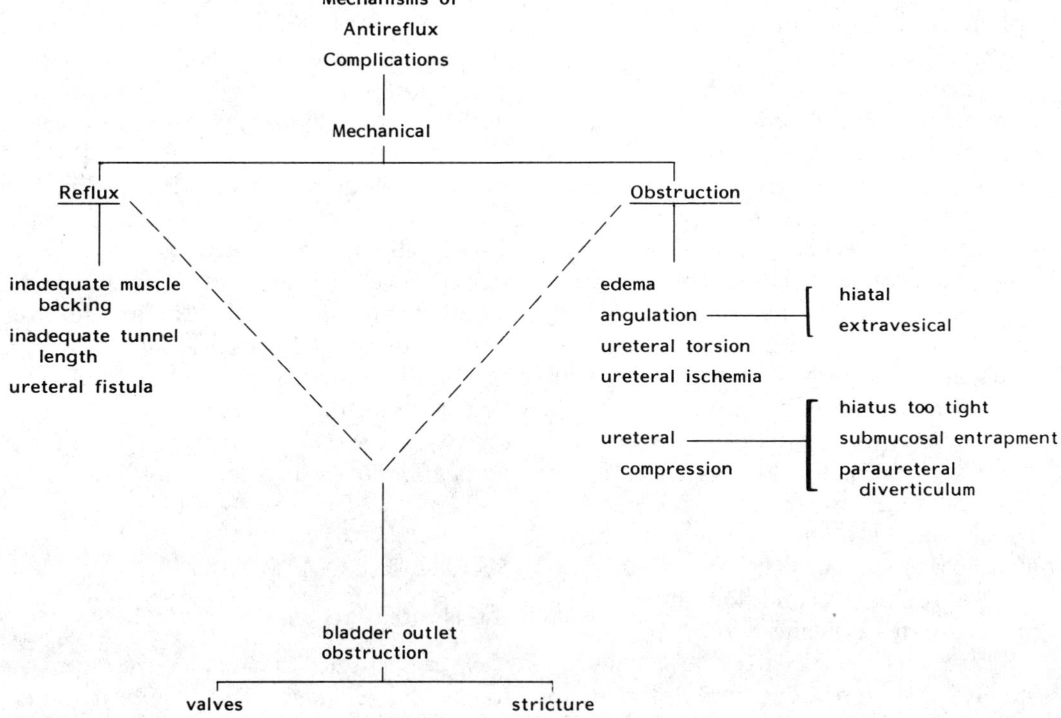

FIG 31–1.
Mechanical reasons for failure of ureteral reimplantation (bladder outlet obstruction may yield both reflux and obstruction).

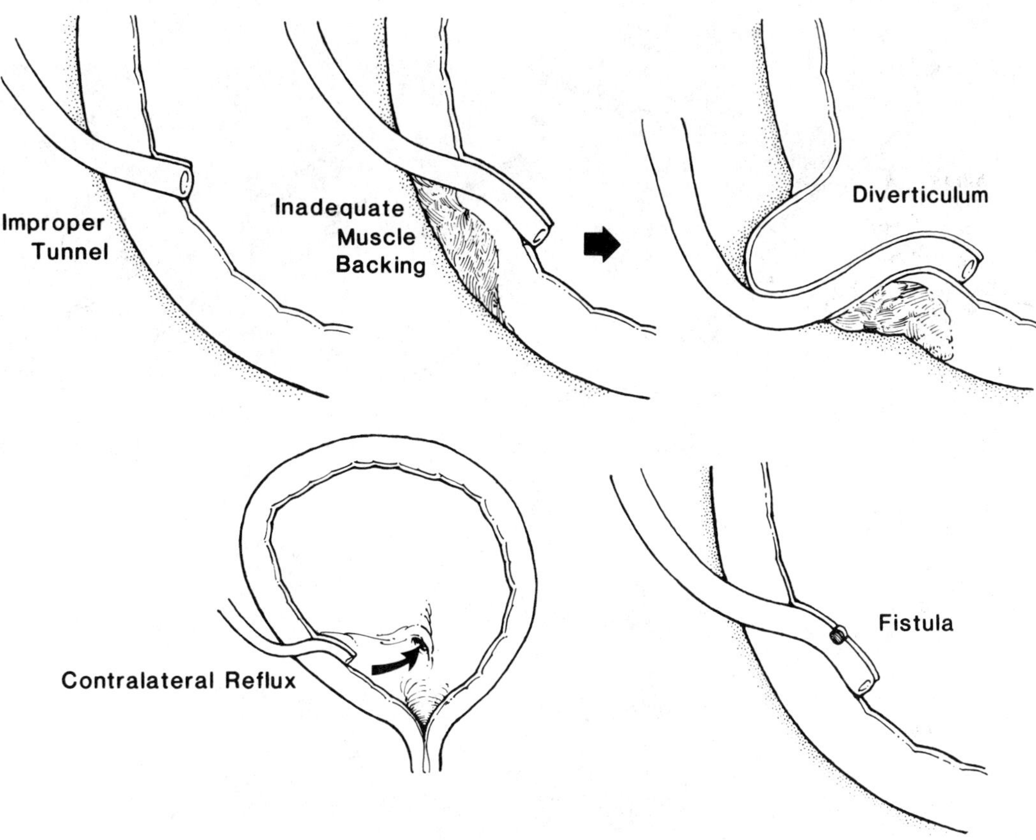

FIG 31–2.
Errors in technique resulting in postreimplantation reflux.

nificant difference, these were done by many different surgeons. Ehrlich reported only a 1.3% persistent reflux rate in 229 ureters by the Cohen technique.[20]

Contralateral *new* reflux developed in 20% of patients in the series reported by Parrott and Woodard (see Fig 31–1).[21] Others have reported a 12% to 14% rate.[19, 20] For example, Ahmed reported a 12.3% contralateral reflux rate, although only one patient required reoperation.[22] Ehrlich, on the other hand, found no instance of contralateral reflux in 41 patients with unilateral ureteral reimplantation by the Cohen technique.[20]

In general, postoperative reflux, whether persistent or new, is apt to be of low grade and to resolve spontaneously. Furthermore, it does not seem to be possible to determine which ureters are at risk for new reflux to develop.[19, 21, 23] We have usually elected to reimplant both ureters.

Ureteral Obstruction.—Postoperative ureteral obstruction as either an early or late event may occur (Fig 31–3). Early obstruction is usually transient secondary to edema or severe bladder spasms caused by the urethral catheter.[16] Bladder catheter drainage for routine reimplantation is now often as short as 24 to 48 hours. In some centers, a ureteroneocystotomy has even been successfully performed without bladder catheter drainage. Severe edema of the reimplantation site, combined with poor dynamics of the proximal ureter, may lead to significant acute postopera-

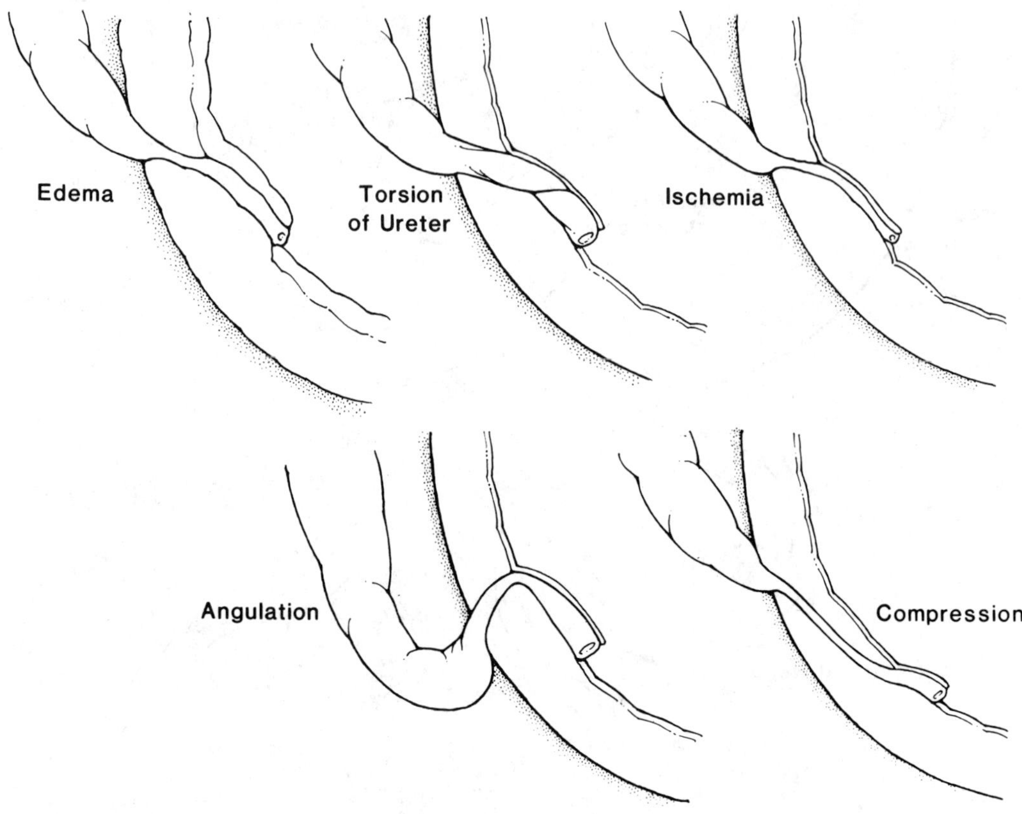

FIG 31–3.
Errors in technique resulting in postreimplantation ureteral obstruction.

tive obstruction in very young patients (1 to 3 months old) and in patients with ureteral dilatation. We routinely leave a 5 F (or 8 F) pediatric feeding tube as a ureteral catheter in all patients under 3 months of age, often in patients with significant ureteral dilatation, and *always* in patients with ureteral tapering.

Late ureteral obstruction is usually more significant. It may be secondary to ureteral angulation extravesically or to a muscular hiatus which has positioned too laterally on the bladder wall. Obstruction may result from twisting of the ureter within its submucosal tunnel or from compression from a paraureteral diverticulum. This latter problem develops if the muscular hiatus is too large. Devascularization of the distal ureter can be caused by excessively aggressive dissection of the ureter without care to preserve the delicate ureteric vessels. This will result in acute and chronic ureteral obstruction. All of these are iatrogenic complications and can be prevented by meticulous technique. A marking suture should be placed prior to ureteral mobilization to prevent ureteral torsion and great care must be taken to preserve the ureteral blood supply. The ureteral mobilization must be adequate to prevent angulation and provide sufficient tunnel length. One should not hesitate to mobilize both intravesically and extravesically if necessary. If a technique requiring a new hiatus is elected, the hiatus must be of adequate size and placed on the immobile portion of the posterior bladder wall to prevent angulation with bladder filling.[17, 24] The ureter must be passed through the new hiatus under direct vision to avoid entering the peritoneum with subsequent bowel injury. The submucosal tunnel must be adequately developed to prevent ureteral entrapment.[16] Postoperative ureteral obstruction is less likely to occur with advancement techniques such as the Glenn-Anderson[25] or the Cohen[26] procedures. With any antireflux technique for the nondilated ureter, this complication should occur in less than 2% of patients.

Diverticulum.—Ahmed recently reported a 17% diverticulum formation rate by the transverse advancement technique (Cohen), but this has not been the experience in our hands.[22] Following intravesical mobilization the muscular hiatus must be carefully closed in reimplantation procedures or reduced in advancement procedures.

Nonmechanical Factors (Fig 31–4).—Postoperative persistent hydronephrosis that may mimic the mechanical problem of either obstruction or persistent reflux may be due to nonmechanical factors. These are most commonly related to bladder dysfunction, i.e., detrusor/sphincter dyssynergia or intrinsic bladder hypertonicity. Persistent hydronephrosis, however, can also be caused by bladder outflow obstruction, such as untreated urethral valves or urethral strictures. High urine volume, as found in patients with tubular defects, and obligate high urine output may also result in postoperative hydronephrosis. Beware of the patient with the history of multiple failed reimplants. This patient should be assumed to have a nonmechanical mechanism to explain the reimplantation failure, until proven otherwise. He/she should be carefully studied. A basic evaluation should include urodynamics (including renal antegrade studies when indicated), careful neurologic evaluation, lumbosacral spine films, and assessment of renal function (including concentrating ability and creatinine clearance). In our clinic, any patient with unsuccessful reimplantation surgery is considered a candidate for such an evaluation.

Infection.—Postoperative urinary tract *infection* occurs either early or late. Immediate postoperative infections generally occur in those patients who were infected at the time of surgery, and they may result in urinary sepsis. All efforts should

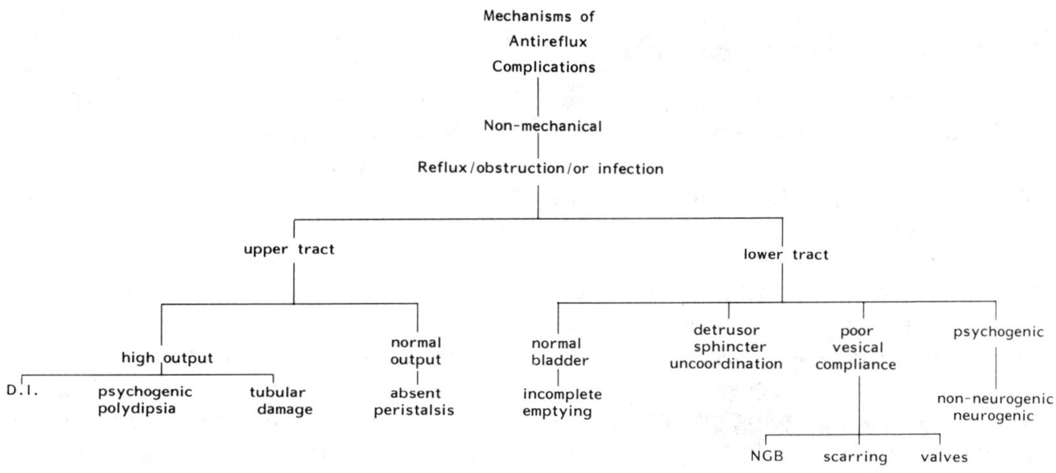

FIG 31–4.
Nonmechanical reasons for failure of ureteral reimplantation (*DI* indicates diabetes insipidus; *NGB*, neurogenic bladder).

be made to sterilize the urinary tract prior to surgery. We maintain patients on postoperative antibiotics a minimum of 4 to 6 weeks after surgery. Late urinary tract infections are not uncommon (occurring in up to 31%).[22, 27] However, Bellinger and Duckett have been quoted as noting only a 4.8% infection rate.[16] Such infections are almost always limited to the lower tract. Bauer et al. noted only a 1.7% pyelonephritis rate.[27] It is important that the patient and family be aware that antireflux surgery may not prevent urinary infection but should help to limit infection to the bladder. Children with recurrent infections before surgery may require close observation and chronic antibiotics after surgery.

Hypertension.—Hypertension is not an indication for antireflux surgery, since it appears to be related to renal scarring and is not prevented by ureteral reimplantation.[16, 28] However, antireflux surgery is not known to worsen hypertension if surgery is otherwise indicated.[28] Transient hypertension postoperatively can be observed in a few patients. We follow such patients closely, since hypertension often develops in them as young adults.

The Dilated Ureter or Megaureter

Surgery for the dilated ureter is technically demanding and complications may occur even when the patient is in the best of hands. Although the technical aspects of megaureter tailoring are the same, no matter what the diagnosis, the need for operative correction and the ultimate success of treatment are determined by establishing the correct diagnosis.[29] Many wide ureters are in fact not obstructed and do not represent an ongoing process of decompensation. Certainly some megaureters diagnosed in early childhood may improve with observation alone.[30]

Megaureters may develop with obstruction at either the ureterovesical junction or bladder outlet with functional bladder outlet obstruction (as with the nonneurogenic neurogenic bladder) or with severe reflux. Massively dilated ureters can also be found in patients with prune-belly syndrome. Furthermore, idiopathic megaureters (nonobstructive, nonrefluxing) are also known to occur. In general, those ureters that are not obstructed and do not reflux can respond to nonoperative therapy such as intermittent clean catheterization. The surgical results with refluxing megaureters can be disappointing. Johnston had 16 successful ureteral taperings and reimplantations in 29 ureters. Persistent reflux was demonstrated in ten ureters, with obstruction occurring in three ureters.[31] In these ureters, ureteral peristalsis is often poor. In contrast, the results of surgical correction of the primary obstructed megaureter are quite good.[17, 29, 30] Kelalis and Kramer noted the results to be almost comparable with those of reimplantation of the nondilated ureter, since these patients usually have a normal bladder and often good ureteral peristalsis.[29]

Iatrogenic Megaureter.—A failed ureteral reimplantation can lead to an iatrogenic megaureter.[29] If the bladder, as determined by urodynamics is normal, reimplantation is indicated. Such surgery, however, is not to be considered trivial. Hendren has warned that repeated extravesical dissection may injure bladder innervation.[17] This complication can be avoided by doing the majority of the dissection intravesically, although one should not hesitate to mobilize the ureter extravesically if necessary. During surgical dissection, care should be taken to preserve the bladder innervation and blood supply and to protect the blood supply of the ureters. When the reasons for a failed ureteral reimplant are not obvious, great care should be taken to evaluate the patient properly and completely.

The megaureter patient, perhaps more so than the patient with a nondilated ureter, is at high risk for nonmechanical complications of reimplantation.

Surgical Technique.—Hendren has beautifully detailed the operative technique for megaureter tapering and reimplantation, and it need not be repeated here.[32] We have been pleased with our results using this method and have not been plagued by devascularization of the tapered ureteral segment, fistula, or ureteral leaks. Potential for these complications, however, is ever present. It is not surprising, therefore, that ureteral folding (rather than partial excision and suturing) has gained widespread popularity since Kalicínski's and, later, Starr's reports.[33, 34] Ehrlich has promoted a ureteral folding technique. He has not noted problems with ureteral bulk, has had no obstruction in 27 ureters, and has had only one patient with persistent reflux.[35, 36] Other advantages of ureteral folding and plication are the shortened time of stent drainage and the decreased need for extensive ureteral dissection. In this regard, we have done ureteral excision and tapering from within the bladder without extravesical dissection in cases of moderate ureteral dilatation. Debate still exists as to what actually happens to the redundant folded portion of the ureters. In general, it seems that nonobstructed nonrefluxing dilated ureter has the potential to diminish in size and tortuosity given time and proper bladder dynamics. It is for this reason that upper tract tapering is rarely necessary.

There are some patients who apparently have irreversible, transmural changes (scarring) in the ureter. Such changes would be found in ureters with chronic infection, as in patients who are severe refluxers or who have had intubated ureterostomies. These ureters do not peristalse when examined under fluroscopy preoperatively and will behave more like "pipes" when tapered and reimplanted. Minimal tunnel resistance leads to partial obstruction, and improper tunnel length leads to persistent reflux. To make things worse, these patients often have altered bladder and urethral dynamics and even renal tubular dysfunction leading to high output states (see chapter 34 on Valves). Urinary reconstruction in such patients is treacherous and difficult, to say the least. Success in this group of patients is relative, but it is dependent on many other factors, such as patient compliance with treatment and compulsive attention by the surgeon to physiologic as well as surgical detail.

Beware of the patient with dilated ureters, high urine output, altered bladder dynamics with or without complete bladder emptying, and/or the absence of peristalsis on fluoroscopy. Such conditions may require much more than "simple" reimplant or megaureter repair and reimplant. For example, a psoas hitch may be necessary to secure better and longer backing to the ureteral tunnel, or, transureteroureterostomy used to achieve effective ureteral length where one ureter is notably short. Intermittent clean catheterization may be necessary to insure complete bladder emptying. Medications (e.g., anticholinergics) and/or bladder augmentation may be necessary to achieve proper bladder compliance/volume. Simply put, consider the dynamics of the total patient. Do not myopically focus on the ureterovesical junction alone, since this will result in disappointment and failure even in the face of adequate surgical execution.

Ureteroceles

As with most disorders of embryogenesis, ureteroceles occur in a spectrum, and consequently, each requires individualized treatment. Ureteroceles may be quite small, involve a single system, and be clinically insignificant ("adult type"). Rarely, these require operative correction because of urinary obstruction or lodging of a stone within the ureterocele. There is little controversy here that simple excision of the ureterocele and reimplantation is in order. In some cases, simple unroofing may be sufficient treatment and will not result in reflux. Kroovand has treated some children by incising the meatus with a flexible electrode or endoscopic scissors. In his experience postincision reflux has been minimal.[37] Such cases present little difficulty.

"Pediatric" Ureterocele.—About twice as common—and certainly more controversial—is the large, "pediatric" ureterocele that is often associated with the upper pole of a duplex system.[38] If the ureterocele is small and does not obstruct the bladder outlet or the contralateral ureter(s), it is often necessary to operate only on the upper tract. If the upper pole parenchyma functions (in about a third or fewer cases), ureteropyelostomy or ureteroureterostomy can be performed along with excision of the upper pole ureter. If the upper pole segment is dysplastic, as is most often the case, upper pole nephroureterectomy is preferable.[30] In either case, the ureterocele only is aspirated, and the distal ureteral stump is left open if *no* reflux is present. In most series, approximately 60% will require no further surgery.[39, 40] Persistent reflux, bladder diverticulum formation, and partial bladder outlet obstruction or recurrent infections may necessitate ureterocele excision as a second-stage procedure. In infants with large ectopic ureteroceles, Kroovand and Perlmutter and others have preferred total one-stage ureterectomy with *extra*vesical ureterocele excision with either upper pole nephrectomy or pyelopyelostomy.[41] They have not found the usual dense common sheath in those with large ureteroceles, so it has been easy to separate the ureters. Diverticulum formation has not been a problem. We think "unroofing" of the ureterocele should be reserved for the sick infant and be considered a temporary drainage measure only.

One-stage complete reconstruction, as proposed by Hendren and Mitchell, has been successful in our hands, resulting in only two clinically insignificant bladder diverticula.[38] This may be exceedingly difficult in the neonate. The risk of reflux following excision of a large ureterocele is much greater than that of routine reimplantation, due to the major muscle defect in the bladder wall. This defect *must* be carefully reconstructed so as to allow adequate muscle backing for reimplantation.

Ectopic Ureterocele.—The ectopic ureterocele extends down through the bladder neck into the urethra. Careless excision may result in bladder neck and/or sphincter injury, leading to incontinence. Great care and effort must be expended to completely dissect out the ureterocele and repair the often-found defect in the posterior bladder wall and bladder neck. The distal rim of an improperly resected or unroofed ureterocele may yield a valve-like obstruction if not removed entirely.[38] After ectopic ureterocele excision, any bladder neck cleft must be reconstructed, lest stress incontinence occur.

Ureteral Reconstruction

Replacement of the ureter with a segment of small bowel has facilitated reconstruction and undiversion in a number of patients with very short or damaged ureters. Debate still exists as to whether it is best to taper and antireflux such ileal ureters or to rely on ureteral peristalsis and permit reflux.[42] Vatandaslar et al.[43, 44] did experiments in dogs which might indicate that an antireflux mechanism may protect the kidneys in such patients. Obstruction, infection, and absorption of electrolytes seem to be the major complications of interposition of a small bowel segment for partial or complete ureteral replacement.

Infection almost invariably reflects

stasis in the bowel ureter and, most commonly, it is secondary to obstruction. Mechanical obstruction can result from excessive tailoring in an effort to create a tunneled reimplant. It may also result from ischemia of the distal portion secondary to the removal of an excessive amount of mesentery to facilitate reimplantation. Midileal ureteral obstruction may also result from a mucosal web. These webs sometimes can be treated by ureteroscopy and fulguration. An acute transition from a dilated ileal ureter can result in a relative obstruction even if the most distal smaller segment is patent, in much the same way that the adynamic segment of a congenital megaureter is obstructive. Stasis in an ileal ureter not only potentiates infection but can also lead to absorption of metabolites from the urine, particularly in the patient with decreased renal function.

Aside from these problems related to mechanical obstruction, similar complications may develop when the ileal ureter is applied to the patient with abnormal bladder and/or urethral function. When an ileal ureter is contemplated, the function of the lower urinary tract must be carefully assessed. Bladder outlet obstruction by either mechanical (such as urethral stricture or valves) or physiologic causes (sphincter-detrusor dyssynergia, nonneurogenic neurogenic bladder, will result in relative obstruction, distention, and stasis in an ileal ureter. Poor bladder compliance, high output states, and incomplete voiding will also result in failure of an ileal ureter, particularly if vesicoileal ureteral reflux is present. The rule of thumb for successful use of the ileal ureter is to make sure there is a compliant reservoir distal to the ileal ureter and that the patient empties this reservoir (bladder) on a regular basis, through voiding or intermittent clean catheterization. Whether or not reflux in this setting is deleterious is still a subject of debate. However, given a choice, we would opt for an antireflux mechanism proximal to the urine reservoir. Furthermore, a tunnel technique is, in our experience, still preferable to a nipple technique.

Unused Bladder

No discussion of complications of ureteral reimplantation would be complete without at least a mention of urinary reconstruction in the previously diverted patient. Ureteral reimplantation is often the cornerstone of an effective undiversion procedure. As such, success or failure rests on the ureteral reimplantation. In such cases, the difficulty of ureteroneocystostomy is compounded by a small, unused bladder and ureters that have often had previous surgeries. These ureters are frequently short, scarred, and aperistaltic. The formula for success, in our opinion, is (1) proper patient evaluation, (2) proper surgical techniques, and (3) adequate follow-up.

Patient Selection and Evaluation.— Preoperative assessment of the bladder and ureters are among the most important elements in proper patient evaluation to insure successful reimplants. The bladder should be cycled, whenever possible, by instilling water or normal saline to pain tolerance two to three times a day. This procedure will often result in bladder enlargement, making reimplantation possible. It will also help to define the potential for continence, make preoperative urodynamics more meaningful, and clearly select those patients willing to follow recommended treatments. Urodynamic evaluation after bladder cycling is essential to successful reimplants. Poor bladder compliance and bladder outlet obstruction are best defined preoperatively, so that surgery and postoperative treatment programs can be properly directed. Fluoroscopic ureteral studies will help to define the dynamic potential of the ureters and the need for tailoring. Renal function and the ability to make concentrated urine must also be defined. Obligate high urine outputs in the face of relative small bladder capacity will commonly lead to failed reimplants, even in the most skillful hands.

Reimplantation Technique.—The surgical technique used for reimplantation depends on the anatomy and physiology. In general, we prefer a long submucosal tunnel with good muscle backing, which often is hard to achieve bilaterally. It is not infrequent, therefore, that this result is best achieved with a single reimplant with psoas bladder hitch and transureteroureterostomy. Technically, preservation of ureteral blood supply, adequate muscle backing and submucosal tunnel length seem critically important. If there is a question about a ureter's viability or degree of scarring, then it should not be used. Furthermore, if a bladder has poor compliance, then augmentation with a bowel patch should be performed at the times of ureteral reimplantation, particularly in the neurogenic bladder patient.

Follow-up, both short- and long-term, can be the difference between successful and failed reimplants in some undiversion patients. We have more than once been surprised to find increasing hydronephrosis in a patient whom we thought was otherwise doing well. Regular radiographic or isotopic studies (6 months to 1 year) make early detection and treatment possible.

Reconstruction Without a Bladder.—Interest in urinary reconstruction in the patient without a bladder and construction of continent urinary reservoirs has rekindled interest in nonrefluxing ureteroenterostomies.[45, 46] Although many recent experiences are limited, Althausen et al.,[47] in a review of colon conduits, clearly showed excellent results from tunneling the ureter into the tinea of large bowel. It has been our experience as well that over 90% of such reimplants in continent urinary reservoir systems are successful. Problems arise when ureters are tapered before such tunneling. Lilien and Camey[48] have recently demonstrated a tunnel technique for small bowel. Kock et al.,[49] on the other hand, propose a nipple technique for a reconfigured ileal reservoir. Hinman,[50] in 1936, wrote a very interesting review of ureteroenterostomy and concluded that the tunnel technique tended to be superior. Use of the ileocecal valve to prevent reflux has, in our hands, been only 50% successful and should be reserved only for massively dilated ureters.

CONCLUSION

Vesicoureteral reflux is one of the more common problems for which the pediatric urologist must provide therapy. Since the discovery of this condition over 30 years ago, the therapeutic pendulum has swung from an aggressive surgical approach to medical management, and then back to the in-between position of the present. The potential for complications by either mode of therapy has therefore been considered. Particular emphasis has been placed on proper patient selection and evaluation. In order to minimize complications, the physician must look beyond the abnormal anatomy of the ureterovesical junction and consider the total patient.

EDITORIAL COMMENT

The chapter includes an excellent discussion of the complications of the medical management of reflux. As indicated, medical management includes the assumption that reflux will resolve with time and that antibiotics can always prevent any urinary tract infection. The pendulum has swung from surgical to medical management and most appropriately needs to return to a more intermediate position. Clearly, patients with higher grades of reflux or noncompliant patients are at higher risk for long-term problems. In addition, the authors stress the importance of evaluation of the total patient, especially the evaluation of bladder dysfunction and voiding dysfunction. The importance of bladder cycling cannot be underestimated in these patients. Before simple ureteral reimplantation, bladder function and continence can be determined as well as the possible need for vesical augmentation at the time of reconstruction.

The standard surgical technical complications are covered in detail. The technique of resection of one of two ureters in a common sheath with a ureteral duplication (as learned from Dr. Hendren) has been described in a paper on the long blind ureteral duplications.* This chapter presents a reasoned approach to the problems of ureteral reimplantation and ureterocele surgery.

REFERENCES

1. Normand C, Smellie J: Vesicoureteric reflux: The case for conversative management, in Hodson J, Kincaid-Smith P (ed): *Reflux Nephropathy.* New York, Masson Publishing Co, Inc, 1979, pp 281.
2. Medical vs. surgical treatment of primary vesicoureteral reflux: A prospective international reflux study in children. *J Urol* 1981; 125:277.
3. Hodson CJ, Cotran RS: *Reflux Nephropathy.* Hospital Practice 1982; 17:133.
4. Winberg J, Claesson I, Jacobsson B, et al: Renal growth after acute pyelonephritis in childhood: An epidemiological approach, in Hodson J, Kincaid-Smith P (ed): *Reflux Nephropathy.* New York, Masson Publishing Co, Inc, 1979, pp 309.
5. Fink JH: Drug-induced hypersensitivity lung disease, in Petersdorf RG, Adams RD, Braunwald E, et al (ed): *Harrison's Principles of Internal Medicine.* New York, McGraw-Hill Book Co, 1983, pp 1523–1524.
6. Ehrlich RM: Risks of long-term Trimethopim-sulfamethoxazole therapy. *Society for Pediatric Urology Newsletter,* April, 1983, p. 22.
7. Elmes PC: Antibacterial drugs used in miscellaneous infections, in Dukes MNG (ed): *Meyler's Side Effects of Drugs.* New York, Elsevier North-Holland, Inc, 1975, vol 8, pp 668–675.
8. Ransley PG: Vesicoureteric reflux, in Williams DI, Johnston JH (ed): *Paediatric Urology.* London, Butterworth Scientific, 1982, pp 151–165.
9. Libertino JA: Adult vesicoureteral reflux, in Johnston JH (ed): *International Prospectives in Urology.* Baltimore, Williams & Wilkins Co, 1984, Chapter 19, pp 241–251.
10. Smellie J, Normand C: Reflux nephropathy in childhood, in Hodson J, Kincaid-Smith J (eds): *Reflux Nephropathy.* New York, Masson Publishing Co, 1979, pp 14–20.
11. Wallace DMA, Rothwell DL, Williams DI: The long-term follow-up of surgically treated vesicoureteric reflux. *Br J Urol* 1978; 50:479.
12. Stecker JF Jr, Read BP, Poutasse EF: Pediatric hypertension as a delayed sequela of reflux induced chronic pyelonephritis. *J Urol* 1977; 118:644.
13. Stickler GB, Kelalis PP, Burke EC, et al: Primary interstitial nephritis with reflux: A cause of hypertension. *Am J Dis Child* 1971; 122:144.
14. Ransley PG: Vesicoureteric reflux: Continuing surgical dilemma. *Urology* 1978; 12:246.
15. Koff SA: Disordered vesicourethral function in the pathogenesis of urinary infection and vesicoureteric reflux, in Johnston JH (ed): *International Perspectives in Urology.* Baltimore, Williams & Wilkins Co, 1984, Chapter 8, pp 67–81.
16. Gibbons MD, Gonzales ET Jr: Complications of antireflux surgery. *Urol Clin North Am* 1983; 10:489.
17. Hendren WH: Complications of ureteral

*Marshall FF, McLoughlin MG: Long blind ureteral duplications. *J Urol* 1978; 120:626.

reimplantation and megaureter repair, in Smith RB, Skinner DG (ed): *Complications of Urologic Surgery: Prevention and Management.* Philadelphia, WB Saunders Co, 1976, pp 151–208.
18. Amar AD: Delayed recurrence of reflux after initial success of antireflux operation. *J Urol* 1978; 119:131.
19. Carpentier PJ, Bettink PJ, Hop WCJ, et al: Reflux: A retrospective study of 100 ureteric reimplantations by the Politano-Leadbetter method and 100 by the Cohen technique. *Br J Urol* 1982; 54:230.
20. Ehrlich RM: Success of the transvesical advancement technique for vesicoureteral reflux. *J Urol* 1982; 128:554.
21. Parrott TS, Woodard JR: Reflux in opposite ureter after successful correction of unilateral vesicoureteral reflux. *Urology* 1976; 7:276.
22. Ahmed S, Tan H: Complications of transverse advancement ureteral reimplantation: Diverticular formation. *J Urol* 1982; 127:970.
23. Snyder HM, Duckett JW: Endoscopic evaluation problems in refluxing orifice in vesicoureteric reflux: The urodynamic evaluation. *Dialogues Pediatr Urol* 1983; 6:3.
24. Hensle TW, Berdon WE, Baker DH, et al: The ureteral "J" sign: Radiographic demonstration of iatrogenic distal ureteral obstruction after ureteral reimplantation. *J Urol* 1982; 127:766.
25. Glenn JF, Anderson EE: Distal tunnel ureteral reimplantation. *J Urol* 1977; 97:623.
26. Cohen SJ: Ureterozystoneostomie eine neve antireflux technik. *Akt Urol* 1975; 6:1.
27. Bauer SB, Wilscher MK, Zammuto PJ, et al: Long-term results of antireflux surgery in children, in Hodson J Kincaid-Smith P (eds): *Reflux Nephropathy.* New York, Masson Publishing, 1979, p. 287.
28. Scott JES: Hypertension, reflux and renal scarring in management of vesicoureteral reflux, in Johnston JH (ed): *Int Perspect Urol* Baltimore, Williams & Wilkins Co, 1984, p. 54.
29. Kelalis PP, Kramer SA: Complications: of megaureter surgery. *Urol Clin North Am* 1983; 10:417.
30. King LR: Ureter and ureterovesical junction, in Kelalis PP, King LR, Belman AB (eds): *Clinical Pediatric Urology.* Philadelphia, WB Saunders Co, 1985, pp 486–512.
31. Johnston JH, Farkas A: The congenital refluxing megaureter: Experience with surgical reconstruction. *Br J Urol* 1975; 47:153.
32. Hendren WH: The dilated ureter, in Eckstein HB, Hohenfellner R, Williams DI (eds): *Surgical Pediatric Urology.* Philadelphia, WB Saunders Co, 1977, pp 218–234.
33. Kaliciński ZH, Kansy J, Kotarbińska B, et al: Surgery of megaureters: Modification of Hendren's operation. *J Pediatr Surg* 1977; 12:183.
34. Starr A: Ureteral plication: A new concept in ureteral tailoring for megaureter. *Invest Urol* 1979; 17:153.
35. Ehrlich RM: Ureteral folding technique for megaureter surgery. *Society for Pediatric Urology Newsletter* May 5, 1982.
36. Ehrlich RM: Editors note on complications of pediatric urologic surgery. *Urol Clin North Am* 1983; 10:422.
37. Kroovand RL: Ureterocele. *Urol Clin North Am* 1983; 10:445.
38. Hendren WH, Mitchell ME: Surgical correction of ureteroceles. *J Urol* 1979; 121:590.
39. Mandell J, Colodny AH, Lebowitz R, et al: Ureteroceles in infants and children. *J Urol* 1980; 123:921.
40. Snow BW, Mitchell ME, Garrett RA: Riley children's hospital, ureteroceles: A 12-year experience. *Indiana Medicine* 1984; 77:522.
41. Kroovand RL, Perlmutter AD: One-stage surgical approach to ectopic ureterocele. *J Urol* 1979; 122:367.
42. Heaney JA, Althausen AF, Parkhurst EG: Ileal conduit undiversion: Experience with tunneled, vesical implantation of tapered conduit. *J Urol* 1980; 124:89.
43. Vatandaslar F, Reid RE, Freed SZ, et al: Ileal segment replacement of ureter. I. Effects on kidney of refluxing vs nonrefluxing ileovesical anastomosis. *Urology* 1984 23:549–558.
44. Vatandaslar F, Reid RE, Freed SZ, et al: Ileal segment replacement of ureter. II. Dynamic characteristics of refluxing, nonrefluxing, and totally tapered ileal ureter. *Urology* 1984; 23:559–564.
45. Mitchell ME, Rink RC: Urinary diversion and undiversion. *Urol Clin North Am* 1985; 12:111.

46. Mitchell ME, Rink RC: Urinary tract undiversion in patients without bladders. Presented at North Central Section, AUA, Hawaii, 1983.
47. Althausen A, Hagan-Cook K, Hendren WH: Non-refluxing colon conduit: Experience with 70 cases. *J Urol* 1978; 120:35.
48. Lilien OM, Camey M: 25-year experience with replacement of human bladder (Camey procedure). *J Urol* 1984; 132:886.
49. Kock NG, Nilson AE, Nilsson LO, et al: Urinary diversion via continent ileal reservoir: clinical results in 12 patients. *J Urol* 1982; 128:369.
50. Hinman F, Weyrauch HM Jr: A critical study of different principles of surgery which have been used in ureterointestinal implantation. *Trans Am Assoc GU Surg* 1936; 29:15.

CHAPTER 32

Complications of Urinary Tract Reconstruction

Terry W. Hensle, M.D.
Kevin A. Burbige, M.D.

Urinary tract reconstruction may be defined as restoration of urinary tract integrity in patients who have either had previous urinary diversions or whose urinary tract has been rendered unusable by previous surgery or underlying disease. Reconstruction of the urinary tract has been popularized over the last decade in both the adult and pediatric population.[1, 2] Long-term favorable results have been published from many centers, including our own.[3, 4] The majority of these reports have involved pediatric and young adult patients who have required reconstruction for a variety of problems including severe obstructive uropathy, myelodysplasia, and bladder exstrophy.[5–7] Although antenatal and neonatal screening of the urinary tract with ultrasound has impacted greatly on any number of urologic conditions, it has not greatly changed our early management of either myelomeningocele, or bladder exstrophy. These two conditions continue to account for the majority of patients undergoing lower urinary tract reconstruction, at least in the younger age group.

Although complications of urinary tract reconstruction have been reported in many individual series, there are few complete compilations of these complications.[8–10] It is hoped that this overview can be useful in avoiding the pitfalls which have been encountered in the past, and provide a safer outlook for the patient undergoing reconstruction. The major focus for avoiding complications in this difficult group of patients involves proper patient selection, technical attention to detail, and impeccable follow-up.

PREOPERATIVE COMPLICATIONS

Perhaps the most important concept in determining the success of urinary tract reconstruction is proper patient selection. Richie and Sacks[8] and others have stressed the need for rational criteria in evaluating patients who are being considered for reconstruction, and artificial parameters for patient selection have been advocated in several areas, including the level of renal function. Although a full evaluation of the patient's renal function and its stability is important in planning reconstructive surgery, there is no absolute cutoff in terms of creatinine clearance that would contraindicate reconstruction. In fact, several patients in our early series with minimal renal function were reconstructed specifically as an adjunct to renal transplantation. Several authors have stressed the importance of bladder capacity and compliance when evaluating patients for undiversion. Kogan and Levitt,[11] as well as Bauer et al.,[12] have defined their criteria for evaluating the bladder of patients being considered for reconstruction; however, it has become clear that defining the urodynamic status of the diverted bladder is of less importance than defining the bladder size and overall anatomy. Although these considerations remain of relative importance, the expanded use of bladder augmentation and bladder replacement has all but eliminated the small or hypertonic bladder as a major contraindication to urinary tract reconstruction.[13]

In terms of patient selection, we feel that there are two major criteria. The first is the ability and willingness of the patient to perform and adhere to a program of clean intermittent catheterization, if indicated. The second is the basic intelligence and motivation of the patient being considered for reconstruction. These two features have proved to be the most important limiting factors in the success and failure of our reconstructed group.

Case 1.—J.S., aged 21 years, presented with a solitary left kidney and a longstanding pyelojejunal conduit. At age 10 months he was noted to have bilateral flank masses and probably an occult neuropathic bladder. At initial presentation, he underwent a left nephrostomy and a Y-V plasty of his bladder neck. Seven years later, a nonfunctioning right kidney was removed, and a left pyelojejunal conduit was created. Following diversion, he experienced multiple bouts of pyelonephritis and a slow, persistent decline in renal function. At presentation for reconstruction, his blood urea nitrogen was 55 mg/dL; serum creatinine, 2.5 mg/dL; and creatinine clearance, 28 mL/min. An excretory urogram demonstrated a poorly functioning hydronephrotic solitary left kidney (Fig 32–1,A) and a voiding cystourethrogram (VCUG) revealed a 6 to 10-cc capacity bladder, no reflux, and a normal urethra. Cystoscopy confirmed no evidence of urethral obstruction, and a retrograde study demonstrated an 8- to 10-cm segment of a distal left ureter (Fig 32–1,B). A percutaneous suprapubic tube was placed in the bladder and hydrodistention was begun. With some difficulty, he was able to hold 200 to 300 mL of fluid; however, he could not empty his bladder completely. The patient was instructed in clean intermittent catheterization (CIC), and despite his reluctance to carry out the procedure, he was felt to be a good candidate for urinary tract reconstruction. Reconstruction involved anastomosis of the left ureter with the tapered jejunal segment, and a long cross-trigonal ureteral neocystostomy (Fig 32–2,A and B). Follow-up radiographic studies done 6 months after reconstruction showed increasing hydronephrosis. A VCUG (Fig 32–3) showed a normal-appearing bladder without reflux. Antegrade and retrograde studies of the kidney and ureter revealed no evidence of obstruction; however, progressive renal deterioration continued. One year after his reconstruction, the patient was admitted to the hospital with urinary tract infection and progressive renal failure, at which time it was noted that he had refused to do CIC at any time during his postreconstructive period. His renal function has continued to deteriorate and at present he is a pretransplantation candidate.

Comment.—This patient represents a classic example of improper patient selection. He was a poorly motivated individual who had marginal renal function at the time of his reconstruction. The rapid deterioration of his upper tracts is clearly related to his reconstruction with increased pressure on compromised kidneys, as well as his unwillingness to perform CIC.

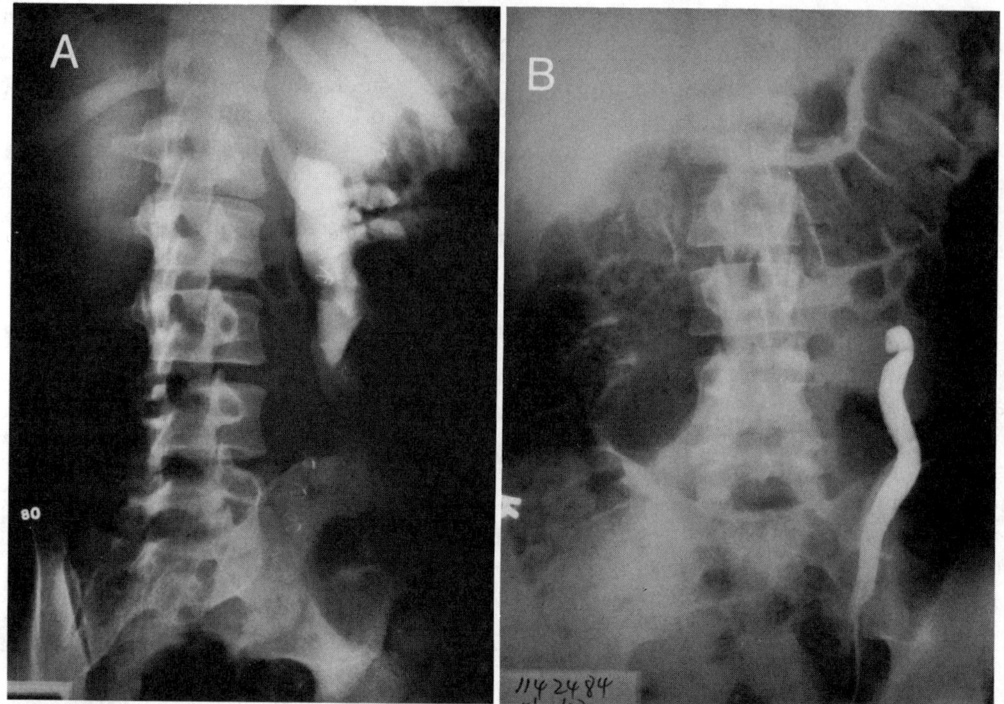

FIG 32–1.
A, preoperative loop study. **B,** preoperative retrograde pyelogram.

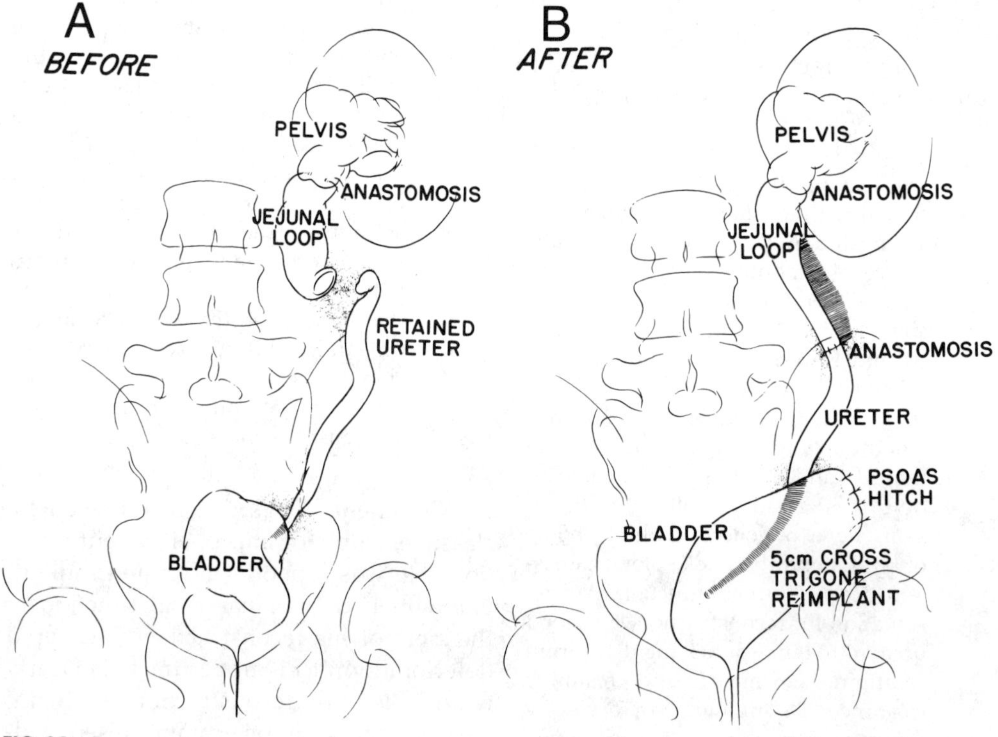

FIG 32–2.
A, preoperative anatomy. **B,** postoperative anatomy.

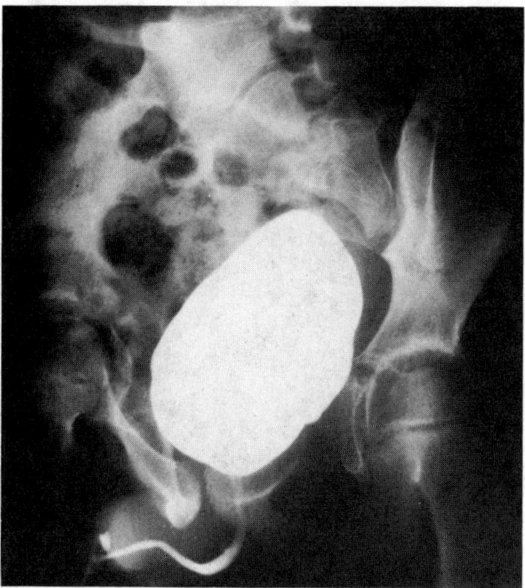

FIG 32–3.
Postoperative voiding cystourethrogram.

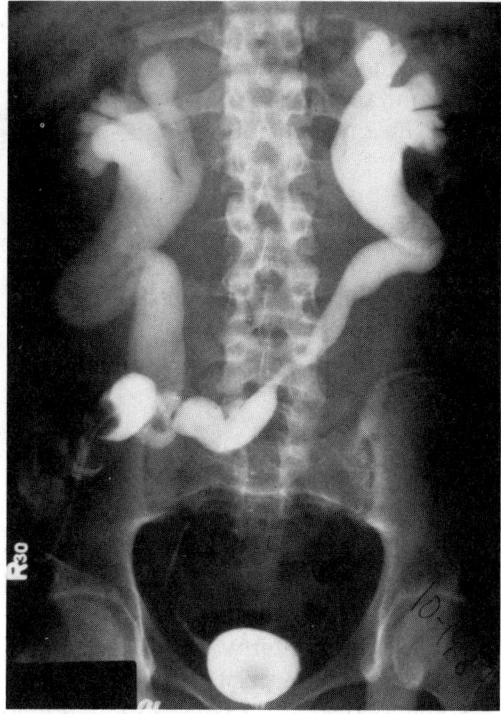

FIG 32–4.
Simultaneous contrast loop study and cystogram to evaluate anatomy available for reconstruction.

INTRAOPERATIVE COMPLICATIONS

Most intraoperative complications can be avoided by accurate identification of the existing anatomy, along with proper exposure of the structures to be reconstructed. Anatomical evaluation should include a preoperative excretory urogram or radionuclide renal scan to define upper tract anatomy and function as well as a retrograde contrast study of the conduit or ureterostomy in a diverted patient to determine ureteral length. This study can be done simultaneously with a voiding cystourethrogram to assess bladder size and ureteral configuration (Fig 32–4). It can also aid in estimating the distance to be bridged between the proximal ureter and bladder.

Renal Complications.—Thorough mobilization of the kidney is often necessary at the time of the reconstruction to gain adequate ureteral length for reimplantation into the bladder. During this mobilization, the renal vasculature is at risk, and renal units have been compromised during this kind of procedure. Care must be taken not to traumatize the renal pedicle and to avoid tension on the renal artery and vein at the time of mobilization or nephropexy.

Ureteral Complications.—Ureteral complications can be categorized as those resulting from inadequate ureteral length and those resulting from stricture or angulation of the reconstructed ureter. The most important of these is the short ureter. Inadequate ureteral length can usually be anticipated preoperatively, thus avoiding intraoperative chaos. A host of techniques are available to compensate for a short ureter such as downward nephropexy, psoas hitch, Boari flap, and transureteroureterostomy.[14]

Bladder Complications.—In the past, the most important contraindication to urinary tract reconstruction was the presence of a high-pressure, fixed-capacity bladder. With the increasing use of intestinal segments for bladder augmentation, this contraindication is no longer absolute. The great majority of the poor results in reported series can be traced directly to postoperative bladder dysfunction. Preoperative identification of the hypertonic fixed-capacity bladder is important in order to plan alternatives and avoid postoperative problems with urinary incontinence, reflux, and progressive upper tract damage.[15]

POSTOPERATIVE COMPLICATIONS

Because so much of our reconstructive effort today involves the use of the bowel segments to create a urinary reservoir, the majority of long-term complications involve problems associated with those reservoirs. Between 1979–1989, ninety-two pediatric and young adult patients underwent some form of urinary tract reconstruction at Babies Hospital, Columbia Presbyterian Medical Center. The complications involved in that series are listed in Table 32–1.

TABLE 32–1.
Complications of Urinary Tract Reconstruction in 92 Patients, 1979–1989

Complication	n
Stone formation	10
Postoperative vesicoureteral reflux	10
Inability to do clean intermittent catheterization postoperatively	5
Urinary incontinence requiring reoperation	5
Small bowel obstruction requiring reoperation	4
Cholelithiasis	3
Spontaneous perforation of augmented bladder	3
Renal deterioration	2
Femoral neuropathy	2
Acute urine leak	1
Acute psychosis (drug-related)	1

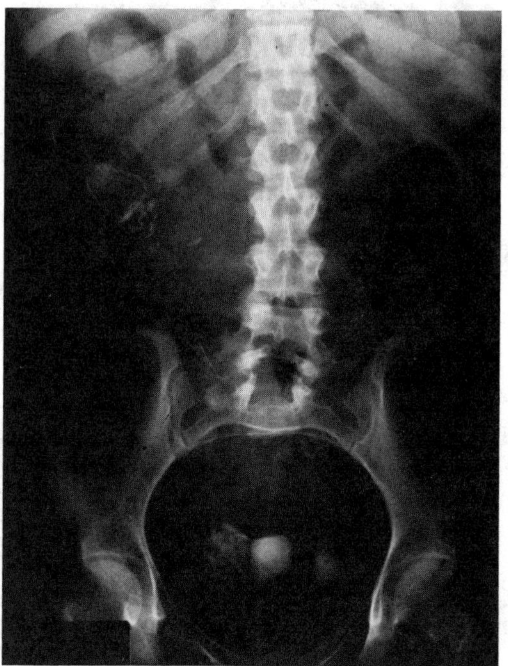

FIG 32–5.
KUB showing three large calculi in an augmented bladder 2 years following reconstruction.

Calculi.—Stone formation has been the most common complication noted in our series, occurring in 10 (11%) of our 92 patients. All 10 of these patients had stones form in a reservoir which had been created either partially or totally from bowel (Fig 32–5). The stones have been 100% struvite in all cases and 2 patients have had stone formation on more than one occasion. Seven of the 10 patients have had endoscopic management of their stones either with electrohydraulic lithotripsy or basket extraction. Three of the patients have required open stone extraction due to the size of the stones (Fig 32–6). Staples have been found imbedded in the stones of 3 patients. This association has been noted previously and staples within the bowel reservoir should be avoided.[16]

Reflux.—Postoperative vesicoureteral reflux has also occurred in 10 patients (11%). Most of this reflux occurred in the

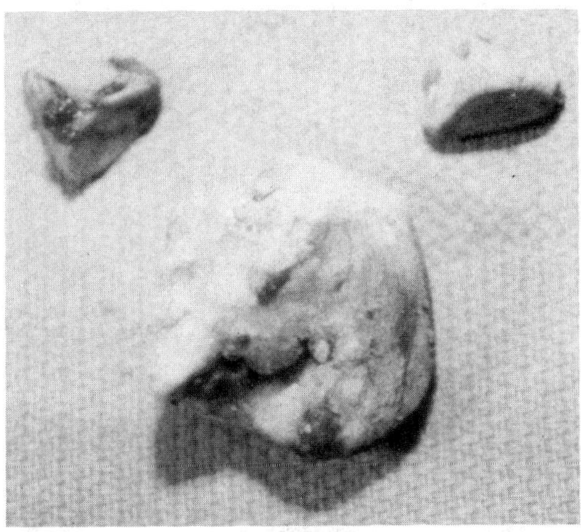

FIG 32–6.
Calculi removed by open cystostomy, the largest measuring 4 × 6 cm.

early part of our experience when we were attempting to use an intussuscepted ileocecal valve as an antireflux mechanism. We along with most others have gone away from the intussuscepted valve mechanism to prevent reflux and now rely on direct reimplantation of the ureter into either native bladder or large bowel segments used for augmentation. Only three of the patients in our series have had reflux using this approach although many are too short-term for accurate assessment. This improved reflux prevention is not only based upon the creation of a submucosal tunnel but also on achieving a large-volume, low-pressure reservoir.

Catheterization.—Five of the patients in our series have been unable to do CIC following reconstruction and an additional five have had postoperative urinary incontinence requiring reoperation. Of the five individuals unable to do CIC, two were unable to catheterize a tapered ileal stoma brought to orthotopic perineal position as part of a modified Indiana pouch continent diversion. One of the patients was unable to catheterize an anterior abdominal wall Koch nipple, and one patient was unable to catheterize a reconstructed Young-Dees urethroplasty; all of these patients required reoperation. One patient for unknown reasons adamantly refused to do intermittent catheterization postoperatively (see Case 1).

The importance of postoperative CIC[17] is so real that patients undergoing reconstruction should be evaluated both for their commitment and their physical ability to perform the procedure. It is not unusual for children, who may be dry for the first time in their lives, to ignore the need to empty the reservoir on a routine basis. We feel very strongly that constant parental supervision, especially in younger children, is necessary to ensure compliance with a proper program of catheterization in the postoperative period.

Incontinence.—In the group of five patients that required reoperation for urinary incontinence three were bladder exstrophy patients, and two were myelomeningocele patients. Four of the five had undergone a Young-Dees urethral lengthening procedure. In order to deal with their postoperative incontinence, two of the patients have had Kropp procedures, which have been successful. Two of the patients had implantation of an artificial urinary sphincter, both of which eroded and led to continent urinary diversion. One patient had a pubovaginal sling which has been effective to date. There are other patients in our series with some degree of postoperative incontinence; however only five of the 92 have required an additional procedure for the problem.

Bowel Complications

Four patients (4%) in our reconstruction group developed small bowel obstruction requiring exploration in the postoperative period. It is of interest that one of those patients developed a small bowel intussusception at a point remote from any area of the surgical procedure. This required a small-bowel resection. One other patient required a small-bowel resection and the other two required simple lysis of adhesions.

Spontaneous Perforation

Spontaneous perforation in an augmented bladder or bowel reservoir has been reported with increasing frequency.[18] Although perforations have been noted in a wide variety of patients whose augmentations have been done with various bowel segments, the common denominator would seem to be patients with impaired sensation such as the myelomeningocele group, the use of a detubularized left colon segment for augmentation, and some history of trauma, albeit minor. Mitchell and his group[19] have reported 16 spontaneous perforations in 231 cases for an overall percentage of 6.1%. Two of his patients have perforated on two separate occasions. It is of interest that of the 14 patients with perforation, 11 were myelomeningocele patients, and only 3 were patients with normal sensation. Eleven of the 14 patients with perforation had sigmoid colon used in their reconstruction, while there were perforations noted in only 1 ileal augmentation and 2 gastric cystoplasties.[19]

In our series, spontaneous perforation has been noted in only three patients (3%). One of these is a child who had a right colon augmentation done in conjunction with placement of an artificial urinary sphincter. Her perforation was directly related to overdistention caused by leaving the sphincter cuff inflated for 2 days without catheterization. The second is a myelomeningocele patient who had undergone a left colon augmentation, and had a spontaneous perforation associated with some mild abdominal trauma (Fig 32–7), and the third was an old sacrococcygeal teratoma patient with a sigmoid

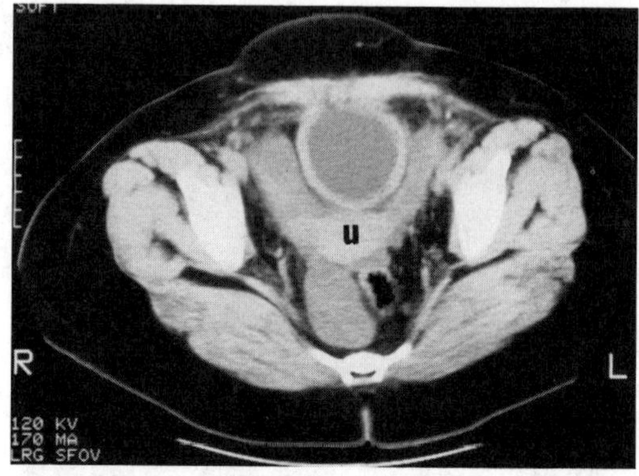

FIG 32–7.
Computed tomography scan in an 18-year-old myelomeningocele patient with spontaneous rupture of her augmented bladder 3 years after reconstruction. The thick-walled bladder is surrounded by a significant urinoma *(u)*.

augmentation and very poor compliance to CIC. We assume that the reason for the relatively low incidence of perforation in our group as compared to other groups might be that our patient population is largely composed of exstrophy patients who do not have impaired sensation. The other important factor is that the majority of our augmentations have been done with detubularized right colon or small bowel rather than left colon. There is no question that increasing attention will be focused on this long-term problem and patients and their primary physicians must be made aware of it.

Carcinoma.—Although there have been no instances of carcinoma noted in the augmented patients in our population, this is another long-term problem which must be recognized.[20] Filmer has documented 13 instances of tumor formation in bowel segments used for augmentation.[21] Nine of the 13 tumors have occurred in ileocystoplasties with 5 of these being adenocarcinoma and 4 having a mixed cell type. Four of the tumors have occurred in large bowel augmentations with adenocarcinoma found in all 4. Although the mechanism is unclear and the

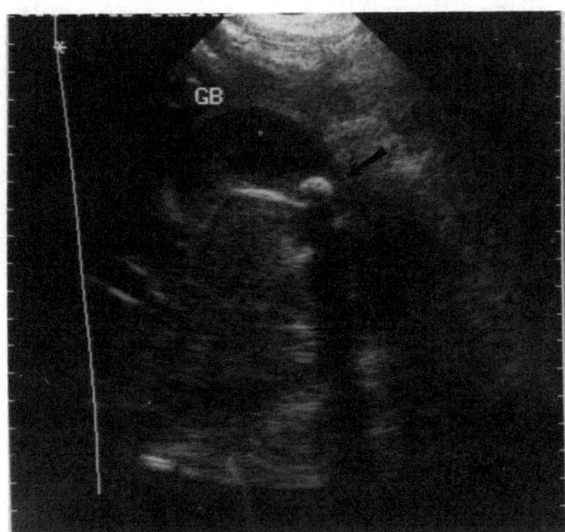

FIG 32–8.
Sonogram of the gallbladder in an 18-year-old female 4 months after urinary tract reconstruction using an ileocecal reservoir. A gallstone with shadowing is demonstrated *(arrow)*.

incidence is low, we must be acutely aware of the long-term potential of this problem.

Metabolic Complications.—Three of our patients have developed symptomatic chololithiasis after their reconstruction (Fig 32–8). There is no immediate explanation for this finding; however, all of the patients were late-adolescent females who had had ileal conduits for more than 15 years, and had their reconstructions done using the right colon and ileocecal valve.

Further metabolic and electrolyte abnormalities have not been a problem for most of the patients in our series. Four patients (4%) have had mild hypochloremic acidosis which has been easily corrected with alkalinization in the postoperative period. Although most published reports have not found any significant metabolic problems,[22] there is at least one other study that suggests long-term severe asymptomatic acidosis despite normal renal function.[23] In addition, McDougal et al.[24] have pointed out a significant degree of bony demineralization in the experimental animal with a longstanding bowel reservoir.

Renal Complications.—One of the most worrisome problems in reconstructed patients is long-term renal deterioration. There was a significant early anecdotal experience with upper tract deterioration when reconstructions were done using small-capacity, high-pressure native bladders. With the increased use of bladder augmentation this problem has been relatively rare. In our series there are two patients who have had significant renal deterioration over time. One of these patients is outlined in Case 1, and his renal failure is very likely related to obstructive uropathy based on his unwillingness to do CIC in the postoperative period. The second patient was an intravenous drug abuser and had evidence of heroin nephropathy at the time of the nephrectomy for end-stage renal disease.

Miscellaneous Complications.—We have seen two patients with femoral neuropathy following reconstructive efforts. Both of these are related to stretching of the femoral plexus during the operation. We do most of our reconstructions in a modified frog-leg position and to avoid this problem care must be taken not to lean on the externally rotated femur. In one patient, the problem was relatively transient, lasting for about 6 months. In the other, however, the problem has persisted over 2 years. We have also had one instance of acute psychosis related to phenothiazine overdose.

CONCLUSION

Urinary tract reconstruction has benefited a vast number of patients with dysfunctional lower urinary tracts caused by congenital abnormalities, previous surgery, or both. Reconstructive efforts have been innovative and continue to evolve.

With this evolution, new and different complications continue to appear, and in order to minimize risk to the patient we must recognize our previously learned lessons. Patient selection is essential in achieving a successful outcome in this group. The patient's neurologic status, urologic anatomy, renal function, and motivation are also important factors in patient selection and correct surgical approach. Close follow-up, however, remains the single most important element in assuring long-term well-being for most of these patients.

EDITORIAL COMMENT

New techniques in urinary tract reconstruction, bladder augmentation, and clean intermittent catheterization have all combined to allow continent urinary tract reconstruction in previously diverted patients. Drs. Hensle and Burbige summarize an extensive experience of over 90 patients. In general, these procedures are well tolerated in the properly selected patient. Clean intermittent catheterization in some patients is mandatory and, as pointed out, complications will ensue if this is not performed. We have had experience with such patients as well. Sometimes it is not always possible to predict patient compliance.

We have also had experience with several bladder perforations. One patient had total bladder reconstruction postcystectomy for cancer. The patient with perforations was receiving chemotherapy, became debilitated, and was unable to stand to void. Overdistention and ischemia of attenuated neobladder wall probably accounted for the perforation.

REFERENCES

1. Hendren WH: Reconstruction of previously diverted urinary tracts in children. *J Pediatr Surg* 1973; 8:135.
2. Dretler SP, Hendren WH, Leadbetter WF: Urinary tract reconstruction following ileal conduit diversion. *J Urol* 1973; 109:217.
3. Hensle TW, Nagler HM, Goldstein HR: Longterm functional results of urinary tract reconstruction in childhood. *J Urol* 1982; 128:1262.
4. Goldstein HR, Hensle TW: Urinary undiversion in adults. *J Urol* 1982; 128:143.
5. Firlit CF, Sommer JT, Kaplan WE: Pediatric urinary undiversion. *J Urol* 1980; 123:748.
6. Perlmutter AD: Experience with urinary undiversion in children with neurogenic bladder. *J Urol* 1980; 123:402.
7. Borden TA, Woodside JR: Urinary tract undiversion in a patient with an areflexic neurogenic bladder, management with intermittent catheterization. *J Urol* 1980; 123:956.
8. Richie JP, Sacks SA: Complications of urinary undiversion. *J Urol* 1977; 117:362.
9. Retik AB, Casale AJ: Complications of urinary undiversion. *Urol Clin North Am* 1983; 10:483.
10. Burbige KA, Hensle TW: The complications of urinary tract reconstruction. *J Urol* 1986; 136:292.
11. Kogan SJ, Levitt SB: Bladder evaluation in pediatric patients before undiversion in previously diverted urinary tracts. *J Urol* 1977; 118:443.
12. Bauer SB, Colodny AH, Hallet M, et al: Urinary undiversion in myelodysplasia: Criteria for selection and predictive value of urodynamic evaluation. *J Urol* 1980; 124:89.
13. Mitchell ME: The role of bladder augmentation in undiversion. *J Pediatr Surg* 1981; 16:790.
14. Hensle TW, Burbige KA, Levin RK: Management of the short ureter in urinary tract reconstruction. *J Urol* 1987; 137:707.
15. McGuire EJ, Woodside JR, Borden TA, et al: Prognostic value of urodynamics in myelodysplastic patients. *J Urol* 1981; 126:205.
16. Heney NM, Dretler SP, Hensle TW, et al: Autosuturing device in intestinal urinary conduits. *Urology* 1978; 12:650.
17. Lapides J, Diokno AC, Silber SJ, et al: Clean intermittent self-catheterization in the treatment of urinary tract disease. *J Urol* 1972; 107:458.

18. Elder JS, Snyder HM, Hulbert WC, et al: Perforation of the augmented bladder in patients undergoing clean intermittent catheterization. *J Urol* 1988; 140:1159.
19. Mitchell ME: Personal communication.
20. Stone AR, Davies N, Stephenson TP: Carcinoma associated with augmentation cystoplasty. *Br J Urol* 1987; 60:236–238.
21. Filmer B: Personal communication.
22. Skinner DG, Lieskovsky G, Boyd SD: Continent urinary diversion: a 5½ year experience. *Ann Surg* 1988; 208:337.
23. Mohler JL: Metabolic acidosis after bladder replacement: Comparison of severity and reversibility in ileal and colon reservoirs. *J Urol* 1988; 139:628.
24. McDougal WS, Koch MO, Shands C III, et al: Bony demineralization following urinary intestinal diversion. *J Urol* 1988; 140:853.

CHAPTER 33

Complications in the Surgical Reconstruction of Classical Bladder Exstrophy

John P. Gearhart, M.D.
Herbert Lepor, M.D.
Robert D. Jeffs, M.D.

Classical bladder exstrophy occurs when the cloacal membrane is not reinforced by an ingrowth of mesoderm. The attenuated cloacal membrane ruptures prematurely, resulting in extrusion of the bladder through the lower abdominal wall defect. The incidence of bladder exstrophy has been estimated at 1 in 10,000 to 1 in 50,000.[1, 2] The surgical management of classical bladder exstrophy represents one of the greatest reconstructive challenges facing the pediatric urologist. Although many reconstructive techniques have been described, a unified approach to the surgical management of this disorder has evolved only recently.

The primary objectives for the surgical management of bladder exstrophy are to obtain (1) secure abdominal wall closure, (2) urinary continence with preservation of renal function, and (3) reconstruction of a functional and cosmetically acceptable penis. These objectives can be achieved following primary bladder closure, bladder neck reconstruction, and epispadias repair or following urinary diversion, cystectomy, and epispadias repair. Historically, both urinary diversion and functional bladder closure have been fraught with complications. The appropriate surgical management for patients with bladder exstrophy requires detailed study and investigation, knowledge of all possible surgical solutions and their results, and a creative team approach to the overall management of the individual patient. It is the purpose of this chapter to examine the complications of the surgical treatment of this condition in order to avoid many of the problems that have occurred in patients treated in the past. We advocate primary functional closure, and therefore we will review a personal series of patients with bladder exstrophy treated at the Johns Hopkins Hospital between 1975 and 1985.

FUNCTIONAL BLADDER RECONSTRUCTION

Historical Perspectives

Hugh Hampton Young reported the first successful functional closure of bladder exstrophy.[4] The patient developed a 3-hour continent interval; however, preservation of renal function was not documented. Marshall and Muecke reviewed 329 functional bladder closures reported in the literature between 1900 and 1966 and determined that urinary continence with preservation of renal function was achieved in only 16 (5%) cases.[5] Dehiscence of the abdominal wall and bladder, urinary fistula, incontinence, persistent reflux, and pyelonephritis frequently resulted in subsequent urinary diversion.

Over the past 20 years, several fundamental modifications in the management of functional bladder closure have contributed to a dramatic increase in the success of this approach. The most significant changes in approaching functional bladder closure have been (1) defining criteria for the selection of patients suitable for functional closure, (2) staging the reconstruction procedures, (3) performing bilateral iliac osteotomies, and (4) reconstructing a competent bladder neck.

Successful treatment of exstrophy by functional closure demands that the potential for success in each child be considered at birth. Bladder size and functional capacity of the detrusor muscle are important considerations in the eventual success of closure. In minor grades of exstrophy that approach the condition of complete epispadias with incontinence, the bladder may appear small; however, acceptable capacity may be demonstrated by observing the bladder bulge when the baby cries or by indenting the bladder with a gloved finger. The elastic and contractile exstrophy bladder that is estimated at birth to have a capacity of 5 mL or more can be expected to develop useful size and capacity following successful closure. Once removed from surface irritation and repeated trauma, the small bladder will enlarge and will gradually increase its capacity. On the other hand, a small fibrotic bladder patch that is stretched between the edges of a small triangular fascial defect without either elasticity or contractility cannot be selected for the usual closure procedure. Bladder augmentation using bowel segments may be required in order to achieve closure in these patients.

The disadvantage of performing the entire surgical reconstruction of bladder exstrophy in a single stage is that a single complication jeopardizes the entire repair. Sweetser et al. first described a staged surgical approach to bladder exstrophy.[6] Bladder closure was performed 4 to 6 days following bilateral iliac osteotomies, and epispadias repair was performed as a separate procedure. A staged approach to functional bladder closure that includes three separate stages (bladder closure, bladder neck reconstruction with an antireflux procedure, and epispadias repair) is currently recommended for most cases of exstrophy reconstruction.[3]

The efficacy of iliac osteotomies is controversial. The primary arguments against osteotomies are that the pubis eventually pulls apart, the penis retracts farther, and continence can be achieved without osteotomies. The advantages of bilateral iliac osteotomies are that reapproximation of the pubic symphysis diminishes tension on the abdominal wall closure and eliminates the need for fascial flaps. Placement of the urethra within the pelvic ring reduces the excessive urethrovesical angle and permits urethral suspension after bladder neck plasty, and reapproximation of the urogenital diaphragm and approximation of the levator ani muscles may aid in voluntary urinary control. It is of note that in the 20 patients referred for secondary bladder closure, 7 had neonatal closure without osteotomy and only 2 of the 20 on their previous closure had undergone pelvic osteotomy.

A major advancement in functional bladder closure was achieving continence without bladder outlet obstruction. Dees modified the Young technique for reconstructing the bladder neck.[7] Specifically, he recommended removing a triangular wedge of tissue from the roof and lateral aspects of the urethra and adjacent bladder neck. The remaining posterior urethral mucosal strip was tubularized and the neourethra was reinforced by the adjacent denuded muscle. Leadbetter modified the Dees procedure by tubularizing a posterior urethral strip 3.5 cm long that included bladder mucosa. The urethra was reinforced with trigonal muscle, and bilateral neoureterocystotomies were performed.[8]

Primary Bladder Closure and Osteotomy

Surgical Technique

The bladder and pelvic ring closure can be carried out without osteotomies, owing to the malleability of the pelvic ring in suitable patients seen within the first 48 hours of life.[9] However, when the separation is unduly wide, or when there is a delay in referral from the time of birth, osteotomies will be required to achieve closure of the pelvic ring. Formerly the osteotomies were performed through bilateral incisions over the sacroiliac region. Recently we have had experience with anterior iliac osteotomy in the closure of both newborns and older patients undergoing reclosure with excellent success. This approach negates the need for turning the child, and the blood loss appears to be less or equal to that of the posterior approach (Fig 33-1). Postoperatively, patients closed without osteotomies in the first 48 hours of life, and patients requiring osteotomies are immobilized by modified Bryant's traction (see Fig 33–1). Traction is maintained for a period of 3 to 4 weeks, allowing firm fibrous healing of the pelvic ring anteriorly. The fibrocartilage of the pubic symphysis is united by a horizontal mattress suture tied anterior to the pubic closure using no. 2 nylon.

The technique for initial bladder closure has previously been described.[10] An incision is made outlining the bladder mucosa and the prostatic plate. The urethral groove is transsected distal to the verumontanum, but continuity is maintained between the thin, mucosa-like, non–hair-bearing skin adjacent to the posterior urethra and bladder neck and the skin and mucosa of the penile shaft and glans. Skin flaps from the area of the thin paraexstrophy skin are subsequently moved distally and rotated to reconstitute the urethral groove, which may be lengthened by 2 to 4 cm (Fig 33–2). Penile lengthening is achieved by exposing the corpus cavernosum bilaterally and freeing the corpora from their attachments to the suspensory ligaments and anterior aspect of the inferior pubic rami. The partially

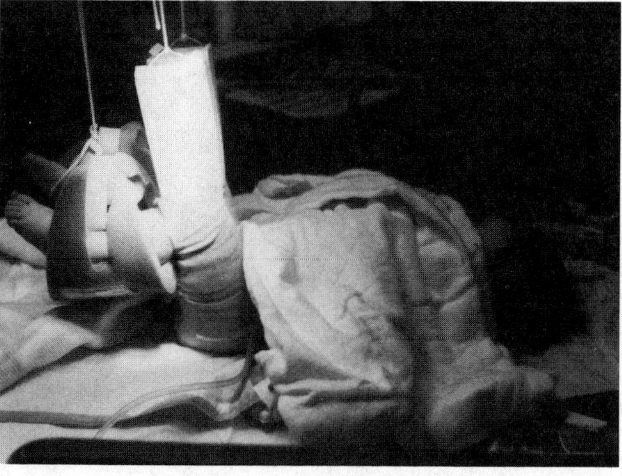

FIG 33–1.
This figure shows a newborn in modified Bryant's traction after initial closure.

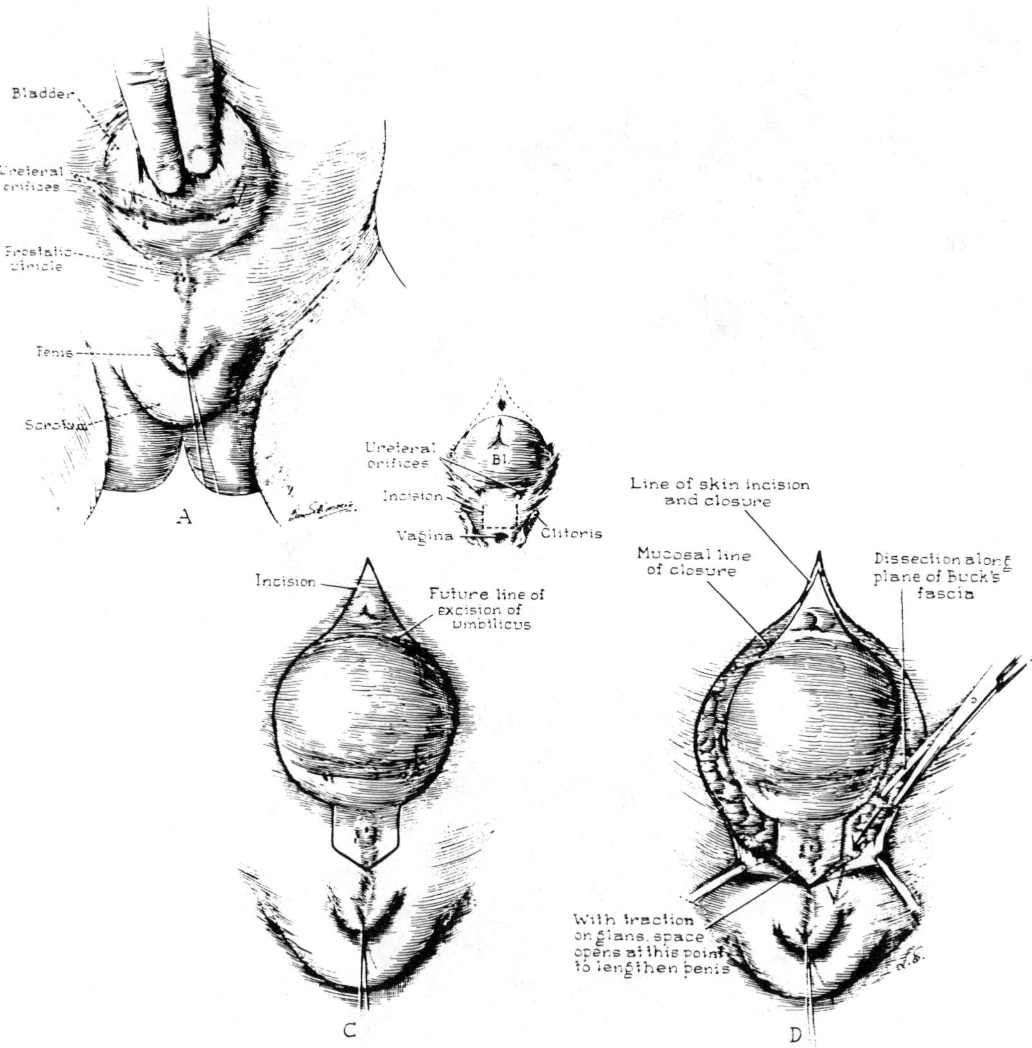

FIG 33–2.
A–D, initial steps in primary bladder closure. *(Continued.)*

mobilized corpora are joined in the midline, and the bare corpora are then covered with flaps of the thin, paraexstrophy skin.

Bladder closure proceeds by excision of the umbilical area. The bladder muscle is then freed from the fused rectus sheaths. A wide band of fibrous and muscle tissue representing the urogenital diaphragm is detached subperiosteally from the pubis bilaterally. The mucosa and muscle of the bladder and posterior urethra are then closed in the midline anteriorly. The posterior urethra and bladder neck are buttressed by the tissues of the urogenital diaphragm. The bladder is drained by a suprapubic Malecot catheter for 4 weeks. The urethra is not stented, in order to avoid pressure necrosis or the accumulation of infected secretions in the urethra. Ureteral stents provide urinary drainage during the 7 days in order to avoid ureteral obstruction and transient hypertension.

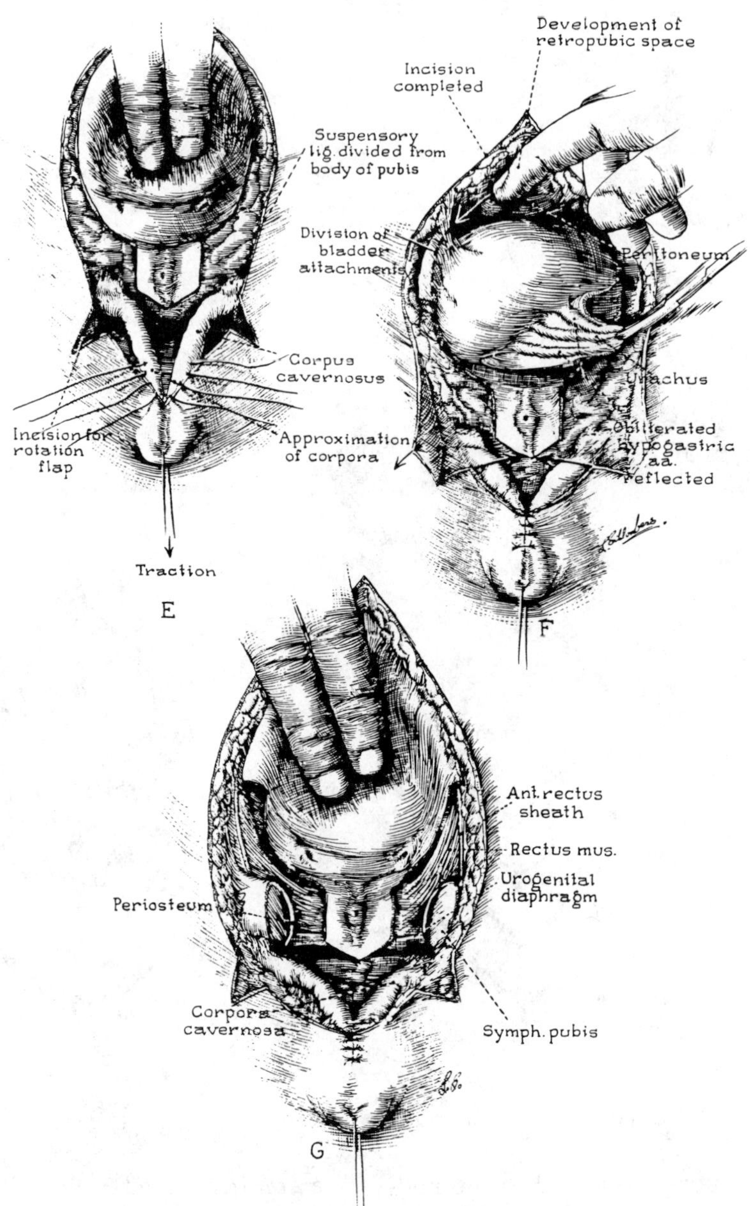

FIG 33–2 (cont.).
E, lateral skin incision allowing rotation of paraexstrophy skin to cover elongated penis. **F,** development of retropubic space in the area of umbilical dissection separating bladder from rectus muscle and sheath. **G,** diaphragm and anterior corpus cavernosum freed from pubis and subperiosteal plane. *(Continued.)*

Results of the Hopkins Series

Fifty of 51 consecutive patients with bladder exstrophy (98%) who were referred to our pediatric urology service prior to any surgical intervention underwent bladder closure during 1975–1985. Partial bladder prolapse occurred in only 2 patients. One patient underwent successful urinary diversion with a colon conduit following an unsatisfactory pri-

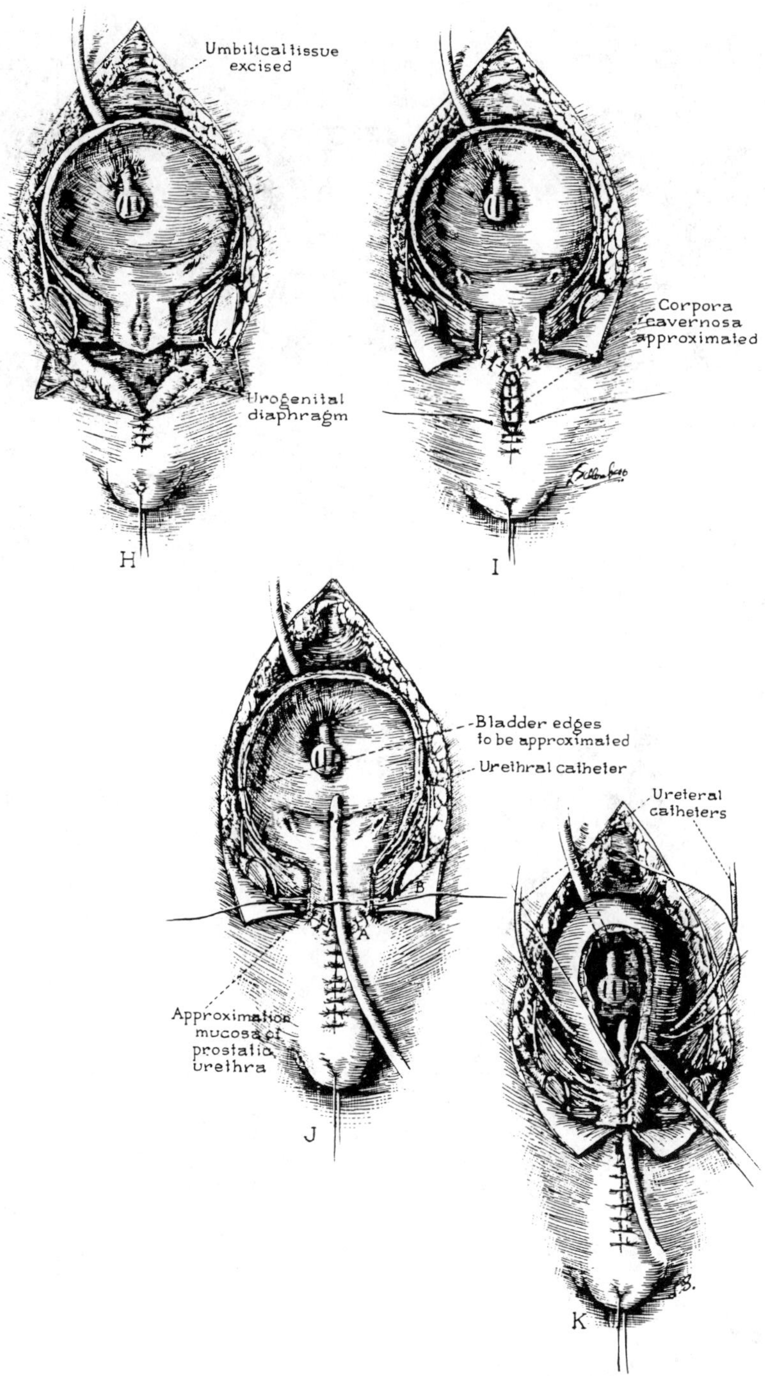

FIG 33–2 (cont.).
H, I, joining prostatic plate to neourethra. **J, K,** initiation of bladder closure. *(Continued.)*

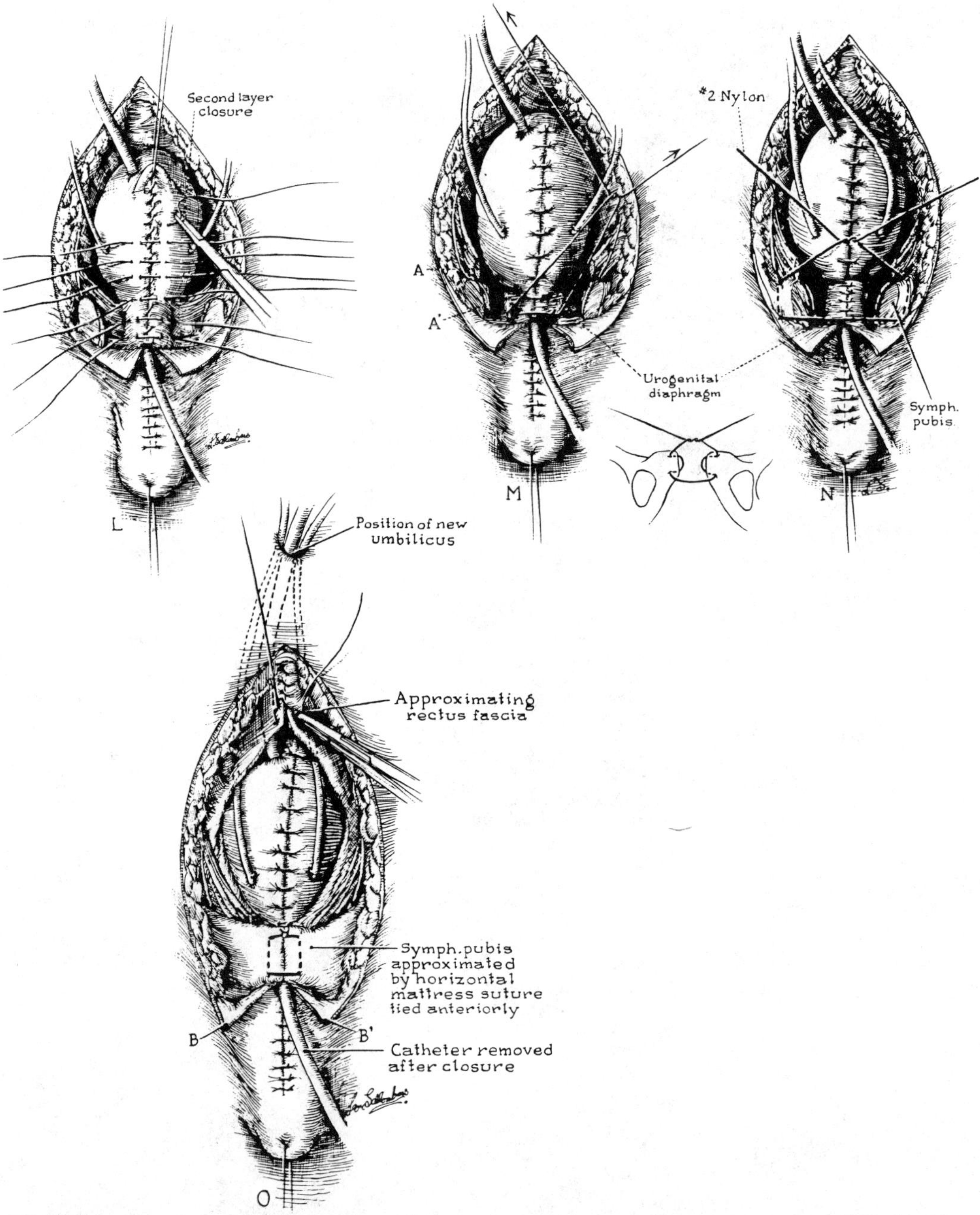

FIG 33–2 (cont.).

L, bladder closure. **M,** urogenital diaphragm is closed with separate layer of sutures. **N,** horizontal mattress suture placed on external surface of symphysis. **O,** catheter removed from closed bladder neck and urethra. (From Harrison JH, Jeffs RD, Lepor H: Management of the exstrophy-epispadias complex and urachal anomalies, in Walsh PC, Gittes RF, Perlmutter AD, et al (ed): *Campbell's Urology,* ed 5. Philadelphia, WB Saunders Co, 1986, vol 2, pp 1895–1899. Used by permission.)

TABLE 33–1.
Complications in 51 Consecutive Bladder Closures

Complication	No.	%
Bladder prolapse	2	4
Unsuccessful primary closure	1	2
Total	3	6

Corrective Surgical Procedures	No.
Repair of bladder prolapse	2
Colon conduit	1
Total	3

mary closure (Table 33–1). These complications required the following surgical interventions: repair of bladder prolapse in 2 patients, and urinary diversion in one patient. Cystolitholapaxy in 3 patients, and urethrotomy in 1 patient. These results represent a significant improvement when compared to a personal series treated between 1959 and 1975.[11] In the former group of 71 patients with bladder exstrophy, bladder dehiscence, prolapse, or fistula following bladder closure developed in 9 patients. In patients undergoing osteotomy prior to bladder closure, exteriorization of the pubic stitch developed in 30%. In 5 patients who underwent neonatal closure without osteotomy there were 3 failures. We attribute the improvement in our more recent series of bladder closures to efforts directed at preventing infection, tissue mobility, and wound tension.[12]

In order to minimize infection, the bladder should be closed as early as possible. During the interval between birth and closure, it is suggested that the bladder be protected with a plastic film such as Saran Wrap, since petroleum jelly, gauze, or diapers adhere and denude the bladder mucosa. The old urine should be washed away liberally with water or body-temperature baths at frequent intervals, and all efforts should be made to minimize the diaper rash and ammonia burn that occurs in this area from contamination with urea-splitting organisms.

At the time of closure, ampicillin and gentamicin are administered preoperatively, and these antibiotics are continued for 5 to 7 days after surgery. The local area is thoroughly washed and cleansed with povidone-iodine (Betadine); this cleansing includes a liberal soaking of the bladder and its interstices. The entire lower half of the body is draped into the operative field so that the pelvic ring can be manipulated at the time of anterior midline closure. An anal plug of gauze should be inserted during the initial preparation to prevent stool contamination during this procedure.

It is our impression that tissue mobility and wound tension also contribute to wound dehiscence.[12] The anterior fixation of the two sides of the pubis after neonatal molding or pelvic osteotomies help to limit the mobility and wound tension. In all of our patients who are not seen immediately after birth, osteotomies are required in order to achieve good midline closure. Neonatal closure has an inherent flaw since the built-in wound distraction lacks the memory of the pelvic bone and tissues of the pelvic girdle. Although the symphysis can be approximated in the neonate, it is still necessary that this anterior approximation be maintained during the healing process. Fixation of the pubic bones is achieved by a suture, and the position of the bones are maintained by the modified Bryant's traction.

Fixation of the coapted pubic bones are provided by heavy horizontal mattress sutures tied on the outside of the closure. Additional heavy nylon sutures may be used in the adjacent rectus fascia. The wire suture that was used previously frequently broke and eroded through the skin. External fixation, plaster casts, wrapping, and so forth have been tried, and it is thought that the distracting muscular forces are minimized by Bryant's traction more effectively.

In order to achieve successful closure, it is also important to control the muscular activity of the child. The entire staff attending the baby must make every effort to ensure that pain, frustration, hunger, and muscle spasm do not produce undue or prolonged activity that defeats the other attempts to provide wound immobility.

Bladder Neck Reconstruction

Timing of Bladder Neck Reconstruction.—Bladder neck reconstruction is performed when the bladder capacity approaches 60 mL, which usually occurs by the time the child is 3 years old. Epispadias repair, however, may precede bladder neck reconstruction if the bladder capacity has not reached 60 mL by the age of 3. In a recent series of 28 patients with small capacities after initial closure, epispadias repair prior to bladder neck reconstruction increased the mean bladder capacity by an additional 57 cc.[13]

Surgical Technique.—The technique for bladder neck reconstruction has previously been described.[10] A U incision is made over the bladder neck, and this incision is extended as a midline bladder cystotomy. Bilateral, crossed trigonal ureteral reimplantations are performed. A midline posterior strip of bladder mucosa, 18 to 20 mm wide and 30 mm long, extending distally from the midtrigone to the prostate or posterior urethra, is selected. The mucosa lateral to the strip is excised. The mucosal strip is tubularized with interrupted sutures, and the adjacent detrusor muscle is overlapped to reinforce the mucosal tube. The anterior aspect of the reconstructed bladder neck is suspended to the rectus fascia and the symphysis in the manner of Marshall-Marchetti-Krantz. Intraoperative urethral pressure profilometry is used to approximate a continence length of 3.5 cm and urethral closure pressure of 60 to 90 cm H_2O when the bladder is distended with 50 mL of saline. A Malecot catheter is introduced into the dome of the bladder through a separate stab incision. No stents or catheters are left indwelling in the newly constructed bladder neck. Pediatric feeding tubes are placed into the ureteral orifices, and the perivesical space is drained with a Penrose drain. The suprapubic catheter is maintained for 21 days and removed if there is no evidence of urinary obstruction. Bladder neck calibration or dilatation may be required before removing the suprapubic catheter if urinary obstruction is identified prior to catheter removal.

Continence and Complications Following Bladder Neck Reconstruction.—Thirty-nine patients have undergone initial bladder neck reconstruction at Johns Hopkins between 1975 and 1985.[3] Urinary continence in a series of patients with classical bladder exstrophy following bladder neck reconstruction is difficult to assess, since perfect urinary control would not be expected in an age-matched control group of patients. We have assessed urinary continence in our exstrophy patients by parental interviews according to average daytime dry interval. Achievement of an average daytime interval greater than 3 hours was considered an excellent surgical result. An excellent surgical result was achieved in 92% in patients assessed by average daytime dry intervals. (Table 33–2). All patients in this series have been followed for a minimum of 1.5 years after bladder neck reconstruction.

TABLE 33–2.
Urinary Continence Following 39 Bladder Neck Reconstructions

Average Daytime Dry Interval		Patients	
Result	Dry Interval (Hr)	No.	%
Excellent	>3	36	92
Satisfactory	1–3	2	5
Poor	<1	1	3

There are several factors that we believe account for our high continence rate. Leadbetter considered the length of the bladder neck to be the most significant factor contributing to achieving continence, and therefore we follow his recommendation of creating a bladder neck approximately 3 cm in length.[8] In addition, bilateral iliac osteotomies are performed at the time of closure, therefore allowing placement of the urethra within the pelvic ring. This maneuver allows for the levator ani and puborectalis muscles to aid in voluntary urinary control. The bladder neck suspension aids in providing static and stress continence. The effectiveness of the bladder neck suspension has been demonstrated intraoperatively, using urethral pressure profilometry.

It is imperative that the mechanism for achieving urinary continence does not compromise renal function. We have evaluated the upper urinary tracts of our patients following bladder neck reconstruction using intravenous pyelograms. Significant upper tract deterioration developed in three patients evaluated by intravenous pyelograms 0.5 to 6.0 years after bladder neck reconstruction.[3]

Complications following bladder neck reconstruction are rare. In our series of 39 consecutive bladder neck reconstructions, postoperative urinary retention developed in 8 patients. The bladder outlet obstruction resolved in all 8 patients following dilatation or prolonged suprapubic catheter drainage.

Epispadias Repair

Male neonates referred to our institution for initial surgical reconstruction undergo penile lengthening and release of chordee at the time of primary bladder closure. Construction of the neourethra, further penile lengthening, and release of chordee are performed approximately 1 year after bladder neck reconstruction. A modified Young urethroplasty is performed when there is sufficient penile skin for construction of the urethra and coverage of the neourethra. Preputial pedicle grafts and full-thickness skin grafts are reserved for the patient with insufficient penile skin.

Surgical Technique.—The technique for urethroplasty has previously been described.[14] The modified Young urethroplasty is begun by placing a nylon suture through the glans, which provides for traction of the penis. Incisions are made over two parallel lines marked previously on the dorsum of the penis that outline an 18-mm strip of penile skin extending from the prostatic urethral meatus to the tip of the glans. Triangular areas of the dorsal glans are excised adjacent to the urethral strip, and glanular flaps are constructed. Lateral skin flaps are mobilized, and a Z incision over the subpubic area permits exposure and division of suspensory ligaments and old scar tissue. The urethral strip is closed in a linear manner from the prostatic opening to the glans over a 10F pediatric feeding tube, using 6-0 polyglycolic acid sutures. The subcutaneous layer is closed with two separate continuous layers of 6-0 polyglycolic acid sutures. The skin is reapproximated with interrupted 5-0 polyglycolic acid sutures. The glans is reapproximated with vertical mattress sutures of 4-0 polypropylene, which are removed in 10 days. The pediatric feeding tube is left indwelling in the neourethra as a stent.

Results of a Personal Series.—A modified Young urethroplasty was performed in 22 of the 24 patients with classical bladder exstrophy undergoing epispadias repair.[14] Fistulas developed in nine patients following epispadias repair: four (17%) closed spontaneously, and five (21%) required surgical closure (Table 33–3). Of the latter five fistulas, four occurred near the corona and one at the midshaft. The corona is the area most deficient in cir-

TABLE 33–3.
Urethral Fistulas Following 24 Epispadias Repairs

Fistulas	Incidence (%)
Surgical closure	5(21)
Spontaneous closure	4(17)
Recurrent	0(0)

cumferential penile skin, and therefore multiple-layered closure at this point over the tubularized urethra is difficult to achieve.

We have attempted to determine whether prior osteotomies, sequence of bladder neck plasty and epispadias repair, hospital of initial treatment, number of prior bladder closures performed, and preoperative androgen stimulation affect the rate of fistula formation. Prior osteotomies appeared to decrease the rate of fistulas that require surgical closure (15% compared to 67% in patients who had not undergone prior osteotomy). The other parameters did not affect the fistula rate.

Most of our patients are preadolescent, and therefore it is too early to evaluate definitively the functional result and potential for fertility. However, personal interviews with several college-age males have shown them to be very sexually well adjusted and performing satisfactorily. The current status of the penile reconstruction was determined indirectly by parental interviews. The angle of the penis at rest was directed downward or horizontally in 83% of the patients. With erections, the penis was deflected upward in 47% of the boys. Some patients with penises that deflected upward during erection may eventually require a Z plasty at the base of the penis to release tethering scar tissue.

URINARY DIVERSION

Ureterosigmoidostomy

The first ureterosigmoidostomy was performed for bladder exstrophy by Simon, and the patient died 1 year later.[15] Early experiences with ureterosigmoidostomies for bladder exstrophy were fraught with complications, which included peritonitis, ureterosigmoid anastomotic strictures, acute and chronic pyelonephritis, stones, intestinal obstruction, incontinence, and hyperchloremic hypokalemic acidosis. The postoperative mortality in a large series of ureterosigmoidostomies performed between 1912 and 1946 was 12.5%.[16] The magnitude of early and late complications following ureterosigmoidostomy for bladder exstrophy was reported in a large personal series of Higgins.[17] The description of a mucosal ureterointestinal anastomosis[18] and, subsequently, an antirefluxing intestinal anastomosis[19] has led to significant improvements in early and late complications following ureterosigmoidostomy.

Spence reviewed the long-term follow-up of 31 exstrophy patients treated with ureterosigmoidostomies.[20] In this carefully followed group of patients, no immediate postoperative deaths occurred, and three subsequent deaths were attributed to the ureterosigmoidostomy. Eleven cases (35%) required subsequent operative procedures for stones, anastomotic strictures, and recurrent pyelonephritis. Of 61 renal units assessed by intravenous pyelography, 41 units (67%) were considered good; 5 units were fair, and 15 units were poor. Major infection developed in 14 patients (23%), and 9 individuals (14%) had absolutely no problems with infection. Although half of the patients developed hyperchloremic acidosis, chronic alkalinization of the urine was rarely required. Despite these complications, 50% of the patients in this series had no complications as measured by excretory pyelogram, infection, blood chemistries, and clinical assessment.

Adenocarcinoma of the colon adjacent to the ureterointestinal anastomosis in an exstrophy patient was initially described in 1948.[21] The risk of adenocarcinoma of the colon developing in exstrophy patients following ureterosigmoidostomy is 100-fold that of the general population.[22] Spence et al. surveyed the literature and identified 35 exstrophy patients who have developed colonic tumors.[23] Twenty-eight of the 35 compiled tumors were malignant, 24 were adenocarcinomas, and approximately half of the adenocarcinomas had metastasized at the time of diagnosis. The course of patients with ureterosigmoidostomies must be carefully studied with either barium enemas or sigmoidoscopy. The true incidence of malignancy following ureterosigmoidostomy is not known, since complete follow-up information is not available in any series. In a review of 90 patients with exstrophy undergoing ureterosigmoidostomy, 5% have developed colonic malignancies to date.[24]

Alternative Methods of Urinary Diversion

Owing to the complications associated with ureterosigmoidostomy, several alternative techniques for urinary diversion for bladder exstrophy have been described. Boyce and Vest reviewed 23 trigonosigmoidostomies, which were followed for a mean interval of 10 years.[25] Renal function was assessed by excretory urography and was thought to be normal in 21 (91%) cases, and stones formed in 2 (9%). Although hyperchloremic acidosis developed in approximately 50%, only a few patients required alkalinization. All children achieved daytime continence, and, overall, 18 (78%) of their cases were considered to be good results.

The Heitz-Boyer and Hovelacque procedure included diverting the ureters into an isolated rectal segment and pulling the sigmoid colon through the anal sphincter muscle just posterior to the rectum. Taccinoli et al. reviewed 21 Heitz-Boyer and Hovelacque procedures for bladder exstrophy in patients whose course was followed for 1 to 16 years.[26] They reported that 20 (95%) of patients had fecal and urinary incontinence, but there were no cases of urinary calculi, electrolyte abnormalities, or postoperative mortality, and 3 (14%) patients developed ureterorectal strictures requiring surgical revision. Isolated cases treated in North America with this approach have resulted in multiple and severe complications.

The early good results with ileal conduit urinary diversion suggested that this technique might be ideal for urinary drainge in bladder exstrophy patients. Unfortunately, significant long-term complications have developed in children who have had ileal conduit diversion.[27] In patients with bladder exstrophy who are expected to have a normal life expectancy, ileal conduit diversion is not acceptable.

Hendren described using colon conduits for urinary drainage in cases of bladder exstrophy.[28] The nonrefluxing ureterointestinal anastomosis represents the primary advantage of the colon conduit. If anal continence is achieved, the ureterocolonic anastomosis is nonrefluxing and there is no upper tract deterioration; the colon conduit may be undiverted into the colon as a colocoloplasty at the age of 4 to 5 years. The long-term assessment of renal function and continence following colon conduit diversion and subsequent colocoloplasty requires further investigation. The initial results reported by Hendren are promising.

Also, the use of continent urinary diversion will certainly have a place in the management of the difficult exstrophy patient. Recent experience at our institution with three of these procedures in patients who had undergone multiple procedures further reinforces the utility of this technique.

BLADDER AUGMENTATION IN THE FAILED EXSTROPHY RECONSTRUCTION

In a recent review of 12 patients with failed exstrophy reconstruction who required bladder augmentation, 8 had dehiscence after initial bladder closure and 9 had at least one prior bladder neck procedure which had failed.[26] Five patients had inadequate bladder volume after initial or subsequent closure and epispadias repair, but the bladder did not adapt to a volume of 50 cc or greater. Seven patients were those whose capacity had failed to improve after bladder neck plasty, but they had a small-capacity bladder and persistent incontinence. Adjunctive procedures were performed at the time of augmentation and included a bladder neck plasty in three patients, one of which was a repeat, and one patient had a transureteroureterostomy and psoas hitch. One patient underwent a Mitrofanoff procedure in association with ileal augmentation and bladder neck closure.

In three patients, an artificial urinary sphincter was placed for continence. The patients selected included an undiversion in which the sphincter was placed around the tubularized bladder, a bladder exstrophy variant in which the sphincter was placed at the upper prostatic level after removing two ectopic ureters from the posterior urethra. The third patient received the sphincter around the failed bladder neck plasty at 5 years of age. Eleven of these 12 patients are continent, although 9 require intermittent catheterization. There were no major complications in this group of patients. Therefore, it is felt that in the failed exstrophy reconstruction, augmentation cystoplasty has provided both prolonged stability of the upper tracts and continence in these patients and has proved to be a successful alternative to diversion in this select group of exstrophy failures.[26]

CONCLUSIONS

Great strides have been made in the surgical management of bladder exstrophy. Although in this chapter we have outlined a rather standard approach for the surgical management of exstrophy, each individual neonate or child requires careful planning and interval follow-up. The planned surgical procedures need to be modified for each patient.

This review of complications emphasizes the complexity of reconstruction for patients with bladder exstrophy. With experienced hands, the surgical results after primary bladder closure, bladder neck reconstruction, and epispadias together are quite acceptable. A review of staged functional closure for bladder exstrophy at the Johns Hopkins Hospital has clearly demonstrated that secure abdominal wall closure, urinary continence with preservation of the upper urinary tracts, and a cosmetically acceptable penis can be achieved without wound dehiscence, with infrequent deterioration of renal function, and with an occasional urethral fistula that requires surgical repair.

EDITORIAL COMMENT

A small bladder capacity was often a difficult problem in some exstrophy patients. Urinary diversion was usually considered. Drs. Gearhart, Lepor, and Jeffs have now utilized bladder augmentation in a few patients successfully, correcting even this most difficult problem. Total genitourinary reconstruction with urinary continence in the exstrophy patient remains one of the more difficult problems in all of urology. The vast majority of these patients can now be reconstructed successfully because of the pioneering efforts of these authors.

REFERENCES

1. Rickham PP: The incidence and treatment of ectopia vesicae. *Proc R Soc Med* 1961; 54:389.
2. Latlimer JK, Smith MJK: Exstrophy clo-

sure: A follow-up on 70 cases. *J Urol* 1966; 95:356.

3. Oesterling JE, Jeffs RD: The importance of a successful initial bladder closure in the surgical management of classical bladder exstrophy: analysis of 144 patients with bladder exstrophy treated at the Johns Hopkins Hospital from 1975 to 1985. *J Urol* 1987; 137:258.
4. Young HH: Exstrophy of the bladder: The first case in which a normal bladder and urinary control have been obtained by plastic operation. *Surg Gynecol Obstet* 1942; 75:729.
5. Marshall VF, Muecke EC: Functional closure of typical exstrophy of the bladder. *J Urol* 1970; 104:205.
6. Sweetser TH, Chisholm TC, Thompson WH: Exstrophy of the urinary bladder: Discussion of anatomic principles applicable to its repair with preliminary report of a case. *Minn Med* 1952; 35:654.
7. Dees JE: Congenital epispadias with incontinence. *J Urol* 1949; 62:513.
8. Leadbetter GW Jr: Surgical correction of total urinary incontinence. *J Urol* 1964; 91:261.
9. Ansell JE: Exstrophy and epispadias, in Glenn JF (ed): *Urologic Surgery.* Philadelphia, JB Lippincott Co, 1983, p 647.
10. Jeffs RD, Lepor H: Management of the exstrophy-epispadias complex and urachal anomalies, in PC Walsh, RF Gittes, AD Perlmutter, et al (eds): *Campbell's Urology* Philadelphia, WB Saunders Co, 1985, p 1882.
11. Jeffs RD: Complications of exstrophy surgery. *Urol Clin North Am* 1983; 10:509.
12. Lowe FC, Jeffs RD: Wound dehiscence in bladder exstrophy: An examination of the etiologies and factors for initial failure and subsequent closure. *J Urol* 1983; 130:312.
13. Gearhart JP, Jeffs RD: Bladder exstrophy: Increase in capacity following epispadias repair. *J Urol* 1989; 142:522.
14. Lepor H, Shapiro E, Jeffs RD: Urethral reconstruction in males with classical bladder exstrophy. *J Urol* 1984; 131:512.
15. Simon J: Ectopia vesicae. *Lancet* 1852; 2:568.
16. Harvard BM, Thompson GJ: Congenital exstrophy of the urinary bladder: Late results of treatment by the Coffey-Mayo method of ureterointestinal anastomosis. *J Urol* 1951; 65:223.
17. Higgins CC: Exstrophy of the bladder: Report of 158 cases. *Am Surg* 1962; 28:99.
18. Coffey RC: Transplantation of the ureter into the large intestine in the absence of a functioning bladder. *Surg Gynecol Obstet* 1921; 32:383.
19. Leadbetter WF: Consideration of problems incident to performance of ureteroureterostomy. Report of a technique. *J Urol* 1955; 73:67.
20. Spence HM, Hoffman WN, Pate VA: exstrophy of the bladder: Long term results in a series of 31 cases treated by ureterosigmoidostomy. *J Urol* 1975; 114:133.
21. Dixon CF, Weisman RE: Polyps of the sigmoid occurring 30 years after bilateral ureterosigmoidostomies for exstrophy of the bladder. *Surgery* 1948; 24:6.
22. Sooriyaarchchi GS, Johnson RO, Carbone PP: Neoplasms of the large bowel following ureterosigmoidostomy. *Arch Surg* 1979; 112:1174.
23. Spence HM, Hoffman WW, Fosmire PP: Tumors of the colon as a later complication of ureterosigmoidostomy of exstrophy of the bladder. *Br J Urol* 1979; 51:466.
24. Bennett AH: Exstrophy of the bladder treated by ureterosigmoidostomies. *Urology* 1973; 2:165.
25. Boyce WH, Vest SA: A new concept concerning treatment of exstrophy of the bladder. *J Urol* 1952; 67:503.
26. Taccinol M, Laurenti C, Rachel T: Sixteen years experience with the Heitz-Hoyer Hovelacque procedure for exstrophy of the bladder. *Br J Urol* 1977; 49:385.
27. Jeffs RD, Schwarz GR: Ileal conduit urinary diversion in children: Computer analysis followup from 2 to 16 years. *J Urol* 1975; 114:285.
28. Hendren WH: Exstrophy of the bladder: An alternative method of management. *J Urol* 1979; 12:527.
29. Gearhart JP, Jeffs RD: Augmentation cystoplasty in the failed exstrophy reconstruction. *J Urol* 1988; 139:790.

SECTION V

Complications of Surgery of the Genitalia and Urethra

CHAPTER 34

Complications of Urethral Valve Surgery

Michael E. Mitchell, M.D.

The potential for complications to occur in the management of young boys with urethral valves is great. This is true not only because posterior urethral valves represent a broad spectrum of pathology and can present with deceptively subtle symptoms, but also because early high-grade urethral obstruction can engender changes throughout the entire urinary tract. Treatment of the patient with urethral valves, therefore, must be directed at the total urinary tract. This perspective represents the major concept of this chapter.

URETHRAL VALVE CLASSIFICATIONS, EMBRYOLOGY, AND PHYSIOLOGY

The classification of posterior urethral valves of Young et al.[1] in 1919 is still generally accepted today. Type I valves are membranous folds that sweep off the urethral crest (crista urethralis) laterally and fuse anteriorly. These type I valves are the most common and, according to Stephens,[2] represent the failure of a membranous extension of the distal wolffian duct to completely resorb. There is the abnormality not only of complete resolution but also possibly of the location of the duct on the cloaca. Both problems could explain the variable spectrum of clinical presentation; there is possible variation in the degree of obstruction and the timing of the obstruction in the developing fetus. Young[3] has proposed an alternative hypothesis which would make valves a müllerian derivation, possibly analgous to the hymen (urethrovaginal folds). If true, urethral obstruction from valves would be possible in the female only if there were severe masculinization of the urethra, as in a urogenital sinus case. Clearly, variation in degree of obstruction is easily accepted as the explanation of the etiology of the spectrum of clinical presentation, but certainly debate exists as to when a valve is not a valve but just a "normal fold."

Timing of the obstruction has recently become of great interest because fetal ultrasonography has been able to define renal hydronephrosis before 20 weeks of gestation. Experimental studies by Harrison and colleagues[4] in the lamb have shown that early second-trimester ureteral obstruction leads to renal dysplasia, as is often observed in severe valve cases. Certainly the mesonephric duct regression would fit with such early timing. What is quite unclear to many authors is why early urethral obstruction in animal models leads only to a patent urachus and no upper tract dysplasia.[5] The association of time of obstruction with the development of renal dysplasia vs. hydronephrosis is still uncertain but of major significance with respect to the potential for renal salvage by in utero decompression. (Complications associated with in utero manipulation are covered in Chap. 27, Complications of Antenatal Intervention, and in utero management will not be discussed further here.)

Type III valves have a similar clinical picture to type I valves but possibly represent a completely different embryologic etiology.[2] These valves are noted as a diaphragm or membrane in the mid- or distal prostatic urethra *not* originating from the urethral crista. This membrane possibly represents the failure of canalization of the urogenital membrane perhaps at roughly the same time as that of the development of type I valves. Because of the similar clinical nature of these valves, they will be considered together; rare differences will be noted in the discussion. Type II valves are folds that sweep proximally from the verumontanum toward the bladder neck. Most urologists believe these are not obstructing and are of historical interest only; they will not be given further consideration herein.

Urethral valves are the most common cause of significant urethral obstruction in young boys. As noted by Hendren,[6] they can present a spectrum of pathology that extends from the acutely ill newborn with renal failure and pulmonary hypoplasia to a young boy with polydipsia, polyuria, and progressive hydronephrosis and renal failure to a healthy teenage boy with enuresis and normal upper tracts.

In the developing human fetus, early obstruction (first trimester or early second trimester) of the urethra can lead to altered renal function, ureteral dilatation, and bladder hypertrophy. All these changes can have major impact on the ultimate function of the urinary tract. In fact, the broad clinical spectrum that is seen in patients with valves reflects, in part, the variable reversibility of these fetal changes. Dramatic improvement in renal function can be noted after relief of obstruction, particularly in the first year of life. However, the amount of dysplasia cannot be altered. Furthermore, altered tubular functions (most commonly a concentrating defect or tubular acidosis) may not improve with time. The ureter, even though "decompressed," may remain dilated because of intrinsic changes (fibrosis) in the wall. The ureterovesical junction can be persistently incompetent, since approximately half of the valve patients reflux as newborns,[7, 8] but half of these correct with valve ablation. Obstruction, as well, can persist at the ureterovesical junction. This is presumably related to bladder wall thickness and fibrosis of the distal ureter. The bladder wall may remain thickened and hypertrophied, resulting in poor bladder compliance, even though all bladder outflow resistance is removed. Failure by the treating physician to appreciate such changes will lead to erroneous procedures and, consequently, complications. A good example of such erroneous procedures is nicely illustrated by the previously intense effort at treating bladder neck obstruction in valve patients, which is now thought to be no longer necessary.[9] It was thought that the persistent upper tract dilatation after valve ablation reflected persistent outflow obstruction—this idea no longer seems to be valid. Another example is reported by Hendren,[8] who describes a young boy referred for obstruction of a solitary left kidney. The child had been treated at age 1 month with transurethral resection of the valves, but because of anuria, the child had a left ureterostomy performed in spite of gross reflux on that side (the right kidney was always nonfunctional and later removed). A reimplant and takedown of the ureterostomy resulted in obstruction and, ultimately, loss of the entire distal left ureter. Reconstruction was made extremely difficult, and several procedures were performed which would have been unnecessary if only the postobstructive diuresis and resultant anuria had been recognized and treated with hydration rather than diversion. Finally, in the subsequent section on the valve bladder syndrome, we will show a number of boys who, even with documented absent outflow obstruction, demonstrate a progressive hydronephrosis and decreased renal function. This syndrome represents a summation of all the possible persistent defects in the urinary tract, including poor renal tubular concentration plus poor ureteral function plus poor bladder compliance and function. If unrecognized, it can lead to multiple procedures and complications and frustrations.

COMPLICATIONS OF THE SURGICAL APPROACH TO URETHRAL VALVES

Newborn

Diagnosis.—About half of the patients with valves are diagnosed when they are newborns with an abdominal mass, anuria, failure to void, or pulmonary hypoplasia.[7, 8] With frequent use of fetal ultrasound, prenatal diagnosis is increasingly possible, permitting early diagnosis and treatment in patients with minimal or no physical findings. Voiding pattern and stream quality are usually poor indications of a problem and, in my experience, have often led to a false sense of security rather than the diagnosis of significant obstruction.

Acute Management.—The acute management of the patient with severe urethral valves must first be directed toward pulmonary, fluid, and electrolyte management. The urinary tract usually can and should be decompressed with an 8F pediatric feeding tube in the urethra. Problems with passing a catheter usually relate to the hypertrophy of the bladder neck and the dilated prostatic urethra. We usually pass the catheter under fluoroscopy when possible or at least obtain a cystogram to make sure the catheter is in the bladder. A Foley catheter is rarely acceptable (its lumen is too small), and an 8 F Foley catheter is usually more difficult to pass than a pediatric feeding tube. Pigtail catheters can work well as long as they are placed properly. If a urethral catheter cannot be passed, then a suprapubic tube can be placed. The urethral catheter that drains intermittently is in the prostatic urethra until proved otherwise.

Surgical Technique.—Catheter drainage is usually necessary or feasible for up to 2 weeks. After the infant is stable, the valves are fulgurated by a transurethral procedure. Surgery is *not* contemplated until renal ultrasound, renal scan (with the bladder open to drainage), and voiding studies have been performed to define anatomy and renal function. We use the technique described by Hendren[8] for the destruction of valves, with the following modifications. Cystoscopy is first performed with the 8 F Storz infant cystoscope. With confirmation of the diagnosis and anatomy, an 8 F Wolf cystoscope that has a 3 F operating channel is then inserted. A 3 F Storz Bugbee electrode is then used to destroy the valve leaflets at 12 o'clock, 5 o'clock, and 7 o'clock. As noted by Hendren, short bursts with cutting current are used to poke the electrode through the valve leaflet; then the electrode and scope are advanced under vision to tear the leaflet. This method avoids sphincter injury and excessive thermal injury to the urethra. I believe this is one reason why we have not had a stricture formation in any patient treated as a newborn with this technique. The catheter is removed at the time of valve ablation.

If the patient voids and has stable or improved renal function we will persist in following such patients, even in the face of severe hydronephrosis and/or reflux. If the patient does well clinically (no infection, good appetite, acceptable weight gain), and renal function improves, we will follow the patient with alternate renal isotope scans and ultrasound. (Intravenous pyelography is useful only in those patients with enough renal function to concentrate the contrast; this still is a gold standard for renal morphology.) The patients that do not follow this course must be evaluated and are usually candidates for surgical intervention.

There are basically two groups that do not do well: (1) the massive refluxers and (2) the patients with apparent ureterovesical obstruction.

Newborns With Reflux.—The patients with massive reflux have such inefficient voiding (double and triple voiding is obviously an impossibility in this age group) that they are effectively in retention and are potential candidates for primary reconstruction as advocated by Hendren.[10, 11] These patients do well with initial catheter drainage but have infection and persistent abdominal distention after fulguration of valve tissue. They represent *very* selected cases. Operative reconstruction should be selected only by a surgeon who feels confident with such surgery. It must not be forgotten that the bladder and ureters of these patients are not necessarily normal. Reimplants should be stented and the stents left in place 10 days to 2 weeks. Follow-up should be meticulous. Perhaps an equally effective approach would be that of Duckett,[12, 13] who decompresses the bladder temporarily with a vesicostomy in those cases that do not do well after fulguration. This treatment would provide time for the ureters to decrease in caliber and the bladder wall to become less hypertrophic.

Newborns With Ureterovesical Obstruction.—The real problem infant is one that does not decompress his upper tracts with catheter drainage. Fulguration alone serves only to decompress distal to the apparent site of obstruction which is usually at the ureterovesical junction. I have treated only three such cases in the past 6 years. Two died of pulmonary hypoplasia and had severe renal dysplasia at autopsy. The initial decompression in such cases should be by percutaneous nephrostomy. Such tubes provide temporary decompression and a mechanism to determine lateralized renal function and access for antegrade perfusion studies.[14] Ureterostomy or pyelostomy diversion is *rarely* necessary but may be reserved for such cases.[15] It must be remembered that with such maneuvers the patient is committed to at least two (or more) operations, the second being perhaps more difficult than primary reconstruction. In patients in whom diversion is anticipated, fulguration of the valves should be postponed until reconstruction. I have seen a number of patients simultaneously diverted and fulgurated who had subsequent development of strictures. Dry ablation of valves should be avoided, since it leads to stricture formation.

Complications of Neonatal Valve Surgery.—Complications from the neonatal treatment of valves are observed. Incomplete ablation may be as frequent as 20% to 30% of cases.[7] Cases with persistent hydronephrosis should have repeat voiding studies and cystoscopy. Stricture formation is uncommon with the technique described above. Furthermore, with the newer pediatric and infant fiberoptic instruments, sphincter injury should not be a problem. There is currently no indication for an open procedure for valve resection. If one feels uncomfortable with a newborn transurethral procedure, then one should refer the patient to a center where the instrumentation and expertise are available or, if this is not possible, consider a temporary vesicostomy.

Upper tract diversion should be reserved only for those rare cases of obstruction unresponsive to lower tract drainage in which the surgeon thinks it unwise to reconstruct the urinary tract primarily. Such patients are uncommon and represent the very difficult end of the valve spectrum. Diversion, when considered, must be done as high as possible, with high ureterostomy or pyelostomy, in order to facilitate proper drainage and undiversion.[8, 15] Urinary tract refunctionalization is quite easy in the patient with vesicostomy, because surgery to correct the offending defect is rarely affected by the takedown of the vesicostomy. This is not true with ureterostomies, which either require operation at both ends of the ureter or staged procedures for refunctionalization. Furthermore, the presence of ureterostomies should not lull the surgeon into a false sense of security. This form of diversion is subject to developing obstruction, is prone to chronic infection, and should be considered a temporary measure of some significant cost.

Valves in the Older Child

Perhaps as many as 50% of the valve cases treated are not diagnosed in the newborn period.[7, 12] The management of urethral valves in the older child may have unique challenges relating to toilet training and to patients previously diverted. Three general groupings will be discussed: (1) patients with severe valves but no previous diagnosis, (2) patients with mild to moderate valves, (3) patients previously diverted because of urethral valves.

Severe Valves Previously Missed

Severe obstructive uropathy caused by urethral valves can escape detection in the newborn period; these patients present at an older age with significant reduction in renal function. Most pediatric urologists are able to recall one or two boys who were "well" and "didn't have any trouble voiding at all!" but who nonetheless were tragically first diagnosed as valve patients because of renal failure. Patients with severe hydronephrosis can sometimes present with subtle symptoms. Although one does not wish to overreact, it is my approach to obtain at least a renal ultrasound study on any boy with daytime and nighttime enuresis (even at age 4–5 years). Included in this group of patients are boys with delayed training, first urinary infection (until puberty), and persistent frequency and urgency, and any patient with polydipsia and polyuria who is not spilling sugar.

Case 1.—Male infant, aged 17 months, was first evaluated shortly after birth because of mild renal failure. He was noted to "wet his diapers regularly" and to "have a good stream." No masses were detected and renal ultrasound was consistent with a small left kidney and poorly visualized right kidney. The renal scan was consistent with poor bilateral function. The voiding study was limited because an attempt at catheterization with a pediatric feeding tube failed, and a suprapubic needle study demonstrated a "small, thick-walled" bladder with extravasation of contrast (Fig 34–1,A). The creatinine stabilized at 2.0 mg/dL and blood urea nitrogen (BUN) at 40 to 50 mg/dL. The child was maintained on Shohl's solution and, aside from two urinary tract infections, seemed to do well over the next year, although the child was thought to be mentally retarded and "a failure-to-thrive patient." At age 17 months he was readmitted with apparent urinary failure and sepsis (BUN of 106 mg/dL, creatinine of 1.8 mg/dL and CO_2 of 15 mg/dL).

The child was treated with aminoglycosides, and the urology service was consulted because of the infection. All studies were repeated. A 24-hour delayed pyelogram demonstrated hydronephrosis on the right (Fig 34–1,B), and a repeat voiding

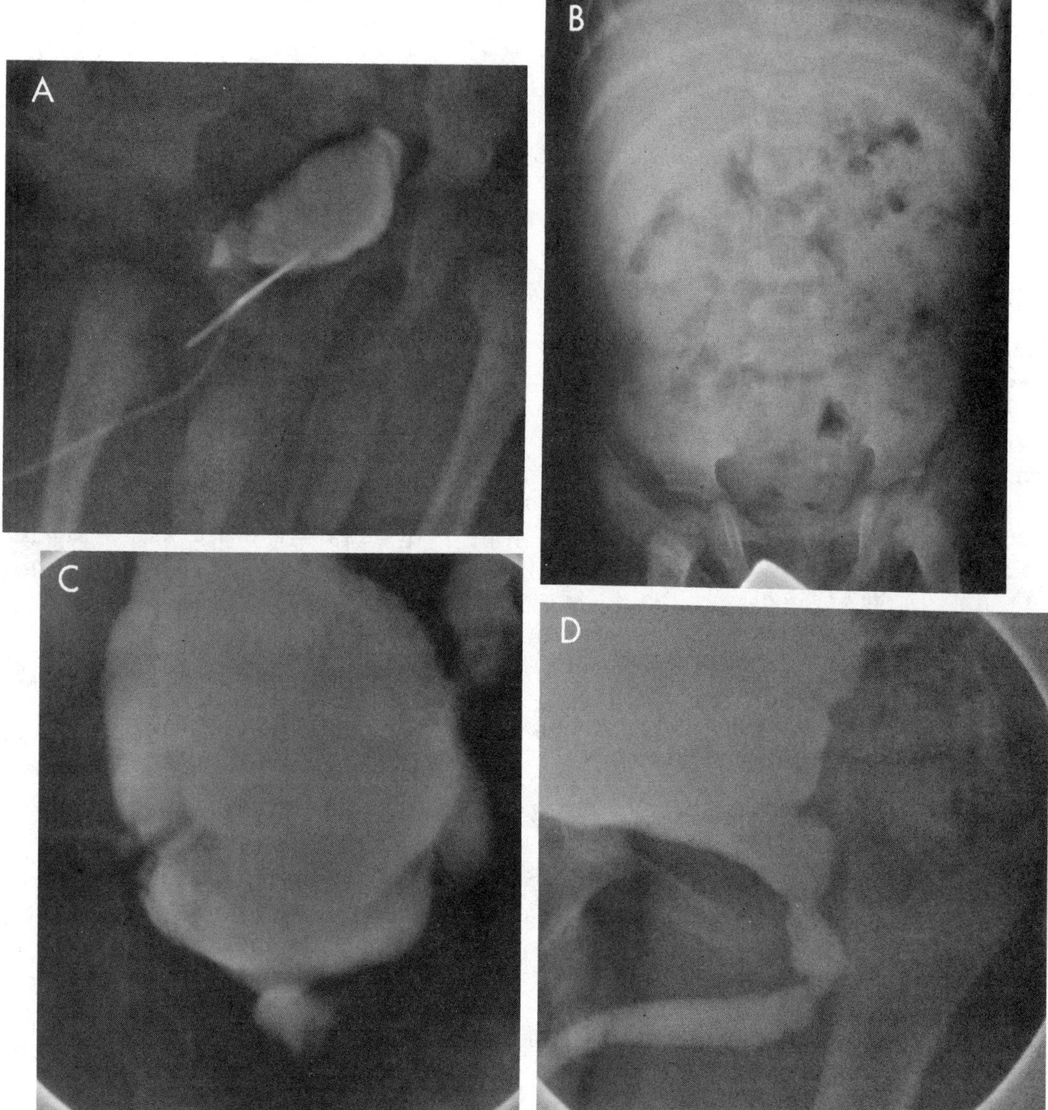

FIG 34–1.
Case 1. **A,** attempted voiding study using suprapubic approach. **B,** intravenous pyelogram, 24-hour film. **C,** repeated voiding study demonstrates a trabeculated bladder and valves (type III). **D,** voiding study after fulguration of urethral valves.

study through a percutaneous suprapubic tube (a catheter could not be passed) demonstrated high-grade bilateral reflux and urethral valves. At cystoscopy, (Fig 34–1,C) large, type III urethral valves were observed, which were fulgurated (Fig 34–1,D). Subsequently, persistent, large, postvoid residuals were noted, and it was believed that voiding efficiency would be improved by correcting the reflux. After treatment of the urinary infection, therefore, the patient underwent an extensive reconstruction (Fig 34–2), which included removal of the nonfunctioning dysplastic left kid-

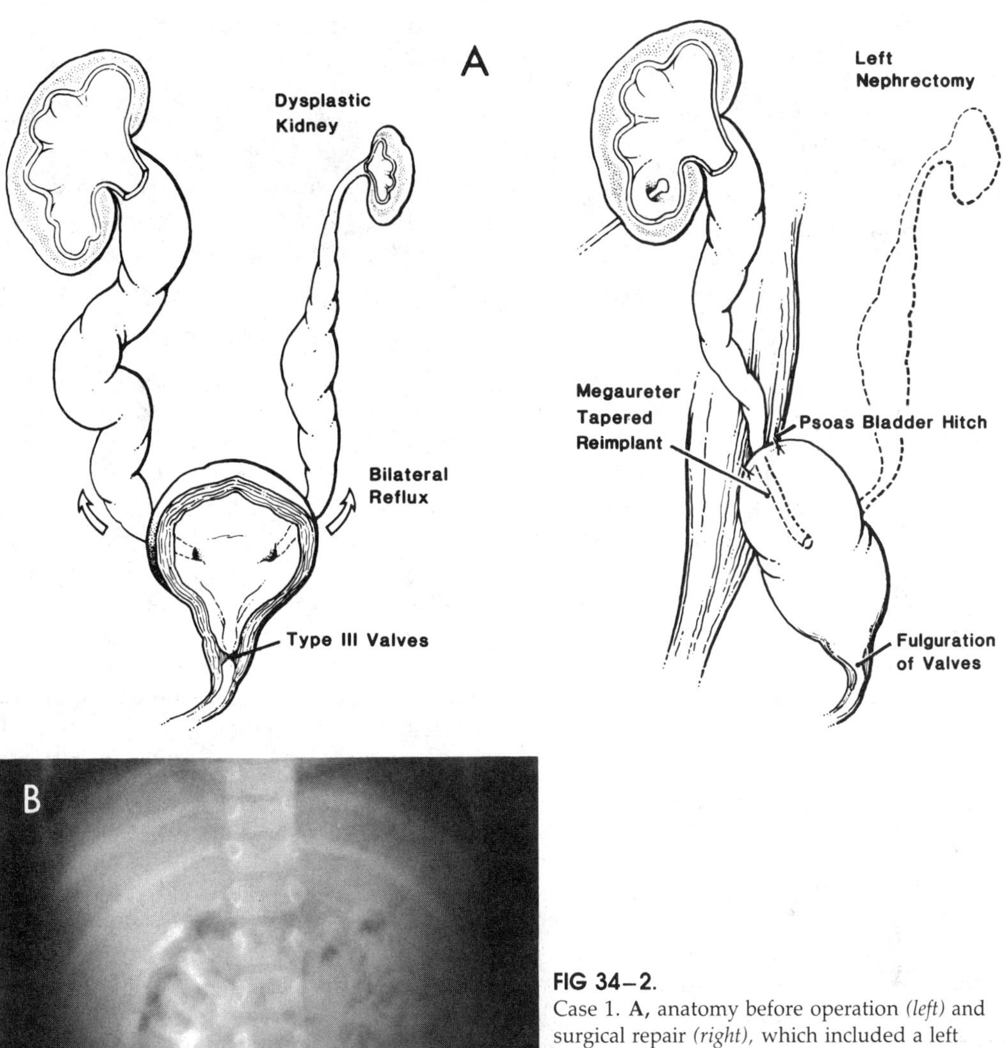

FIG 34–2.
Case 1. **A,** anatomy before operation *(left)* and surgical repair *(right),* which included a left nephroureterectomy, right megaureter taper and reimplant, and fulguration of valves. **B,** intravenous pyelogram after reconstruction and nephrostomy drainage prior to removal of nephrostomy tube.

ney and ureter, partial distal excision (15 cm) of the right ureter, ureteral tapering, and reimplant with psoas bladder hitch. Because of the significant renal failure and questionable nature of the bladder, a nephrostomy tube was left in place for an extended period (3 months). In the 5 years since surgery, renal function has remained stable (creatinine clearance:

55 mL/min/1.73 m^2). The patient requires Shohl's solution for renal tubular acidosis and has been very slow to toilet-train because of nephrogenic diabetes insipidus. His daily urine output is stable at 3 to 4 L/24 hr. The child still has nocturnal enuresis but is dry during the day with frequent voiding. Bladder function on anticholinergics has been acceptable in the face of high-volume urine production.

Comments.—The diagnosis of urethral valves was tragically missed in the newborn period in spite of extensive testing. Difficulty with urethral catheterization and infection should have alerted the physicians to pursue a diagnosis other than bilateral dysplasia. As mentioned previously, type I valves present difficulties with catheterization because of hypertrophy of the bladder neck. Type III valves can present difficulties with passing a catheter through the membrane. This patient did well after reconstruction until toilet training was initiated. Because of the frequent poor bladder compliance and high urine output in these patients, toilet training represents a period of major problems. This is true not only because of the obligate frequency of voiding and accidents but also because of the potential risks to the upper tracts. (These complications will be covered in the section, Valve Bladder Syndrome.) What has proved to be most frustrating to me in dealing with such patients is the inevitable human aspects of the situation: Little boys who make a large volume of urine and who are cajoled to void frequently either don't and dribble, or void infrequently and have accidents, or void frequently but *do not empty*. They are capable of complete voiding but simply do not take the time or effort. Anticholinergics (oxybutynin chloride [Ditropan], propantheline bromide [Pro-Banthine]), although being the ideal medication, may serve to make the situation worse. It takes an *extreme* effort on the part of the parent and physician to achieve dryness and protect the upper tracts in these patients. These complications of toilet training probably explain why diversion was such a popular method of handling these patients in the past, but nonetheless I am convinced, that diversion creates more problems than it solves.

Mild Valves

Boys with mild valves usually do not represent a major problem for the physician. By definition, significant upper tract changes are not found, presumably because the urethral obstruction is partial. Difficulties in management center around voiding dysfunction, such as daytime and nighttime wetting. Fulguration of the valve leaflets in these patients usually resolves the symptoms, but such patients sometimes require anticholinergic medication as well. Prostatitis and epididymitis in young boys may indicate mild valves. It is this group that has been the object of some debate as to when the "normal urethral folds" become physiologically significant enough to be called valves. Some of these patients will exhibit some "old" changes of the upper tracts, which seems to suggest that the nature of valve obstruction diminishes with growth. It is almost as if the valve leaflets remain fixed, so that with urethral growth the relative obstruction decreases.

Previously Diverted Patients With Valves

The previously diverted patient with valves presents all the problems of a nondiverted valve patient plus those of reconstruction and undiversion. The scope of this chapter does not permit the enumeration of potential problems in undiversion (see Chap. 18, Complications of Urinary Diversion), but a few of the particular problems as related to valves will be demonstrated in Case 2. Undiversion is predicated on the effective relief of bladder outflow obstruction. One must diligently prove the effective ablation of the urethral valves and make sure the urethra is without stricture and functional.

Case 2.—Man, aged 24 years, presented with a solitary hydronephrotic kidney drained by end-cutaneous ureterostomy. He was diverted at a young age for "either urethral valves or neurogenic bladder dysfunction." Because of stomal and appliance problems he was reevaluated and considered for undiversion. Our evaluation disclosed an intelligent, well-motivated young man with a massively hydronephrotic right kidney which drained through an end-cutaneous ureterostomy, which periodically became obstructed. The bladder drained through a vesicostomy. Bladder cycling did not result in a significant increase in bladder volume (50–75 cc). The patient did not leak but was unable to void. Although his serum creatinine was 1.3 mg/dL and his clearance 64 mL/min, he had poor ability to concentrate urine and his urine output averaged 3.5 to 6 L/24 hr. The undiversion procedure in the patient was based on this high urine output (Fig 34–3). At cystoscopy, tightly adherent type I valves were fulgurated. The left ureteral segment was reimplanted, and a right-to-left transureteroureterostomy constructed. The bladder was enlarged with a cecal cap. He tolerated the procedure well and is now 5 years post-

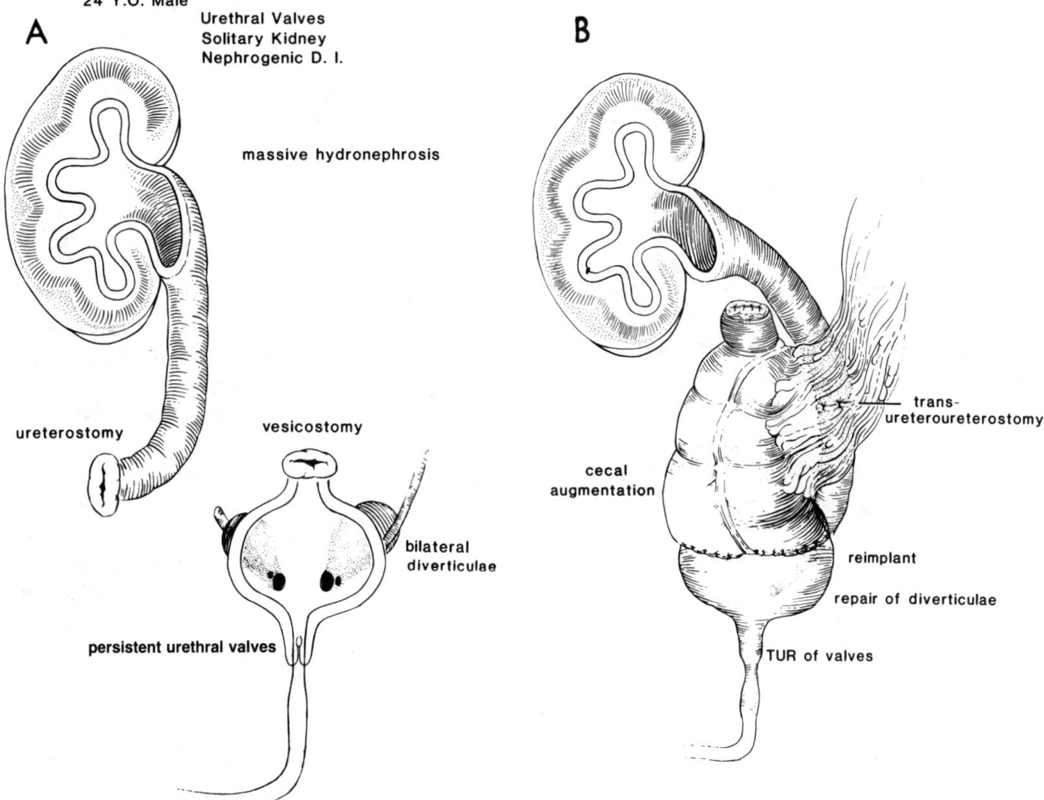

FIG 34–3.
Case 2. **A,** anatomy before surgery included a single hydronephrotic kidney with severe concentrating defect. Persistent urethral valves were present. The bladder was small with cellules and diverticula. **B,** reconstructed urinary tract with a cecal augmentation.

undiversion. Renal function has remained stable, and he voids to completion, is dry, and feels well.

Comment.—This patient demonstrated not only persistent valves but also a severe defect in tubular function with high urine output. Undiversion was successful only because the bladder outflow was relieved, and the bladder capacity (postoperatively, 650 cc) was increased appropriately. Undiversion without adjustment for this high urine output would have been a disaster.

Valve Bladder Syndrome

The components of this problem have been mentioned previously in this chapter. Although this section deals with the most difficult valve patients, many boys with valves may have one or all of the components of this syndrome. Several years ago,[16] we reviewed our severe valve cases (53) and found this problem to be present in six (11%). These six patients all demonstrated persistent or progressive hydroureteronephrosis in the face of no proven outflow problems, gradual loss of renal function, polydipsia and polyuria, and urinary frequency. They also usually had nocturnal enuresis and a tendency to constipation. The mechanism of these problems is felt to be dependent on three problems: (1) severe renal tubular dysfunction, resulting in high urine output and often acidosis; (2) ureteral dysfunction related to massively dilated ureters that either no longer move in peristalsis or fail to have effective peristalsis because of dilatation; and (3) bladder dysfunction that relates to poor bladder compliance and a learned insensitivity to increased intravesical pressure.

Case 3.—Boy, aged 3 years, was diagnosed as having urethral valves and bilateral hydronephrosis when he was evaluated for a urinary tract infection (Fig 34–4,A). He underwent a transurethral resection of valves. Because there was no subsequent resolution of the hydronephrosis, bilateral loop cutaneous ureterostomies were performed at age 3½ years. A repeat cystoscopy demonstrated minimal residual valve tissue, which was resected. At age 4, the patient's ureterostomies were taken down, and at age 5, bilateral ureteroneocystostostomies were performed with tapering of the distal ureters.

He did not do well, and at age 6, because of increasing hydroureteronephrosis shown by intravenous pyelography and an increase in serum creatinine from 0.6 mg/dL to 1.2 mg/dL, bilateral nephrostomies were placed. At age 7, because of resolution of the hydronephrosis and because antegrade perfusion (nephrostogram) studies demonstrated no obstruction of flow into the bladder (bladder catheter open), the nephrostomies were removed.

At age 8, hydronephrosis was massive, and repeat antegrade perfusion (Whittaker flow) was thought to be consistent with obstruction of the distal right ureter. Vesicoureteral reflux to the kidney was noted on the left. The creatinine clearance had dropped from 38 mL/min/1.73 m^2 to 19mL/min/1.73 m^2. A left ureteral reimplant and right-to-left transureteroureterostomy were performed. At age 8½, the patient noted little clinical improvement. He was still wetting day and night and voided every 20 to 30 minutes. Persistent bilateral massive hydronephrosis was noted on pyelography (Fig 34–4,B). Cystometry showed a small, contracted, poorly compliant bladder. Repeat antegrade study demonstrated no obstruction to flow into the bladder with the bladder empty. As the bladder filled, the perfusion pressure reflected the rapidly increasing intravesical pressure. A suprapubic tube was left in the bladder, with minimal resolution of hydronephrosis.

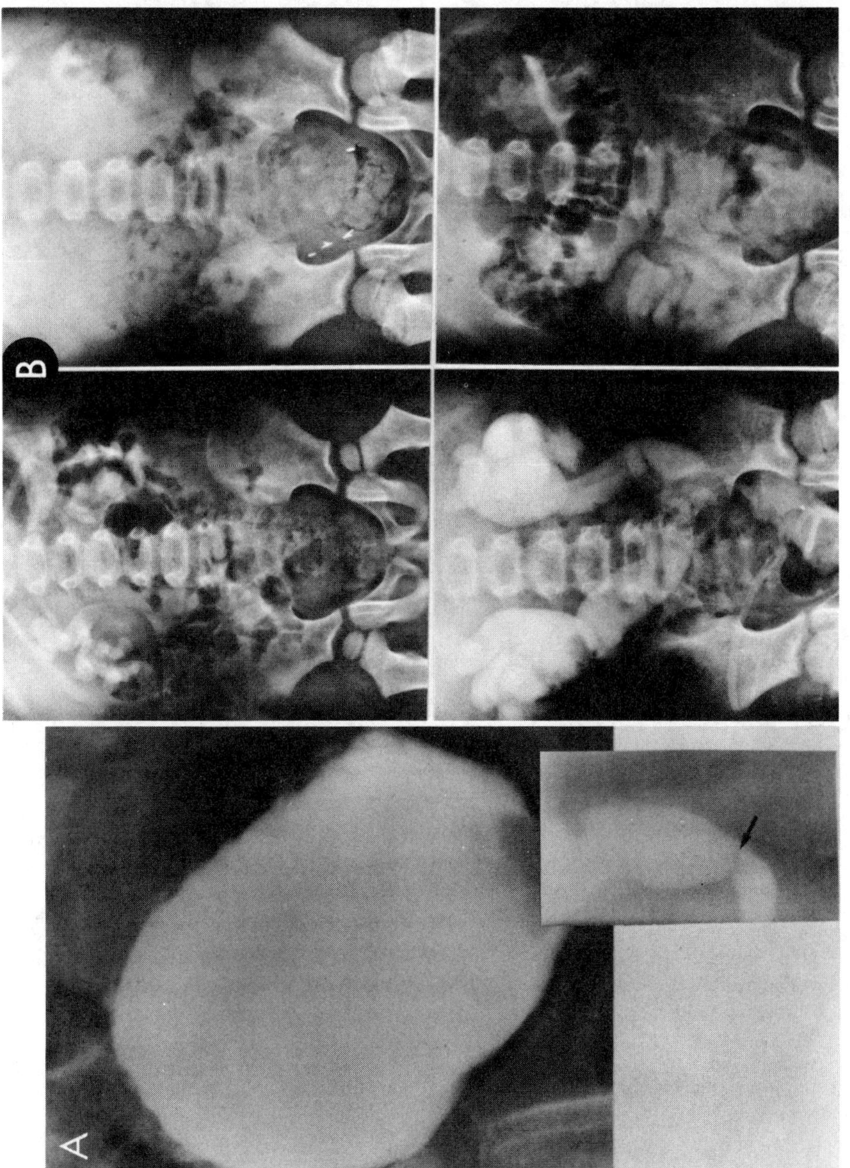

FIG 34–4.
Case 3. **A,** voiding urethrogram at time of initial diagnosis. *Arrow* in inset demonstrates type I valves. **B,** serial intravenous pyelogram studies demonstrate some improved renal function during diversion *(upper left)* but progressive loss after undiversion *(upper right)*. After reconstruction, function improved with suprapubic tube drainage *(lower left)*. Function stabilized after augmentation *(lower right)*.

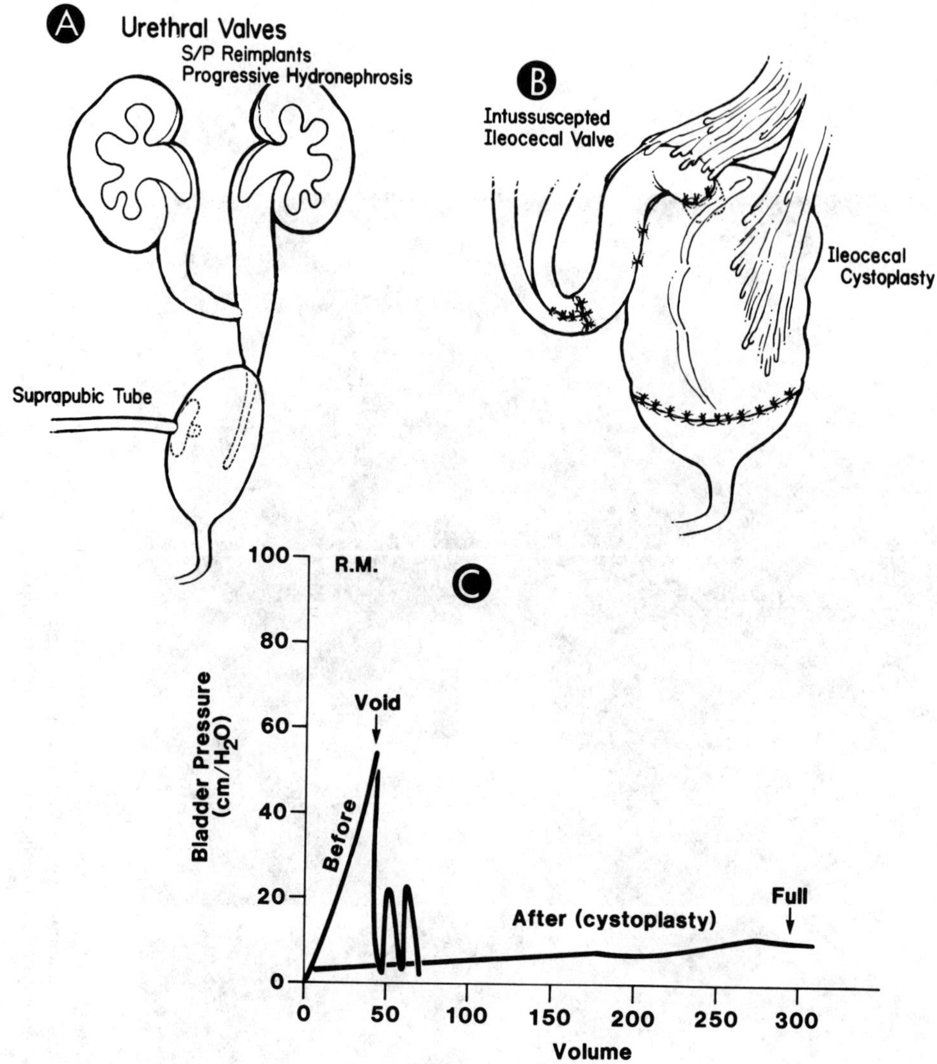

FIG 34–5.
A, anatomy after reconstruction; patient (9-year-old boy) is wet and has progressive hydronephrosis without suprapubic drainage. **B,** augmentation provides volume and compliance and daytime continence. **C,** urodynamics demonstrate a small, poorly compliant bladder, which changes with augmentation cystoplasty.

At age 9, an ileocecal cystoplasty was performed in which the ureters were anastomosed end-to-end with the terminal ileum and the intussuscepted ileocecal valve served to prevent reflux (Fig 34–5). At age 9½, he was treated for acute myelogenous leukemia during which he remained free of infection. He voided every 2 to 3 hours, although the specific gravities of his urine were persistently 1.010. The urine output was invariably 50 to 80 mL/hr in spite of fluid restriction. For almost 3 years, renal function was stable at 25 mL/min/1.73 m^2, and he was dry during the day but wet at night. Ultimately, however, after a bone marrow transplant he succumbed to a graft-vs.-host reaction.

Comment.—This tragic case represents all the components of the valve bladder problem.

Components of the Urethral Valve Syndrome

Renal.—The obligate high output of these patients can present a major problem, but most significantly it must be recognized before undiversion and preferably before toilet training. These patients cannot concentrate urine, even when fluid is restricted. This, in fact, makes postoperative management difficult, because urine output can have no relation to state of hydration. If one waits for urine output to drop off, one may have a seriously dehydrated patient. These patients will not respond to antidiuretic hormone (ADH) and will not respond to saline depletion (thiazide therapy). Often patients with severe concentrating defects will have renal tubular acidosis, but this is not absolute. Creatinine clearance may be depressed, but serum creatinine may be normal and not reflect the severe tubular deficit.

Ureter.—As in the case example, the ureters of these patients can be severely dilated and scarred (either from infection, surgery, or chronic distention). Unless I see active peristalsis with fluroscopy, I assume the ureters are incapable of acting as anything but a pipe. Flow must be, therefore, *down* a pressure gradient. High intravesical pressure or high tunnel resistance can lead to progressive renal damage.

Bladder.—It is well known that the bladder of the valve patient is thick-walled and hypertrophied with cellules and diverticula. Physiologically, these bladders sometimes behave worse than they look. The major problem is with compliance. That is, with filling, the bladder distends with increasing pressure. It is not so much the size but the pressures generated that is the important factor. Furthermore, these patients learn to *tolerate* very *high* intravesical pressure so that they can hold more and void less frequently. Is is interesting (Fig 34–6) to observe the pain threshold change with treatment. For example, whereas a patient may be able to tolerate 50 cm H_2O intravesical pressure without pain before treatment, with therapy bladder discomfort may be noted at an intravesical pressure

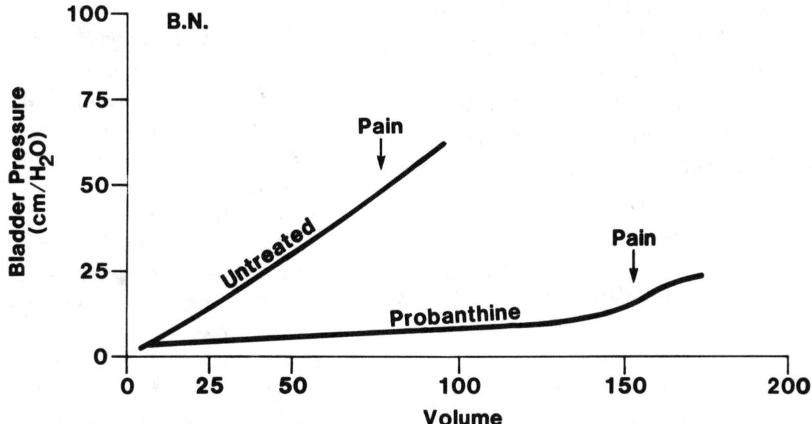

FIG 34–6.
Cystometrogram on patient with urethral valves and valve bladder. Before treatment with anticholinergics, patient had poor bladder compliance and felt pain only at high intravesical pressure. After treatment, however, improved compliance was noted and pain was noted at significantly lower intravesical pressures.

of 5 to 10 cm H_2O. This is a good sign therapy is working.

Treatment

Management of a patient with all or some of the components of this syndrome is necessarily dependent first on the recognition of the problem. Unfortunately, little can be done with the renal component short of making sure that the storage capacity of the lower urinary tract is adequate to handle the volume created. Furthermore, if acidosis is noted, augmentation of the urinary tract with bowel will increase absorption and make acidosis worse. This problem can be treated with oral sodium bicarbonate. If ureteral peristalsis is present, then ureteral tapering may be very effective in restoring a "ureteral pump." A fixed, scarred ureter should not be extensively tapered, since obstruction may result. The mechanism would be similar to that noted in the adynamic segment of a megaureter. The bladder component seems to be most amenable to therapy. With anticholinergic therapy (oxybutynin or propantheline), significant improvement in bladder compliance occurs in most cases. Furthermore, as mentioned previously, painful sensation on filling is noted at lower pressures. Some patients are exquisitely sensitive to anticholinergic medication, possibly because they become used to voiding with high intravesical pressure. Such patients initially will have a marked inability to empty and must be watched carefully. Prior to toilet training many of these patients will be quite stable. With the development of urinary continence, problems may develop, because the patients are working against a high-volume poorly compliant system.

Therefore, during toilet training, urodynamic assessment and anticholinergic therapy must begin. Those patients who do not respond to medication may be candidates for bladder augmentation. In such cases, I presume the patient will require intermittent clean catheterization to empty the bladder.

Boys with urethral valves present a spectrum of disease resulting in a wide variety of challenges and potential for complications. Unlike other forms of bladder outflow obstruction in older patients, such as from stricture or prostatic enlargement, where correction of the obstruction results in cure, congenital urethral valves present unique problems which relate to dysfunction throughout the urinary tract. Success in treatment often relates to the correct recognition and management of these problems.

EDITORIAL COMMENT

Dr. Mitchell appropriately emphasizes the clinical spectrum of posterior urethral valve patients. The newborn can present with severe hydronephrosis or an older child can present with mild enuresis. We have seen three adults present with posterior urethral valves, including one patient with symptoms similar to prostatitis.* Two other patients were renal transplant candidates because their posterior urethral valves were never recognized. One patient had normal bladder function following destruction of the urethral valves in spite of having a urinary diversion for over 20 years.

The understanding of all of the abnormalities in the urinary tract are essential in the total management of posterior urethral valve patients. As Dr. Mitchell indicates, urinary diversion usually creates more long-term problems than it solves. It is important to recognize the valve bladder syndrome, which includes high-output renal failure, poorly functioning, dilated ureters, and high-pressure, noncompliant bladders. If these potential problems are recognized and

*Mueller SC Marshall FF: Spectrum of unrecognized posterior urethral valves in the adult. *Urology* 1983; 22:139.

anticipated, the patient will have a more successful result.

REFERENCES

1. Young HH, Frontz WA, Baldwin JC: Congenital obstruction of the posterior urethra. *J Urol* 1919; 3:289.
2. Stephens FD: *Congenital Intrinsic Lesions of the Posterior Urethra in Congenital Malformations of the Urinary Tract.* New York, Praeger Publishers, 1983.
3. Young BW: *Lower Urinary Tract Obstruction in Childhood.* Philadelphia, Lea & Febiger, 1972.
4. Glick PL, Harrison MR, Adzick SN, et al: Correction of congenital hydronephrosis in utero IV: In utero decompression prevents renal dysplasia. *J Pediatr Surg* 1984; 19:649–657.
5. Tanagho EA: Persistent ureteral dilatation following valve resection. *Dialogues Pediatr Urol* 1982; 5:4.
6. Hendren WH: Posterior urethral valves in boys, a broad clinical spectrum. *J Urol* 1971; 106:298–307.
7. Cass AS, Stephens FD: Posterior urethral valves; diagnosis and management. *J Urol* 1974; 112:519.
8. Hendren WH: Complications of urethral valve surgery, in Smith RB, Skinner DG (eds): *Complications of Urologic Surgery.* Philadelphia, WB Saunders Co, 1976, pp 303–335.
9. Duckett JW: Anomalies of the urethra, in *Campbell's Urology.* Philadelphia, WB Saunders Co, 1978, pp 1635–1662.
10. Hendren WH: A new approach to infants with severe obstructive uropathy. Early complete reconstruction. *J Pediatr Surg* 1970; 5:184.
11. Hendren WH: Posterior urethral valves management. *J Urol* 1973; 110:682.
12. Duckett JW: Current management of posterior urethral valves. *Urol Clin North Am* 1974; 1:471.
13. Duckett JW: Cutaneous vesicostomy in infants and children. *Urol Clin North Am* 1974; 1:484.
14. Whitaker RH: The ureter in posterior urethral valves. *Br J Urol* 1973; 45:395.
15. Johnston JH: Temporary cutaneous ureterostomy in the treatment of advanced congenital urinary obstruction. *Arch Dis Child* 1963; 38:161.
16. Mitchell ME: Valve bladder syndrome. Presented at the North Central Section of the American Urological Association, Hamilton, Bermuda, 1980.

CHAPTER 35

Complications of Hypospadias Surgery

Boyd H. Winslow, M.D.
Bert Vorstman, M.D.
Charles J. Devine, Jr., M.D.

Hypospadias is a congenital disorder in which the urethral meatus opens not at the tip of the glans penis but more proximally, between the ventral glans and the perineum. The etiology of this condition is a failure of closure of the embryonic urethral tube. Hypospadias-like conditions may occur as the result of meatotomy, circumcision accidents, or erosion from a longstanding catheter.

The incidence of hypospadias is approximately 1 in every 300 male births; in the majority of these cases the urethral meatus is found on the distal shaft and there is some degree of distal chordee. The goals of reconstructive surgery for this condition are to produce a penis that is straight when erect, has a urethral opening at the tip of the glans, and is cosmetically appealing. Properly performed, surgery for hypospadias achieves normalization of both form and function. We prefer to carry out genital reconstructive surgery in children within a few months of their second birthday. In this age group we observe little if any detrimental psychologic effect due to hospitalization, especially when we utilize preoperative counseling, parental rooming-in, and modern nursing supportive techniques.

This discussion will focus on the surgical complications of hypospadias repairs and not on the possible medical complications common to all surgical procedures. Female hypospadias will not be covered in this chapter. We will first categorize the surgical complications and then discuss the various preventive measures, including nonsurgical aspects of their treatment.

To achieve the desired repair of hypospadias through reconstructive surgery, thorough preoperative evaluation, precise surgical technique, and appropriate postoperative care are required. All new and reoperative cases warrant a preoperative evaluation to assess any associated anatomical anomalies,[1, 2] either congenital or acquired.

Strict adherence to fundamental principles of meticulous, systematic, delicate tissue-handling techniques is mandatory. Measures to prevent infection and to provide appropriate urinary diversion are also necessary. Reoperative cases and hypospadias "cripples" appear to be at greater risk for postoperative infection. Therefore, secondary repair should be attempted only 6 months or more after any failed surgery to ensure that inflammation and/or infection have resolved, wounds have healed, and the tissues have returned to their normal pliable state.

PREOPERATIVE EVALUATION

Initial evaluation of all patients includes a thorough history, physical examination, observation of the urinary stream during voiding, and microscopic examination of the midstream urine sample. The surgeon must seek details regarding the methods and complications encountered during previous attempts at surgical repair. He must also inquire about symptoms of voiding dysfunction, incontinence, and urinary tract infections and observe the straightness of the erection. The physical examination focuses on the genitalia: the size of the phallus, position and adequacy of the meatus, presence of chordee, skin scarring, urethrocutaneous fistulas, and penoscrotal transposition. We inspect the entire course of the urethra before, during, and after the patient's voiding effort to look for evidence of a diverticulum. Even if a bulge cannot be felt, we suspect a diverticulum when compression of the urethra after voiding produces significant dribbling. We note the caliber and direction of the stream and whether there is any spraying. If the patient strains during voiding, he may be experiencing outflow obstruction. We also note in the physical examination the location of hairless skin. If the child is prepubertal, we look at the father's hair distribution to help us find appropriate donor sites in the patient for skin grafts.

A midstream urine specimen is sent for analysis and culture. If the urine is infected, the patient is started on antibiotics preoperatively.

All of our patients undergo preoperative ultrasonic evaluation of the kidneys and upper urinary tracts. This noninvasive procedure has a high degree of sensitivity and allows us to diagnose any associated renal lesions and/or hydroureteronephrosis.[2]

Patients with undescended testis, partial penoscrotal transposition, severe hypospadias, or utricular abnormalities must be carefully evaluated to define a possible underlying intersex problem.[3] Appropriate investigations would then include a peripheral blood specimen for karyotype, serum follicle-stimulating hormone (FSH), luteinizing hormone (LH), and testosterone, and urinary 17-hydroxycorticosteroids and 17-ketosteroids and then possibly a genital skin biopsy to evaluate 5α-reductase and androgen receptor content. In some patients it is necessary to proceed with laparoscopy and/or exploratory laparotomy and gonadal biopsy or excision before proceeding with hypospadias surgery. Patients with hypospadias and severe microphallus may be better served through gender reassignment.

OPERATIVE TECHNIQUE

Our evaluation and planning continue after the induction of anesthesia. Urethroscopy with an 8 F. pediatric cystoscope is carried out in all of our patients, including hypospadias cripples. We inspect the urethra all the way to the bladder neck, noting the presence of utricular abnormalities, which are more common with severe hypospadias cases. Failure to recognize an enlarged utricle can allow faulty placement of the urethral catheter in the utricle rather than in the bladder.[4] We have also diagnosed coexisting type I urethral valves and congenital bulbourethral strictures in hypospadiac patients, which we have incised at the time of surgery. In order to avoid recurrent stricture formation in the urethra that is thus treated, we recommend that a stent or catheter be kept in place until shortly before normal voiding is resumed.

In reoperative hypospadias cases, urethroscopy is done to exclude coexisting acquired abnormalities of the urethra, such as strictures, diverticula, and folds, which might act as valves during voiding. These lesions can occur distal to fistulas and can promote recurrence of fistulas after repair. The presence of hair-bearing skin in the neourethra may require excision and repeat urethroplasty in order to achieve a successful result without recurrent infections and calculus formation. Unexpected abnormalities necessitate surgical improvisation in some cases.

After the urethroscopy we place a 5-0 silk dorsal glans traction suture to allow penile manipulation and immobilization. Furthermore, traction on the dorsal suture, when combined with digital pressure to the dorsum of the phallus, affords excellent control of bleeding.

We plan our skin incisions carefully before actually cutting.

Appropriate incisions should provide optimum exposure for correction of chordee, urethral reconstruction, and penile skin coverage.[5] The proposed incisions are outlined with a marking pen prior to cutting. These incisions usually take the form of a flip-flap or a circumscribing incision around the urethral meatus with an extension of the incision distally to circumscribe the glans (Fig 35–1). After exposure, chordee is corrected.[6] It is of the utmost importance that urethroplasty not be performed until penile straightness is confirmed with an artificial erection. The artificial erection[7] test is performed repeatedly during the dissection to correct chordee. In order to avoid devastating complications, we check at each artificial erection that physiologic saline only is used for the infiltration. Maneuvers that may be used to achieve a straight phallus have been outlined.[8]

Construction of the neourethra may be achieved by using a flap of penile skin or a full-thickness tube graft from genital or extragenital skin. We do not use split-thickness skin grafts for our urethroplasties, since stricture formation may result if insufficient dermis is taken with the graft. The use of hair-bearing skin—for example, scrotal or perineal skin—is not advised, since it is likely to result in a hairy neourethra that is susceptible to infections and urethral stones. However, the midline of the scrotum can afford a strip of

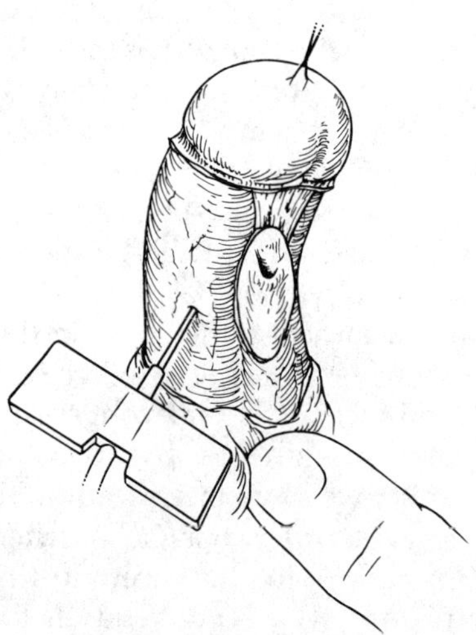

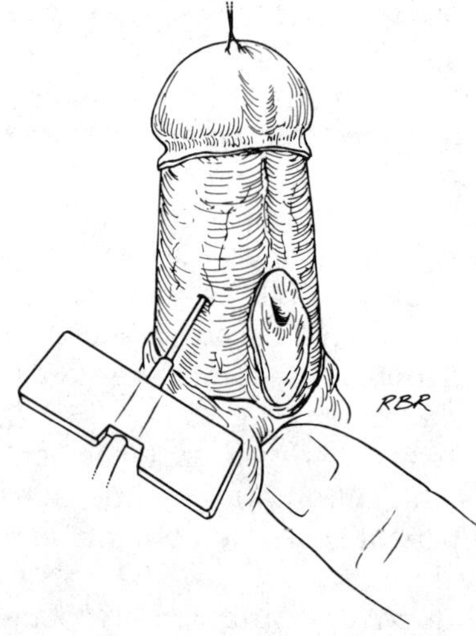

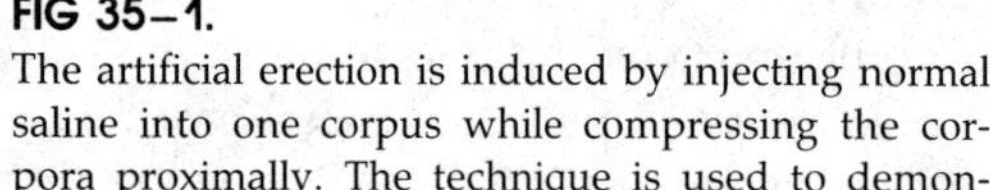

FIG 35–1.
The artificial erection is induced by injecting normal saline into one corpus while compressing the corpora proximally. The technique is used to demonstrate the extent of chordee after exposure of the corpora and also to confirm the straightness of the penis after the various maneuvers to correct chordee.

hairless skin for urethral reconstruction in many cases. Alternatively, hair-bearing skin may be depilated prior to use. It is important to outline the width and length of the flap or graft required to construct the neourethra to the glans tip and to err on the generous side. Spatulated (elliptic) anastomoses of the neourethra to the native urethra allow contraction of the anastomosis over a greater length than does an end-to-end circular anastomosis, thereby reducing the incidence of symptomatic stricture formation. Surgical trauma can be minimized by delicate tissue handling with fine forceps and skin hooks and meticulous pinpoint hemostasis with bipolar cautery.

The viability of flaps must be zealously protected. There must be no tension at suture lines. If there is any question of flap viability, intravenous fluorescein should be used to test the blood flow.[9] The recommended dose of fluorescein is given only after a test dose is used to exclude hypersensitivity reactions. After 5 to 10 minutes of injecting the full dose, the penile skin and flaps are inspected under an ultraviolet lamp. The well-perfused areas fluoresce, while poorly perfused areas have a mottled appearance. The absence of any fluorescence means that the tissue has an inadequate blood supply to survive. Recently, we have utilized the Fluoroscanner (Santa Barbara Technologies) to evaluate flap perfusion during and after surgery in a more objective fashion.

Suturing of the neourethra is accomplished with 6-0 Polydioxanone suture (PDS, Ethicon) or Vicryl sutures (Ethicon) placed in a subcuticular fashion to invert epithelial edges into the lumen. Failure to remove epithelium from the wound edges will result in inclusion cysts and/or promote fistula formation. The use of optical loupes or the operating microscope may enhance surgical technique.[10] The watertightness of the anastomosis can be checked by injecting methylene blue–dyed saline through the meatus. Additional sutures may be required to close any leaks demonstrated after this technique.

The bladder is then filled through a small feeding tube in the urethra, and a 10 F or 12 F percutaneous suprapubic catheter is inserted immediately prior to the urethral reconstruction. A small soft silicone urethral stent (10 F) is placed in the neourethra, extending just proximal to the anastomosis. The urethral stent is secured to the dorsal glans traction suture at the end of the procedure. Those repairs using a flap of penile skin have a feeding tube catheter stent for urinary diversion.

The surgical dressing we usually select is Bioclusive (Ethicon). The Bioclusive is applied *without tension* as a circumferential dressing to the penile shaft including the glans. This dressing serves as a semiocclusive wrap to contain edema and minimize the chance of suture line disruption. A cotton dressing is applied around the outside of the Bioclusive and is soaked with iced saline for the first 48 hours postoperatively to reduce pain and swelling. The cotton is contained within a cylinder of Microfoam tape (Ethicon) until the patient is calm after anesthesia. This cotton dressing is changed every 8 hours or so, using sterile technique.

POSTOPERATIVE CARE

Small children must have their lower limbs restrained as needed postoperatively to prevent turning onto the repair site. The foot of the bed is elevated for the first 48 hours postoperatively, and the patient is kept supine to minimize further genital edema. The reconstructive site is protected by a bed cradle, and the patient remains at bed rest for 3 to 5 days. Pain is controlled with acetaminophen and codeine. Preoperative and postoperative antibiotics are used prophylactically to prevent wound and urinary tract infections.

The Bioclusive dressing is removed on about the sixth day with the help of sitzbaths. Povidone-iodine (Betadine) baths are encouraged once the urethral stent is removed on the fifth postoperative day. For those patients who have undergone a flip-flap urethroplasty, a suprapubic catheter is not inserted and an 8 F feeding tube serves as a catheter and stent. A voiding trial is instituted on the fifth postoperative day for patients who have undergone a flip-flap reconstruction or a fistula repair. For tube grafts or tubed flaps, the voiding trial is performed at 10 to 14 days postoperatively or later, depending on the amount of edema and apparent extent of wound healing.

Gentle meticulous meatal toilet and obturation are an integral part of the postoperative management. The meatal region is cleansed with half-strength peroxide and kept soft with Neosporin ointment (bacitracin zinc-neomycin sulfate-polymyxin B sulfate). The tip of the Neosporin Ophthalmic tube is used for periodic meatal obturation for about 4 weeks after the urethral stent has been removed.

The management of hypospadias cripples embodies all of the techniques delineated above and of course requires improvisation.[5] Although treatment must be individualized, we prefer to correct all problems in a one-stage reconstructive procedure if possible. Failure to correct chordee is a common cause for failed repair in those patients referred to our unit, and we have developed a systematic approach to the surgical treatment of chordee in these hypospadias patients.[8]

EARLY COMPLICATIONS

Hemostasis.—Hemostasis is an important aspect of hypospadias surgery and is best achieved through accurate pinpoint cautery. The semiocclusive dressing, Bioclusive, helps to minimize postoperative bleeding and contain edema. We no longer use subcutaneous infiltration of lidocaine (Xylocaine) with epinephrine, since it appears to result in rebound bleeding postoperatively. Most hematomas will be obvious at the completion of surgery, and optimal treatment is evacuation of the hematoma and reassessment of hemostasis. A Mini-vac drain may be left in the wound at the completion of all hypospadias operations, and certainly one should be left if a wound has been reexplored for bleeding. The Mini-vac drain is constructed by using a 21-gauge scalp vein set, removing the Luer-lock end, cutting holes in the tubing, and inserting the needle end into a vacuum blood tube (Fig 35–2). Failure to treat a hematoma after genital reconstruction may compromise blood flow to skin flaps or inhibit inosculation (ingrowth of vessels) of skin grafts after urethral reconstruction.

Wound Infections.—Wound infections can usually be prevented by administering prophylactic antibiotics, pHisoHex (an emulsion containing hexachlorophene) genital scrubs preoperatively, povidone-iodine skin preparation in the operating room, delicate tissue handling, and excision of any devitalized tissue noted during the procedure. We do not prepare the urethra preoperatively with povidone-iodine or use topical antibiotics. A suspected abscess or infected hematoma is managed by incision and drainage to allow healing by secondary intention. Postoperatively the wound is cleansed with povidone-iodine sitz baths and half-strength peroxide soaks three or four times a day. When infection is suspected, cultures of the wound are taken for organism identification and antibiotic sensitivities. The presence of infection may promote local tissue necrosis, scarring, and formation of fistula and stricture. Purulence emanating from the neourethra during the period of urinary diversion should be treated with irrigations of half-strength peroxide.

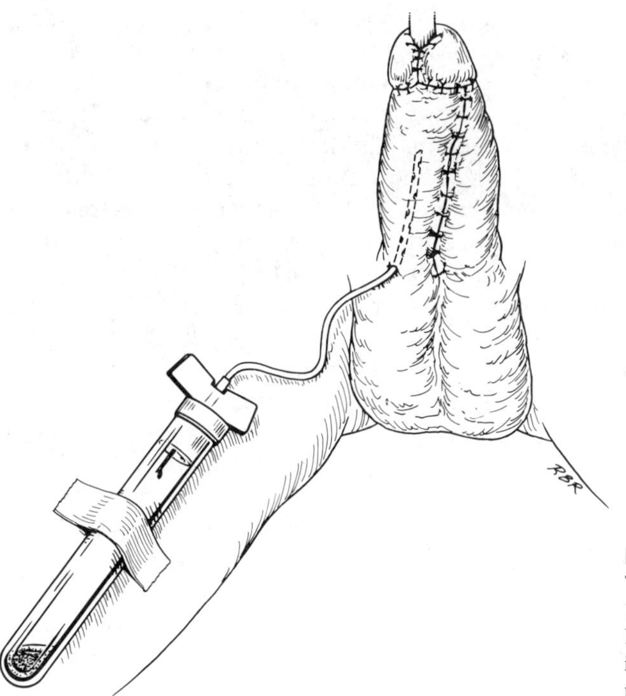

FIG 35–2.
The Mini-vac drain is constructed from a 19-gauge butterfly needle with the Luer-lock end cut off. Extra holes are cut in the side of the plastic tubing. The needle end is inserted in a vacuum tube.

Ischemia.—We attempt to avoid potential ischemia of flaps by preserving underlying fascia during dissection, by creating flaps of appropriate dimensions, and by avoiding suturing under tension. If we doubt the viability of a flap during surgery, we inject intravenous fluorescein and assess the amount of fluorescence of the area in question under the ultraviolet light or Fluoroscanner. Inadequate fluorescence at the distal margins of flaps probably indicates inadequate vascularity and impending flap necrosis. Those portions that do not fluoresce should be trimmed. On occasion, an alternative flap design or skin coverage may be required. If the neourethra has been constructed from a preputial flap, its vascularity can be assessed by evaluating the fluorescence of the meatus after reconstruction. Sometimes, after we have constructed the neourethra from a flap, we find the vascularity to a portion of remaining penile skin is compromised. At these times, rather than discarding the flaps, we remove the subcutaneous tissue and apply the poorly perfused skin as a full-thickness skin graft for penile coverage.

If a flap blanches when sutured, excessive tension has been placed on the flap, and its vascularity will therefore be diminished. When the distal margin of a flap does not bleed, it is likely to undergo marginal necrosis because of its poor vascularity. The distal ends of such flaps should be trimmed until the edges bleed. Sometimes poor flap perfusion may be secondary to hypotensive anesthesia and due to vasoconstriction from an inadequately heated operating room. If a flap shows poor vascularity by any of these criteria, its survival should not be left to chance, but rather it should be reconstructed. Of course, in some cases one need only remove the subcutaneous tissue and divide the flap at its base to create a full-thickness skin graft. The wings of the glans also may become ischemic due to suturing under tension or excessive surgical trauma. Necrosis of the tips of the wings of the glans is likely to result in fistula formation. Rarely, flap vascularity may be compromised by a semiocclusive dressing such as Bioclusive. If the Bioclusive dressing is suspected to be at fault, it should be incised along its length but can be left in situ. Flap ischemia is not always full thickness; at times only the superficial skin will be involved and begin to blister. At this stage it is important to keep the flap moist and soft with xeroform gauze or Neosporin ointment to prevent dessication that may progress to full-thickness loss. Completely demarcated ischemic areas may require surgical debridement.

Catheter Problems.—Catheter problems should be infrequent if the catheter is appropriately placed and secured. For flip-flap repairs or fistula repairs we normally use an 8F feeding tube through the neourethra and secure it with the dorsal glans traction suture. This tube then serves to drain the bladder and stent the neourethra. These patients do not require suprapubic urinary diversion, since they generally undergo a voiding trial on the fifth or sixth postoperative day. Patients who have undergone tubed full-thickness skin grafts, tubed flaps, or more extensive genital surgery will require insertion of a percutaneous suprapubic catheter. A stent is also left in the neourethra. With careful suturing, neither the suprapubic catheter nor the stent is likely to be dislodged prematurely. If a catheter does come out early, we do not encourage reinsertion in the early postoperative period. Blind manipulation of the neourethra can disrupt suture lines and may destroy a new skin graft. In these situations, we would choose to divert the urine by means of a suprapubic Cystocath placed in the operating room under anesthesia.

Catheter obstructions are uncommon but generally can be relieved by irrigation. Poor drainage raises the possibility of extravesical percutaneous placement of the catheter, in which case a cystogram is advisable. Rarely, the tip of a suprapubic catheter may slip beyond the bladder neck and result in drainage through the urethra. Partial withdrawal of the tube solves the problem immediately. In most patients bladder spasms occur secondary to catheter stimulation of the bladder or trigone. At times these spasms may induce transient hematuria. It is important to achieve satisfactory control of bladder spasms for two reasons: first, to avoid excessive patient movement due to pain that could damage the repair, and second, to avoid high-pressure extravasation of urine through the urethroplasty wound which may result in fistula or stricture formation. We control postoperative spasms routinely with oxybutynin supplemented by belladonna and opium (B&O) suppositories. Adequate hydration seems to diminish bladder spasms. We have seen complications from these medications, although they are unusual. Oxybutynin, of course, results in xerostomia and facial flushing in some patients. With B&O suppositories, the anticholinergic effects may result in ileus. When such an ileus occurs, the dosage of the drugs must be reduced or stopped. Prior to the voiding trial, these drugs must be stopped, since they can inhibit bladder emptying. To minimize these drug side effects and high-pressure voiding through the repair site as a consequence of bladder catheterization, a recent report suggests the use of a "splint."[11] This split stent sits in the urethra across the repair site and allows the patient to void immediately postoperatively.[11]

Edema and Wound Disruption.—Postoperative edema is usually consequent to surgical trauma and can result in disruption of suture lines. This increase in wound tension brought on by a large amount of edema may interfere with local blood supply and healing. If wound disruption becomes evident after removal of the Bioclusive dressing, the skin edges can be reapproximated with Steristrips. In general, edema and wound disruption may be avoided by delicate tissue handling, tying knots securely, using fine sutures, and by distributing shearing forces through the use of subcutaneous sutures. The sudden onset of edema late in the postoperative course may be due to urine extravasation and/or infection. In reoperative cases edema may become more pronounced because of venous or lymphatic obstruction.

Patients should not be allowed to become constipated, since straining may cause engorgement of the phallus and disruption of the delicate urethral repair. It is not uncommon for a small amount of urine to be squirted through the neourethra or through the stent when the patient is having a bowel movement. Therefore, part of our routine postoperative regimen is a nonconstipating diet and a stool softener.

Leg Pain.—An unusual complication after hypospadias surgery is the onset of severe lower limb pain in the first or second postoperative day. The pain affects both legs and appears to be a spasm involving all the muscle groups in the legs. It is believed to be brought about by the patient's voluntary immobilization of his hips and lower limbs to diminish genital and bladder pain caused by movement of the catheter. This limb spasm phenomenon affects the 5- to 6-year-old group and can be cured within 48 hours by gentle passive physiotherapy to the legs.

Psychiatric Disturbance.—Psychiatric disturbances can complicate the early postoperative course in older children who have undergone multiple reconstructive attempts. As with all complications, these problems are better treated by anticipation and preoperative psychologic counseling. Nonetheless, on occasion we have to ask for de novo psychologic counseling for children so afflicted.

LATE COMPLICATIONS

We define *late complications* as those that appear after the voiding trial.

Fistula.—A common complication is urethrocutaneous fistula, which occurs in about 15% of patients after hypospadias surgery.[12] Fistulas usually present within the first 24 hours after the initiation of voiding and are located along the ventral aspect of the penis where a healing wound overlies the neourethra. Sometimes fistulas may be suspected prior to the voiding trial when an area of inflammation or wound breakdown is noted along the ventral penile shaft. Common factors in the genesis of postoperative fistulas are ischemia of the tissues used to construct the neourethra or its skin coverage, wound infection, failure to invert the epidermis into the lumen, and the use of nonabsorbable or excessively traumatic suture materials. Other factors that may play a role in the development of fistulas are meatal crusting and glanular and meatal edema. Fistulas rarely develop in nonobstructed cases. Meatal crusting can be minimized by a regimen of frequent gentle meatal toilet with half-strength peroxide and Neosporin ointment.

When the patient voids against an obstruction, there is an increase in the intraurethral pressure, which then blows out a weak spot in the healing wound. More than one stream will be noted during the patient's voiding effort, and examination of the penis will reveal a ventral urethrocutanecus fistula. Some patients find that they need to sit to void since they are unable to direct their stream. Fistulas vary in size, in some cases amounting to a large defect in the urethral wall, while in others appearing as a pinpoint leak. Patients who have a percutaneous suprapubic catheter can have their urinary diversion period extended for several days in an attempt to encourage closure of the fistula. In our experience, closure after a period of further urinary diversion is unusual. In those patients who do not have a suprapubic catheter in situ, we do not usually recommend placement of a catheter in order to bypass the fistula. Further damage to the neourethra may be precipitated in attempting catheter placement in an anxious, unanesthetized child.

Certain measures may help to promote closure of postoperative fistulas. Precise application of silver nitrate to the small fistula may cause it to granulate and close. In some patients whose fistula margins are clean, we recommend applying Steristrips to the penile skin to approximate the edges after insuring meatal patency. Older children with small fistulas are instructed to void while occluding the fistula with a finger. In general we have noted that fistulas are more likely to close if the neourethra is constructed from a flap rather than a graft. No attempt should be made to resuture the fistula in the early postoperative period, since the inflammatory process will be exacerbated. If the fistula has not healed by 6 months or more, we elect to close it surgically.

The technique of fistula repair depends upon the number, position and size of the fistula(s). Small fistulas may be excised and closed, while larger fistulas may be excised or closed by rotation flaps, flip-flaps, or Y-V advancement techniques (Fig 35–3). Before attempting repair of the fistulas, distal urethral obstruction needs to be corrected, whether it be due to stricture or meatal stenosis. We prefer to examine the distal urethra cystoscopically. If no obstructive lesions are found, we inject methylene blue–dyed saline into the urethra to identify any occult fistulous tracts. The fistula is then circumscribed with a knife, and the wound edges are elevated with skin hooks. Further mobilization of the fistulous tract is then undertaken by dissecting through the dartos layer and identifying the neck of the fistula. We excise redundant fistula tract and then pass a small sound through the fistula along the dorsal wall of the urethra in the direction of the meatus. By this technique, we have identified intraurethral flaps that might have produced obstruction and recurrent fistula formation. The edges of the fistula are then reapproximated with running subcuticular sutures of 6-0 or 7-0 PDS, inverting the epithelium in a watertight fashion. The wound is closed in layers over the fistula closure. If ventral penile skin is deficient after fistula closure, skin may be advanced from the dorsum, where grafting may be utilized more safely. The use of multiple layers may be important in fistula closure. We use a small feeding tube to stent the urethra and to drain the bladder after repair of larger fistulas. Urinary diversion can be omitted after small fistula closures. Larger fistulas can be treated with a flip-flap or a rotation flap of local penile skin. A large flap may be advanced to cover more than one fistula. Strictures immediately distal to fistulas must be treated at the time of closure. In some cases, we have augmented the urethral caliber at the site of a distal stricture with the same skin flap that is used to cover the fistula. Alternatively, a fistula associated with a more severe urethral stricture may be treated simultaneously with a patch graft urethroplasty.

Stricture.—Factors that promote stricture formation are poor design of the neourethra, tissue ischemia, tension on the repair, inappropriate repair of an existing stricture, trauma from a large catheter or stent, or secondary infection in the repair. Patients or their parents may note a diminution in the caliber of the stream or the onset of urinary tract infections as the presenting features of a stricture. Rarely, a patient may develop urinary retention. If the stricture is at the level of the meatus, our initial management is to perform periodic dilatations. The regimen is comparable to that used in the postoperative period already mentioned. Stric-

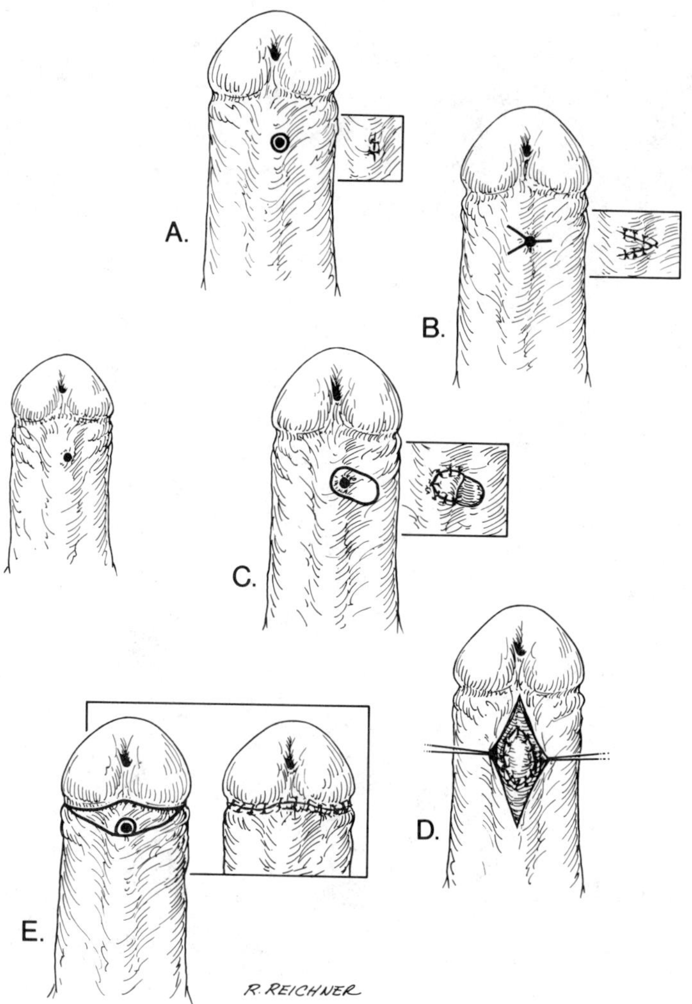

FIG 35–3.
Methods of repair of fistulas after hypospadias repair. A distal shaft fistula is demonstrated. Methods of repair include circumscribing incision with excision of the tract and closure of the urethra and skin in separate layers **A,** Y-V advancement after excision and closure of the fistula **B,** repair of the urethral defect with a local penile skin flap **C, D,** a larger urethral defect is repaired with a full-thickness patch graft. **E,** a small subcoronal fistula is excised and closed, and shaft skin is advanced to cover the defect.

tures not responding to dilatation require further evaluation with retrograde urethrography and/or cystoscopy. We have treated short urethral strictures with visual internal urethrotomy (Fig 35–4). The optical urethrotome has not proved satisfactory for the long-term correction of strictures in tube grafts. It may, however, correct a stricture that has formed in a flap neourethra. Dense strictures and longer deeper strictures that have not responded quickly to dilatation are treated with penoscrotal or perineal urethrostomy followed by a delayed reconstructive procedure 6 months or more after the initial attempt at repair.

Most strictures occur within 6 months in the region of the anastomosis. Prevention of stricture formation then requires satisfactory surgical design that uses spat-

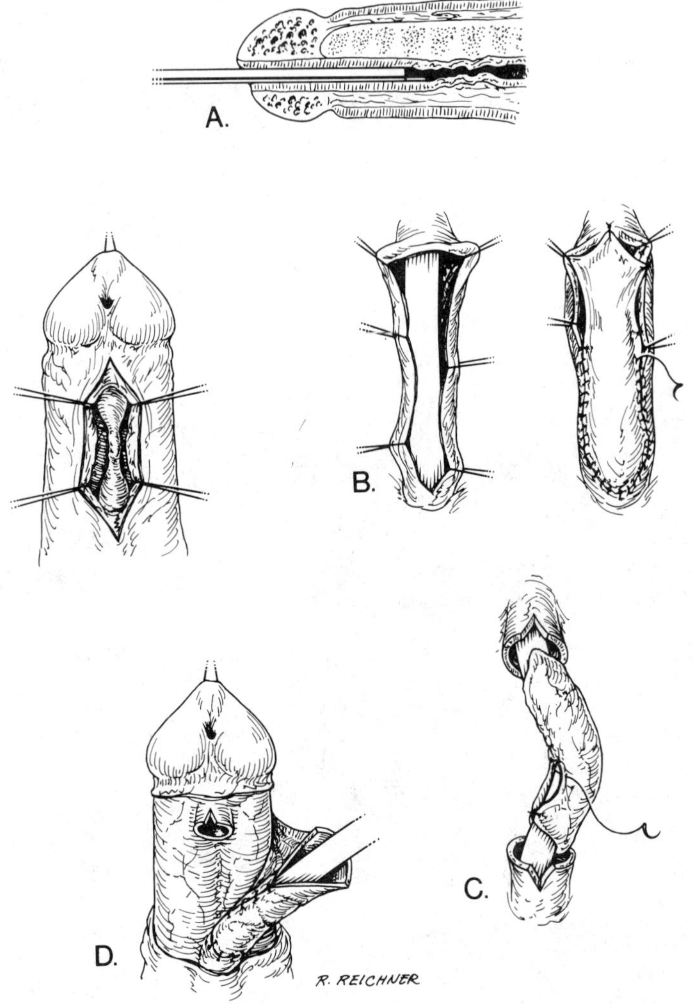

FIG 35–4.
Methods of treatment for stricture after hypospadias repair. A stricture in the neourethra is demonstrated. **A,** visual internal urethrotomy is demonstrated. **B,** the stricture has been opened and a full-thickness patch graft is applied. **C,** the stricture is excised and a full-thickness tube graft is interposed. **D,** a flap of penile skin is fashioned into a tube and interposed.

ulated anastomoses and an adequate amount of tissue to give satisfactory initial caliber to the neourethra. Split-thickness skin grafts, because they lack dermis, have a propensity to contract and therefore should not be used in urethral reconstruction. The techniques used to repair strictures include patch grafts, full-thickness tubed skin grafts, and flaps from penile skin. Since strictures are often found in association with other complications, such as fistulas or diverticula, the technique for stricture repair may require modification to allow correction of the associated complications. Sometimes the neourethra is completely strictured, and the urethroplasty needs to be redone. One procedure that may have an increased propensity for stricture formation is tunneling of the neourethra through the glans without creating glans wings. To avert this problem, it is important to

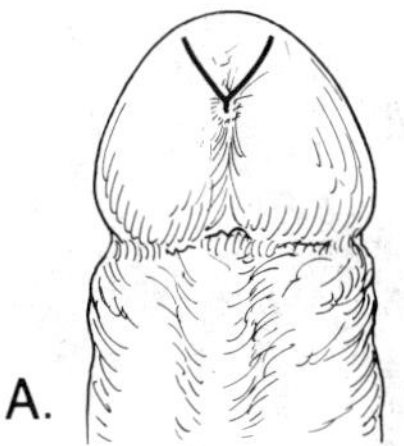

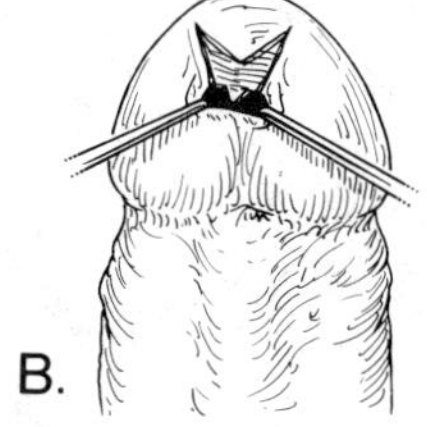

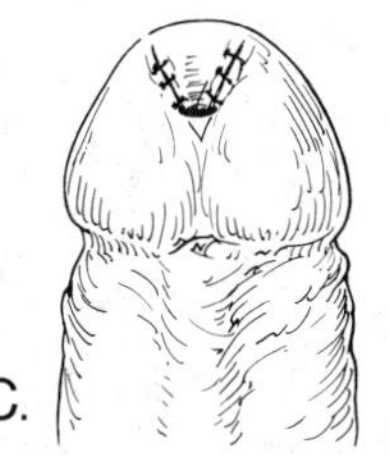

FIG 35–5.
Meatal stenosis following hypospadias surgery is repaired by means of a dorsal V-flap advancement. **A,** the incision; **B,** the undermined V-flap and dorsal urethrotomy; **C,** the V-flap advanced to widen the dorsal urethra.

excise a small core of the glans in the creation of the tunnel. Some meatal stenoses do not respond to dilatation and may be treated by surgical meatoplasty, using either ventral penile skin or Y-V advancement of dorsal glans epithelium into the meatus (Fig 35–5).

Diverticula.—Diverticula (sacculation or aneurysmal dilatation) of the neourethra may arise secondary to distal urethral or meatal narrowing or a decrease in glanular pliability. These tissues may be unable to expand during voiding, subsequently increasing intraurethral pressure. If a urethrocutaneous fistula does not develop, then the increased pressure during voiding may dilate an area of the penile neourethra. A lack of supporting corpus spongiosum may increase the tendency for diverticular formation, but this is unlikely, considering the low incidence of postoperative diverticula after hypospadias repair. A diverticulum may appear in the native urethra if there is a marked step-off in diameter between the native urethra and neourethra. The diverticular tissue can appear relatively well vascularized and elastic and therefore suitable for use in the repair.

Patients with urethral diverticula may notice an increase in the caliber of the urethra during voiding and often complain of postvoid dribbling because of late drainage of pooled urine from the diverticulum. These patients can minimize their dribbling by milking the urethra empty at the end of voiding. Stagnant urine may increase the chance of urinary tract infection. Long-standing diverticula may become infected and may contain stones which can then erode and cause fistula formation.

In our general approach to diverticulum repair, a ventral penile incision is made and the diverticulum exposed (Fig 35–6). The diverticulum is then opened and a flap fashioned from the diverticular tissue to be advanced distally to enlarge the strictured area (Figs 35–7 and 35–8).[13] Redundant diverticular tissue is excised. An alternative to this approach that has been described involves imbrication of the diverticular tissue.[14] This procedure appears to provide a satisfactory buttress to the neourethra but may prove inadequate if distal urethral resistance remains uncorrected.

Residual Chordee.—Residual chordee is a frequent cause of failed hypospadias repair. This complication will decrease with appropriate use and interpretation of the artificial erection. We utilize the artificial erection test after each step in our dissection to verify our achievement of a straight phallus. Residual chordee can be corrected through a systematic approach. In most cases, the previous operative site can be reexposed, and dysgenetic scar tissue can be excised from the ventral aspect of the corporal bodies. Correction of

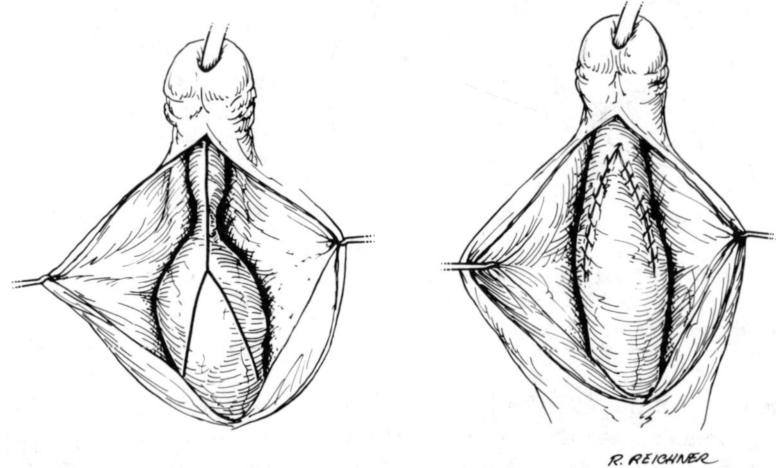

FIG 35–6.
Urethral diverticulum after hypospadias surgery Y-V advancement to correct a stricture distal to diverticulum.

chordee may require elevation of the neourethra, sometimes an exacting task. If the artificial erection at this stage indicates residual curvature, we do not usually proceed to division of the urethra.

Our next step is a sagittal incision of the restrictive tissues in the intercorporal septum (Fig 35–9). This incision releases some of the additional midline dysgenetic tissue, allowing the corporal bodies to rotate outward and straighten the phallus. Further dysgenetic tissue and scar tissue exposed by this maneuver are excised.

Persistent chordee after these steps is due to the tethering effect of the neourethra, and we will then mobilize the urethra completely. If we find at this point that the neourethra is bowstringing, we divide it (Fig 35–10). If chordee is again demonstrated after this step, we know that we are dealing with inadequacy of the tunica albuginea of the corporal bodies. To correct mild to moderate residual chordee, we perform a dorsal plication by excising an ellipse of tunica albuginea at the point of maximum penile curvature[8] (Fig 35–11). An incision is made laterally in Buck's fascia and the neurovascular bundle is elevated from the dorsal tunica. Prolene stay sutures are placed laterally on each corporal body at the point of maximal curvature. We estimate the size of the ellipse to be excised by applying traction to the stay sutures while producing an artificial erection and simultaneously pushing the penis straight. This technique produces a fold in the dorsal tunica and, when marked, identifies the ellipse of tunica to be removed. The ellipse is excised and the edges of the defect closed with a running 5-0 PDS suture. Although this technique corrects the chordee, it may decrease slightly the length of the dorsal aspect of the penis.

For severe residual ventral chordee, correction may require dermal grafting, which would lengthen slightly the ventral aspect of the penis. The dermal graft is usually taken from the area adjacent to the anterior superior iliac spine[8] (Fig 35–12). To harvest such a graft, we de-epithelialize a measured area by freehand cutting through the epidermis and develop the plane between the epidermis and dermis with a no. 10 blade. Once the dermis is excised, it is defatted to a thickness of about 1 mm. Closure of the skin in the region of the donor site is easily accomplished, because it is relatively loose. A ventral transverse incision is made in

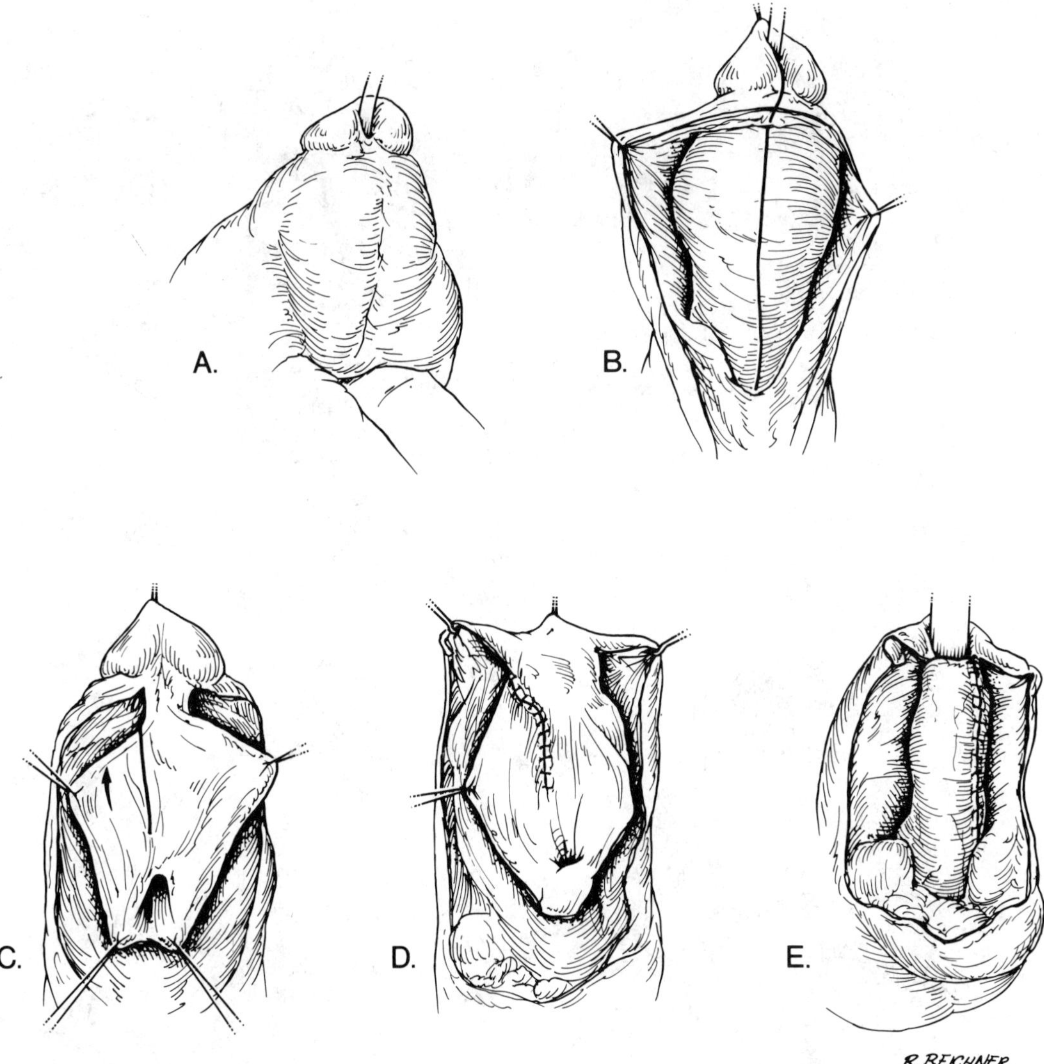

FIG 35–7.
Large diverticulum after urethroplasty in hypospadias cripple. **A,** dilated ventral penis. **B,** exposure of diverticulum and division of glans. **C,** proposed incision to create flap of diverticular tissue. **D,** flap advancement to augment submeatal stricture. **E,** completed urethroplasty.

the tunica albuginea at the point of maximal penile curvature. This incision allows the edges of the tunica to spring apart and the corporal bodies to straighten. The incision extends to the lateral margins of the corpora. The edges are undermined slightly to expedite suturing of the graft tissue. The size of the dermal graft is about one and one-half times the size of the defect created. The dermal graft is placed fat side down and secured with continuous 6-0 PDS in a running, locking, watertight suture. When a dermal graft has been used in the repair, a skin graft should not be used for urethroplasty or skin coverage if it will be in direct contact with the dermal graft. Two grafts in juxtaposition will not become vascularized. In some situations it is necessary to delay the urethroplasty until a later date. A ure-

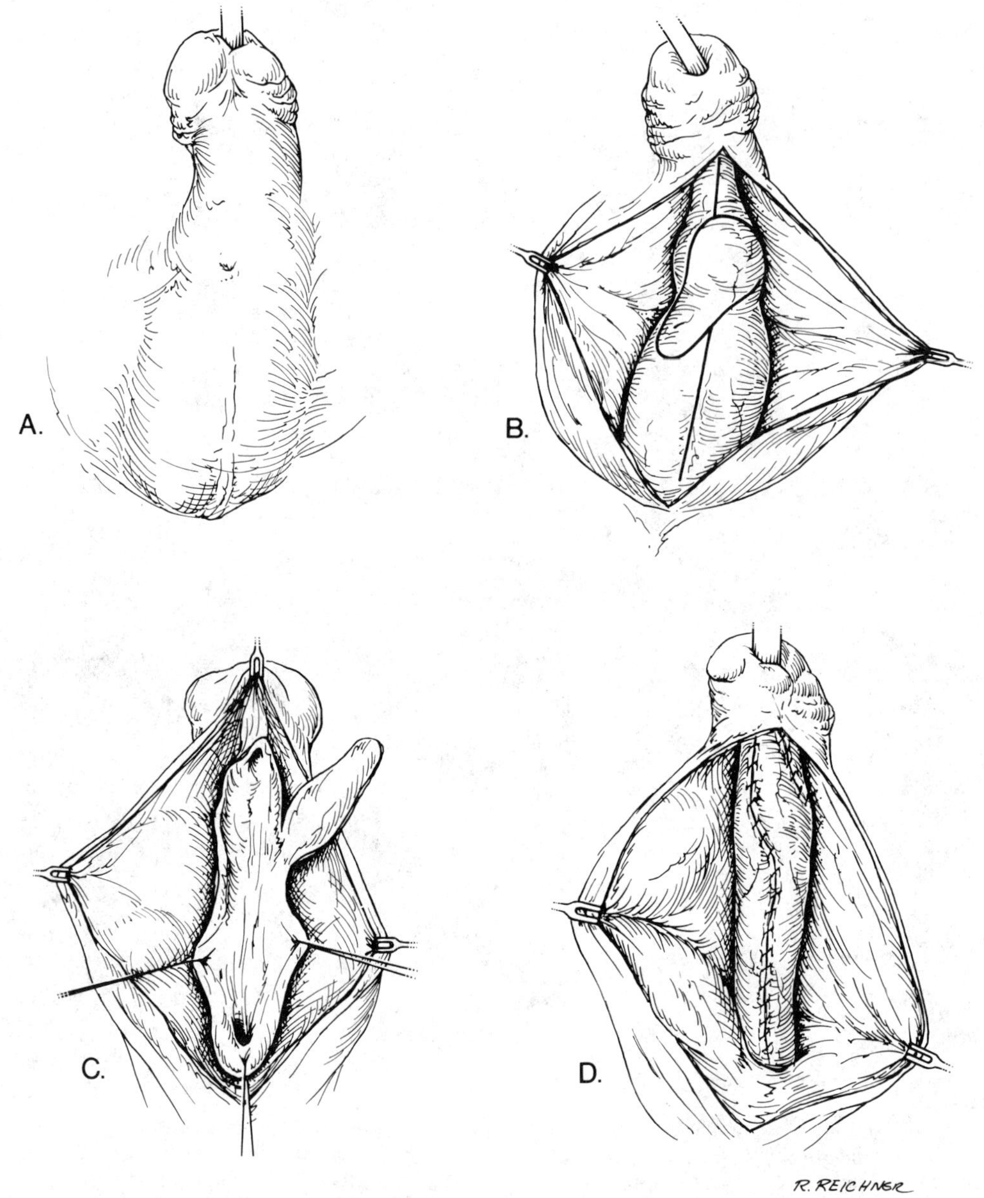

FIG 35–8.
Diverticulum and urethral stricture after hypospadias repair. **A,** dilated ventral penis. **B,** skin and fascial layers are dissected, and proposed lines of incision are marked on urethral diverticulum. **C,** incision with development of flap from diverticular tissue. **D,** completed urethroplasty.

throplasty may be completed with a flap, however, if there is sufficient penile skin. Similarly, penile skin coverage in these cases must be achieved with flaps, perhaps from the scrotum. If the cosmetic result of such penile coverage is unsatisfactory, revisions may be made after a period of 6 months.[15]

Hair in the Neourethra Lumen.—If hair-bearing skin is used for a urethroplasty, the patient may eventually experi-

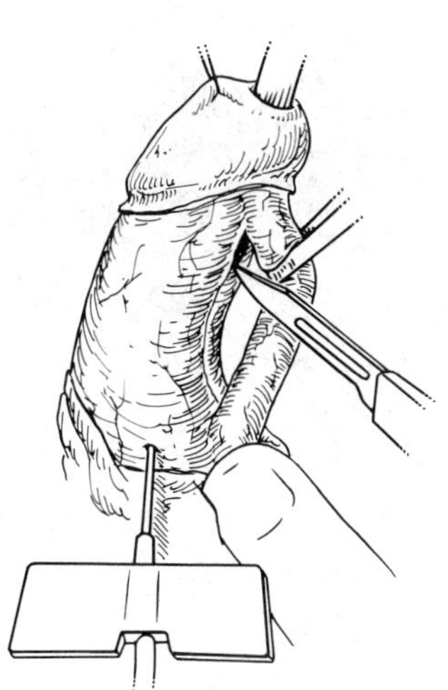

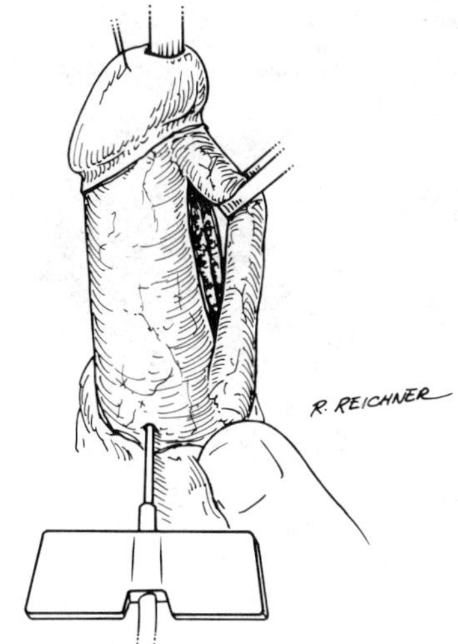

FIG 35–9.
Correction of chordee persistent after resection of dysgenetic tissue. The intercorporal septum is incised while an artificial erection is maintained. This figure depicts chordee without hypospadias.

ence the complication of hair within the lumen of the neourethra. In severe cases the hair can protrude from the meatus, presenting as a urethral beard. Urinary tract infections and stone formation may occur, particularly if there is pooling of urine in the neourethra. When urethral hair is associated with recurrent infections, the affected neourethra is best excised and repaired with hairless skin. Ide-

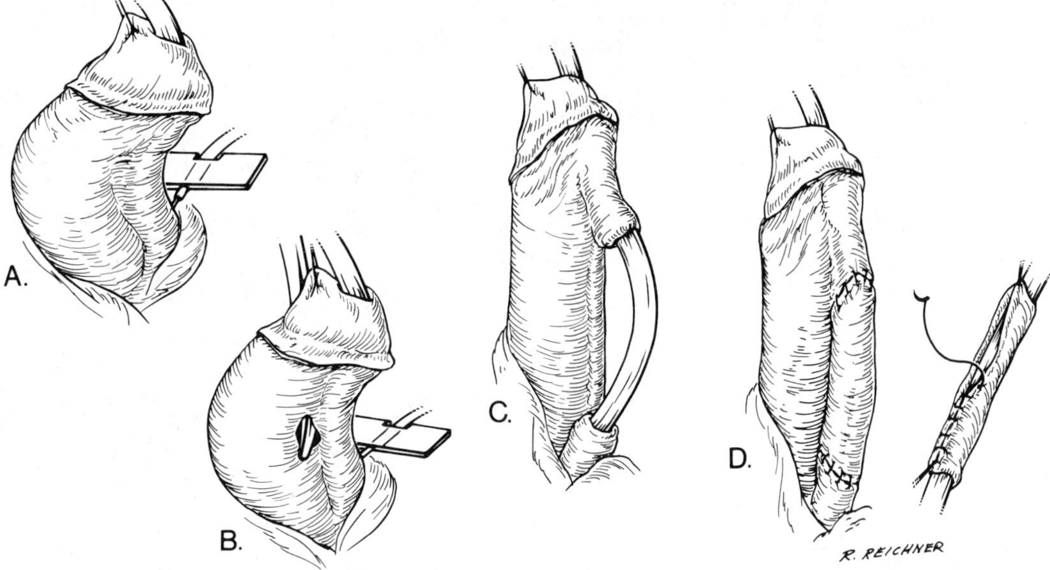

FIG 35–10.
The congenitally short urethra. In this very rare condition, resection of dysgenetic layers and mobilization of the urethra have not resulted in a straight phallus. Therefore, the urethra is divided, and a full-thickness tube graft urethral repair is performed.

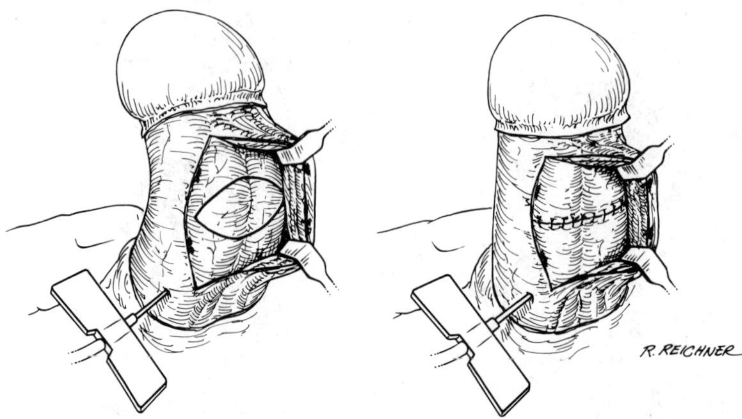

FIG 35–11.
Excision of an ellipse of dorsal tunica albuginea in persistent chordee. Note that the dorsal neurovascular bundle has been carefully reflected after a lateral incision in Buck's fascia.

ally, the neourethra is constructed from distal penile skin. If this skin is unavailable, other hairless portions of the body may be used. The midline of the scrotum tends to be hairless and may be used in the urethroplasty as a flap or a graft.

Urinary Tract Infections.—Persisting or recurrent urinary tract infections with or without hematuria after hypospadias surgery usually imply a urethral stricture. Most strictures, as we have mentioned, will manifest within 6 months. All infections will respond to an appropriate antibiotic regimen. After treatment, further investigation of the urethra will be required to ensure adequate patency. Depending upon the clinical circumstances, the evaluation should include uroflowmetry, retrograde urethrography, and/or cys-

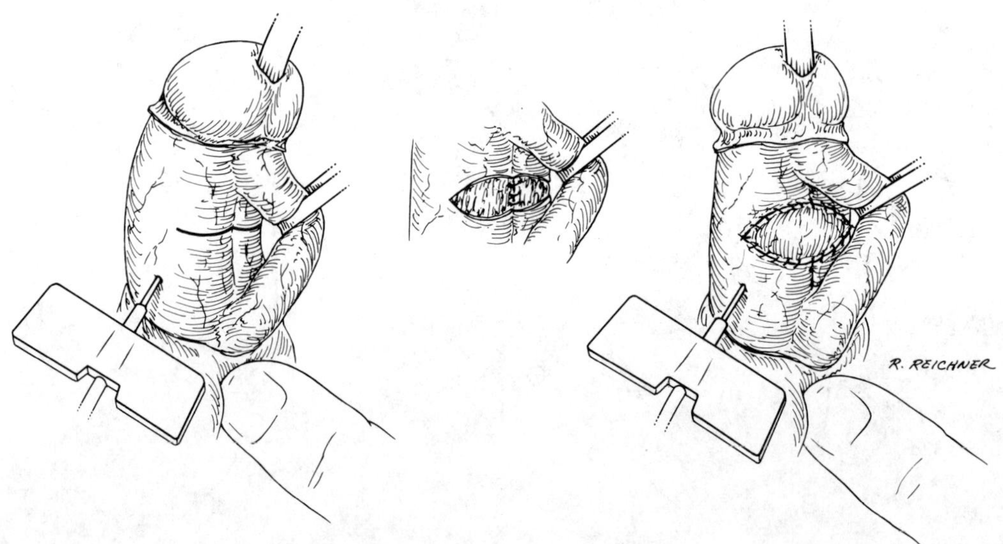

FIG 35–12.
In chordee without hypospadias, when other measures have failed to produce straightness, a transverse incision in the ventral tunica at the point of maximum curvature will allow straightening of the phallus. The defect is repaired with a dermal graft.

toscopy. Treatment of the strictures has already been discussed. Epididymoorchitis and/or prostatitis may occur in conjunction with strictures and infections involving the neourethra.

Loss of Erection.—The loss of erection after hypospadias surgery has been rare in our experience. In the pediatric patient, there is a chance that penile nerve regeneration can take place after trauma to the dorsal neurovascular bundle. In the adult patient who has undergone multiple attempts at hypospadias repair, we perform nocturnal penile tumescence testing and have the patient and his sexual partner counseled by our sex therapist preoperatively. In the majority of cases with an impotence problem, the defect is functional in nature.[8] If in the adult it proves to be organic, we elect to treat the impotence with a penile prosthesis at a later date.

Penile Torsion.—Penile torsion may occur as a consequence of the manner in which penile skin has been reapproximated to the glans. Penile torsion may be prevented by rotating the penis to the anatomical position before final approximation of the penile skin to the coronal margin. The preputial flap urethroplasty techniques may produce torsion by turning the penis to the side of the vascular pedicle. Penoscrotal transposition may occur secondary to hypospadias reconstructions in which there was a shortage of skin for shaft coverage. Scrotal tissue engulfing the base of the penis may be excised or recessed by carrying out a V-Y plasty at a later date.

Cosmetic Problems.—Dissatisfaction with the cosmetic appearance of the penis after hypospadias surgery has been noted, generally in the hypospadias cripple population. A patient who complains about the deviation or spraying of the stream should undergo careful examination for redundant meatal skin tags that can be corrected surgically. There may be recurrent or residual chordee and/or penoscrotal tethering and webbing. Other cosmetic problems involve the color mismatch of skin grafts, scarring of the glans, retrusion of the meatus, or redundant neourethral tissue at the meatus. Although many of these cosmetic defects can be improved by revisional surgery, we have found that in some cases dissatisfaction was related to deep-seated psychologic concerns which should have been managed concurrently by the sex therapist.[15]

ACKNOWLEDGMENT

We would like to extend our gratitude to Marilyn Anderson, R.N., our genitourinary reconstructive nurse, for her caring nature, her attention to detail, and her ability to counsel.

EDITORIAL COMMENT

This chapter reflects the extensive experience of the authors in hypospadias surgery, especially in patients with complications of hypospadias surgery. The step-by-step approaches to recurrent chordee, stricture, fistulas, infection, and skin loss are all outlined in detail. The use of microsurgical techniques, including magnification, microinstruments, bipolar cautery, and fine PDS suture are all adjuncts that will improve the overall results in hypospadias surgery. The PDS suture is a monofilament absorbable suture that represents a significant improvement over the older, braided absorbable sutures. Last, as was stated, any patient with even a small amount of glanular hypospadias and undescended testis should be investigated for intersex.

REFERENCES

1. Devine CJ Jr, Franz JP, Horton CE: Evaluation and treatment of patients with failed hypospadias repair. *J Urol* 1978; 119:223.
2. Fallon B, Devine CJ Jr, Horton CE: Congenital anomalies associated with hypospadias. *J Urol* 1976; 116:585.
3. Rajfer J, Walsh PC: The incidence of intersexuality in patients with hypospadias and cryptorchidism. *J Urol* 1976; 116:769.
4. Gonzalez-Serva L, Stecker JF Jr, Devine CJ Jr, et al: Lower urinary tract morphology in patients with hypospadias, in Kogan SJ, Hafey ESE (eds): *Clinics in Andrology,* Vol 7, *Pediatric Urology*. Boston, Martinus Nijhoff Publishers, 1981.
5. Horton CE, Devine CJ Jr: A one stage repair for hypospadias cripples. *Plast Reconstr Surg* 1970; 45:425.
6. Devine CJ Jr, Horton CE: Hypospadias repair. *J Urol* 1977; 118:188.
7. Gittes RF, McLaughlin AP III: Injection technique to induce penile erection. *Urology* 1974; 4:473.
8. Vorstman B, Devine CJ Jr: Penile torsion, bent penis and Peyronie's disease, in Lipshultz (ed): *BIMR Urology,* vol 4, *Andrology*. Stoneham, Mass, Butterworth, in press.
9. McCraw JB, Myers B, Shanklin KD: The value of fluorescein in predicting the viability of arteriolized flaps. *Plast Reconstr Surg* 1977; 60:710.
10. Gilbert DA, Devine CJ Jr, Winslow BH, et al: Microsurgical hypospadias repair. *Plast Reconstr Surg* 1986; 77:460–467.
11. Mitchell ME, Kulb TB: Hypospadias repair without a bladder drainage catheter. *J Urol,* in press.
12. Horton CE, Devine CJ Jr, Graham JK: Fistulas of the penile urethra. *Plast Reconstr Surg* 1980; 66:407.
13. Winslow BH, Vorstman B, Devine CJ Jr: Urethroplasty using diverticular tissue. *J Urol* 1985; 134:552.
14. Walker D: Urethral diverticula after hypospadias repair. *Soc for Pediatr Urol Newsletter* July 20, 1984.
15. Vorstman B, Devine CJ Jr., Horton CE: Current hypospadias techniques. *Ann Plast Surg,* in press.

CHAPTER 36

Complications of Orchidopexy

Jack S. Elder, M.D.
Fray F. Marshall, M.D.

The complications of orchidopexy fall into two groups: the complications of the surgical procedure and the complications of cryptorchidism itself or delayed orchidopexy.

COMPLICATIONS OF SURGERY

Anesthesia, Outpatient Surgery.—Orchidopexy is usually performed as an outpatient procedure. In a recent review of orchidopexies performed in 1984, 99 of 103 (96%) were performed in an outpatient setting.[1] Adequate preoperative evaluation of these children remains important for anesthesia considerations. The anesthetic risk is never zero, especially in very young children, but as long as adequate precautions are taken, outpatient surgery is safe, as well as economical. In general, children over 6 months of age with an American Society of Anesthesiologists' Physical Status of 1 or 2 may undergo outpatient general anesthesia with minimal chance of anesthetic morbidity. Contraindications to outpatient orchidopexy include prune-belly syndrome, congenital heart disease, and preexisting conditions that affect respiratory function such as asthma and bronchopulmonary dysplasia. Administration of a caudal block by the anesthesia staff or infiltration of the incision with bupivacaine or lidocaine allows the child to awaken from anesthesia with minimal discomfort. While it might be assumed that children undergoing an intraperitoneal dissection for testicular mobilization will develop an ileus, we have found that some of these patients may be discharged on the day of surgery. However, some children will need to be admitted if they experience nausea and vomiting from traction on the spermatic cord, severe discomfort, respiratory distress, or develop significant inguinal or scrotal swelling. There is no evidence that early ambulation associated with outpatient orchidopexy results in increased complications such as testicular retraction or hematoma.

Recurrence of Undescended Testis/Inguinal Hernia.—Testicular retraction usually results from an inadequate orchidopexy. The steps in a typical orchidopexy include testicular mobilization, division of the cremasteric attachments to the testis and spermatic cord, high ligation of the hernia sac, and retroperitoneal dissection, in which the external spermatic fascial attachments to the cord are divided. In selected cases, the floor of the inguinal canal must be taken down with division of the inferior epigastric artery and vein to allow the testicular artery to assume a more direct path to the scrotum. Placement of the testis in a dartos pouch

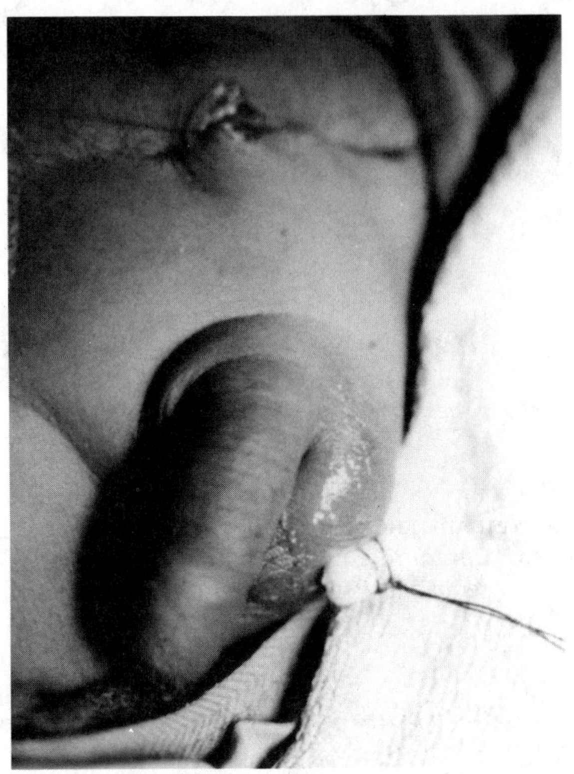

FIG 36–1.
A second-stage orchidopexy in a patient with prune-belly syndrome was successful in placing the testis within the scrotum.

secures the testis in the scrotal wall, reduces the likelihood of testicular retraction, and allows the testis to be palpated easily.[2] It is important to close the neck of the scrotum following placement of the testis in the dartos pouch. Some surgeons place a fixation stitch between the testis and scrotal wall or use an external bolster for temporary fixation (Fig 36–1). Testicular atrophy did not occur in any of the 27 orchidopexies that Pryn[2] originally described with the subdartos pouch.

In most cases of recurrent undescended testes, there has been an inadequate dissection of the spermatic vessels high in the retroperitoneum. Failure to dissect the hernia sac off the spermatic cord usually results in postoperative retraction of the testis, but may also cause a clinically apparent hernia. Furthermore, if the sac is torn or incompletely ligated, a recurrent indirect hernia may result. It is also possible that a hernia that appears following orchidopexy may actually represent a direct inguinal hernia rather than an indirect inguinal hernia.

If the patient has had a previous attempt at orchidopexy, a second attempt often is successful, as several authors have described.[3, 4] Maizels et al. reported 36 boys with a previously failed orchidopexy.[5] At reexploration, retroperitoneal dissection was necessary in 12 of the 16 testes that were proximal to the external ring, and in most cases division of the floor of the inguinal canal was necessary for successful secondary orchidopexy. In two boys orchiectomy was performed. At follow-up, all testes were situated in the scrotum and none became atrophic. Thus, a second attempt at orchidopexy should be attempted.

Vascular Injury and Injury to the Vas Deferens.—During the dissection of the hernia sac off the spermatic cord, injury to the spermatic vessels can occur. Sometimes injecting saline may elevate the processus vaginalis and help with the dissection. If the surgeon is familiar with pediatric procedures and operates with gentle care, the incidence of vascular injury is low.

Injuries or division of the vas deferens can also occur at this time. Sometimes these injuries are not appreciated until later, when the patients discover they have fertility problems. We have seen adult patients who have had a testis become atrophic from mumps orchitis and then were found to have a contralateral occluded vas from an earlier inguinal dissection. We have performed successful microsurgical transvasovasotomy or transvasoepididymostomy in treating this complication (see Chapter 24, Complications of Microsurgery). If transection of the vas is discovered during an orchidopexy, immediate microsurgical vasovasostomy probably should be performed.

Vascular injury can occur more commonly in a patient with a nonpalpable undescended testis. If, after exploration of the inguinal area, no testis is seen immediately, an intraperitoneal incision will usually identify the testis at the internal ring. An intraabdominal testis may be more difficult to place into the scrotum, and vascular injury is more likely to occur as a result.

If the testis is intraabdominal and does not appear to be likely to reach the scrotum by conventional techniques, a Fowler-Stephens orchidopexy can be performed with division of the testicular artery, allowing perfusion of the testis through the deferential artery.[6] If one is considering a Fowler-Stephens procedure, the vas deferens should not be skeletonized or else the collateral arterial supply will be disrupted. Therefore, it is important to leave the peritoneal attachment to the vas intact. In approximately 20% to 30% of cases, testicular atrophy occurs, secondary either to arterial injury or spasm. To improve the success of this procedure, Ransley et al. have proposed staging the operation, ligating the testicular artery in situ during the first stage, and 6 to 12 months later, after the collateral blood supply presumably has developed, performing a standard Fowler-Stephens orchidopexy.[7] Silber and Kelly[8] have recommended a microvascular anastomosis to the inferior epigastric vessels as an alternative and have been successful. In children with prune-belly syndrome there can be tremendous difficulty in obtaining adequate length of the spermatic cord to place the testis within the scrotum. However, if the orchidopexy is done within the first 2 to 3 months of life, frequently it is possible to place the testes within the scrotum.[9] These patients are still very likely to be infertile because of their prostatic and vasal abnormalities, but the testes may develop more normally.

If inguinal dissection reveals only a vas deferens that appears to end blindly, the dissection should not necessarily stop, because there may be nonunion of the epididymis and testis or a long looped vas. It is necessary to identify both the vessels and the vas deferens and look for any testicular tissue[10] (Fig 36–2). When the vessels and vas appear to end in a nubbin of tissue, this tissue may represent a detached epididymis and the testis still may be present.[10] The surgeon should be aware that epididymal abnormalities occur in as high as one third of patients with an undescended testis[11] (Fig 36–3).

Lastly, male fetuses exposed to diethylstilbestrol (DES) appear to have a higher-than-normal incidence of cryptorchidism and epididymal abnormalities.[12] If a history of DES exposure is elicited, careful inspection of the epididymis at the time of orchidopexy is indicated because of the implications of impaired testicular growth and fertility.

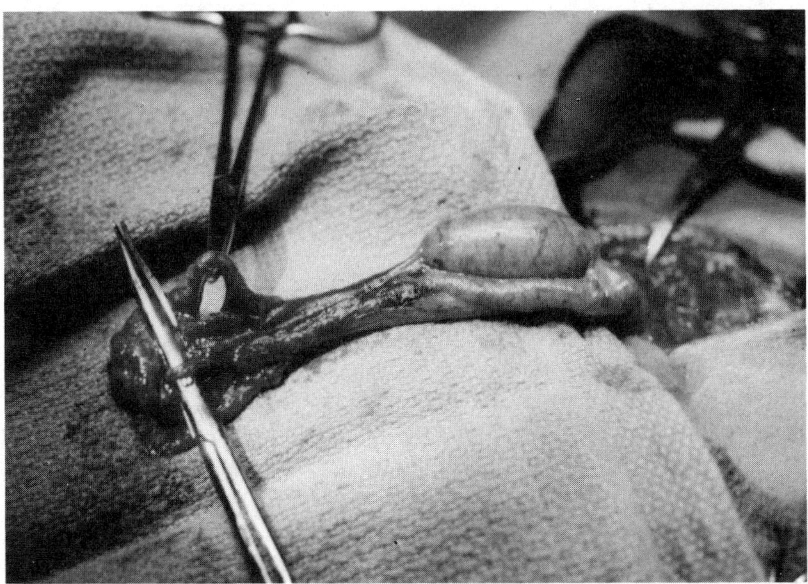

FIG 36–2.
The scissors are placed under a long looped vas that extended far below the testis at the time of orchidopexy.

Atrophic Testes.—If a testis becomes atrophic from a vascular insult, it is sometimes necessary to remove it because of pain. Although atrophic testes may generate reasonable levels of serum testosterone, the cosmetic appearance may cause concern. The newer silicone prostheses feel very similar to a normal testis and give a normal cosmetic appearance.[13] On the other hand, if a small testicular prosthesis is placed at an early age, it may be necessary to change this prosthesis in the future. If there is unilateral atrophy and the testis has been removed, assurance from the physician will usually calm any fears of the parents. A testicular prosthesis can always be placed at a later time if the patient has continued concern about his physical appearance.

Wound Infection, Hematoma.—As in any surgery there can be problems with infection and hematoma, although these problems appear to be relatively rare and are usually handled in the standard fashion with any necessary drainage procedures and utilization of antibiotics.

COMPLICATIONS OF CRYPTORCHIDISM OR DELAYED ORCHIDOPEXY

Histologic Abnormalities.—In the 1700s John Hunter recognized that if the testis were left within the abdomen it would not develop normally. In 1926 Moore[14] described the deleterious effects of temperature if the testis was kept within the abdomen of the guinea pig. Spermatogenesis appeared to stop after 3 weeks, but some recovery could be demonstrated if the testis was returned to the scrotum. By light microscopy, in the human, an undescended testis cannot be distinguished from a normal testis for 12 months.[15] However, by 2 years of age, the mean number of germ cells in the undescended testis decreases and is significantly less than in the normal testis.[15, 16] Other findings include progressive loss in the size of the seminiferous tubules and peritubular hyalinization and fibrosis. Mengel et al. showed that the cryptorchid testis never has a normal spermatogenic pattern while in an undescended posi-

EPIDIDYMAL ABNORMALITY

	PATIENTS
A. *A Agenesis of epididymis-vas deferens*	*1 patient*

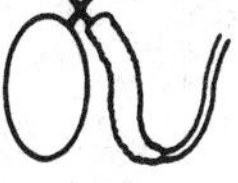

B. *Atresia, loss of continuity between:*	
1. Head of epididymis and testis	*2 patients*

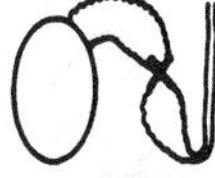

2. Mid-epididymis	*1 patient*

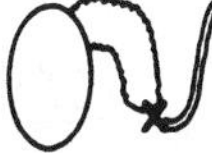

3. Tail of epididymis	*5 patients*

C. *Loop or Elongated Epididymis*	*6 patients*

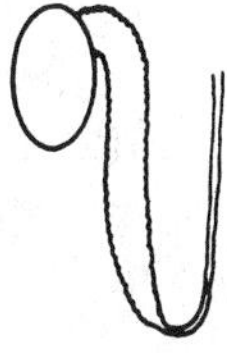

TOTAL: 15 patients

FIG 36–3.
Of 42 undescended testes in 32 patients, 15 (36%) had epididymal abnormalities. A description of the epididymal abnormalities is shown. (From Marshall FF, Shermeta DW: *J Urol* 1979; 121:341. Used by permission.)

tion.[17] By electron microscopy, interstitial fibrosis has been demonstrated as early as 1 year of age.[18] Whether orchidopexy alters these acquired changes is uncertain. Kiesewetter and associates studied 29 patients with bilateral undescended testes, initially performing a unilateral orchidopexy and testis biopsy.[19] Six to 12 months later, contralateral orchidopexy and bilateral testis biopsies were performed. Fifty-two percent of the testes showed moderate or marked improvement in spermatogenesis when compared with the original biopsy.

Some of the testicular changes may be related to epididymal abnormalities. As was demonstrated in a prospective study,[11] 36% of patients with cryptorchidism had significant abnormalities of the epididymis, including many with atresia. If the atresia occurs in the caput epididymidis, there may be subsequent testicular atrophy. This finding has been demonstrated in an ACI rat model,[20] in which testicular atrophy occurs at the time of puberty.[21]

The optimal age for orchidopexy has been debated over the years. In 1962 Scott stated that the testis should be repaired before age 10 years.[22] The recommended age has steadily decreased and orchidopexy has been recommended before age 5[23] and, most recently, by 2 years of age.[17, 24] Since microscopic pathologic changes are present in the cryptorchid testis by 1 to 2 years of age, and because spontaneous descent of the testis does not occur beyond 1 year of age, orchidopexy is recommended when the child is 12 to 18 months old. In this young age group the testis and structures in the spermatic cord are extremely delicate, and orchidopexy technically is somewhat more difficult than in older boys. Whether the complication rate from orchidopexy is higher in this young population is unknown.

Infertility.—There is less precise information on the fertility of patients with an undescended testis (Table 36–1). In a review by Chilvers et al. of 27 papers that reported fertility following treatment for a unilateral undescended testis, 31% of patients had oligospermia and 14% had azoospermia.[25] In those who had undergone surgery for bilateral cryptorchidism, 31% had oligospermia and 42% had azoospermia. Thus, patients undergoing surgery for bilateral cryptorchidism have a significantly poorer prognosis for fertility than those with a unilateral undescended testis.

More important than the semen analysis is the paternity rate. In men who have undergone orchidopexy for a unilateral undescended testis the paternity rate is 65% to 80% (see Table 36–1), compared with an expected 85% to 90% in the normal adult male population. In men treated for bilateral cryptorchidism, only 50% to 60% report reproduction.

If the orchidopexy is performed earlier in life, patients may be more likely to be fertile. There are eight long-term studies that have reported the age at the time of orchidopexy. In general, until recently, most orchidopexies have been performed at 4 or 5 years of age or later, after pathologic changes in the testes have begun to occur. Chilvers and co-workers found that fertility (defined by semen analysis) was similar in patients treated before and after 8 years of age.[25] However, to date, there is only one long-term follow-up study of patients undergoing orchidopexy before age 2 years. In this report, Ludwig and Potempa[34] found that patients who had an orchidopexy during the first 2 years of life had an 87.5% fertility rate. If the operation was performed between ages 3 and 4, the fertility rate dropped to 54%, and if the operation was performed after puberty, only 14% of the patients were fertile. The perfect prospective study that includes long-term follow-up with semen analysis and paternity has not yet been performed.

Cancer.—The association of undescended testis and testicular tumors was made in the nineteenth century. Over 40 years ago, Campbell[35] reported a 4% to 12% incidence of testicular tumors in undescended testes, and Gilbert and Hamilton[36] reported that 12% of over 7,000 cases of testicular carcinoma occurred in undescended testes. The abdominal testis is four times more likely to become malignant than an inguinal testis. There are no data that orchidopexy diminishes the potential for malignancy. However, having the testis in a scrotal position allows early detection of a testicular mass, and it is important that families of boys with an undescended testis be counseled that malignant degeneration may occur, not only in the cryptorchid testis but also in the contralateral descended testis.

Recently, occult carcinoma in situ has been described in testes many years following orchidopexy. The natural history of carcinoma in situ of the testis is that 50% develop invasive tumor growth within 5 years.[37] Patients at particular risk include men with a small testis or oli-

TABLE 36–1.
Fertility in Patients With Unilateral Undescended Testis Following Orchidopexy*

Source	Cases	Age at Operation (yr)	Fertility (Favorable Semen Analysis) Usually >60 Million/CC)			Successful Reproduction		Comment
			No. of Patients	Condition	%	No.	%	
Hansen (1949)[26]	36	Not given	14	Normal	38			Group of patients with untreated unilateral undescended testis with similar semen analysis
			10	Slightly depressed	27			
Mack (1953)[27]	23	—	4	Normal	17	—		—
			11	Somewhat impaired	47			
Hand (1956)[28]	12	Not given		—		11/12	92	12/15 patients (80%) with untreated unilateral undescended testis had children
Scott (1962)[22]	3	Prepubertal	3	Normal	100	—		Summarized literature to that time: 91/119 (76%) unilateral undescended testis patients had good sperm counts or paternity
Hortling et al. (1967)[29]	19	1–14	14	Normal	73	8/42 pregnancies in group of patients with good semen analysis		—
Albersen et al. (1971)[30]	14	Prepubertal mean age 11	13	Normal	93	—		Favorable semen analysis in 7 patients treated successfully with hCG; all patients came from an original series of 400
Atkinson (1975)[31]	42	2.5–14		Not given		32/42	76	8/18 patients (44%) with bilateral undescended testes had children
Lipshultz et al. (1976)[32]	29	4–12	18	>25 million/cc		7/10 married	70	—
			11	<25 million/cc				
Bar-Maor et al. (1979)[33]	46	All 6	39	25 million/cc	85			—

*From Marshall FF, Elder JS: *Cryptorchidism and Related Anomalies* New York, Praeger, 1982, p 61. Used by permission.
hCG = human chorionic gonadotropin.

gospermia and those with a history of cryptorchidism who have developed a testicular tumor on the opposite side. Many patients with intersex and cryptorchidism are at significant risk for the development of gonadal neoplasms, but the incidence differs with the type of defect. At greatest risk are patients with mixed gonadal dysgenesis, in whom gonadal neoplasms develop in approximately 25%, both in the streak gonad and in the testis. Gonadoblastoma and seminoma are the most common histologic types. Another intersex condition in which there is an increased risk of gonadal neoplasia is complete testicular feminization, and in this disorder, bilateral gonadectomy should be performed.

In a postpubertal male, if there is a small atrophic testis, especially intraabdominal, it should be removed, since it is unlikely to provide any significant spermatogenesis and has a higher risk of carcinoma. The patient will function satisfactorily with a normal contralateral testis. If orchidopexy is performed, it may not provide any greater protection for development of carcinoma, but it certainly allows for a more accurate examination.

Bilateral Impalpable Testes.—If both testes are nonpalpable, an attempt should be made to localize them. Computed tomography scans and magnetic resonance imaging can be utilized to locate nonpalpable testes. In a prepubertal child, if the gonadotropins are elevated, the child may have anorchia.

Torsion.—When there is a lack of posterior fixation of the testis, torsion of the testis can occur, and it is well recognized that it can occur in an undescended testis.[38] When torsion occurs in a cryptorchid testis, there is a high association of malignancy.[39] As many as 25% in a general series or 64% of adult cryptorchid patients with torsion have been reported to have tumors. Diagnosis may be more difficult, especially if the testis is impalpable.

Hernia and Trauma.—An indirect inguinal hernia is almost always present with an undescended testis. High ligation of the sac is an essential part of any orchidopexy. If the hernia is clinically evident in an infant with cryptorchidism, repair before 1 year of age is necessary. Both the herniorrhaphy and the orchidopexy should be performed at the same time, because it may be difficult to bring the testis down if only the hernia is repaired initially.

One of the most common sites of undescended testis is the superficial inguinal pouch. The testis is more fixed in this area and, as a result, is more susceptible to trauma. Some of these ectopic testes lie near the pubic symphysis and may be easily traumatized. Athletic teenagers may have more symptoms related to these undescended or ectopic testes.

Failure of Hormonal Therapy.—The theoretical basis for the use of hormonal therapy to stimulate testicular descent is that normal descent of the testis is androgen-mediated. Accordingly, human chorionic gonadotropin (hCG), which is similar in structure to luteinizing hormone (LH), has been used to stimulate the Leydig cells to produce testosterone and possibly induce testicular descent. In carefully controlled studies, however, the success rate in the treatment of the true undescended testis with hCG in only 6%.[40] On the other hand, when it is suspected that a testis is retractile, hCG 3,000 IU may be administered by intramuscular injection weekly for 4 weeks. One week after the final injection, the patient is reexamined. If the testis has "descended" into the scrotal sac, then it is probably retractile. However, the child should be reexamined 6 months after completion of hormonal therapy to reassess the exact location of the testis. If it has returned to an apparent undescended position, then an orchidopexy should be performed. More recently, there has been considerable interest in the use of natural gonadotropin-releasing hormone (GnRH) to induce testicular descent. Administered as a nasal spray, it must be given three times daily for 4 to 6 weeks. To date, nearly 30 clinical trials have been reported. In uncontrolled studies using intranasal GnRH, approximately 50% of patients reportedly have had testicular descent.[41] However, in double blind studies, only 8% to 20% of testes have descended with GnRH.[40, 42, 43] In follow-up examinations, the testes often have returned to their original position, necessitating orchidopexy.

REFERENCES

1. Siegel AL, Snyder HM, Duckett JW: Outpatient pediatric urological surgery: Techniques for a successful and cost-effective practice. *J Urol* 1986; 136:879.
2. Pryn WJ: The maintenance of maldescended testicles within the scrotum using a dartos pouch. *Br J Surg* 1972; 59:175.
3. Gross RE, Replogle RL: Treatment of the undescended testes. Opinions gained from 1967 operations. *Postgrad Med* 1963; 34:266.
4. Persky L, Albert DJ: Staged orchidopexy. *Surg Gynecol Obstet* 1971; 132:43.
5. Maizels M, Gomez F, Firlit CF: Surgical correction of the failed orchidopexy. *J Urol* 1983; 139:955.
6. Fowler R, Stephens FD: The role of testicular vascular anatomy in the salvage of the high undescended testis. *Aust NZ J Surg* 1959; 29:92.
7. Ransley PG, Vordermark JS, Caldamone AA, et al.: Preliminary ligation of the gonadal vessels prior to orchidopexy for the intra-abdominal testicle: A staged Fowler-Stephens procedure. *World J Urol* 1984; 2:266.
8. Silber SJ, Kelly J: Successful autotransplantation of an intraabdominal testis to the scrotum by microvascular technique. *J Urol* 1976; 115:452.
9. Woodard JR, Parrott TS: Reconstruction of the urinary tract in prune belly uropathy. *J Urol* 1978; 119:824.
10. Marshall FF, Weissman RM, Jeffs RD: Cryptorchidism: The surgical implications of nonunion of the epididymis and testis. *J Urol* 1980; 124:560.
11. Marshall FF, Shermeta DW: Epididymal abnormalities associated with undescended testis. *J Urol* 1979; 121:341.
12. Cosgrove MD, Benton B, Henderson BE: Male genitourinary abnormalities and maternal diethylstilbestrol. *J Urol* 1977; 117:220.
13. Elder JS, Keating MA, Duckett JW: Infant testicular prostheses. *J Urol* 1989; 141:1413.
14. Moore CR: Biology of the mammalian testis and scrotum. *Q Rev Biol* 1926; 1:4.
15. Huff DS, Hadziselimovic F, Duckett JW, et al: Germ cell counts in semithin sections of biopsies of 115 unilaterally cryptorchid testes: The experience from the Children's Hospital of Philadelphia. *Eur J Pediatr* 1987; 146(suppl 2):S25.
16. Hedinger CE: Histopathology of undescended testes. *Eur J Pediatr* 1982; 139:266.
17. Mengel W, Heinz AJ, Sippe WG II, et al: Studies on cryptorchidism: A comparison of histological findings in the germinative epithelium before and after the second year of life. *J Pediatr Surg* 1974; 9:445.
18. Mininberg DT, Rodger JC, Bedford JM: Ultrastructural evidence of the onset of testicular pathological conditions in the cryptorchid human testis within the first year of life. *J Urol* 1982; 128:782.
19. Kiesewetter WB, Shull WR, Fetterman GH: Histologic changes in the testis following anatomically successful orchidopexy. *J Pediatr Surg* 1969; 4:59.
20. Marshall FF, Ewing LL, Zirkin BR, et al: Testicular atrophy associated with agenesis of the epididymis in the ACI rat. *J Urol* 1982; 127:155.
21. McCullough R, Marshall FF, Berry SJ, et al: The influence of epididymal agenesis in the development and maturation of the testis: Experimental model and clinical correlations. *Urol Res* 1984; 12:165.
22. Scott LS: Fertility and cryptorchidism. *Proc R Soc Med* 1962; 55:1047.
23. Numanoglu I, Kokturk I, Mutaf O: Light and electron microscopic examinations of undescended testes. *J Pediatr Surg* 1969; 4:614.
24. Elder JS: The undescended testis: Hormonal and surgical management. *Surg Clin North Am* 1988; 68:983.

25. Chilvers C, Dudley NE, Gough MH, et al: Undescended testis: The effect of treatment on subsequent risk of subfertility and malignancy. *J Pediatr Surg* 1986; 21:691.
26. Hansen TS: Fertility in operatively treated and untreated cryptorchidism. *Proc R Soc Med* 1949; 42:645.
27. Mack WS: Discussion on male infertility. *Proc R Soc Med* 1953; 46:840.
28. Hand JR: Undescended testis: Report of 153 cases with evaluation of clinical findings, treatment and results followed up to 33 years. *J Urol* 1956; 75:973.
29. Hortling H, de la Chapelle A, Johansson CJ, et al: An endocrinologic follow-up study of operated cases of cryptorchidism. *J Clin Endocrinol Metab* 1967; 27:120.
30. Albersen JZ, Bergada C, Cullen M: Male fertility in patients treated for cryptorchidism before puberty. *Fertil Steril* 1971; 22:829.
31. Atkinson PM: A follow-up study of surgically treated cryptorchid patients. *J Pediatr Surg* 1975; 10:115.
32. Lipshultz LI, Camino-Torres R, Greenspan CS, et al: Testicular function after orchiopexy for unilateral descended testes. *N Engl J Med* 1976; 295:15.
33. Bar-Maor JA, Nisan S, Lernau OZ, et al: Orchiopexy in cryptorchidism assessed by clinical, histological and sperm examinations. *Surg Gynecol Obstet* 1979; 148:855.
34. Ludwig G, Potempo J: Der optimale Zeitpunkt der Behandlung des Cryptorchismus. *Dtsch Med Wochenschr* 1975; 100:680.
35. Campbell HE: Incidence of malignant growth of the undescended testicle. *Arch Surg* 1942; 44:353.
36. Gilbert GB, Hamilton JB: Incidence and nature of tumors in ectopic testes. *Surg Gynecol Obstet* 1940; 71:731.
37. Skakkebaek NE, Berthelsen JG, Muller J: Carcinoma-in-situ of the undescended testis. *Urol Clin North Am* 1982; 9:377.
38. Johnston RH: The undescended testis. *Arch Dis Child* 1964; 40:113.
39. Riegler HC: Torsion of intra-abdominal testis. An unusual problem in diagnosis of the acute surgical abdomen. *Surg Clin North Am* 1972; 52:371.
40. Rajfer J, Handelsman DJ, Swerdloff RS, et al: Hormonal therapy of cryptorchidism: a randomized, double-blind study comparing human chorionic gonadotropin and gonadotropin-releasing hormone. *N Engl J Med* 1986; 314:466.
41. Hadziselimovic F: Testicular development, in Gillenwater JY, Grayhack JT, Howards SS, et al (eds): *Adult and Pediatric Urology.* Chicago, Year Book Medical Publishers, 1987, p 1932.
42. Karpe B, Eneroth P, Ritzen EN: LH-RH treatment in unilateral cryptorchidism: effect on testicular descent and hormonal response. *J Pediatr* 1983; 103:892.
43. Keizer-Schrama SMPF deM, Hazebroek FWJ, Drop SLS, et al: Double-blind, placebo-controlled study of luteinising-hormone–releasing-hormone nasal spray in treatment of undescended testes. *Lancet* 1986; 1:876.

Index

M

Q

R

U